PSYCHOGERIATRICS:
An International Handbook

Manfred Bergener, M. D., is Professor of Psychiatry at the University of Düsseldorf and Director of the Rheinische Landesklinik of Cologne. He has served as President of the Clinical Section of the German Association of Gerontology since 1980. Currently, he is President of the International Psychogeriatric Asssociation. Dr. Bergener's publications include over 200 contributions to psychiatric journals, as well as several books and monographs. His research interests include Psychiatry, Gerontopsychiatry, Psychopharmacology, Drugs and the Aged Patient, and the Organization of Psychiatric Services (in both hospitals and day hospitals).

PSYCHOGERIATRICS:
An International Handbook

Manfred Bergener, M.D.
Editor

SPRINGER PUBLISHING COMPANY
New York

Copyright © 1987 by Springer Publishing Company, Inc.

All rights reserved

No part of this publication may be reproduced, stored in a retrieval system, or transmitted in any form or by any means, electronic, mechanical, photocopying, recording, or otherwise, without the prior permission of Springer Publishing Company, Inc., 536 Broadway, New York, NY 10012

87 88 89 90 91/ 5 4 3 2 1

Library of Congress Cataloging-in-Publication Data

Psychogeriatrics: an international handbook.

   Includes bibliographies and index.
   1. Geriatric psychiatry. 2. Aged—Mental health services. I. Bergener, Manfred. [DNLM: 1. Mental Disorders—in old age.   WT 150 P9725
RC451.4.A5P776   1987   618.97'689   87-9615
ISBN 0-8261-5070-5

Printed in the United States of America

Contents

Foreword by Carl Eisdorfer   ix

Preface   xi

PART I   Basic Dimensions of Aging

1   Human Longevity   3
Leonard Hayflick

2   Molecular Biological Aspects of Aging   12
Werner E. G. Müller, Michael Bachmann, and Heinz C. Schröder

3   Sociological Dimensions of Gerontology   43
Leopold Rosenmayr

4   Psychological Aspects and Disorders Associated with Aging   75
Lawrence W. Lazarus

5   Psychosomatic Problems in Geriatrics   96
Joep M. A. Munnichs

PART II   Diagnostics

6   New Perspectives in the Classification and Diagnosis of Psychiatric Disorders in Late Life   109
Sir Martin Roth

7   Multidimensional Assessment in Geriatric Psychiatry   136
M. Robin Eastwood and Sandra Corbin

8   Brain Hemodynamic and Metabolic Approaches in Senile Cerebral Impairment Related to Dementia   148
Willy J. Dekoninck

9	Noninvasive Diagnostic Techniques to Study Age-Related Cerebral Disorders Steven B. Waller and Edythe D. London	172
10	Electrophysiologic Methods for Assessing Sleep Disorders in the Elderly Horst W. Ebeling	194

PART III Psychogeriatric Disorders

11	Epidemiology of Psychogeriatric Disorders Michael Shepherd	215
12	Depression, Alcoholism, and Other Functional Syndromes Felix Post	223
13	Organic Brain Syndrome Kazuo Hasegawa and Akira Homma	251
14	Hypertension and Stroke Yukito Shinohara	285
15	Senile Dementia of the Alzheimer's Type Barry Reisberg, Steven H. Ferris, Mony J. deLeon, Thomas Crook, and Nathaniel Haynes	300

PART IV Strategies of Treatment

16	The Interface Between Internal Medicine and Psychogeriatrics Hannes B. Stähelin	337
17	Nutrition and the Elderly Bertil Steen	349
18	Drug Therapy in the Elderly—Biochemical, Pharmacological, and Clinical Considerations Christof Hesse and Kevin O'Malley	362
19	Psychotherapy in Advanced Age Götz Kockott	377

PART V Care and Services

20 Rehabilitation and Long Term Care in the Elderly   407
    Jean Wertheimer

21 The Psychogeriatric Day Hospital: Definition,
    Historical Development, Working Methods,
    and Initial Efforts in Research   432
    *Manfred Bergener, Erhard U. Kranzhoff, Joachim Husser, and
    Valentin Markser*

22 Evaluation and Effectiveness in Psychogeriatric
    Services: An Economic Perspective   449
    Robert G. Jones

PART VI Research

23 Innovations in Psychogeriatrics: Interdisciplinary
    Research   475
    Ewald W. Busse

24 Current Developments in Psychogeriatrics in the
    United States   488
    Sanford I. Finkel

PART VII Humanistic Perspectives

25 Education for Death   503
    Robert Kastenbaum and Reinhard Schmitz-Scherzer

26 Learning to Accept Death: Dealing with
    Terminally Ill and Dying Patients   518
    Manfred Bergener

27 Outlook   525
    Manfred Bergener

Index   531

Foreword

by Carl Eisdorfer

As the editor of this work suggests, the emerging concerns with defining geriatrics as a branch of medicine presents us with a challenge. It therefore also represents an opportunity. Gerontologists have developed a particular appreciation for the bio-psycho-social nature of adaptation in later life. Indeed, while we understand that heterogeneity is among the most conspicuous hallmarks of aging, we must also appreciate that the aged have at least one important similarity, that is, their eventual increased vulnerability.

Clinicians, whether physician or social worker, understand that alterations in interpersonal or adaptive functioning are likely to be caused by an apparent social disruptive or obvious physical disease occurring in the life of the individual. Greater insight and understanding, however, is needed to appreciate that apparent changes in one domain, either social, psychological, or biological, may be caused by and are assuredly influenced by (often undetected) unresolved problems in another domain. Indeed, what is germane is the near universality of the bio-psycho-social nature of all human adaptive function. Of considerable saliency for those of us who are concerned with the capacity of the aged to adapt is the effect of aging as a process in altering the balance. Because the aging process is hardly understood, our ability to appreciate the subtle nuances of its effect on pathology and adaptive capacity is necessarily confounded. Data compel us to accept that clinical outcome is a function of the bio-psycho-social interaction in the patient and to recognize that the ongoing aging process is substantially determined by a similar complex of genetic, biologic, environmental, psychological, and socioeconomic factors (just to name a few). It therefore seems accurate, to borrow a descriptive phrase from another domain, to conclude that in trying to develop a scientific and humanistic geriatric psychiatry we are dealing with a riddle wrapped in an enigma shrouded in more of the same. Yet, we know that over the past decades there have been monumental strides ranging from a firmer understanding of the genetics of manic depressive illness and aspects of Alzheimer's disease to clinical psychopharmacology and brain chemistry through a fuller appreciation of the cognitive strengths of older persons and the effective roles of exercise and nutrition in improving functional adaptive capacity.

This volume presents a full appreciation of the importance of the complex interactions stemming from the aging process. It includes important basic approaches to the biological, psychological, and social aspects of aging in its opening section. Subsequent chapters cover a range of salient issues in the emerging field of geriatric psychiatric disorders, from the more technologic to a range of clinical, structural, and interpersonal issues affecting clinical care. By bringing to this volume a large international group of outstanding clinicians and scholars, Professer Bergener has played an important role in advancing the dialogue across continents in the service of improved understanding of the complex multifactorial nature of cognitive and emotional disorders in later life. In addition, this volume provides useful technical information on diagnosis and management of the patient. In his introduction, Professor Bergener makes an appeal for reactions to this work, which may be "taken into consideration in future projects." In the open spirit of that request, this writer can only add a supportive second and endorse the sentiment that as data and insights emerge from the widest range of laboratories, clinics, and sensitive observation throughout the world, they will come together to enhance the quality of caring and thus the quality of life for those whom we attempt to serve.

CARL EISDORFER, Ph.D., M.D.
Professor and Chairman
Department of Psychiatry
School of Medicine
Director, Center for Adult
  Development and Aging
University of Miami
Miami, Florida

Preface

Numerous congresses and symposia in recent years have focused on current issues in geriatrics, especially in psychogeriatrics. What emerged repeatedly during the many lively discussions at these meetings was the question regarding the methodological prerequisites and the characteristics of geriatrics as an independent medical discipline. This recurrent theme stimulated the genesis of this volume, a project involving more than two years of intensive preparation. The contributions here attempt to provide an overall assessment of geriatrics. This assessment includes a review of the body of knowledge; the research methodologies; the possibilities and limitations of the available diagnostic instruments; the difficulties in the nosological coordination and the diagnostic classification of specific disease processes; and the treatment possibilities within the context of psychogeriatrics. Much consideration is given to geriatric care within an institutional context. In addition, trends in geriatrics research are highlighted, and the difficulties involved in the application of such research to the hospital and private practice settings are thoroughly discussed.

In view of the profusion of knowledge and the rapid developments in psychogeriatrics, the editor realized from the outset that it would be impossible to achieve a complete, up to date assessment of the state of this discipline. Nevertheless, the contributors attempt to present a critical examination of the current state of knowledge in a well-balanced and comprehensive manner. All readers are invited to contribute their criticisms and suggestions, which may in turn be taken into consideration in future projects on related topics.

Psychogeriatrics is no longer a mere "hobby" of a few experts, whose primary specialty could be psychiatry, internal medicine, neurology, surgery, orthopedics, or gynecology, for example. Today, psychogeriatrics presents a challenge to medicine and especially to geriatrics, which is growing steadily in importance and attention. Based on the principles of gerontology and on the application of interdisciplinary methodology, a modern medical specialty has been established which, in the same manner as psychosomatics, could have considerable consequences for other medical disciplines. The first few chapters in this volume illustrate that proper application of psychogeriatrics depends upon the interdisciplinary cooperation of biology, psychology, and sociology.

A comprehensive theory of aging would therefore take into consideration not only the complexity and multidimensionality of the aging process itself, but also the relevant medical, psychological, sociological, and economic factors. Such a theory recognizes that aging is a developmental process equally affected by physiological, psychological, and social factors. Further advances in geriatrics and particularly in psychogeriatrics will depend not so much on preoccupation with diagnoses or with specific disease systems, but rather on a medical concept that includes the cultural and social roots of medicine, with the patient in the center of this new model.

Practitioners of psychogeriatrics have long been aware that, although it is possible to cure many ailments through conventional treatment, the personal contact and communication necessary for total healing are often missing in such treatment. The human rapport tends to get lost in the depersonalized atmosphere of the hospital and under the pervasive dominance of medical technology. The holistic approach to the patient calls for the renewed recognition of the essential element of communication; it acknowledges that there is an additional human dimension beyond the physical, chemical, biological, physiological, and morphological, a dimension that cannot be comprehended from the perspective of causal determination. Multidimensional diagnostics and treatment as defined here presuppose the existence of a much more interdisciplinary mentality, as well as the further development of suitable practical strategies for interprofessional cooperation.

As a helping science, medicine has derived its standards from a theory of social action. Without such a theory founded on a practical-theoretical framework, medicine will not be prepared to cope with the needs and challenges of tomorrow. Physicians need to become more aware of the social mission of medicine, thereby reintegrating it into the total life experience. Psychogeriatrics as conceived here can lead the way in this endeavor.

MANFRED BERGENER

Acknowledgments

I wish to express my gratitude to all the contributors for their participation in this very challenging undertaking. For many, such involvement was possible only at the expense of other obligations and responsibilities. Thanks are also due to the publisher, Dr. Ursula Springer, who spared no effort to ensure that this volume met the highest expectations in every respect. Her publishing expertise effectively tackled many problems that arose along the road to publication. My heartfelt appreciation is expressed to Dr. Springer for invaluable collaboration and support.

MANFRED BERGENER

Contributors

Michael Bachmann, Ph.D.
Department of Applied Molecular Biology
Johannes Gutenberg University
Mainz, West Germany

Manfred Bergener, M.D.
Rheinische Landesklinik
Cologne, West Germany

Ewald W. Busse, M.D.
Department of Psychiatry
Duke University Medical Center
Durham, North Carolina

Sandra Corbin, M.D.
Clarke Institute of Psychiatry
Toronto, Canada

Thomas Crook, Ph.D.
Center for Studies of the Mental Health
  of the Aging
National Institute of Mental Health
Rockville, Maryland

Willy J. Dekoninck, M.D., Sc.D.
Geriatric and Psychogeriatric Units
Centre Hospitalier Universitaire de
  Montigny
Montigny-le-Tilleul, Belgium

Mony J. deLeon, Ed.D.
Geriatric Study Program
Department of Psychiatry
New York University Medical Center
New York, New York

M. Robin Eastwood, M.D.
Clarke Institute of Psychiatry
Toronto, Canada

Horst W. Ebeling, M.D.
Rheinische Landesklinik
Cologne, West Germany

Steven H. Ferris, Ph.D.
Geriatric Study Program
Department of Psychiatry
New York University Medical Center
New York, New York

Sanford I. Finkel, M.D.
Department of Psychiatry
Northwestern University Medical School
Chicago, Illinois

Kazuo Hasegawa, M.D.
Department of Psychiatry
St. Marianna University School of Medicine
Kawasaki, Japan

Leonard Hayflick, Ph.D.
Center for Gerontological Studies
University of Florida
Gainesville, Florida

Nathaniel Haynes, Ph.D.
Geriatric Study Program
Department of Psychiatry
New York University Medical Center
New York, New York

Christof Hesse, Ph.D.
Rheinische Landesklinik
Cologne, West Germany

Akira Homma, M.D.
Division of Psychiatry
Tokyo Metropolitan Institute of
  Gerontology
Tokyo, Japan

Joachim Husser, M.D.
Rheinische Landesklinik
Cologne, West Germany

Robert G. Jones, Ph.D.
Department of Health Care of the Elderly
The University of Nottingham
  Medical School
Nottingham, United Kingdom

Robert Kastenbaum, Ph.D.
Adult Development and Aging Program
Arizona State University
Tempe, Arizona

Götz Kockott, M.D.
Psychiatrische Klinik
Technical University of Munich
Munich, West Germany

Erhard U. Kranzhoff, Dipl. Psychol.
Rheinische Landesklinik
Cologne, West Germany

Lawrence W. Lazarus, M.D.
Rush-Presbyterian-St. Luke's Medical
  Center
Chicago, Illinois

Edythe D. London, Ph.D.
Addiction Research Center
National Institute on Drug Abuse
Baltimore, Maryland

Valentin Markser, M.D.
Rheinische Landesklinik
Cologne, West Germany

Werner E. G. Müller, Ph.D.
Department of Applied Molecular Biology
Johannes Gutenberg University
Mainz, West Germany

Joep M. A. Munnichs, Ph.D.
Department of Social Gerontology
Katholieke Universiteit
Nijmegen, The Netherlands

Kevin O'Malley, M.D., Ph.D.
Department of Clinical Pharmacology
Royal College of Surgeons in Ireland
Dublin, Ireland

Felix Post, M.D., F.R.C.P., F.R.C. Psych.
The Bethlehem Hospital and
The Maudsley Hospital
London, United Kingdom

Barry Reisberg, M.D.
Geriatric Study and Treatment Program
Department of Psychiatry
New York University Medical Center
New York, New York

Leopold Rosenmayr, Ph.D.
Ludwig Boltzmann Institute for Social
  Gerontology and Life Span Research
Vienna, Austria

Sir Martin Roth, M.D.
Department of Psychiatry
Cambridge University Clinical School
Cambridge, United Kingdom

Reinhard Schmitz-Scherzer, Ph.D.
Soziale Gerontologie
Gesamthoschule Kassel
Kassel, West Germany

Heinz C. Schröder, Ph.D.
Department of Applied Molecular Biology
Johannes Gutenberg University
Mainz, West Germany

Contributors

Michael Shepherd, M.D.
Institute of Psychiatry
London, United Kingdom

Yukito Shinohara, M.D.
Department of Neurology
Tokai University School of Medicine
Bohseida, Isehara, Japan

Hannes B. Stähelin, M.D.
Geriatric Clinics
Kantonsspital and Felix-Platter-Spital
Basel, Switzerland

Bertil Steen, M.D., Ph.D.
Vaernheim Hospital
Lund University
Malmö, Sweden

Steven B. Waller, Ph.D.
Department of Pharmacology and
   Physiology
University of South Dakota
Vermillion, South Dakota

Jean Wertheimer, M.D.
Service Universitaire de Psychogériatrie
Hôpital Psychogériatrique
Prilly, Switzerland

PART I
Basic Dimensions of Aging

1
Human Longevity

Leonard Hayflick

The common belief that the triumphs of modern biomedical research have lengthened the human life-span is not supported by either vital statistics or biologic evidence. There is no proof that the maximum human life-span has changed from what it was several hundred thousand years ago. No authentic record exists to confirm that a human ever lived longer than about 115 years (Bureau of the Census, 1981).

Medical achievements in this century simply have allowed more people to reach what appears to be the fixed upper limit of the human life-span. That is, life expectation has increased but life-span has not. Successful prevention and treatment of illnesses that formerly led to many deaths in the early years are yielding life tables that are simply becoming more rectangular (Fig. 1.1). In many privileged countries, one can now expect to grow old, which is a relatively new phenomenon.

THE BIOLOGICAL LIMIT ON LIFE-SPAN

The fact that a limit exists on human or animal life-span is not only apparent from actuarial data but is also demonstrable at the fundamental level of the cell itself. The discovery that normal human and animal cells have a limited capacity to divide or function both in vitro and in vivo has added considerable weight to the thesis that there is an intrinsic biologic limit on life-span (Hayflick & Moorhead, 1961; Hayflick, 1965; Hayflick, 1980).

This limit, presumed to be genetically determined for each cell, has been frequently misunderstood. The basis for this misunderstanding is the observation that normal tissue transplanted from one host to another, as the first host ages, often survives longer than the life-span of the host species

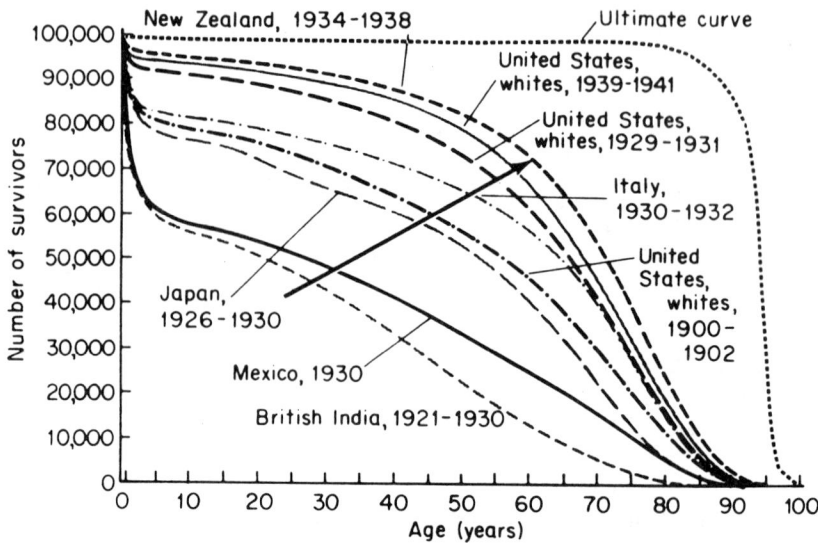

FIGURE 1.1 Human survival curves for various countries and times reveal that as medical care and hygiene improve, fewer deaths occur in the earlier years. This has the effect of rectangularizing the survival curves, as depicted by the direction of the arrow. Elimination of all causes of death attributable to pathology and accidents would result in the hypothetical ultimate curve. Here individuals would die only from the normal physiological decrements that lead to age changes or what were once called "natural causes." (Adapted from Comfort, 1956.)

(Harrison, 1973; Daniel & Young, 1971). Some have interpreted this to mean that the finite capacity of normal cells to function and divide in vitro, which lasts no longer than about one year, is not expressed in vivo. There is ample evidence that transplants of normal cells do survive longer than cultured cells taken from the same species, however, the cells in the grafted tissue still have a limited capacity to be grafted seriatim. The misunderstanding arises because of the failure to appreciate the fact that cells in tissue transplants undergo far fewer population doublings per unit period time than do cultured cells. If the normal cells in a transplant divided at the same rate that they do in vitro, the recipient animal would bear a transplant many times its size in a few months, and that simply does not happen. Cells in transplants simply do not replicate as frequently as they do in vitro nor is the size of the dividing pool of cells as large. Homeostatic constraints on rate of cell division and numbers of dividing cells in the pool prevent most cells from dividing in vivo. These constraints do not operate in vitro so that most cells divide and function until their finite limit to do so is reached (Hayflick, 1965, 1980).

The behavior of transplanted tissues is very much like that of cultured cells that are incubated at temperatures lower than the common 37°C. Under these conditions, cultured normal cells will still undergo the expected number of population doublings, but they will occur over a longer period of time. The number of population doublings that a normal fetal human cell strain will undergo is about 50 (Hayflick & Moorhead, 1961). This represents a biomass of about 20 million tons. The 50 population doublings generally occur over a period of 10 or 12 months when cultured cells are incubated at the ideal temperature of 37°C. However, if the cultures are incubated at lower temperatures, the time necessary for a population to double will be increased and the calendar time over which the 50 doublings occur will be extended.

An extreme example of this condition would be a temperature lowered to the point where cell division does not take place at all. The temperature of cryogenic storage of cells in liquid nitrogen (−196°C) is a good example. Under these circumstances normal human cells could be considered immortal because that storage temperature has not reduced the viability of our normal human diploid cell strain, WI-38, for 23 years (Hayflick, unpublished 1985). There is no reason to believe that WI-38 will not survive indefinitely at this temperature. Nevertheless, this is not a tenable argument for the immortality of humans, just as the survival of a viable transplant beyond the life-span of an animal is not an argument for the potential survival of functionally normal cells beyond that animal's known life-span. Normal human or animal somatic cells simply have not been shown to replicate continuously even under ideal physiological conditions for periods of time in excess of the life-span of the animal studied.

THE RECTANGULAR CURVE

More than sixty years ago the leading gerontologist, Raymond Pearl apparently was first to recognize that with the elimination of deaths in the early years, survival curves constructed over intervals were becoming more rectangular (Pearl, 1940) (Fig. 1.1). This phenomenon was subsequently discussed by Comfort (1956), by Kohn (1971), and by Hayflick (1973, 1974). More recent discussions of the meaning of this curve and its interpretation for future geriatric planning has met with considerable controversy (Fries, 1980, 1983, 1984; Fries & Crapo, 1981; Manton, 1982; Myers & Manton, 1984; Schneider & Brody, 1983).

Fries argues that the continued rectangularization of human survival curves in developed countries is compressing the period of time in which mortality occurs in later life. Thus, the increase in life expectation is approaching the fixed life-span, resulting in a compression of those years in which mortality is most likely to occur. This is interpreted by Fries (1980) to mean that (1) the number of very old people will not increase, (2) the average period of diminished vigor will decrease, (3) chronic diseases will occur in a smaller proportion of the total life-span, and (4) this will result in a reduction in the need for medical care in the elderly. Since the future allocation of health resources could be influenced by these conclusions they merit further consideration.

Schneider and Brody (1983) interpret the rectangularization of survival curves diametrically opposite to that of Fries. They argue that (1) the number of very old people is increasing rapidly, (2) the average period of decreasing vigor will increase, (3) chronic diseases will occupy a larger proportion of the life-span, and (4) requirements for medical care will increase in later life. Schneider and Brody (1983) go on to say, "One important cornerstone to Fries' predictions is that there is a genetically defined human life-span that we are rapidly approaching." They cite the work of Hayflick and Moorhead (1961) in which we established the finite ability of normal human cells to proliferate and function in vitro, as the evidence that Fries uses to support his belief that there is a genetically defined program.

Schneider and Brody (1983), state that ". . . it has been amply demonstrated that some replicating cell populations have life-spans that far exceed the replicative life-span of the parent organism, often by several fold." They site the work of Harrison (1973) and Daniel and Young (1971) in support of their contention. The fact that grafted normal tissue may survive longer than cultured normal cells from the same species is a spurious argument against a genetically determined program. Transplanted tissue simply has a much smaller pool of replicating cells, and those cells that do replicate do so at a different rate than occurs in vitro. (This has been discussed more fully in the previous section.) The essential point is that when normal cells are cultured or transplanted, they have a finite ability to replicate and function. A genetically determined program, as championed by Fries, is still therefore quite tenable.

The evidence for a genetically determined life-span is significant even in the absence of compelling in vitro evidence for a finite life-span. The wide range of life-spans for each animal species provides some evidence for this: a fruit fly is old in 30 days, a mouse in 30 months, and a human in 75 years. When deaths in young members of these species are eliminated, survival curves reveal a remarkable constancy in time of death that is characteristic for each species. If this constancy was not at least partly attributable to a chronometer, probably located in information containing molecules, one would expect random appearances of old animals in each species over a much broader span of time.

Schneider and Brody (1983) argue that there is no evidence that "natural death" can occur without disease because no functional decline associated with aging "... is compromised sufficiently, even at extreme ages, for death to result in the absence of disease. Therefore the compromised physiology of the elderly still requires a specific pathologic insult ... for death to occur." There is much confusion on this important point that arises from the blurred distinction between death attributable to natural causes, and death attributable to pathological processes. It is further compounded by the fact that death attributable to "natural causes," once frequently written on death certificates, is no longer common. Physicians in more recent years apparently have felt that to write "natural causes" on a death certificate, even when the cause of death is truly unknown, is an admission of ignorance and hence undesirable in an enlightened scientific era. Thus cardiac arrest, pulmonary infarction or some other "acceptable" cause is a far more professionally acceptable cause of death when the real reason is unknown. The impact that this nonmedically based, sociologically determined phenomenon has had on the statistics of true causes of death in the past fifty or so years can only be speculated upon. Thus, one of the most significant triumphs of biomedical research in the twentieth century has in fact been the resolution of deaths previously attributable to "natural causes."

Despite the magnitude of this achievement, the scientific literature describing the resolution of "natural causes" of death is nowhere to be found. The extraordinary modesty of the discoverers of the cure for, if not the cause of, "natural causes" has apparently persuaded them not to publish their findings. The mystery is further compounded when one considers that this monumental accomplishment occurred without grant support.

The term "natural causes" represents the very category that should be defined "death in the absence of disease." Functional decline does occur during aging as Schneider and Brody (1983) admit, but they conclude that a specific pathologic insult is required to administer the coup de grace. The fact that functional decline is recognized to occur as are pathological insults implies that a distinction can be made between the two concepts. I believe that this distinction although subtle, is nevertheless crucial. Functional decline is believed to be a normal process. Pathology is not a normal process. The subtlety is that the normal process of functional decline increases the vulnerability to pathology which is not a normal process. As a consequence of this it is just as likely that the causes of death written on death certificates of the elderly are all in error, including those attributable to accidents.

The true causes of death among the aged are normal functional decrements that increase vulnerability to a pathologic process. Thus, whatever is written on the death certificates of the aged should be preceded with the disclaimer that whatever the ultimate cause of death might be, the penultimate cause is a normal loss of function. Schneider and Brody (1983) argue that ". . . the compromised physiology of the elderly still requires a specific pathologic insult, such as pulmonary edema or pulmonary infarction, for death to occur." They provide no evidence for this statement. Their belief that it is true probably is based on the questionable assumption that since virtually all death certificates of the aged contain a cause of death attributable to a pathology, natural causes or loss of function alone cannot be the ultimate cause. Their reasoning is circuitous because the fact that deaths attributable to natural causes do not appear on death certificates does not mean that they do not occur.

It is very likely that a significant number of deaths among older people should be attributed to loss of the function in a vital organ and not to an unproven pathology. Even those causes of death among the elderly that are reported to be accidental bear some scrutiny in this context. If the ultimate cause of death was a fall or a failure to avoid an approaching vehicle the penultimate cause was normal loss of function in which such normal decrements as reduced reaction time, presbyopia or presbycusis actually led to the accident. A younger person probably would have escaped death under similar conditions because those normal decrements would not have been manifest.

RESEARCH DIRECTIONS IN GERONTOLOGY

The above discussion leads inevitably to a consideration of the goals of gerontological research. If cardiovascular diseases, which are now the leading cause of death in the United States and other developed countries, are successfully eliminated approximately 12 years of additional life can be expected (Table 1.1). If cancer, the second greatest cause of death, is eliminated, about 2 years of additional life expectancy will result. The net increase in life expectancy at birth achieved in the United States from 1900 to 1950 was almost 20 years. This increase resulted from the decrease in the large number of deaths that occurred before the age of 65. However, the gain in life expectancy at 65 and 75 years of age from 1900 to 1969 was, respectively, only 2.9 and 2.2 years.

What would be the effect on human longevity and human life-span in a world in which all causes of death reported on death certificates (not "natural causes") were totally eliminated (Table 1.1)? The effect on human longevity would be a realization of the ultimate rectangular curve (Fig. 1.1), where citizens would live out their lives free of the fear of premature death, but with the certain knowledge that their normal physiologic decrements would result in death on or about their 100th birthday.

These concepts force the conclusion that the disease oriented approach to medical research might increase life expectation but will have little impact

TABLE 1.1 Gain in Expectation of Life at Birth and at Age 65 Due to Elimination of Various Causes of Death (1969–71)

Cause of death	Gain (in years) in expectation of life if cause was eliminated	
	At birth	At age 65
Major cardiovascular-renal diseases	11.8	11.4
Diseases of the heart	5.9	5.1
Cerebrovascular diseases	1.2	1.2
Malignant neoplasms[a]	2.5	1.4
Motor vehicle accidents	0.7	0.1
All accidents excluding motor vehicles	0.6	0.1
Influenza and pneumonia	0.5	0.2
Diabetes mellitus	0.2	0.2
Infectious and parasitic diseases	0.2	0.1
Tuberculosis	Less than 0.05	

[a]Including neoplasms of lymphatic and hematopoietic tissues.

Source: Greville, T. N. E. (1976). U.S. life tables by causes of death: 1969–71. In *U.S. decennial life tables for 1969–71,* Vol. 1, No. 5. U.S. Public Health Service, National Center for Health Statistics.

on increasing the human life-span. If such an increase is desirable, and there is considerable doubt that it is, one must first separate the disease related causes of death from the age-dependent normal physiologic decrements that give rise to the manifestations of old age. The diseases of old age are simply superimposed on these normal physiologic decrements but must be separately regarded to consider ways of increasing the human life-span. Although age-associated physiologic decrements surely increase vulnerability to disease, the fundamental causes of death are not pathologies, but the physiologic decrements that make their occurrence more likely.

Biomedical research has focused its goals almost exclusively on the pathologies that cause death. Scant attention has been paid to the underlying causes of biologic aging, that is the functional decrements that increase vulnerability to pathology. Unless more attention is paid to these fundamental biologic causes of aging, the most likely fate of all of us who are fortunate to become old will be death on or about our 100th birthday.

PROSPECTS FOR INCREASING HUMAN LONGEVITY

There are two ways in which the efforts of biomedical research can be expected to extend human longevity in the next 25 years. The first is to reduce or eliminate the major causes of death. For most developed countries, this would mean eliminating cardiovascular diseases and cancer. In the developing countries (and in some areas of developed countries), life expectancy can be extended by the simple expedient of motivating the political and economic infrastructure to provide citizens with the necessary food, hygienic conditions, and medical care that are commonplace in most developed countries. The results of reducing the effect of minor diseases in developed countries will be minimal. For example, in the United States, if tuberculosis were completely eliminated, the gain in life expectation at birth would be less than 0.05 year (Table 1.1). Thus it could be argued that if an increase in life expectation becomes the main goal of biomedical research in the developed countries, all such research should be directed toward the elimination of the two major causes of death. This position, although less than humane and not likely to attract many adherents, is nonetheless the most logical conclusion to be drawn from life-table studies and the projections dealt with in Table 1.1.

The second way in which biomedical research can affect human longevity is to address itself specifically to the underlying normal physiological decrements that increase vulnerability to pathology and death. This approach does not directly concern itself with efforts to increase human life expectation but is aimed at extending what appears to be a fixed life-span.

One measure of current efforts put forth toward these two approaches are the funds spent in the United States on cardiovascular disease and cancer research. They are about twenty times greater than the funds spent in biogerontology. It is also probable that the number of researchers, and consequently the amount of effort, in both of these areas also differs by twentyfold. Consequently, the likelihood that any significant increase in human longevity will occur in the next 25 years depends on significantly better cure rates for cardiovascular diseases or cancer, or both, and significant advances in our understanding and ability to manipulate the biological clocks that set a maximum life-span for each species.

If potential success in either of these endeavors can be measured by the current attitudes and priorities of the biomedical research establishments in the United States and elsewhere, then clearly the search for cures for cardiovascular disease and cancer is more likely to affect human longevity than is biogerontological research. A further conclusion is that by resolving these two diseases a maximum of 14 years of additional life expectation can be attained, but with successful efforts to increase the life-span itself, no fixed end-point is ruled out. Furthermore, the resolution of the two leading killers will in no way reverse or halt the decline in normal physiological decrements that are characteristic of old age, whereas efforts to increase life-span could lead to such a reversal. Clearly, research in cardiovascular diseases and cancer should not be stopped, but if our goal is to maximize opportunities to effectively increase human longevity, then our current priorities are seriously out of balance. If this imbalance continues unchanged, there is little likelihood that the research accomplishments of a handful of underfunded biogerontologists will ever increase the human life-span.

REFERENCES

Bureau of the Census. (1981). Population characteristics of the United States. Age, sex, race and Spanish origin of the population by regions, divisions, and states. Supplementary reports, 1980 census of population.

Comfort, A. (1956). *The biology of senescence.* New York: Holt, Rinehart and Winston, Inc.

Daniel, C. W., & Young, L. J. T. (1971). Influence of cell division on an aging process: life-span of mouse mammary epithelium during serial propagation in vivo. *Exp. Cell Res., 65,* 27–32.

Fries, J. F. (1980). Aging, natural death, and the compression of morbidity. *New Eng. J. Med., 303,* 130–135.

Fries, J. F. (1983). The compression of morbidity. *Milbank Memorial Fund Quarterly/Health and Society, 61,* 397–418.

Fries, J. F. (1984). The compression of morbidity: Miscellaneous comments about a theme. *The Gerontologist, 24,* 354–359.

Fries, J. F., & Crapo, L. M. (1981). *Vitality and aging: Implications of the rectangular curve.* San Francisco: W. H. Freeman.

Harrison, D. E. (1973). Normal production of erythrocytes by mouse marrow continuous for 73 months. *Proc. Natl. Acad. Sci. USA, 70,* 3184–3188.

Hayflick, L. (1965). The limited in vitro lifetime of human diploid cell strains. *Exp. Cell Res., 37,* 614–636.

Hayflick, L. (1973). The biology of human aging. *Am. J. Med. Sci., 265,* 433–445.

Hayflick, L. (1974). The strategy of senescence. *The Gerontologist, 14,* 37–45.

Hayflick, L. (1980). Cell aging. In C. Eisdorfer (Ed.), *Annual review of gerontology and geriatrics.* New York: Springer Publishing Co.

Hayflick, L., & Moorhead, P. S. (1961). The serial cultivation of human diploid cell strains. *Exp. Cell Res., 25,* 585–621.

Kohn, R. R. (1971). *Principles of mammalian aging.* Englewood Cliffs, NJ: Prentice-Hall.

Manton, K. G. (1982). Changing concepts of morbidity and mortality in the elderly population. *Milbank Memorial Fund Quarterly/Health and Society, 60,* 183–244.

Myers, G. C., & Manton, K. G. (1984). Compression of mortality: Myth or reality? *The Gerontologist, 24,* 346–353.

Pearl, R. (1940). *Introduction to medical biometry and statistics* (3rd ed.). Philadelphia: Saunders.

Schneider, E. L., & Brody, J. A. (1983). Aging, natural death, and the compression of morbidity: Another view. *New Eng. J. Med., 309,* 854–856.

2
Molecular Biological Aspects of Aging

Werner E. G. Müller, Michael Bachmann, and Heinz C. Schröder

INTRODUCTION

A finite life-span is a common feature of all multicellular eukaryotic organisms. The mean life-span can vary and is strongly influenced by the environment. The maximal life span is a species constant and controlled genetically and/or epigenetically. Aging is a physiological process which proceeds in multicellular eukaryotes and is caused by a phase-specific readout of genetic information. It was calculated (Cutler, 1976) that if the four most serious diseases and dysfunctions were eliminated today, the gain in the expectancy of life would be 10.9 years for cardiovascular-renal diseases, 5.9 years for heart diseases, 1.3 years for vascular diseases affecting the central nervous system, and 2.3 years for malignant neoplasms. These diseases are the result of the complex array of dysfunctions in older individuals. Hence, an elimination of one disease will not extend the maximal life-span but would create another disease. Aging and differentiation of multicellular organisms are two terms describing the same biologic events. The speed of these processes is cell and/or tissue specific with the exception of cells of the germ line. Germ cells are immortal (Medvedev, 1981b) compared to aging of somatic cells. Besides the experimentally unproven possibility that the germ cells are less error prone with respect to DNA, RNA, and protein synthesis,

We are indebted to Ms. Renate Steffen for her excellent technical assistance since 1975. This work was supported by a "Deutsche Forschungsgemeinschaft" grant (Mu 348/7–5; Schr 277/2-1).

these cells are provided with an exceptional mechanism for rejuvenation which occurs during meiotic recombination and repair. During the haploid stage of gametogenesis these cells are under a strong selective pressure which results in the elimination of those germ cells which have a reduced viability. These processes seem to protect germ cells against endogenous and exogenous lesions and alterations.

To understand the genetic basis of aging, it must be stressed that taking place during evolution from prokaryotic to eukaryotic organisms was an increase in the complexity of intracellular compartmentalization. In addition to the existence of the nucleus, eukaryotes are distinguished from prokaryotes by the presence of a specialized membrane system which partitions the cell into functionally distinct compartments. In eukaryotes the DNA is sequestered in the nucleus and delimited by the nuclear envelope. This double membrane isolates DNA replication and RNA transcription and processing from protein translation (reviewed by Müller et al., 1984). Due to this higher compartmentalization, and the complex enzymic control mechanisms associated with it, the phase-specific gene realization during development and aging in eukaryotic cells is not only controlled on the replicational level but also on the transcriptional, posttranscriptional, and translational levels (Fig. 2.1). It even appears that among the levels of control mentioned, the predominant regulatory and stage-determining control processes occur during the maturation pathway of heterogeneous nuclear RNA (hnRNA; primary transcript), and messenger RNA (mRNA). This view is supported by the fact that whereas in prokaryotes the extent of expression of a particular gene is indicated by the concentration of the primary transcript (identical to the concentration of the mRNA), in eukaryotes only the concentration of the functional mRNAs in the polyribosomal complex (not the concentration of the primary transcripts) is a measure of the efficiency of gene realization. With this background, a description of the genetic basis of aging cannot be restricted to age-dependent alterations on the level of DNA but has to be extended to changes on the levels of RNA and protein as well.

REPLICATION

The genetic information of all organisms is encoded in their DNA. This macromolecule is embedded in a highly organized way of increasing complexity in the chromatin (nucleosomes → superbeads → supercoiled loops) (Robinson et al., 1982). The DNA sequence, with some few exceptions, is identical in all cells of a given multicellular organism. It is an essential requirement that after division of a cell the daughter cells are

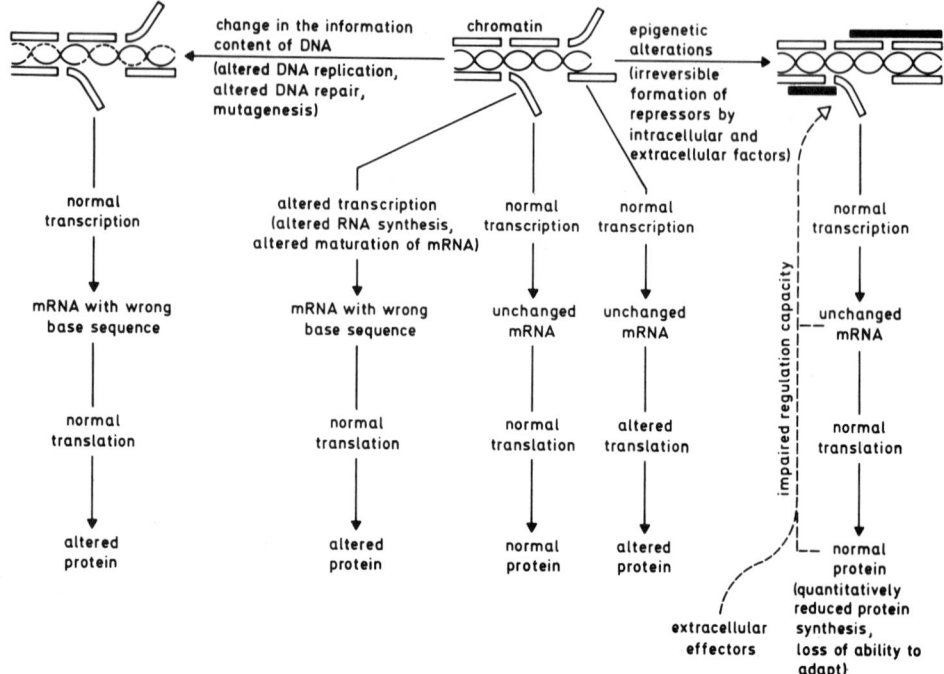

FIGURE 2.1 Molecular biologic theories to explain aging.

supplied with an identical and undamaged set of DNA molecules. In contrast, those cells that have lost the ability to divide at a specific stage during development, require intact DNA only in those stretches which are transcribed; the amount of this DNA fraction can be estimated to be less than 1%. The implication is that cells which have retained their proliferation capacity (mitotic cells) must be provided with more efficient systems to repair DNA than postmitotic cells, which are blocked at a restriction point in their cell cycles.

Today it is well established that a series of different physical and chemical influences, originating both in the organism and in the environment, permanently modify the DNA (reviewed by Gensler & Bernstein, 1981; Zahn, 1983) (Fig. 2.2). Most of these alterations do not become genetically manifest because they are repaired by several distinct DNA repair systems.

Oxygen radicals have been thought to be the major cause of damage of DNA (Sinex, 1977), also resulting in the modulation of the developmental pathways in the direction of cancer and aging (Ames, 1982). Oxygen-anion radicals ($\cdot O_2^-$) are formed from molecular oxygen after an uptake of one electron; this process is induced during photosensitization and radiation. The radicals are also produced in macrophages (Fridovich, 1975). The

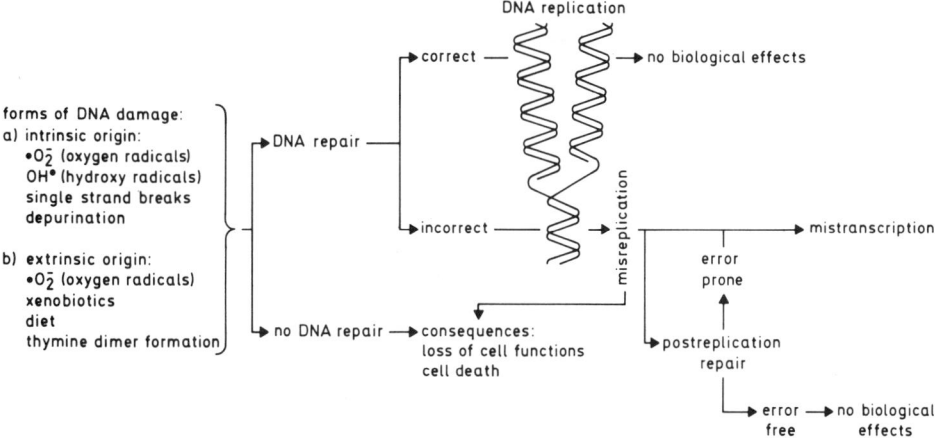

FIGURE 2.2 Effect of various forms of DNA damage on gene realization.

oxygen radicals can interact either directly with the macromolecules, or after their conversion to hydroxy radicals according to the Haber-Weiss reaction. Uptake of electrons by oxygen can also result in the formation of peroxide, another aggressive and destructive agent. The fact that these radicals only rarely interact with DNA and RNA has to be attributed to the enzyme superoxide dismutase, which disproportionates or dismutates the superoxide radicals to hydrogen peroxide (Fig. 2.3) before they reach their target macromolecules. It is interesting to note that on a molar basis this enzyme is present in some organs in an 100,000-fold excess compared to the existence of oxygen radicals (Borek & Troll, 1983). Moreover, the level of superoxide dismutase was shown to correlate positively with the longevity during primate evolution (Tolmasoff et al., 1980). Ames et al. (1981) proposed that uric acid and ascorbic acid are two further strong antioxidants which scavenge singlet oxygen, hydroxyradicals, and oxoheme oxidants formed in vertebrates, in a nonenzymatic way (Fig. 2.4). The authors proposed that it was the innovation of an increased level of uric acid that caused an increase in life-span and a decrease in age-specific cancer rates during primate evolution (Ames, 1982). The ability to synthesize ascorbic acid was lost in primate evolution at about the same time uric acid levels increased.

Xenobiotics and allelochemicals are further agents of potential damage to DNA. Among them the polycyclic aromatic carbohydrates are known to induce a series of enzymes, the mixed-function oxygenases, which convert these water-insoluble compounds into their water-soluble derivatives. Some of them are electrophilic and have the potential to react with macromolecules (Heidelberger, 1975) and thereby can cause cancer and aging

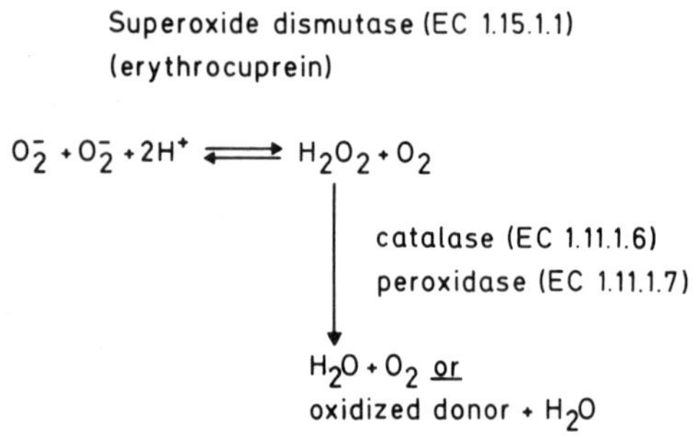

Superoxide dismutase (EC 1.15.1.1)
(erythrocuprein)

$$O_2^- + O_2^- + 2H^+ \rightleftharpoons H_2O_2 + O_2$$

catalase (EC 1.11.1.6)
peroxidase (EC 1.11.1.7)

$$H_2O + O_2 \text{ or}$$
$$\text{oxidized donor} + H_2O$$

FIGURE 2.3 Detoxification of oxygen radicals by superoxide dismutase and catalase or peroxidase.

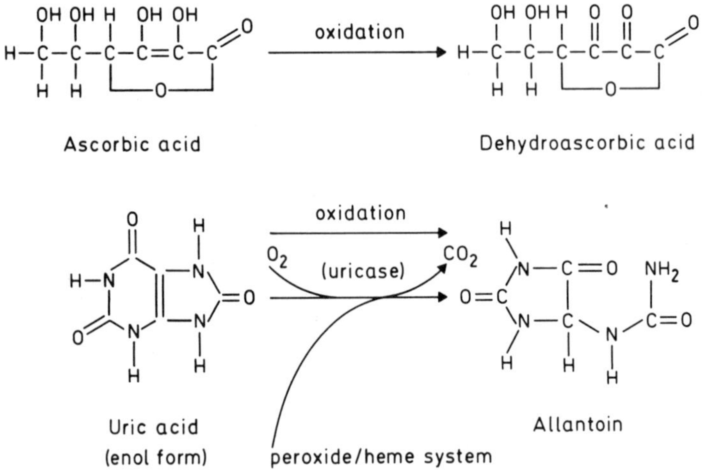

Ascorbic acid → (oxidation) → Dehydroascorbic acid

Uric acid (enol form) → O_2 (uricase) / peroxide/heme system → CO_2 + Allantoin + NH_2

FIGURE 2.4 Nonenzymatic detoxification of singlet oxygen and radicals by the antioxidants ascorbate and urate.

(Huberman & Sachs, 1977). These agents react not only with nucleic acids but also with some key enzymes, whose specific activities were determined to decrease in correlation with age (Rothstein, 1977).

Many toxic chemicals are present in our diet, which have been identified as mutagens, teratogens, and carcinogens (Ames, 1983); e.g., the genotoxic theobromin in tea and chocolate, and the genotoxic agents quercetin, quinones, safrole and fucocoumarines in homeopathic teas. It remains to be studied however, to what extent these agents influence the mean life-span. Further well studied injuries to DNA occur with the introduction of single-strand breaks, the depurination and oxydation of the deoxyribofuranose ring, and the formation of intrastrand thymine dimer (reviewed by Zahn & Müller, 1975).

Several DNA repair systems (excision repair system that removes the mispaired or damaged bases from DNA; apurinic acid repair system) are available in the cell to repair damaged DNA before it is replicated (Fig. 2.2). Of importance were the findings (Hart & Setlow, 1974) that the capacity of fibroblasts from placental mammals to repair DNA damage induced by ultraviolet light varies by at least 8-fold and is directly proportional to the life-span of the species from which the tissue is derived. However, even in the repair-proficient cells, DNA damage accumulates with time (Wilkins & Hart, 1974). Since the repair capacity of a given cell line remains constant over the life-span of a culture (Clarkson & Painter, 1974), it appears that the extent of DNA damage remains constant with age as well as being species-dependent (Hart et al., 1975). This would mean, according to a simplified explanation, that such species with lower DNA repair capacities accumulate genetic damage more rapidly than others with higher DNA repair capacities. Nonetheless, some of the remaining incorrect DNA sequences are replicated. These misreplicated sequences do not necessarily lead to mistranscribed RNA, since the injuries to DNA can be repaired by the postreplication repair system (Painter, 1970) either correctly or incorrectly.

The consequences of DNA lesions may lead to loss of cell function and death, due to an accumulation of single-strand nicks and gaps that occur with age (Chetsanga et al., 1977). These events could become crucial especially in the brain owing to its lower DNA repair capacity compared to other organs (Gensler, 1981). However, in a subsequent study Dean and Cutler (1978) did not find any age-dependent accumulation of S_1-sensitive DNA sites in the livers of aged mice. In one thorough study, Zahn (1983) isolated highly purified DNAs from human muscle (equals postmitotic tissue) and determined their number of single-strand nicks after treatment with three different single-strand-specific deoxyribonucleases. The material came from donors 35 to 86 years of age. The results revealed no significant correlation between accumulation of nuclease-sensitive DNA sites and the age of the donor. However, the correlation between age and the standard deviation of the molecular weight was found to be significantly different. These findings do not support the error catastrophe theory of Orgel in its original version (1963). It is more likely that the rate of error, also in the DNA, converges to a stable terminal point (Edelman & Gallant, 1977; Orgel, 1970), resulting in a slowdown of the biosynthetic and biodegrading pathways.

Nevertheless, the observed increase of the standard deviation of the molecular weight of DNA with age implies a steady gain of changes in the structure and integrity of this macromolecule (Zahn, 1983). Consequently, it is not surprising that the DNA, also embedded in its proteinaceous organization lattice, displays age-dependent changes. By a series of studies

(Jacobs et al., 1963; Puvion-Dutilleul & Macieira-Coelho, 1983) it became experimentally well established that the number of chromosome abberations (trisomy and errors during somatic recombination) increase with age (Sinex, 1977). In this context the findings of Puvion-Dutilleul and Macieira-Coelho (1983) are important, since they revealed a close age-correlated increase of chromatin alterations in fibroblasts taken from in vivo and in vitro model systems, as well as in those from donors with the Werner syndrome.

The organization of DNA, histones, and nonhistone chromatin proteins to the functional chromatin complex occurs along fixed hierarchies. The first level is the winding of the DNA into bead-like particles (nucleosomes), composed of the histones H2A, H2B, H3, and H4. The second level of organization is the formation of 30-nm helical chromatin fibers from a series of nucleosomes by the help of histone H1. The final packing to chromosome fibers occurs in the presence of nonhistone proteins that constitute the scaffold of the chromosomes. Von Hahn and Verzár (1963) found that the interaction between the protein components of the chromatin and the DNA is stronger in older animals compared to younger ones. During aging, the portion of DNA-bound protein that is resistant to SDS, urea, and pronase treatment steadily increases (Müller & Zahn, 1979). Later findings, excellently reviewed by Medvedev (1981a), revealed no marked age changes of the chromatin with respect to the pattern of H1, H3, H2B, H2A, and H4. However, a marked increase of one subtype of H1 histone, H1°, which appears in nondividing cells only (Panym & Chalkley, 1969), was observed during aging of rats (Medvedev et al., 1978; Sinex, 1977). This increase of H1° is correlated with the decrease of both H1a and H1b subfractions (Smith & Johns, 1980). Other well-confirmed changes had not been detected in chromatin; therefore, Medvedev (1981) formulated the theory that "the interaction between DNA and chromatin proteins is not age constant."

In spite of the slight age-correlated changes in the structure of the chromatin hitherto observed, marked differences exist in the function of DNA in the chromatin complex, isolated from animals of different age. We (Müller, Rohde, et al., 1975) observed that the template activity of DNA in chromatin from quail oviduct for exogenous RNA polymerase strongly decreases age-dependently. The finding that the fidelity of the genuine enzyme of DNA replication, the DNA polymerase, decreases with age (Linn et al., 1976) was of similar interest. However, the latter finding cannot be generalized for all aging systems, as demonstrated by Fry et al. (1981). The specific activities of the two major DNA polymerases (α and β) were determined to decrease age-dependently (Müller & Zahn, 1979).

Taken together, two qualitatively different age-correlated changes occur on the level of DNA (Fig. 2.1): first, irreversible formation of repressors in the chromatin complex, and second, changes in the information content of DNA, due to altered DNA replication, altered DNA repair, and mutagenesis. The interplay of these factors could contribute to the loss of genetic code, the loss of readout device, or the loss of conditions for readout as formulated by Strehler (1976). The ultimate biologic consequence of these changes is a slowing down of protein synthesis (Adelman, 1971).

TRANSCRIPTION

The four RNA species—transfer RNA (tRNA), messenger RNA (mRNA), ribosomal RNA (rRNA), and small nuclear RNA (snRNA)—are transcribed in eukaryotes by different RNA polymerases. RNA polymerase I is responsible for the formation of the large rRNA molecules; RNA polymerase II transcribes the genes that code first for proteins (formation of mRNA), and second for some snRNA species, while RNA polymerase III synthesizes tRNAs and the small 5S rRNA. In prokaryotic organisms, mRNAs are transcribed in most instances from polycistronic transcriptional units and translated as such even before the transcriptional process has been completed. In contrast to prokaryotic mRNA, the primary gene transcript of eukaryotes, the heterogeneous nuclear RNA (hnRNA), must be modified by a series of posttranscriptional processing steps before it can leave the nucleus as translationally active mRNA (Fig. 2.5). As in prokaryotes, eukaryote tRNAs and rRNAs derive from larger precursor RNAs.

These new molecular biologic facts that emerged during the last 10 years devaluate a series of previously performed age-dependent studies on the level of transcription because most of them did not consider the dissection of gene expression processes in transcription and posttranscription. There is no question that the template activity of DNA in the chromatin complex for the overall transcription process reduces age-dependently; many published data support this view (Müller, Rohde, et al., 1975; Berdyshev, 1976). These observed changes always parallel a simultaneous change in the histone and nonhistone composition of chromatin. Moreover, in some reports it is documented that the overall rate of synthesis of both total and polyadenylated RNA significantly decreases with age (Semsei et al., 1982), the endogenous nucleotide pool decreases age-relatedly (Bolla & Miller, 1980), and perhaps even the extractable activities of those enzymes that catalyze the RNA synthesis are reduced during the aging process (Müller et al., 1976).

The observed impairment of efficiency of gene realization on the level of transcription can be operationally attributed to changes in the matrix (DNA, chromatin), and in the enzymic machinery (RNA transcription complex). In thoroughly performed studies (Johnson & Strehler, 1972; Johnson,

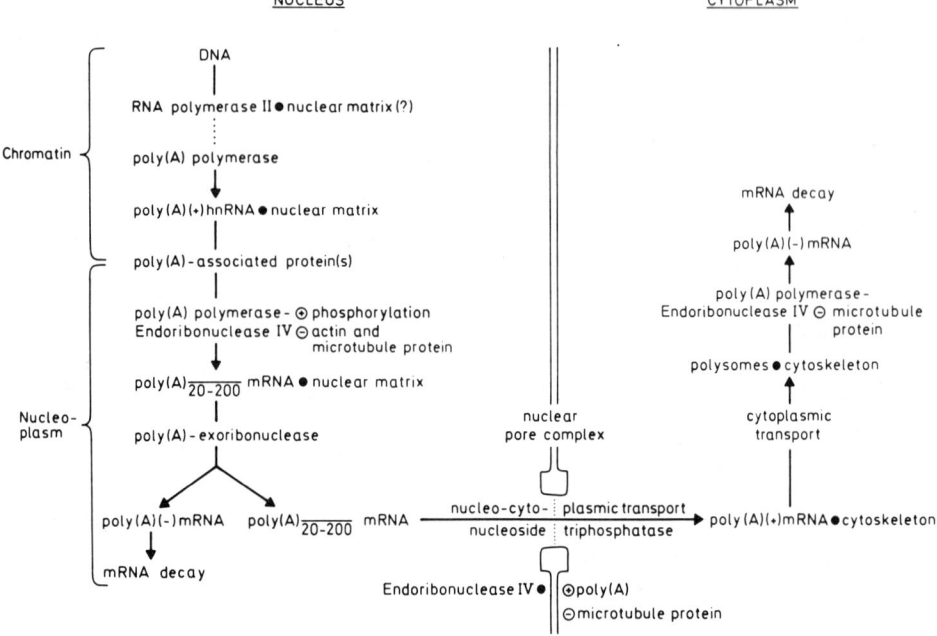

FIGURE 2.5 Diagram illustrating mechanisms for intranuclear and intracytoplasmic transport and metabolism of mRNA and its precursors. +, Activation of enzyme activity; −, inactivation of enzyme activity; ●, complex formation (Müller et al., 1985).

Chrisp, et al., 1972) the hypothesis was tested to determine if tandemly duplicated regions of the DNA, for example, those coding for rRNA, become functionally inactive during aging. It was postulated that these regions separate from each other and are subsequently stabilized in self-complementary loops within single strands. This re-annealing occurs in an out-of-register manner resulting in the formation of a "sense" strand and a "nonsense" strand. Then the remaining DNA loop is enzymically excised, a process that ultimately leads to a loss of information in both DNA strands. In an experimental attempt to prove this hypothesis, the degree of redundancy of the tandemly duplicated rRNA genes was determined in various tissues of dogs of different ages. The results revealed a selective loss of DNA coding for this product especially in postmitotic organs (brain, muscle, heart). This result has been confirmed in subsequent studies of human myocardium which revealed a similar decrease in hybridizable rDNA loci per cell (Johnson et al., 1975). If this finding can be generalized then it appears to be plausible that the reduction of the number of functional rRNA genes with age, together with age related functional alteration during ribosome assembly (Vandenhaute et al., 1983), significantly contributes to a slowdown of overall protein synthesis.

POSTTRANSCRIPTION

The information contained in the mRNA is encoded in the transcriptional unit and is transcribed by RNA polymerase II into hnRNA. The transcriptional unit is framed by a control region (a sequence that is essential for expression of the gene) and a termination region (a sequence beyond the 3'terminus of the primary hnRNA). The control region and the TATAAT sequence are only recognition sites for RNA polymerase II and are not transcribed. The RNA start site (initiation site) is located 25 to 30 nucleotides upstream (in the 5' direction) from the TATAAT sequence. Initiation has been shown to be controlled either negatively (e.g., T-antigen-mediated shut off of early SV40 transcription) or positively (e.g., in the case of hormonally controlled genes) (Darnell, 1982). The primary transcripts of eukaryotic mRNA contain, besides the coding RNA sequences (exons), long insertions of noncoding RNA sequences (introns). While the 5' terminus of the primary mRNA transcript corresponds to the initiation site of transcription, no definite termination site for the 3' terminus of the hnRNA has been identified. However, it is already proven that transcription proceeds beyond poly(A) addition sites. Furthermore, only a portion of the initiated RNA transcripts are completely synthesized; a considerable number of them stay at a premature stage (Acheson, 1978). It remains a future task to elucidate the actual transcriptional rates of different genes and their changes during aging.

The discovery that mRNA transcripts are interrupted by noncoding RNA sequences came unexpectedly. Today it is well established that most eukaryotic mRNAs are composed of several coding sequences located separately in the genome. They are joined to each other during RNA processing (= RNA splicing). This pathway is a complicated, multistep process (Fig. 2.6) which is involved in the development (Slater et al., 1974), and aging of an organism and is prone to physiological and pathological influences. The latter aspect has been studied for the first time in the quail oviduct model (Müller, Zahn, & Arendes, 1979). In this work, and in subsequent investigations, the question was raised whether the efficiency of polyadenylation of hnRNA (one step during mRNA processing) correlates with aging or even directly influences the observed age-dependent gene realization.

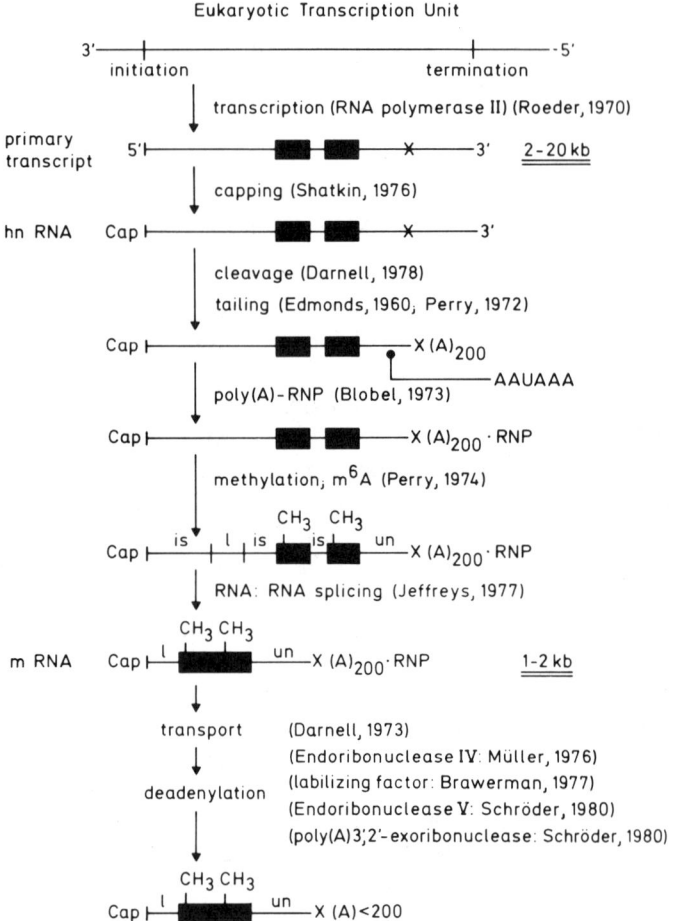

FIGURE 2.6 Model describing the processing steps in nonhistone mRNA biosynthesis (Müller et al., 1983). *Wide bar* = coding region; *narrow* bar = noncoding region. x, Initiation site of polyadenylation; un, untranslated region; l, leader sequence; is, intervening sequence (= intron) (Müller et al., 1985).

hnRNA-Ribonucleoprotein Particle Assembly

Like DNA, all RNA species are packed to form regular higher-order structures. In contrast to prokaryotic systems, the mRNA precursors of eukaryotes become associated with a specific set of proteins to form the hnRNP particles with sedimentation coefficients as high as 200 to 300S (Samarina et al., 1981). These large complexes are composed of monomeric units, termed informofers, which sediment at 30S. Recently, Economidis et al. (1983) succeeded in identifying the proteins that build up these particles. They demonstrated that six proteins (M_r 32,500–42,500) interact with one another through protein–protein contacts to form a core. This preassembled unit interacts subsequently with hnRNA in such a way that RNA remains localized on the surface of the informofer cores. In a further functionally important step the hnRNP particles become associated with the nuclear matrix (Comings et al., 1981)(Fig. 2.5), which provides the organizational platform for the following enzymic modification processes.

Capping and Methylation

Most hnRNPs are modified at the 5' end (Shatkin, 1976). This modification is termed cap formation (Fig. 2.6) and is catalyzed by four to six different enzymes (Perry, 1981).

A second very early modification step is the methylation of internal adenylate residues at the N^6 position (Perry et al., 1974). The function of internal base methylation is not clear; however, based on the fact that m^6A residues are conserved during RNA processing (Chen-Kiang et al., 1979) and on additional inhibition studies (Stoltzfus et al., 1982), it is suggested that these nucleotides play a positive role in splicing and/or confer some resistance to ribonucleases on the mRNA.

Poly(A) Addition

Most eukaryotic mRNAs, from sponges (Müller et al., 1983) to humans, carry a polyadenylic acid sequence [= poly(A)] of 50 to 250 AMP residues at the 3' end (Carlin, 1978). This highly conserved sequence has been detected also during the initial stage of synthesis of some histone mRNAs (Ruderman et al., 1977). As described above, transcription proceeds beyond the poly(A) addition sites. This fact implies first that a nucleolytic cleavage process precedes polyadenylation, and second that the poly(A) site selection is a transcriptional event. One signal for the initiation of poly(A) addition is the AAUAAA sequence, which is usually 10 to 30 nucleotides upstream from the poly(A) initiation site (Proudfoot et al., 1976). This sequence, however, does not seem to be essential for the poly(A) polymerization process alone.

The metabolism of the poly(A) segment of mRNA is well understood on the enzymic level. The poly(A) anabolic enzyme(s)—the poly(A) polymerase(s)—have been isolated from both nucleus (Edmonds et al., 1976) and cytoplasm (Tsiapalis et al., 1975) of higher eukaryotic cells. In contrast to the RNA polymerases, the poly(A) polymerase synthesizes poly(A) in a template-independent reaction. Likewise it is well documented that the activity of this enzyme is modulated by a protein kinase (Schröder et al.,

1983). All poly(A) catabolic enzymes known so far have been detected and purified by us: endoribonuclease IV (Müller, 1976), endoribonuclease V (Schröder, Dose, et al., 1980), and 2', 3'-exoribonuclease (Schröder, Zahn, et al., 1980).

Because the chain length of the poly(A) segment of mRNA is not genetically determined, we have to conclude that it is the result of a tuned interrelation between the poly(A) metabolic enzymes. It has been shown by a series of studies that these enzymes respond to altered physiological conditions and neoplasia. Focusing on this topic, Jacob and Rose (1978) have summarized data on the level of poly(A) polymerase activity. We will discuss here the alterations of the activities of poly(A) anabolic and poly(A) catabolic enzymes during aging.

The balance between the poly(A) metabolic enzymes changes during the development of the organism. We have studied extensively the age-correlated alterations of poly(A) metabolism of mRNA in quail oviduct. It was established that during the proliferation phase of this organ, initiated in immature animals by estrogen and gestagen hormones, the activity of the extractable poly(A) polymerase remains unchanged, while the level of poly(A) nuclease activities alters in response to the stimuli (Müller, Totsuka, et al., 1975). Detailed analysis of the enzyme activities in mature and old oviducts revealed that the activities of the extractable endoribonuclease IV and poly(A) polymerase remain unchanged after progesterone treatment in both age groups, however, the levels of both enzymes are significantly higher in oviducts from old animals (Müller et al., 1980). Furthermore, there is a large difference between the levels of poly(A)-specific 2', 3'-exoribonuclease in mature and old animals. First, in mature animals the enzyme level is low (22 units/mg DNA tissue), compared with the enzyme level in older animals (75 units/mg DNA tissue), and second the activity of the exoribonuclease drops in mature animals after progesterone treatment, while in older animals it increases by 30% after a five day progesterone treatment.

These enzymic data suggest that during aging the poly(A) segment of mRNA (in the steady state) decreases in size. To test this hypothesis, analytical studies were performed (Bernd, Bathe, et al., 1982). They revealed that the size of the poly(A) segment of mRNA from old oviducts is shorter (average size: poly(A)$_{70}$) compared to that present in mRNA from mature oviducts (poly(A)$_{130}$). This result supports the hypothesis in a clear-cut manner. Recently we succeeded in quantifying the amount of oligo(A) fragments formed in vivo (Schröder et al., 1983). Extracting these fragments from oviducts of mature and old animals we found that the amount of low molecular weight oligo(A) fragments gradually decreases during aging of the animals. This result can be explained by the experimentally supported assumption that due to the higher content of poly(A) catabolic enzymes, oligo (A) fragments, once formed, are rapidly degraded in organs of older animals. These examples show that the activities of poly(A) metabolic enzymes are correlated with the physiological state of the organism, and hence are also dependent on the developmental stage of the animal.

The size of the poly(A) segment in different mRNAs has an uneven distribution. The size is dependent on the cell function and the length of the mRNA species (Goto et al., 1981). Consequently, it has been concluded that the poly(A) termini in some mRNA species are cleaved more rapidly than in others (Morrison et al., 1979). Moreover, evidence has been presented that a shortening of the poly(A) region of mRNA occurs in the absence of de novo protein synthesis (Merkel et al., 1976). Therefore, it appears that the equilibrium between poly(A) catabolic and poly(A) anabolic events is actively controlled and this state might be essential for the function of poly(A) to ensure the stability of some mRNA species. There are two mechanisms that may play major roles in the maintenance of this steady state. These are protection of the poly(A) segment by poly(A)-associated proteins against attack by poly(A)-specific nucleases, and control of enzymic polyadenylation by actin and tubulin. Both mechanisms have been experimentally demonstrated by us (Müller et al., 1978; Schröder et al., 1982).

Splicing

The splicing process occurs in the nucleus by a mechanism that is not yet fully understood, and usually follows poly(A) addition (Fig. 2.6). Compared to the polyadenylation process, which is completed within a few minutes (Weber et al., 1980), splicing of hnRNA is slow and requires approximately 20 minutes (Nevins, 1979). The introns are removed by a stepwise elimination process that may involve formation of "branch" intermediates with a 2'-5'-phosphodiester bond (Wallace & Edmonds, 1983). So far the removed introns have never been isolated, which suggests that these RNA fragments are degraded rapidly. In spite of great efforts, no progress has been made toward constructing an in vitro splicing system composed of purified enzymes and nucleic acids. We therefore approached this problem in a different way postulating (Bachmann, Zahn, et al., 1983) first, that the splicing enzymes [endoribonuclease(s) and RNA ligase(s)] are particle-bound, and second, that their activities must be modulated by specific RNA sequences. Based on the speculation (Bina et al., 1980) that the poly(A) tail of mRNA facilitates splicing by alignment of the splicing sites of mRNA precursors, we searched for an endoribonuclease that displays the following properties: (1) hydrolyzes base-specifically, (2) is particle–bound, (3) functions endonucleolytically, (4) binds to specific RNA sequences without degrading them, and (5) is modulated by poly(A). We have now identified and purified such an enzyme which has been named endoribonuclease VII (Bachmann, Zahn, et al., 1983). This novel enzyme was found to be poly(U) and poly(C) specific and to be bound to nuclear 45S particles which are composed of RNA and ten major proteins, one of which, P74, is the enzyme itself. Endoribonuclease VII cleaves poly(U) endonucleolytically, forming oligo$(U)_{12}$ fragments with 3'-OH and 5'-P termini. Its most prominent property is its high affinity for poly(A).

The assumption that Ul snRNA is essential for the splicing process gave us the impetus to search for enzyme activities which are associated with Ul snRNP particles. Previous reports have already indicated the presence of poly(A) polymerase (Niessing & Sekeris, 1973), a nonspecific endoribonuclease (Niessing & Sekeris, 1970), and an endoribonuclease specific for double–stranded RNA (Rech et al., 1979) in the hnRNP complex. By chromatography on lupus antibody affinity columns we succeeded in identifying a base-specific endoribonuclease (Bachmann, Trautmann, et al., 1983). In sodium dodecyl sulfate polyacrylamide gels the RNP preparation obtained showed a protein pattern typical for snRNP, four major polypeptides (M_r: 42,000, 13,500, 11,500, and 10,800), and two minor polypeptides (M_r: 29,000 and 26,000). Moreover, the particles had the characteristic sedimentation coefficient of 12S.

On the assumption that both the poly(A) segment of the hnRNA and the Ul snRNP particles are involved in splicing, the investigation of the two described nucleases associated with the splicing complex may contribute to the understanding of the splicing mechanism at the enzymic level. Considering the fact that poly(A) catabolic processes predominate over poly(A) anabolic reactions in cells of old animals, we postulate that during aging there is a reduced capability to form a splicing complex, and there is a lower overall processing efficiency due to lower activity of the poly(A)-regulated endoribonuclease VII.

It is generally agreed that nucleocytoplasmic transport of poly-(A)(+)mRNA occurs through nuclear pore complexes (Webb et al., 1981). The nuclear pore complexes are not simple holes but are composed of eight granular components—fibrils present in concentric and traversing arrangements, and an inner annular granule (Franke, 1974). The inner annular granules are associated with intranuclear fibrils, and it appears that the nuclear envelope and nuclear pore complex are structurally linked to the nuclear matrix. Poly(A)(+)mRNA is exported from nuclei as ribonucleoprotein (Webb et al., 1981). Theoretical calculations suggest (Clawson & Smuckler, 1982) that the 170–220 nm long mRNA (Dubochet et al., 1973) in a RNP particle is exposed on the particle surface. The nuclear export of such particles with diameters of about 20 nm (Dubochet et al., 1973) through the nuclear pores (diameter of the water-filled cylindrical channel, 9 nm; length, 15 nm)(Paine et al., 1975) is not explainable by simple diffusion. Therefore, it is not surprising that mRNP release is a specific energy-dependent process, as suggested by the work of Klein and Afzelius (1966). Since the studies of Maul and Baglia (1983) it seems established that a nucleoside triphosphatase (NTPase) is envelope-associated, perhaps near the pore complexes; this enzyme was assumed to be involved in mRNA release. In more recent studies a reciprocity has been observed between the NTPase activity and RNA transport with regard to kinetics, to substrate behavior, and to effects of activators (cAMP) and inhibitors (thioacetamide and CCl_4)(Agutter et al., 1979b; Clawson et al., 1980).

Very recently we succeeded in characterizing the processes involved in the enzyme-directed translocation of mRNA through the nuclear pore (Bachmann et al., 1984). Based on detailed enzyme data, we propose a new model to explain the nucleocytoplasmic and NTPase-mediated transport of poly(A)(+)mRNA (Fig. 2.7). It is a modification of the general energy-transduction scheme introduced by Hill (1969). In step 1, ATP binds to the phosphorylated "carrier" S~P. This binding results in a conformational change of SNP to *SNP (step 2); *S~P, is a better enzyme for ATP hydrolysis than SNP. The splitting of phosphate from ATP (step 3) results in a conformational change from *S~P to S~P. According to Hill, and supported by our experimental data, ADP has a low affinity to S~P and dissociates from the "carrier" (step 4). The overall reaction velocity of this

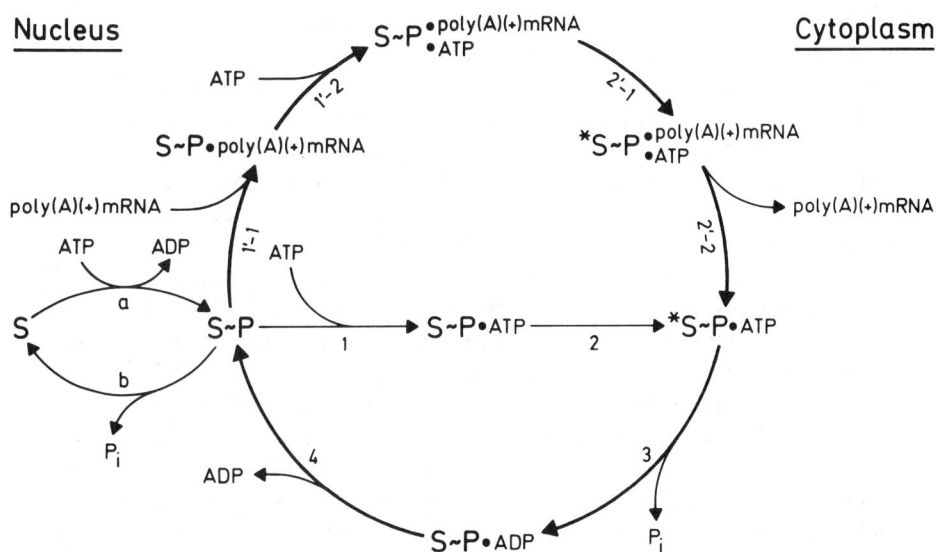

FIGURE 2.7 Scheme for energy transduction by nuclear envelope nucleoside triphosphatase. The two "carrier" conformations are depicted as *S~P and *S~P. (Müller et al., 1985).

nucleoside triphosphatase cycle is accelerated if the system is coupled with the poly(A)(+)mRNA molecule to be transported. According to experimental data (McDonald & Agutter, 1980; Bernd, Schröder, et al., 1982), poly(A)(+)mRNA binds preferentially to S~P rather than to S (step 1'–1). In step 1'–2 ATP binds to the S~P·poly(A)(+)mRNA complex which leads to a conformational change in the "carrier" from S~P to *S~P (step 2'–1). ATP in this complex causes a release of poly(A)(+)mRNA (step 2'–2), in accordance with the results of McDonald and Agutter (1980). This transition is analogous to the ATP-induced change in myosin conformation. It is not clear that the ATP and the poly(A)(+)mRNA must bind to the same polypeptide. "S~P" could be a lamina component (possibly lamina B) which binds ATP, and it could be mechanically coupled through the lamina to a poly(A)(+)mRNA binding protein, X, in the pore complex. In this proposed model for nucleoside triphosphatase-mediated mRNA transport no dephosphorylation of the "carrier" occurs. This means that, in contrast to the model described earlier (Agutter, 1980), phosphorylation (step a), and dephosphorylation (step b), of the "carrier" are distinct reactions, which proceed independently from the nucleoside triphosphatase cycle. Phosphorylation and dephosphorylation of the "carrier" only modulate its affinity to poly(A)(+)mRNA and ATP as shown earlier (Bernd, Schröder, et al., 1982).

In a recent study we demonstrated that the activity of the NTPase in quail oviduct and liver alters during development and responds to estrogen and progesterone treatment of young animals (Bernd et al., 1983). The experiments revealed that the NTPase activity in nuclear ghosts from liver did not change markedly between the different age groups and remained unaffected by estrogen (DES) and progesterone. In contrast, the activity of the oviduct enzyme alters during hormone-induced cell proliferation and differentiation. The activity in untreated immature preparations was determined to be 0.29 μmol/h $\times$ 10^8 ghosts. During estrogen-induced cell proliferation and differentiation the activity increased dramatically and reached, after 6 days of treatment with DES, a value of 2.2 μmol/h $\times$ 10^8 ghosts. Concomitant administration of progesterone resulted in only a slight additional increase. The maximal activities reached in hormone-treated immature animals remained at this level during the mature age phase. However, during the transition from mature to old animals, the activity dropped to 1.1 μmol/h $\times$ 10^8 ghosts. These data show a close correlation between the extents of ovalbumin and avidin syntheses and the level of NTPase. During hormone-induced cell proliferation and differentiation, the stimulatory potency of poly(A) on the oviduct enzyme decreased to 6% in young animals after 6 days of hormone treatment, and to 7% in the case of mature animals. The enzyme from old animals responded only very slightly to the presence of poly(A) (4%). The experiments with the liver enzyme revealed no obvious age changes.

On the basis of this experimental background and the finding that (with the exception of histone mRNAs) nuclear mRNAs lacking the poly(A) sequence are not transported across the nuclear envelope (Latorre & Perry, 1973), we ascribe to the nuclear envelope-associated NTPase a crucial role in the determination of frequency distributions of translationally active mRNAs. It seems reasonable to assume that the age-dependent decrease of overall protein synthesis is partially due to an impaired transport of mRNP from nucleus to cytoplasm, first because of a reduced capacity of poly-(A)(+)mRNA to bind to the specific translocation sites in the pore complex [due to a shorter size of the signal sequence "poly(A)"], and second, because of a reduced nucleocytoplasmic transport rate of mRNA (due to a lower NTPase activity).

Using the quail oviduct system, we have obtained the first experimental evidence that the efficiencies of the posttranscriptional modification processes (polyadenylation and splicing) and of the mRNA transport mechanism decrease during aging (Fig. 2.8). On all the different levels control processes occur, resulting in an inactivation and degradation of RNA transcripts; these processes positively accelerate during aging in a tissue-specific

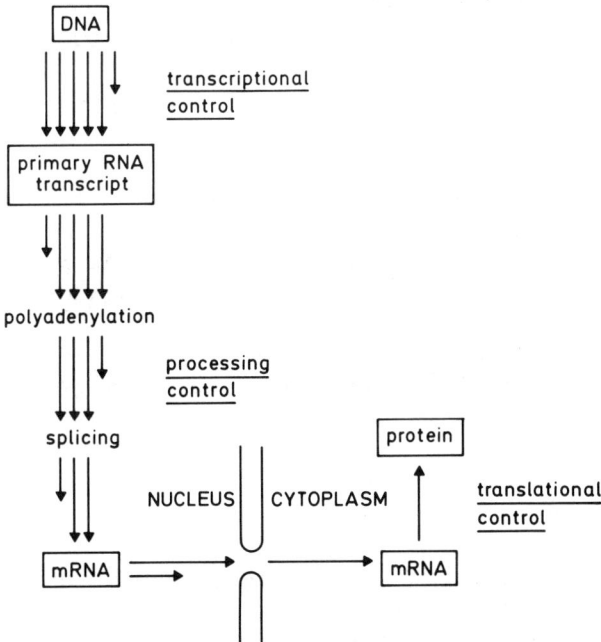

FIGURE 2.8 Control systems govern gene expression in multicellular eukaryotes. The number of arrows indicates the relative amounts of RNA transcripts (Müller et al., 1985).

manner. In conclusion, aging and ultimate death may be viewed by molecular biologists as the result of (1) a change in the genetic program, (2) a coding error or point mutation in DNA, (3) an impaired control of transcription and *posttranscription,* (4) a reduced *transport* of mRNA, and/or (5) a protein missynthesis.

TRANSLATION

Changes occurring in the structure of DNA and RNA do not always result in nonsense in protein synthesis (Fig. 2.1). Eukaryotic cells are provided with an enzymic machinery to repair damaged DNA on the level of pre– and postreplication (Hart & Trosko, 1976) and to exclude misprocessed mRNA on the levels of splicing (Esumi et al., 1982) and nucleocytoplasmic translocation (Villarreal & White, 1983). Nevertheless, a series of reports has been published (reviewed by Andron & Strehler, 1973; Gershon, 1979) demonstrating that several proteins (especially enzymes) are altered during aging. As examples, the enzymes enolase and phosphoglycerate kinase from nematodes, and the enzyme superoxide dismutase from rats show a reduced catalytic ability in old animals compared to young animals (Rothstein, 1977). The observed changes have been grouped under random alterations and nonrandom alterations (Medvedev, 1976). Both types of changes cause conformationally and functionally impaired proteins, the result of which is an inactivation or decrease of specific activities of enzymes or of other regulatory or structural proteins.

Random alterations can be caused by translation of mRNA with an erroneous nucleotide sequence, resulting in errors of amino acid sequence (Fig. 2.1) [e.g. treatment of fibroblasts with the mutagen 5-fluorouracil causes the synthesis of glucose-6-phosphate dehydrogenase displaying an increased thermolability (Lewis, 1976), which reflects a change in the amino acid sequence of this enzyme]. In addition, age-dependent impairment of protein synthesis machinery may be due to a malfunction of the ribosomes themselves (Vandenhaute et al., 1983) (Fig. 2.1). Alterations could also be the result of random modifications occurring during posttranslational modification of proteins, for example, during glycosylation of correctly synthesized proteins or by protein oxidation, deamination, and acetylation (Strehler, 1977).

Nonrandom alterations in proteins are, for example, the formation of cross linkages in fibrous proteins (Kohn, 1971) or the aggregation with other macromolecular or cellular components. The formation of the age pigment lipofuscin is classified in this group; it has been shown to result from the accumulation of autooxydation of lipid components of lysosomes and other membranous cell organelles. A clear age-correlated acceleration of these two processes could be demonstrated. The fibrous collagen becomes progressively more insoluble and less responsive to mechanical stress, with the loss of some of its flexibility (Hall, 1967). This change is primarily due to the formation of new intermolecular bonds which are often termed "cross-links." Concerning lipofuscin, Strehler et al. (1959) demonstrated a linear increase in the amount of the age pigment in the myocardium, with the rate of accumulation being about 0.3% of the total heart volume per decade.

Very often a declining functional capacity in any given organ system is coupled with a decrease in protein synthesis and/or changes in turnover rates. Based on these correlations, Adelman (1971) suggested that age-dependent modifications in the ability to synthesize certain protein species in response to endogenous and exogenous stimuli may be a general biochemical expression of aging. Strehler (1977) concluded from theoretical kinetic considerations that only a few kinds of changes cause the accumulation of altered proteins. Even if age-correlated changes of the content and/or the specific activity of enzymes are not always the rule (Rothstein, 1977), the available experimental data showing an increase of defective proteins with age as well as an age-correlated change in protein content indicate that the occurrence of these alterations and the aging process itself are at least linked phenomena.

CONCLUSION

Based on intense molecular biological research during the last 40 years it is now experimentally well established that all processes of life are genetically controlled. This fact implies that all phenotypical manifestations during development and aging can be traced back to specific readout processes on the level of DNA. However, this does not necessarily mean that a change in the genetic program is the sole cause of development and aging. Gene expression (realization) in multicellular eukaryotes is complex and is controlled not only on transcriptional, posttranscriptional (reviewed by Müller et al., 1985), and translational levels (reviewed by Strehler, 1977), but also on the level of nucleocytoplasmic transport of mRNA (reviewed by Müller et al., 1985). In a eukaryotic cell fewer than 10% of the DNA sequences are ever transcribed and only a portion of them codes for structural proteins. Furthermore, never more than 25% of the hnRNA molecules synthesized are processed to functional mRNA. Even more surprising is the fact that a single gene may give rise to different protein products. It appears to be unlikely that the extension of the maximal life-span (which occurred, for example, in the family *anthropomorphidae* during the last 3 million years) is due to dramatic genetic changes (Cutler, 1976). In experimental studies it was shown that the composition of some structural genes in humans is practically identical with those in chimpanzees (King & Wilson, 1975).

Considering these facts, a description of the aging process can only rely—given the present state of knowledge—on those theories that take into account that the aging process in multicellular eukaryotes is universal, progressive, harmful (in the physiological sense), and intrinsic (Strehler, 1977).

Somatic Mutation Theory

This attractive theory originated with Failla (1958) and Szilard (1959) who suggested that the aging process is primarily initiated and maintained by mutation or chromosomal damage. They assumed that the elementary step in the process of aging is an "aging hit" which "destroys" a chromosome of the somatic cell in the sense that it renders inactive all genes carried on the chromosome. This assumption implies that the two homologous chromosomes in a given somatic cell are damaged by hits at the same sites, or that only one chromosome has suffered a hit at a site at which the homologous chromosome carries a deleterious recessive allele. In subsequent years this theory was criticized for a variety of reasons. It was objected to as being inconsistent with the observation of a high fertility of consanguineous marriages because the two individuals should be burdened, according to the theory, with a very high degree of faults (Maynard Smith, 1959). It also appears relatively unlikely that a single hit renders ineffective all the genes of a chromosome. Moreover, if the rates of gene mutation in somatic cells and in germ cells are approximately similar, then the extent of damage in the chromosome would be too small to account for aging (Maynard Smith, 1962). Strehler (1977) came also to the conclusion that somatic mutations or chromosomal abberations accumulating with age are not significant factors in determining the longevity of eukaryotes. They are only contributing factors in the control of the aging process. However, this assessment must be corrected after the presentation of direct, experimentally supported cause–effect relationships between DNA damage and aging, which demonstrates the dominant mode of genetic deterioration with age.

Error Catastrophe Theory

This theory was built on the basis of the idea that inaccuracy in the translational (Orgel, 1963, 1970) and transcriptional apparatus (Hart & Setlow, 1974) led to a slow loss and deterioration of genetic information stored in DNA, RNA, and protein. This theory implies as its major component that the errors that led to changes in the informational content of these macromolecules initiated a self-perpetuating process that resulted in an error catastrophe.

It is experimentally well proven that age-caused errors occur in DNA, DNP, RNA, and protein (reviewed by Medvedev, 1976). However, these errors created during the formation of mistranslated proteins were found not to cause an enhancement of the overall error rate with age (Edelman & Gallant, 1977). Furthermore, there is increasing evidence that demonstrates that many enzymes do not undergo age-correlated changes (Kahn et al., 1977) and, if they are changed, that these changes are primarily due to posttranslational modifications (Gershon, 1979). The major weakness of this hypothesis is that no causal relationship between reduced enzyme activities and physiological aging could be demonstrated (Holliday, 1975).

Codon Restriction Theory

Based on a series of observations, Strehler (1976) postulated, in an openminded way, that the genetic off-switches ultimately responsible for aging operate at the translational rather than the transcriptional level. This view took into consideration that in contrast to prokaryotic systems, the operon-type selective derepression or repression contributes only very little to eukaryotic ontogeny or gene expression. As an alternative, Strehler and coworkers (Bick & Strehler, 1972; Strehler, 1977) proposed the codon restriction model to understand control of development and aging.

Triplet nucleotides in the mRNA code for amino acids. The meaning of a given triplet nucleotide (codon) is deciphered by specific transfer RNAs (tRNAs) which recognize with their anticodon sequences the codon. Some amino acids have only a single codon, while others have up to six different codons. This means that, as calculated by Strehler (1977), any given amino acid sequence for a typical protein subunit containing about 100 amino acids can be symbolized by about 10^{40} different sequences. Consequently, the possibility exists that the kind of proteins produced at a given time by a given cell type may be restricted to only those messages containing exclusively "words" the cell is also competent to translate. This concept implies first that a given cell is provided with mechanisms that restrict the codon-decoding capacity in such a way that only a limited group of messages is translated; second, that different groups of code "words" are untranslatable at different times in development; third, that the array of codons translatable may either facilitate its own continued function or be expanded as a cell moves from one stage to another, and fourth, that the capacity to translate particular ensembles of codons confers the capacity to synthesize substances which inhibit the translation of specific codons (Strehler, 1977).

This theory is supported in part by a series of experimental findings, for example, transcription is not necessary for the control of early stages of development (Davidson & Britten, 1973), the tRNA aminoacylation profiles of extracts of different eukaryotic tissues from the same individual show significant differences (Bick & Strehler, 1971), and aminoacylase extracts from senescing tissues contain inhibitors that specifically inhibit certain aminoacylations but not others (Bick & Strehler, 1972). In view of later findings (Gurdon et al., 1971) that, for example, hemoglobin messages can effectively be translated in heterologous cell systems, the codon restriction theory in its original version (Strehler et al., 1971) does not appear to be sufficient any longer to explain development and aging on the molecular level. However, it is still a valuable theoretical model because it considers for the first time the fact that gene realization in eukaryotic cells is controlled by restriction mechanisms that do not function during transcription but at later stages in the informational flow system. This view was later adopted by the authors (Müller et al., 1985) for the assumption that programmed development and aging are controlled on the level of posttranscription.

Hypothesis of Aging and Life Maintenance Processes

Between 1972 and 1976, Cutler developed a novel unifying hypothesis on the nature of the aging process. This hypothesis is based on the likely assumption that all aging processes are the result of, first, the existence of an inherent finite life-span of the components which make up an organism and, second, the manifestation of harmful pleiotropic effects of an otherwise beneficial reaction. The two intrinsic processes lead to a time-dependent accumulation of damages. The different animal species have unique life-spans. The age at which the last animal dies has been found to be remarkably independent of a wide range of different living conditions (Comfort, 1964). This age is called maximum life-span potential (MLP) and in mammals ranges from 1.5 years (voles) to 110 years (man).

One major characteristic of aging is the progressive decline with time of the maximum reserve capacity of most physiological functions of an organism. It is interesting that in spite of substantial differences in life-span, correlated with different rates of loss of physiological functions, species express dysfunctions qualitatively and temporally in a similar manner. Therefore, it appears (Cutler, 1976) that mammalian species age in a qualitatively similar manner and perhaps by similar processes but at different rates. This idea implies a type of regulatory mechanism that governs aging rate. Cutler (1972) assumes that only a few common primary aging processes exist in mammals, because of the observation that mammalian species with different MLP age in a qualitatively similar manner. It appears to be possible to even predict the MLP for many mammals from knowledge of either maturation age (Cutler, 1975), brain and body weight (Cutler, 1975), the extent of UV repair (Hart & Setlow, 1974), or the degree of metabolic activity of chemical carcinogenic agents (Schwartz, 1975) measured in fibroblast cells in tissue culture. The most convincing evidence for a primary aging process, governed by a low genetic complexity of factors, came from the finding that MLP evolved at an unusually high rate (Cutler, 1975). For example, during the evolution of modern man, the increase in MLP was estimated to be 14 years per 100,000 years, and to have involved not more than 0.5% of the functional genes.

These ideas suggest that aging effects are caused primarily by a direct modification of a few regulatory genes. Hence, an increase of MLP of mammalian species may be possible mainly by utilizing the same processes that have resulted in the present life-span, although in a better life-maintaining form. The working hypothesis (Cutler, 1976) implies that first mammalian aging processes arose as a natural by-product of otherwise useful metabolic reactions (for example, the presence of natural crosslinking agents as O_2^- or $HO^\bullet$), and second, that the different aging rates are mainly the result of different timing and degree of expression of only a small fraction of common life maintenance processes.

Efforts in the field of molecular gerontology were made in the past (as summarized in this review) to elucidate those age-dependent alterations in the informational flow system of a cell (Fig. 2.1) that are believed to be small in their biochemical extent, yet, on the other hand, display a profound effect on the overall function of an organism. Those changes include age-dependent physical (e.g., Hahn, 1970; Müller & Zahn, 1979) and transcriptional (Müller, Rohde, et al., 1975; Medvedev, 1981a, b) changes in chromatin, a decrease in fidelity of ribosomal protein synthesis (Ogrodnik et al., 1975), and the presence of and age-dependent increase in abnormal protein (Gershon & Gershon, 1976).

During evolution some mechanisms developed that now protect the species against the harmful pleiotropic effects of certain physiological reactions, which result in the above-mentioned damages to DNA, RNA, and proteins and thereby support a lengthening of life-span, and cause a decrease in age-specific cancer rates. These protective mechanisms include:

- the enzyme superoxide dismutase (Tolmasoff et al., 1980)
- the selenium-containing enzyme glutathione peroxidase (Pryor, 1981)
- the radical scavengers in the lipid portion of the cell (e.g., α-tocopherol) (Pryor, 1981)
- the radical scavengers in the aqueous phase (e.g., ascorbic acid and uric acid)(Ames et al., 1981)
- the DNA repair system (Hart & Setlow, 1974)

- control systems involved in posttranscription and transport of mRNA (Müller et al., 1985)

It is assumed that these systems ensure the integrity of the structure as well as the function of DNA and RNA, the primary macromolecules involved in the informational flow system of the cell, and hence maintain the physiological activity potential of the genes to be expressed.

REFERENCES

Acheson, N. H. (1978). Polyoma virus giant RNAs contain tandem repeats of the nucleotide sequence of the entire viral genome. *Proc. Natl. Acad. Sci. USA, 75,* 4754–4758.

Adelman, R. C. (1971). Age-dependent effects in enzyme induction: A biochemical expression of aging. *Exp. Gerontol., 6,* 75–88.

Agutter, P. S. (1980). Influence of nucleotides, cations and nucleoside triphosphatase inhibitors on the release of ribonucleic acid from isolated rat liver nuclei. *Biochem. J., 188,* 91–97.

Agutter, P. S., McCaldin, B., & McArdle, H. J. (1979). Importance of mammalian nuclear-envelope nucleoside triphosphatase in nucleocytoplasmic transport of ribonucleoprotiens. *Biochem. J., 182,* 811–819

Ames, B. N., Cathcart, R., Schwiers, E., & Hochstein, P. (1981). Uric acid provides an antioxidant defense in humans against oxidant-and radical-caused aging and cancer: A hypothesis. *Proc. Natl. Acad. Sci. USA, 78,* 6858–6862.

Andron, L., & Strehler, B. L. (1973). Recent evidence on tRNA and tRNA acylase-mediated cellular control mechanisms: A review. *Mech. Ageing Develop., 2,* 97–116.

Bachmann, M., Bernd, A., Schröder, H. C., Zahn, R. K., & Müller, W. E. G. (1984). The role of protein phosphokinase and protein phosphatase during the nuclear envelope nucleoside triphosphatase reaction. *Biochem. Biophys. Acta, 773,* 308–316.

Bachmann, M., Trautmann, F., Messer, R., Zahn, R. K., Meyer zum Büschenfelde, K. H., & Müller, W. E. G, (1983). Association of a polyuridylate-specific endoribonuclease with small nuclear ribonucleoproteins, which had been isolated by affinity chromatography using antibodies from a patient with systemic lupus erythematosus. *Europ. J. Biochem., 136,* 447–451.

Bachmann, M., Zahn, R. K., & Müller, W. E. G. (1983). Purification and properties of a novel pyrimidine-specific endoribonuclease termed endoribonuclease VII from calf thymus that is modulated by polyadenylate. *J. Biol. Chem., 258,* 7033–7040.

Berdyshev, G. D. (1976). Age-dependent changes of in vitro transcription activities of animals. *Interdiscipl. Topics Gerontol., 10,* 70–82.

Bernd, A., Batke, E., Zahn, R. K., & Müller, W. E. G. (1982). Age-dependent gene induction in quail oviduct, XV. Alterations of the poly(A)-associated protein pattern and of the poly(A) chain length of mRNA. *Mech. Ageing Develop., 19,* 361–377.

Bernd, A., Schröder, H. C., Leyhausen, G., Zahn, R. K., & Müller, W. E. G. (1983). Alteration of activity of nuclear-envelope nucleoside triphosphatase in quail

oviduct and liver in dependence on physiological factors. *Gerontol., 29*, 394–398.
Bernd, A., Schröder, H. C., Zahn, R. K., & Müller, W. E. G. (1982). Age-dependence of polyadenylate stimulation of nuclear-envelope nucleoside triphosphatase. *Mech. Aging Develop., 20*, 331–341.
Bick, M. D., & Strehler, B. L. (1971). Leucyl transfer RNA synthetase changes during soybean cotyledon senescence. *Proc. Natl. Acad. Sci. USA, 68*, 224–228.
Bick, M. D., & Strehler, B. L. (1972). Leucyl-tRNA synthetase activity in old cotyledons: Evidence on repressor accumulation. *Mech. Ageing Develop., 1*, 33–42.
Bina, M., Feldmann, R. J., & Deeley, R. G. (1980). Could poly(A) align splicing sites? *Proc. Natl. Acad. Sci. USA, 77*, 1278–1282.
Bolla, R. I., & Miller, J. K. (1980). Endogenous nucleotide pools and protein incorporation into liver nuclei from young and old rats. *Mech. Ageing Develop., 12*, 107–118.
Borek, C., & Troll, W. (1983). Modifiers of free radicals inhibit in vitro the oncogenic actions of X-rays, bleomycin, and the tumor promoter 12-O-tetradecanoylphorbol 13-acetate. *Proc. Natl. Acad. Sci. USA, 80*, 1304–1307.
Carlin, R. K. (1978). The poly(A) segment of mRNA: (1) Evolution and function, and (2) the evolution of viruses. *J. Theor. Biol., 71*, 328–338.
Chen-Kiang, S., Nevins, J. R., & Darnell, J. E. (1979). N-6-methyl-adenosine in adenovirus type 2 nuclear RNA is conserved in the formation of messenger RNA. *J. Molec. Biol., 135*, 733–752.
Chetsanga, C. J., Tuttle, M., Jacobini, A., & Johnson, C. (1977). Age-associated structural alterations in senescent mouse brain DNA. *Biochim. Biophys. Acta, 474*, 180–187.
Clarkson, J. M., & Painter, R. B. (1974). Repair of X-ray damage in aging WI-38 cells. *Mutation Res., 23*, 107–112.
Clawson, G. A., James, J., Woo, C. H., Friends, D. S., Moody, D., & Smuckler, E. A. (1980). Pertinence of nuclear envelope nucleoside triphosphatase activity to ribonucleic acid transport. *Biochem., 19*, 2748–2756.
Clawson, G. A., & Smuckler, E. A. (1982). A model for nucleocytoplasmic transport of ribonucleoprotein particles. *J. Theor. Biol., 95*, 607–613.
Comfort, A. (1964). *Aging: The Biology of Senescence*. New York: Holt Rinehart and Winston.
Comings, D. E., & Peters, K. E. (1981). Two-dimensional gel electrophoresis of nuclear particles. In H. Busch (Ed.). *The Cell Nucleus* Vol. 9, (pp. 89–118). New York: Academic Press.
Cutler, R. G. (1972). Transcription of reiterated DNA sequence classes throughout the lifespan of the mouse. *Adv. Gerontol. Res. 4*, 219–321. New York: Academic Press.
Cutler, R. G. (1975). Evolution of longevity and the genetic complexity governing aging rate. *Proc. Natl. Acad. Sci. USA, 72*, 4664–4668.
Cutler, R. G. (1976). Nature of aging and life maintenance processes. *Interdiscipl. Topics Geront., 9*, 83–133.
Darnell, J. E. (1982). Variety in the level of gene control in eukaryotic cells. *Nature, 297*, 365–371
Davidson, E. H., & Britten, R. J. (1973). Organization, transcription and regulation in the animal genome. *Quart. Rev. Biol., 48*, 565–613.
Dean, R. G., & Cutler, R. G. (1978). Absence of significant age-dependent increase of single stranded DNA extracted from mouse liver nuclei. *Exp. Gerontol., 13*, 287–292.

Dubochet, J., Morel, C., LeBleu, B., & Merzberg, M. (1973). Structure of globin mRNA and mRNA-protein particles. Use of dark-field electron microscopy. *Europ. J. Biochem., 36,* 465–472.

Economidis, I. V., & Pederson, T. (1983). Structure of nuclear ribonucleoprotein: Heterogeneous nuclear RNA is complexed with a major sextet of proteins in vivo. *Proc. Natl. Acad. Sci. USA, 80,* 1599–1602.

Edelman, P., & Gallant, J. (1977). On the translation error theory of aging. *Proc. Natl. Acad. Sci. USA, 74,* 3396–3398.

Edmonds, M., & Winters, M. A. (1976). Polyadenylate polymerases. *Prog. Nucleic Acids Res. Molec. Biol., 17,* 149–179.

Esumi, H., Takahashi, Y., Sekiya, T., Sato, S., Nagase, S., & Sugimura, T. (1982). Presence of albumin mRNA precursors in nuclei of analbuminemic rat liver lacking cytoplasmic albumin mRNA. *Proc. Natl. Acad. Sci. USA 79,* 734–738.

Failla, G. (1958). The aging process and carcinogenesis. *Ann. N.Y. Acad. Sci., 71,* 1124–1135.

Franke, W. W. (1974). Nuclear envelopes. *Phil. Transact. Roy. Soc. Lond. B., 268,* 67–93.

Fridovich, I. (1975). Superoxide dismutases. *Ann. Rev. Biochem., 44,* 147–159.

Fry, M., Loeb, L. A., & Martin, G. M. (1981). On the activity and fidelity of chromatin-associated hepatic DNA polymerase-β in aging murine species of different life spans. *J. Cell. Physiol., 106,* 435–444.

Gensler, H. L. (1981). Low level of UV-induced unscheduled DNA synthesis in postmitotic brain cells of hamsters: Possible relevance to aging. *Exp. Gerontol., 16,* 199–207.

Gensler, H. L., & Bernstein, H. (1981). DNA damage as the primary cause of aging. *Quart. Rev. Biol., 56,* 279–303.

Gershon, D. (1979). Current status of age altered enzymes: Alternative mechanisms. *Mech. Aging Dev., 9,* 189–196.

Gershon, D., & Gershon, H. (1976). An evaluation of the "error catastrophe" theory of aging in the light of recent experimental results. *Gerontology, 22,* 212–219.

Goto, S., Buckingham, M., & Gros, F. (1981). Length of the polyadenylated sequence in cytoplasmic ribonucleic acid isolated from fetal calf myoblasts differentiating in vitro. *Biochem., 20,* 5449–5457.

Gurdon, J. B., Lane, C. D., Woodland, H. R., & Marbaix, G. (1971). Use of frog eggs and oocytes for the study of messenger RNA and its translation in living cells. *Nature, 233,* 177–186.

Hahn, H. P. von(1970). Structural and functional changes in nucleoproteins during the aging of the cell. *Gerontologia, 16,* 116–128.

Hall, D. A. (1967). The aging of connective tissue. In *Aspects of the Biology of Aging,* pp. 101–126. New York: Academic Press.

Hart, R. W., & Setlow, R. B. (1974). Correlation between deoxyribonucleic acid excision repair and life-span in a number of mammalian species. *Proc. Natl. Acad. Sci. USA, 71,* 2169–2173.

Hart, R. W., Setlow, R. B., Gibson, R. E., & Hoskins, T. L. (1975). DNA repair: A possible control mechanism for cellular aging. *Abstr. 10th Int. Congr. on Gerontology,* Jerusalem.

Hart, R. W., & Trosko, J. E. (1976). DNA repair processes in mammals. *Interdiscipl. Topics Gerontol., 9,* 134–167.

Heidelberger, C. (1975). Chemical carcinogenesis. *Ann. Rev. Biochem., 44,* 79–129.

Hill, T. L. (1969). A proposed common allosteric mechanism for active transport, muscle contraction, and ribosomal translocation. *Proc. Natl. Acad. Sci. USA, 69,* 267–274.

Holliday, R. (1975). Testing the protein error theory of aging: A reply to Baird, Samis, Massie, and Zimmerman. *Gerontologia, 21,* 64–73.

Hubermann, E., & Sachs, L. (1977). DNA binding and its relationship to carcinogenesis by different polycyclic hydrocarbons. *Int. J. Cancer, 19,* 122–127.

Jacob, S. T., & Rose, K. M. (1978). RNA polymerases and poly(A) polymerase from neoplastic tissues and cells. In H. Busch (Ed.), *Methods in Cancer Research* (Vol. 14, pp. 191–241). New York: Academic Press.

Jacobs, P. A., Brunton, M., & Brown, C. W. (1963). Change of human chromosome count distributions with age: Evidence of a sex difference. *Nature, 197,* 1080–1081.

Johnson, L. K., Johnson, R. W., & Strehler, B. (1975). Cardiac hypertrophy, aging and changes in cardiac ribosomal RNA gene dosage in man. *J. Mol. Cell. Cardiol., 7,* 125–133.

Johnson, R., Chrisp, C., & Strehler, B. (1972). Selective loss of ribosomal RNA genes during the aging of post-mitotic tissues. *Mech. Aging Develop., 1,* 183–198.

Johnson, R., & Strehler, B. (1972). Loss of genes coding for ribosomal RNA in aging brain cells. *Nature, 240,* 412–414.

Kahn, A., Guillouzo, A., Cottreau, D., Marie, J., Bourel, M., Boivin, P., & Dreyfus, J. C. (1977). Accuracy of protein synthesis in in vitro aging. Search for altered enzymes in senescent cultured cells from human livers. *Gerontology, 23,* 174–183.

King, M., & Wilson, A. C. (1975). Evolution at two levels in humans and chimpanzees. *Science, 188,* 107–116.

Klein, R. L., & Afzelius, B. A. (1966). Nuclear membrane hydrolysis of adenosine triphosphate. *Nature, 212,* 609.

Kohn, R. R. (1971). *Principles of Mammalian Aging.* Foundations of Developmental Biology Series. Englewood Cliffs, NJ: Prentice-Hall.

Latorre, J., & Perry, R. P. (1973). The relationship between polyadenylated heterogeneous nuclear RNA and messenger RNA: Studies with actinomycin D and cordycepin. *Biochim. Biophys. Acta, 335,* 93–101.

Lewis, C. M. (1976). Cellular aging and the accumulation of altered protein. *Interdiscipl. Topic Gerontol., 9,* 198–208.

Linn, S., Kairis, M., & Holliday, R. (1976). Decreased fidelity of DNA polymerase activity isolated from aging human fibroblasts. *Proc. Natl. Acad. Sci. USA, 73,* 2818–2822.

Maul, G. G., & Baglia, F. (1983). Localization of a major nuclear envelope protein by differential solubilization. *Exptl. Cell Res., 145,* 285–292.

Maynard Smith, J. (1959). A theory of aging. *Nature, 184,* 956–958.

Maynard Smith, J. (1962). Review lectures on senescence, I. The causes of aging. *Proc. R. Soc. London B, 157,* 115–127.

McDonald, J. R., & Agutter, P. S. (1980). The relationship between polyribonucleotide binding and the phosphorylation and dephosphorylation of nuclear envelope protein. *FEBS Lett., 116,* 145–148.

Medvedev, Z. A. (1976). Error theories of aging. In D. Platt (Ed.), *Alternstheorien* (pp. 37–46). Stuttgart: Schattauer Verlag.

Medvedev, Z. A. (1981a). Chromatin proteins and cellular aging. In W. E. G. Müller, & J. W. Rohen (Eds.), *Biochemical and Morphological Aspects of Aging* (pp. 125–148). Wiesbaden: Steiner Verlag.

Medvedev, Z. A. (1981b). On the immortality of the germ line: Genetic and biochemical mechanisms: A review. *Mech. Ageing Develop., 17,* 331–359.

Medvedev, Z. A., Medvedeva, M. N., & Robson, L. (1978). Tissue specificity and age changes of the pattern of H1 group of histones in chromatin from mouse tissues. *Gerontology, 24,* 286–292.

Merkel, C. G., Wood, T. G., & Lingrel, J. B. (1976). Shortening of the poly(A) region of mouse globin messenger RNA. *J. Biol. Chem., 251,* 5512–5515.

Morrison, M. R., Brodeur, R., Pardue, S., Baskin, F., Hall, C. L., & Rosenberg, R. N. (1979). Differences in the distribution of poly(A) size classes in individual messenger RNAs from neuroblastoma cells. *J. Biol. Chem., 254,* 7675–7683.

Müller, W. E. G., Agutter, P., Bernd, A., Bachmann, M., & Schröder, H. C. (1985). Role of post-transcriptional events in aging: Consequences for gene expression in eukaryotic cells. In M. Bergener, M. Ermini, & H. B. Staehelin (Eds.), *The 1984 Sandoz Lectures in Gerontology* (pp. 21–57). London: Academic Press.

Müller, W. E. G., Arendes, J., Zahn, R. K., & Schröder, H. C. (1978). Control of enzymic hydrolysis of polyadenylate segment of messenger RNA: Role of polyadenylate-associated proteins. *Europ. J. Biochem., 86,* 283–290.

Müller, W. E. G., Bernd, A., & Schröder, H. C. (1983). Modulation of poly(A)(+)mRNA-metabolizing and transporting system under special consideration of microtubule protein and actin. *Molec. Cell. Biochem., 53/54,* 197–220.

Müller, W. E. G., Rohde, H. J., Zahn, R. K. & Löhr, J. (1975). Alternsabhängige Avidin-Induktion: Änderungen auf dem Transkriptionsniveau. *Akt. Gerontol, 5,* 625–638.

Müller, W. E. G., Rohde, H. J., Zahn, R. K., & Löhr, J. (1976). Alternsabhängige Avidin-Induktion, IV. *Akt. Gerontol., 6,* 469–476.

Müller, W. E. G., Totsuka, A., Kroll, M., Nusser, I., & Zahn, R. K. (1975). Poly(A) polymerase in quail oviduct. Changes during estrogen induction. *Biochim. Biophys. Acta, 383,* 147–159.

Müller, W. E. G., & Zahn, R. K. (1979). Age-dependent gene induction in quail oviduct, VII. *Mech. Aging Develop. 9,* 527–534.

Müller, W. E. G., Zahn, R. K., & Arendes, J. (1979). Age-dependent gene induction in quail oviduct, IX. *Mech. Aging Develop., 10,* 315–324.

Müller, W. E. G., Zahn, R. K., & Arendes, J. (1980). Age-dependent gene induction in quail oviduct, X. Alterations on the post-transcriptional level (enzymic aspect). *Mech. Aging Develop., 14,* 39–48.

Müller, W. E. G., Zahn, R. K., Schröder, H. C., & Arendes, J. (1979). Age-dependent enzymatic poly(A) metabolism in quail oviduct. *Gerontol., 25,* 61–68.

Nevins, J. R. (1979). Processing of late adenovirus nuclear RNA to mRNA. Kinetics of formation of intermediates and demonstration that all events are nuclear. *J. Molec. Biol., 130,* 493–506.

Niessing, J., & Sekeris, C. E. (1970). Cleavage of high-molecular weight DNA-like RNA by a nuclease present in 30-S ribonucleoprotein particles of rat liver nuclei. *Biochim. Biophys. Acta, 209,* 484–492.

Niessing, J., & Sekeris, C. E. (1973). Synthesis of polynucleotides in nuclear ribonucleoprotein particles containing heterogeneous RNA. *Nature New Biol., 243,* 9–12.

Ogrodnik, J. P., Wulf, J. H., & Cutler, R. G. (1975). Altered protein hypothesis of mammalian aging processes, II. *Exp. Gerontol., 10,* 119–136.
Orgel, L. E. (1963). The maintenance of the accuracy of protein synthesis and its relevance to aging. *Proc. Natl. Acad. Sci. USA, 49,* 517–521.
Orgel, L. E. (1970). The maintenance of the accuracy of protein synthesis and its relevance to aging: A correction. *Proc. Natl. Acad. Sci. USA, 67,* 1476.
Paine, P. L., Moore, L. C., & Horowitz, S. D. (1975). Nuclear envelope permeability. *Nature, 254,* 109–114.
Painter, R. B. (1970). The action of ultraviolet light on mammalian cells. In A. C. Giese (Ed.), *Photophysiology* (pp. 169–189) New York: Academic Press.
Panym, S., & Chalkley, R. (1969). A new histone found only in mammalian tissues with little cell divisions. *Biochim. Biophys. Acta, 37,* 1042–1049.
Perry, R. P., & Kelley, D. E. (1974). Existence of methylated messenger RNA in mouse L cells. *Cell, 1,* 37–42.
Proudfoot, N. J., & Brownlee, G. E. (1976). 3'Non-coding region sequences in eukaryotic messenger RNA. *Nature, 263,* 211–214.
Pryor, W. A. (1981). *Free Radicals in Biology.* New York: Academic Press.
Puvion-Dutilleul, F., & Macieira-Coelho, A. (1983). Aging dependent nucleolar and chromatin changes in cultivated fibroblasts. *Cell Biol. Int. Rep., 7,* 61–72.
Rech, J., Brunel, C., & Jeanteur, P. (1979). HnRNP from HeLa cells contain a ribonuclease active on double-stranded RNA. *Biochem. Biophys. Res. Comm., 88,* 422–427.
Robinson, S. I., Nelkin, B. D., & Vogelstein, B. (1982). The ovalbumin gene is associated with the nuclear matrix of chicken oviduct cells. *Cell, 28,* 99–106.
Rothstein, M. (1977). Recent developments in the age-related alteration of enzyme: A review. *Mech. Aging Develop., 6,* 241–257.
Ruderman, J. V., & Pardue, M. L. (1977). Cell-free translation analysis of messenger-RNA in echinoderm and amphibian early development. *Develop. Biol., 60,* 48–68.
Samarina, O. P., & Krichevskaya, A. A. (1981). Nuclear 30S RNP particles. In H. Bosch (Ed.), *The cell nucleus,* Vol. 9 (pp. 1–48). New York: Academic Press.
Schröder, H. C., Dose, K., Zahn, R. K., & Müller, W. E. G. (1980). Isolation and characterization of the novel polyadenylate- and polyuridylate-degrading endoribonuclease V from calf thymus. *J. Biol. Chem., 255,* 5108–5112.
Schröder, H. C., Schenk, P., Baydoun, H., Wagner, K. G., & Müller, W. E. G. (1983). Occurrence of short-sized oligo(A) fragments during course of cell cycle and aging. *Arch. Gerontol. Geriatr., 2,* 349–360.
Schröder, H. C., Zahn, R. K., Dose, K., & Müller, W. E. G. (1980). Purification and characterization of a poly(A)-specific exoribonuclease from calf thymus. *J. Biol. Chem., 255,* 4535–4538.
Schröder, H. C., Zahn, R. K. & Müller, W. E. G. (1982). Role of actin and tubulin in the regulation of poly(A) polymerase-endoribonuclease IV complex from calf thymus. *J. Biol. Chem., 257,* 2305–2309.
Schwartz, A. G. (1975). Correlation between species life span and capacity to activate 7,12-dimethylbenz(a)anthracene to a form mutagenic to a mammalian cell. *Exp. Cell. Res., 94,* 445–447.
Semsei, I., Szeszák, F., & Nagy, I. Zs. (1982). In vivo studies on the age-dependent decrease of the rates of total and mRNA synthesis in the brain cortex of rats. *Arch. Gerontol. Geriatr., 1,* 29–42.
Shatkin, A. J. (1976). Capping of eukaryotic mRNAs. *Cell, 9,* 645–653.

Sinex, F. M. (1977). The molecular genetics of aging. In C. E. Finch & L. Hayflick (Eds.), *Handbook of the biology of aging* (pp. 37–62). New York: Van Nostrand Reinhold Comp.

Sinex, F. M., & Ingram, P. H. (1977). Modification of chromatin in aging rats. *The Gerontologist, 17* (No. 5, Pt. II), 119.

Slater, I., & Slater, D. W. (1974). Polyadenylation and transcription following fertilization. *Proc. Natl. Acad. Sci. USA, 71,* 1103–1107.

Smith, B. J., & Johns, E. W. (1980). Histone H1°, its location in chromatin. *Nucleic Acids Res., 8,* 6069–6079.

Stoltzfus, C. M., & Dane, R. W. (1982). Accumulation of spliced avian retrovirus mRNA is inhibited in S-adenosylmethionine-depleted chicken embryo fibroblasts. *J. Virol., 42,* 918–931.

Strehler, B. L. (1976). Elements of unified theory of aging: Integration of alternative models. In D. Platt (Ed.) *Alternstheorien* (pp. 5–36). Stuttgart: Schattauer Verlag.

Strehler, B. L. (1977). *Time, cells, and aging.* New York: Academic Press.

Strehler, B. L., Hirsch, G., Gusseck, D., Johnson, R., & Bick, M. (1971). The codon-restriction theory of aging and development. *J. Theor. Biol., 33,* 429–474.

Strehler, B. L., Mark, D., Mildvan, A. S., & Gee, M. (1959). Rate and magnitude of age pigment accumulation in the human myocardium. *J. Gerontol., 14,* 430–439.

Szilard, L. (1959). On the nature of the aging process. *Proc. Natl. Acad. Sci. USA, 45,* 35–45.

Tolmasoff, J. M., Ono, T., & Cutler, R. G. (1980). Superoxide dismutase: Correlation with life-span and specific metabolic rate in primate species. *Proc. Natl. Acad. Sci. USA, 77,* 2777–2781.

Tsiapalis, C. M., Dorson, J. W., & Bollum, F. J. (1975). Purification of terminal riboadenylate transferase from calf thymus gland. *J. Biol. Chem., 250,* 4486–4496.

Vandenhaute, J., Claes-Reckinger, N., & Delcour, J. (1983). Age-related functional alteration of mouse liver ribosomes. *Experiment. Gerontol., 18,* 355–363.

Villarreal, L. P., & White, R. T. (1983). A splice junction deletion deficient in the transport of RNA does not polyadenylate nuclear RNA. *Molec. Cell. Biol., 3,* 1381–1388.

Wallace, J. C., & Edmonds, M. (1983). Polyadenylated nuclear RNA contains branches. *Proc. Natl. Acad. Sci. USA, 80,* 950–954.

Webb, T. E., Schumm, D. E., & Palayoor, T. (1981). Nucleocytoplasmic transport of mRNA. In H. Busch, Ed. *The cell nucleus* Vol. 9, (pp. 199–248) New York: Academic Press.

Weber, J., Blanchard, J. M., Ginsberg, H., & Darnell, J. E. (1980). Order of polyadenylic acid addition and splicing events in early adenovirus mRNA formation. *J. Virol., 33,* 286–291.

Wilkins, R. J., & Hart, R. W. (1974). Preferential DNA-repair in human cells. *Nature, 247,* 35–36.

Zahn, R. K. (1983). Measurement of the molecular weight distributions in human muscular deoxyribonucleic acid. *Mech. Aging Develop., 22,* 355–379.

Zahn, R. K., & Müller, W. E. G. (1975). Alternsabhängige Veränderungen an informationstragenden Makromolekülen. *Verh. Dtsch. Ges. Path., 59,* 3–20.

3
Sociological Dimensions of Gerontology

Leopold Rosenmayr

When dealing with the elderly, be they healthy and active or frail and dependent, one should keep in mind that they act and suffer as individuals who hold a certain status in the society in which they live. Depending on whether they are wealthy or poor, powerful or weak, educated or illiterate, their knowledge and money will command a certain amount of respect socially. But, in addition, in the society in which they live, the various phases of life—childhood, adolescence, young and mature adulthood, mid-life, and early and late senescence— are also socially evaluated. Historical studies and comparisons teach us that the later phase of life in particular has gone through great variations of evaluation. The reason for this variety is that not only the image but also the social reality of older age depended and still depends on structural economic changes, and also on ideological and value changes.

Older people feel and more or less vaguely know what society thinks about them. These evaluations are "internalized," and thus become, in individually varying degrees, part of their self-images. It is therefore important that the medical doctor or psychiatrist, the psychologist or social worker become familiar with the historico-social structures and values that furnish at least part of the material for self-evaluation. These structures transmit to the individuals the securities or anxieties which thus become part of the lives of patients and clients.

In modern times the plethora of motives and conditions makes it very difficult to demonstrate how the age status is built by society. Therefore, in my effort to demonstrate the societal foundation of the evaluation of age and of older individuals, I refer back to early mankind, even to animal society. This makes it easier for me to show that the social position (status, prestige, and power) of the old should be viewed primarily as an element of the total social structure—its ways to produce and to consume, to learn, to communicate, and to develop value preferences.

By studying animal sociology one may examine systemic social effects that are derived from societies with relatively little cultural superstructures, where the biological impulses lead to activities and equilibria. Biosociological research on animal behavior shows that the social organization of a species has direct influence on the organism. Thus, it is not only the organism that needs (for its early phases of development, its nurturing, protection, learning to survive, etc.) a certain social infrastructure. The mode of interaction and the whole social network of a species has feedback effects on the evolutionary profile of the organism. The social organization and association has somatic consequence. My emphasis on sociobiology and early human society in describing the unfolding of the social dimension in aging in this chapter should be understood as an attempt to underline sociosomatic perspectives.

If I am able to show—and I think the reader will recognize it—that social organization has a direct impact on the organism from an evolutionary point of view, then this may serve as an argument that the classical psychosomatic perspective will have to be extended in order to include sociosomatic elements. In short, my discussion here, although it leads to prehistoric and ethnographic data and dwells on them rather extensively, is just another line of arguing for the power of the social structure (and its dynamics) in defining the organic and psychological conditions of aging in individuals.

My aim is to elaborate theoretical views of the sociology of aging in order to make them applicable to a social medicine of aging and a sociosomatic geriatrics. Elsewhere I have tried to describe perspectives of indepth psychology, particularly psychoanalytics, in trying to understand intergenerational relations within the family and in aging couples and friendships (Rosenmayr 1983a, 1983b). Here my approach is more directly sociological and historical. In the final sections (pp.67–71) I attempt to outline some fundamental convictions and value models of Western culture and their impact on the status of the old

Gerosociology encompasses an almost infinite variety of topics including family and intergenerational relations, retirement, housing problems of the elderly, work, and leisure. In general, gerosociology is the study of practically all major problem areas of society, among them the economic and health needs of the elderly and all forms of deficiency and neglect. I will not list them all here—they may be taken from the existing handbooks (Birren & Schaie, 1984) and the multitude of textbooks. Instead, I will examine briefly several questions:

- What are some elements of a theoretical language that enable the social scientist to study the relationships of the individual to society in view of the aging and developmental processes of the second half of life? (See following sections, pp. 45–51.)
- What is the sociobiological basis for an integrated gerosociology? (Pages 51 through 57 deal with the status of old individuals in primate society and emphasize the significant changes in the value of the old in the transition from pre-human or anthropoid societies to early humankind. It is thought that for the medical scientist and the psychiatrist the frontier-area of the sociobiology of aging may be of particular interest.)
- What are the factors in nonliterate ("primitive") societies, described by ethnography and ethnosociology, that constitute the high prestige of the old? (See pp. 57–65.)
- What are some reasons for a decline in the status of the old in early Western society? Religious and philosophical egalitarianism relativize the special position of the old and transform them into objects for care. The sciences support the notion of exchange which turns out to be unable to balance off the needs of a vastly grown subpopulation of older and old people. With reference to what concepts does modern social science analyse the social position of older people?
- (Pages 66 through 71 inform the medical scientist and practitioner of the great social and historical plasticity within the evaluation of old people. Also discussed are two major concepts, namely, "exchange" and "self" to briefly orient the reader to a mode of analysis that combines a perspective of society with a view of the individual.)

THEORETICAL ELEMENTS OF GEROSOCIOLOGY

The sociologist studies how aging, development, and fulfillment are shaped by technology and modes of production, by the changing man–environment relation, and by models of culture, meaning, and self-interpretation. Sociologists are concerned with the impact of social structures and their power in distributing and allocating material and cultural goods and resources, how they in fact are allocated to age groups and the social, economic, and cultural subgroups of these age groups. Sociologists explain and interpret life history, aging, and development according to variables of social structure and cultural conditions. In spite of a rapid growth of sociological studies on aging some topics and areas remain neglected for reasons which might be worthy of study in themselves.

Dyads, like married couples or friends, have hardly been studied under developmental aspects. The fullfledged longitudinal study of small institutionalized groups like families still present great methodological and organizational difficulties for social research. This is true particularly if such research goes beyond general sociodemographic comparative surveys of changing patterns of household, marriage, and family composition. Most data on marital relations in later life are data from and on individuals and much less on the processes of mutuality and the changes resulting therefrom. However, aging, development, and mutual fulfillment in longstanding relations among individuals, the change in creativity, gratification, and the intensity of connection with each other are necessary and promising areas of future research. Only recently elements of ideology, culture, and religion have received more attention in their significance to guide the self-interpretation of individuals as they face problems and decisions in the second half of life.

Sociologists disagree on the question of which points of view and angles sketched here should be given preference. Agreement may be better on the need of a systems approach to the individual's relationship to the environment, to other individuals, to the social structure, and to culture, if aging and development are to be studied. A systems approach has the advantage of permitting the interrelation of various disciplines, and to some extent can even connect natural with social sciences, and both with medicine.

Such a systems approach, however, will vary according to the sociologist's views on the decisive dimensions and variables of social structures and social relations. Another question is how wide these perspectives should be opened toward other disciplines in the human, social, and cultural sciences. The majority of sociologists follow a more classical perspective which focuses on the analysis of roles and status of the elderly. I propose a more risky and to some extent less "conclusive" sociocultural, pluridisciplinary, interpretative approach, related to but not exclusively based on "hard data."

Interdependency, cohesion, exchange, and integration of individuals and groups of greatly different ages, especially in intergenerational relations (an important sub-area of a life-course oriented social gerontology), need a plurality of disciplines to avoid reductionism. A systems approach to human society, individual interaction, and relationships, from our point of view, would have to link perceptions and interpretations of reality to the position of the perceiver within the system. This is one of the reasons why history and culture (through which the human self perceives) need to be studied. Seniority, for example, coupled with age to some extent, is a status or an element in a status system viewed and defined under the impact of cultural influences and values. The gerontologist or life-course scientist in my view has to understand that individuals, families, groups, and institutions live and develop by interpreting their age notions and evaluations in view of their cultural heritages and cultural changes. In this sense the systems' approach has to be supplemented by looking at individuals and groups from a historical perspective. This means that the uniqueness of each life history, cohort, or generational participation must be considered. The sociological perspective of aging must, however, also include an appreciation of biological and genetic conditions of the organism, and of the health and economic needs of individuals and groups, needs that these individuals and groups feel and claim vis-à-vis the society they live in.

From a sociologist's point of view aging may be defined as a sequential change, following certain general and at least partially irreversible biologically and medically definable tendencies with a wide range of cultural, social, psychological, and biological variety. In order to explore this definition let us first look at aging from the point of view of the individual's relations to environment and then at the organization of society responding to the existence of various groups of older people.

Each living system needs environmental support. Loss of energy and material losses of the system must be compensated. In order to establish equilibrium an input of energy is needed for survival. Equilibria and processes of equilibration undergo certain systematic shifts in time. The establishment of homeostasis varies biologically, according to the complexity of the system. Biological aging is characterized by processes of loss and, at least partially, recovery of homeostatic equilibria. In biological aging as demonstrated by some cases of cell maturation, we already find a succession of equilibrium shifts: each maturation stage has a particular equilibrium state appropriate for its functioning. The capacity to regenerate varies greatly according to subsystems of the organism. If some biologically important elements are lost they can sometimes be replaced in a "natural" way; sometimes they cannot. Irreversibility is an important characteristic of aging. Therefore, it is one of the strategic tasks of life-course science to define the frontiers of irreversibility and to explore possibilities to narrow them. Another task is to compensate for losses due to irreversible processes, or to describe the means to permit acceptance of the effects of irreversible change.

Loss in sociopsychological terms is a paradoxical notion, it may mean personal gain; for example, a person in late midlife can decide to abandon a powerful position or a long established field of activity in order to select withdrawal to focus on more internalized, self-oriented, and self-determined activities. What may appear to be a loss from the point of view of the person's established practices may be (may have the "meaning" of) a sort of liberation from the point of view of the actor himself (and of others), and might be termed "yield." In order to "yield," higher order values must be accepted that permit one to live with losses or even willingly renunciate.

Sometimes the motivation for yielding may be gained by the conviction that stabilization in the sense of peace or happiness may only be obtained by "structural overbalancing," or by giving more than receiving (Rosenmayr, 1978c). This means that the decision-making individual is willing to accept an even long-term imbalance of gratification. Intergenerational cooperation needs phases of overbalancing; yet other relations like friendship or love in the richness of exchange also include nonmeasured mutual "yielding."

CHARACTERISTICS OF THE SYSTEMS APPROACH TO GEROSOCIOLOGY

In order to proceed further and to conceptually unfold the pluridisciplinary sociological perspective, I will note here some differences between biological and social systems:

1. Biologically, the living system (organism) may be functionally defined from a certain maximum or optimum point of view. The notion of maturity has a simpler meaning in a biological context: it implies a point from which no further growth is possible. Decline alleviated by some form of restitution is the only conceivable further process after biological maturity has been achieved. In a sociocultural reality, however, where processes of intellectual and cultural information gathering and learning, and self-expression take on a central importance, no functional maximum, saturation, or full maturation point can be determined, certainly not in any general way. Any human and social maturity definition is uncertain and depends on the values predefining the criteria applied for attributing "maturity" to observed phenomena.

2. All homeostatic systems are balance-oriented. For reasons of psychological continuity and well-being, complex adaptive systems like the human personality tend toward the achievement of balance. Unlike simpler homeostatic systems, human personalities need a multitude of interconnected balance areas and sequences of equilibration, that is, "stages" of development (e.g., stages of consciousness and of bodily sensations for the discovery and fulfillment of needs). To generalize with regard to stages in adult life is a highly hypothetical gesture and, if not taken as such, tends to deteriorate from the suggestive level to a deplorable reification.

3. In spite of a tendency toward psychological balance a certain amount of imbalance, for example, stress and a variety of stimulations interrupting (routine-) behavior, is necessary for the development of innovative attitudes. Development in complex adaptive systems requires the permission or even the search for a destruction of older forms. The capacity to change is as

much a capacity necessary for the survival of the system as is the homeostatic faculty.

4. The complex adaptive organization of the human personality, in order to allow change and development, disposes of the memory that permits the turning back of the experience of the individual upon himself by means of generalized symbols taken or transmitted from various levels of culture. This "reflexiveness" and thus connection with culture is a special characteristic of human aging, a necessity for human development, and a prerequisite of fulfillment. In relation to one's own history, memory also refers to the history of the cohort and to "history at large." Aging has been defined as "an index of events which occur at different points of time" (Bengtson, 1973, p. 15). It seems necessary to insist on the "exploration" of these events, their repercussions and effects on the individual, which may be called experiences. This in turn favors and increases "reflexiveness" and expands it over more than mere cognitive elements. If it takes on forms of exposure, experience may lead to emotional and deeply effective "existential" reflexiveness. Such existential concern and awareness are more likely to cause or facilitate human change than mere cognitive speculation.

5. Complex adaptive systems, unlike simple homeostatic systems, are goal-oriented and based on planned cooperative action. Thus they are capable not only of recording the past, but also of utilizing experience for an organization of the future, for example, by developing life plans and projects. They are irreplaceably necessary for individuals in changing, as competitive societies are built on individual achievement and/or a multiplicity of offers and opportunities in a pluralist system. Anticipation of structured action plus capability for planned revision go beyond mere responses to competitiveness. They may furnish understanding of many conflicts and contradictions in aging and human development. Evaluation of past achievements in the light of newly visualized standards and plans for the future are the special contributions that consciousness may offer to a homeostatic balance. Taking into account the feedback of discrepancies between past achievements and future expectations is particularly important for understanding aging and development from a sociological point of view.

6. A person with a differentiated consciousness and an extended perception of emotions and motives may be characterized by a certain need for self-expression. The production, reception, and interpretation of symbols are often connected with needs for self–expression and encounter. Esthetic values of beauty and harmony are special homeostatic elements; their perusal must be considered as an important activity for the stabilization of the system. Happiness, that is, the feeling connected with fulfillment, is a special element necessary for human development.

SOCIOLOGICAL AND CULTURAL CONDITIONING OF AGING, DEVELOPMENT, AND FULFILLMENT

Human personalities, with their complex adaptive characteristics, constitute society in cooperative and antagonistic relations, in organizations and institutions. Orientation and integration occur through values and symbols over long stretches of individual time throughout the life course, or over social and cultural time (cohorts, generations, regional, and global history).

The key question of a sociology of aging is how to relate the individual, acting in a social and cultural context within and under the conditions of social structures, to the biological changes of the human organism which occur over time. We ought to go one step further and say that the sociologist must pay special attention to profiles of aging, development, and fulfillment according to the socially significant factors of income, education, occupational group, and other factors such as ethnicity, cultural tradition, and life-style, including cultural evaluations of time.

To give an example, a change-oriented and innovation-based society tends to underscore a continuance of activity. It is a paradox that, on the one hand, modern time is considered to be fugitive and overly precious yet, on the other hand, time spent to perform an activity is valued comparatively little. Periods of social time spent in certain groups or institutions were highly valued by traditional society; therefore the seniority principle was used as a measuring stick. Modern society with its system of social mobility and learning honors quickness and readiness to change. However, postindustrial society is rediscovering that continuity is a necessary element of a self-determined rhythm of development and fulfillment. (Meditation, e.g., looks at time in a different way.) It may be expected that the change to postmodern values will underline the need for personal creativity as different from mechanical and prefabricated innovation. Such a change in cultural values may ultimately influence the evaluation of time and, furthermore, increasingly honor the capacity to wait, "to let grow," and to develop, and may effect the status of older people in society. The acceptance by the aging individual of a more active self-definition and a creativity-oriented attitude will condition this gain in status. It is the task of the sociologist to venture an early diagnosis of developments of the Zeitgeist. In addition, the sociologist may offer concepts for the analysis of historically emerging phenomena.

Self-reflexiveness is one of the important basic characteristics of the human personality as-a-system. This relation is based on an accompanying self-consciousness (self-knowledge) and emotional ties to oneself, including several forms and levels of (revised) narcissism. Self-acceptance and self-defense are of central importance in social and environmental conflicts in which the elderly must fight with the environment as well as with the young, including their own children. Technological and scientific change tends to devalue the older person, but if an older person can demonstrate creativity and his or her own contributions to the immediate social environment and to society at large, this will tend to enhance the status of the old.

A sociological gerontology must refer to the socioeconomics of a society that determines fertility and death. The societal aging process and the rhythm or cycle of fertility and mortality cause social order and social norms to react to these cycles. The various types of aging and reproductive and survival systems, are connected with societies and cultures in different ways. One of the major tasks of the life-course scientist will be to sharpen a perception of the social variety and the cultural necessity of the individual and social responses to aging. There is no single "general" path of aging, and no general model of societal and political reaction to the system of reproduction and mortality. Therefore, the fertility-mortality system is an outcome of, as well as an influential factor in, determining the development of society. An interrelation exists between individual and "population aging," inasmuch as, for example, the proportion of older people in a society, the predominance of their needs, the resulting welfare systems, their lifestyles are additional conditions of the general social value climate of the society. General evaluations that stem from society's reaction to mass aging leave traces on the self-definition of older people.

ELEMENTS OF A SOCIOBIOLOGICAL GERONTOLOGY

Before we study the human personality as a goal-oriented actor and complex adaptive system, and its aging, development, and fulfillment, and before we deal with the impact of human economy and culture on the definition of age criteria and norms, we turn to the evolutionary self-regulation of the position of the older individuals in animal society.

The biosocial organization of a species determines the chance of survival of the organism. The life-span, the capacity to regenerate, the rearing of the brood, etc., all depend on the structural design of the organism, its complexity, and ability to react. However, the evolutionary development of the organism is also a function of the biosocial organization of that particular species to which the individual organism belongs. The biosocial organization must be considered not only as something external to the organism but as a basis for a chance of survival and for a propagation of the individuals and the species to which they belong. The biosocial organization of the species becomes the implementing tool for the goals prescribed by the genetically circumscribed biological individual. Environment is experienced and coped with by the individual not only together with, but also through (e.g., under the guidance of) other individuals. Age groups are differentiated as aspects and expressions of the organization of animal society. The limits that define these groups are constituted and modified for the purpose of the survival of the biological group. Some examples may serve to demonstrate this.

Protection is the first consideration. If socially highly organized primates such as baboons find themselves in an environment where they lack their usual protection against specific enemies, the baboons aggregate in a special way. Young males often perform something like an escort function in which they protect the troop against attack from outside by the formation of a defensive ring around the troop. The young males are exposed at the edge of the troop to ferocious animals for the purpose of selection or evolution within the species. Assuming that those that are more able will have the greater chance of surviving at the edge, the principle of selection can take effect.

In baboon society well-defined age group limits prevail. As long as the young females are not in a state of rut they are covered by the peripheral young males. With the onset of rut the females mate exclusively with their unit leader, a fully grown male. This has important hereditary consequences. Those that survive the hardship of their youth to become adult males and unit leaders with a "harem" also become the main genetic transmittors (Campbell, 1976). After remaining at the top of power and acting as "unit leader" for a certain time, the fully grown and experienced male's physical power begins to deteriorate (e.g., he loses his teeth). The leadership of the harem is then taken by another individual. An old baboon that has lost his harem may be recognized and respected for his special qualities. He may leave the troop to go "stalking" for a lion, find one without being detected himself, return to the troop, and then lead the troop in a detour around the lion to an appropriately protected sleeping place (Kummer, 1968). For such functions he receives a "place of honor" within the troop. Old baboons without harems sometimes form subgroups within the troop. The baboons have a tendency to respect such old experienced males and grant them a leading position. They do this even if the old are practically toothless and can no longer substantiate their physical aggression in interindividual conflict any more. Leadership positions that impose the role of protector and scout may be held by old baboon males well beyond the period when as unit leaders they controlled "harems." These positions are then based on specialized functions, and no longer on the central biologically important leadership of "harems."

Charles Darwin discovered that old animals enjoy an incredibly high standing in the pack. Animal behavior studies now show this in great detail. We know that the strongest rutting-stag does not dare revolt, but follows when the old animals lead (in particular outside the rutting time). "Problem solving" for the benefit of the whole group is a function separate from biological reproduction. Although the latter is fought over violently, the "problem solving" position of the individual older male animal beyond the reproductive conflict is accorded independently of the status definition, as an outcome of such conflict.

The situation is similar with other species that have been studied intensively over decades (Lorenz, 1977). With wild fowl the old gander serves as a type of ombudsman and holds a position of responsibility and leadership. Grey geese are led on by the older mother animals flying at the head of the flock. Security and safety however, are provided by the old ganders; there are about five or six that have this security function in a flock of approximately one hundred geese. The old ganders stand with their heads high up and their backs to the flock until the next cover is reached. Because their aggressive and overalert functions vis-à-vis the environment have made them afraid of each other the "security seniors" of the flock avoid one another. The mutual relationships among old members of the flock are difficult to study because contact is hardly achieved. If they suddenly meet eye to eye while feeding, they pretend not to have seen each other and leave in different directions. They circle around the flock as guards aware of danger and how to approach it. Their warning threshold, however, is particularly low (Lorenz, 1977).

Sociobiological studies of the life-course permit the generalization that dominance-orders are based on two principles: the power of territorial defense connected with sexual competence and domination; and memory, along with the alertness and prevailing motor skill, that makes it functional to the group for scouting and defense. We may thus assume that in order to provide functions of leadership sociobiologically, there exists a species-preserving purpose for longevity beyond fertility. Longevity permits the accumulation of learned content useful for survival of the species.

CHANGES IN INFORMATION TRANSFER ALTER THE STATUS OF THE OLD

The more highly developed animal individual requires a prolonged period of parental protection for an extended learning period. Intergenerational support in terms of feeding, protection, and learning feedback processes are necessary for the offspring to acquire the "knowhow" and fitness to survive. Prolonged learning from parents leads to improved chances of survival. This has been shown experimentally for three consecutive mammalian generations (Wilson, 1975).

Some species require a high learning potential and a large store of experience for the maintenance of evolutionary efficiency. From the point of view of the biological group not only reproduction but also experience-induced achievements have to be socially guaranteed. This means that experienced individuals as well as the learning phases of the young must be supported. The "prestige" of old individuals in leadership functions preserves them. Youth and old age, although in conflict, complement each other, and the life-phase of "maturity" is a necessary one, at least for a minority. Biosociological progress is based on a gain of experience which then becomes effective through selection. From the acquired "knowledge" of older individuals the group may profit, mainly to enhance survival chances. The status of the old is preserved by the group also for the further accumulation of experience in other individuals. By giving others a chance to imitate their behavior, the old become distributors of knowledge.

In human society principles for effective accumulation and diffusion of information differ widely from those that are effective in animal society. The differences concern the scope of as well as ways of passing on information. With man we find a special type of "sharing" of information. Middle- and long- range information transmission in animal society is steered by genetic transmissions and by selection principles. Through action and planned organizations human society accumulates its own body of information which can be circulated and augmented largely independent of genetic factors. When an invention is created, not only the inventor's genetic offspring participate thereby—as would be the case with a mutation—but principally the whole of society. We may call this the horizontal scheme of information dissemination, different from the two types of vertical schemes, namely the genetic and the seniority-based social transfer of information. The horizontal transfer leads to a new type of organization and community in human culture. The typical sharing of human information reduces the value of the accumulation of knowledge based on seniority. In comparison with highly developed animal society, horizontal (or peer-oriented) information sharing in human society relativizes but does not abolish the prerogatives of the old. Longevity receives a definite and respected place in early human society, particularly in nonliterate and later in many types of traditional literate societies based on structures of kinship.

Older individuals become functional in the transmission of the learning contents of tradition and to some extent in the application of learning content to new situations. The scope of knowledge typical for the old varies in quantity and content. The new horizontal principle of information dissemination changes the information system and flow. Feedback loops of practices and techniques generally no longer need vertical testing over long periods of time through transmission and selective control. They are tested through the established cultural channels of information and direct and quick processes of application to reality. Innovation is characterized by a separability from biologic sequence, and the role of accumulated "knowledge" in older individuals has to be assessed and defined for each stage of culture and evolution. Strategic inheritance no longer proceeds from generation to generation but is extended by a cultural tradition that is open to innovation. We find in human society a new type of transmission of knowledge and capabilities through integrated systems of culture which generate special aspirations. To internalize at least part of cultural knowledge and capacity older individuals must protect long phases of learning for the young. Inversely, protection is needed for the elderly who pass on the content of learning. This social protection of the old by the young, however, is far less general than the amount of protection, information and instruction given by elders to the young. A minority of the old protects itself by not yielding its power function or by retaining at least some form of control. High positions are attributed to and recognized by older individuals who contribute significantly to collective survival. Yet no special elder group solidarity is observed as is the case for solidarity of the brood. It appears to be a particular feature of human society that if a certain level of compensation for protection is reached, then not only do the old protect the young by their knowledge and survival techniques, but in return the old are (in varying and lesser degrees) protected by the young.

COHESION AND SEPARATION OF GENERATIONS: THE "RED LAMP OF INCEST" SEEN FROM A LIFE-COURSE PERSPECTIVE

The complicated incest problem arises with several species of highly developed mammals, the offspring of whom need a longer learning phase. Adolescents reach sexual maturity while still needing to remain within the family. Defense against incest already shows itself among primates (Fox, 1980), and among human beings it is further elaborated (Lévi-Strauss, 1949). If the learning phase makes it possible to drive the young away, and if the continuous fight for the sexually mature females is to be avoided, the result must be to introduce rules and sanctions. The prohibition of incest protects the older generation from the younger one, and vice versa. The "classical" sociocultural incest explanation looked upon the incest taboo as a defense mechanism against patriarchal superdominance (Freud, 1913). It may now be viewed as mutual protection and regulation allow for transgroup exchange of marriage partners permitting the unfolding of culture. An extended period of protection that places human offspring under parental control, and thus phases of initiation for the young (Fox, 1980), considerably increase the chance for individual and collective survival and development. Since the early stages of hominization, humans, compared to many other animals, have been bodily weak, and have always been endangered and threatened by their environment. Human survival chances lay in being a polyvalent adaptor, and in ecological "plasticity."

It was by experience, swift passing on of information, and innovations (development of tools and well-adapted social networks) that humans pushed ahead in the midst of threats and dangers of the development of a "superspecies." For this spectacular "upward mobility of mankind" longevity was needed. The establishment of a social order that granted a relatively high although ambivalent status to older individuals was instrumental in enabling this longevity. For the genesis of homo sapiens the higher life expectancy (accessible only to a minority in the early phases of the development of mankind) was a necessary condition. Early human normative systems defended the old according to the Codex Hammurabi, the Mosaic Decalogue, and many other regulations of Early Judaism. The first of the commandments that refer to obligations vis-à-vis humans (after the three commandments relating to God) exhort the young to extend care to their parents:

> Honour thy father and thy mother: that thy days may be long upon the land which the Lord thy God giveth thee. (Exodus 21.12)
>
> Ye shall fear every man his mother, and his father, and keep my sabbath I am the Lord your God. (Leviticus 19.3)

This very clearly indicates the necessity for the normative imposition of and thus support for the obvious insufficient readiness of the young to compensate for what they have received. When it was written and codified, culture became an important instrument for political and spiritual leaders, and the incest taboo no longer needed to be included in the basic commandments. The exhortation not to reject an aging parent (in spite of family and clan-based social organization) needed to be given high priority in the codification of the sacred law. This codification seems to indicate that the development of human culture had reached a point where an important amount of horizontal distribution of knowledge through peers and contemporaries outside the family had developed. The influence and power of vertical intergenerational information from the elders and the dependency on them had obviously weakened already.

As larger groups in human society made the transition from the system of hunting and gathering to the pastoral system they also established specific forms of division of labor, and defined age group structures became rooted therein. (The development of life phases, e.g., the prolongation of childhood, is connected with the division of labor, as will be shown later.) The principle should be stated here that the higher the qualifications needed for survival and its dynamic evolution in production systems, the longer and more differentiated must be the training and education of the young for progressive survival. For the human race biology offers still another aspect of plasticity in the life course.

Corresponding to the potential expansion of the period of youth for learning purposes is the expansion of the postfertile late parental phase. The biological resources for self-maintenance of the human female are not exhausted with the end of her fertility. The phenomenon of menopause differentiates humans from all other mammals (Comfort, 1964). For the history of humankind the postprocreative phase in women has had a species-preserving function to serve evolution. A human mother may bear children up to the end of her fertile phase; fifteen years following the end of this phase are necessary to ensure that the last child is capable of surviving. To protect this child the mother has to survive well beyond fertility. To live a considerable time beyond the reproductive age, in the form of a full-fledged postprocreative life-phase, is unique to humans. Biological dysfunction becomes socially functional and meaningful from the point of view of the cultural learning aspect.

LONGEVITY AND LEARNING CHANCES IN EARLY HUMAN CULTURE

Comparisons between primates and man have led researchers to conclude that for early human society the aged made unique contributions to the survival of a culture as "repositories of experience and wisdom" (Campbell, 1976). We may also draw the conclusion that the aged who were rich in their capacity to give advice, increased the chances of survival for their group. Longevity was a function of leadership in a culture that was basically stable, but barely maintaining economic survival.

Among animals the shaping of life-phases is based on the evolutionary interplay of genetic structure, learning, and selection. Among human beings, it is derived from the purposeful transmission of information and knowledge, on which cooperative division of labor is based. Socially communicable knowledge furthered the division of labor, and the latter in turn pressed for new social learning. Division of labor based on learning may be seen as a specific type of "evolution." Traditional learning was intergenerational, that is, the accumulation of knowledge was based on longevity.

Just as the "extrauterine year," the first year of the life of humans, is a continuation of pregnancy by social means in order to endow a human being with the full capacity to survive, so, too, the postprocreative late phase in human life offers special chances for human survival and development of the species. Homo sapiens is characterized by his "Weltoffenheit"—his "openness to the world" or adaptive plasticity—which is (Portmann, 1976) supported by an intergenerational social organization.

With the increase in the scope of planning in early human history, experience and memory became highly valued. Storage of information is useful for planning and gains in importance for survival. One part of the power of the older individuals lay in their information surplus, which allowed them an increased hold on the continuity of relationships. The unfolding of the personality and its capacities in human development is therefore connected with the specific character and institutionalization of human longevity. The granting of status to the old in primate as well as in early human society is clearly connected with the specialized (and to some extent restricted), yet real and functional contribution of the old to the group, horde, or tribe to which they belong.

CULTURAL LEADERSHIP FUNCTION OF THE OLD IN NONLITERATE SOCIETIES

We have studied the position of the old in animal society with particular reference to primates where the comparison with human society seems most meaningful. We have also tried to understand features of hominization and the role older individuals played in the development of early man in general, and homo sapiens in particular.

We now turn to a different phase of our evolutionary cultural approach and study the structure and meaning of culture that is coupled with a nondynamic and nonexpansive subsistence economy of sedentary people as it developed out of the more casual food collection and hunting of the earliest human economy. In studying such nonliterate societies based on subsistence economies we again find that the old fulfill a protective function. Yet this protection of the old of the group, family, and tribe goes far beyond control of the visible environment, like scouting or warning, found to be so important in various types of animal society.

The protective function of the old leaders in human society includes magical, cosmological, and religious relationships to the other world. This nonvisible world, however, is an integral part of the whole culture. Where modernization has not broken the cosmological belief system, the economy and survival of society are strongly influenced by magical practices. The central function of the old in this type of preliterate society is to assist the animistic cosmological cycle, the most explicit form of which is ancestor worship.

According to the prevailing division of labor in many preliterate (African) societies it is the task of the old to satisfy the ancestors. Because they are less active in the fields, the old have the time to occupy themselves with ancestor worship. This "rational" explanation, however, certainly does not give the whole picture. A minority of the old profit from a higher degree of initiation. Secret forms of psychological and medical practices, magical techniques, as well as special powers of self-control and endurance, predispose the old to spiritual leadership functions like counseling and ancestor liturgy. Clans and tribes form social units with defined hierarchies and the old, being closest to the ancestors, are at least potentially the highest in social rank. Their position is guaranteed by the system, yet they are its spiritual and most frequently also its economic and "political" (e.g., communal) leaders. Some anthropologists affirm that traditional African societies make no significant distinction between deceased ancestors and living elders, and argue that differential and respectful behavior toward both is a reflection of a gerontocratic system, in which the young must honor and obey seniors (Kopytoff, 1971; Mendosa, 1976). In return, ancestors and elders protect the young, particularly within the descent group where the young hold a liminal position. Thus the position of the elders not only involves privileges of respect but also contains special obligations.

Most studies agree that there is a close relationship between ancestor worship and a high respect for older people. According to the basic structure of an animistic cosmology, ancestors act as mediators in prayer and wishes. They act as intermediaries between the living and a supreme yet unknown God (Schweeger-Hefel, 1980). Animistic cosmological belief systems vary; some make sharp distinctions between ancestors and deities, while with others there is more continuity. Ancestors are worshipped in particular places such as small simple shrines built from stone, wood, and twigs and found in the vicinity of houses and villages. If ancestors are venerated then they will better pass on the prayers of the living to the unknown and feared deity.

THE COSMOLOGICAL CYCLE OR THE RETURN OF THE ANCESTORS

If we venture a comparison between the status of the aged in societies with a cosmological, magical world view, and the status of the aged in modernized, particularly industrial cultures, we find that the old in a cosmological society reinforce and intensify this world view, whereas the old in modernized societies are outside the centers of culture (Eisenstadt, 1974).

It is this close link between the status of the aged and cultural coherence in societies with cosmological, magical world views which causes the fundamental differences between their position and the position of the aged in modern societies. We shall later discuss the most recent changes toward postmodern features of culture which include increased chances for improvement in the status of the old.

Linked with nondynamic subsistence economies of sedentary peoples without developed urban centers the cosmological aspect is basic for nonliterate cultures. Animistic magical cosmological cultures unify the visible and comprehensible with the invisible and presageable, representing a circular and repetitive process.

Myths and rites are transmitted from one generation to the other. They "repeat" the past and continue it in the cyclical order of the repetition of mythological storytelling and ritual celebrations. Repetition is also strongly emphasized by the return of ancestral souls.

The cosmological cycle is represented here in a diagram. The cycle applies, in its basic form, to various African cultures (Kabawasa, 1982) which place emphasis on the reentry of ancestors.

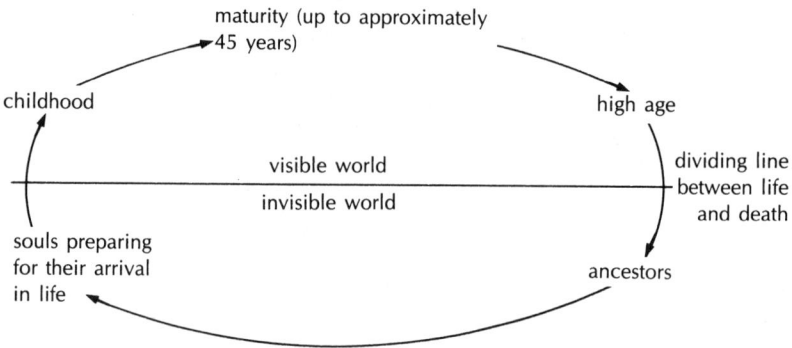

FIGURE 3.1 The cosmological cycle in the animistic magical unity of the visible and the invisible world.

Many African people were firmly convinced that physically dead ancestors who were properly worshipped, would be given sustenance to live on spiritually, and would return one day under certain ritual conditions to reside in new-born children. Thus the cosmological animistic cycle of birth, growth, gaining of experience, becoming old, dying, reentering life, aging, etc., is closed. Cosmological animism makes for the unity of the cycle. The relationship between the physical and the spiritual during the life course can be shown in a diagram, the shaded parts represent the physical aspects and the white parts the spiritual aspects of life.

Sociological Dimensions of Gerontology

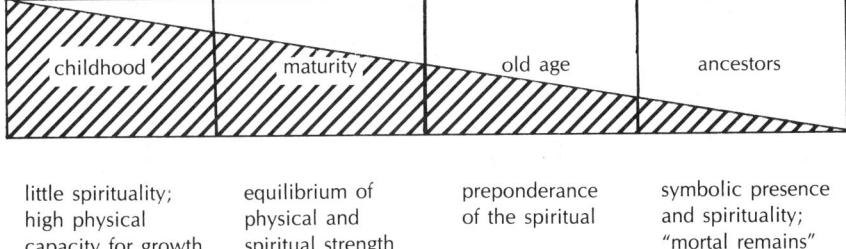

FIGURE 3.2 Development stages of the physical/spiritual aspects of life.

Some African cultures are based on lifelong processes of initiation. Such an order of initiation exists at least for a strategic minority of societies and groups; it defines stages of increasing degrees of enlightenment about the secrets of life. The renewal and repetition of exercises and rites of initiation play an important role also later on in life. Initiation acts of circumcision and excision are performed on children and youth. Initiation as a stepwise enlarging of secret knowledge, often also framed by test periods and rituals, extends far into adulthood with many traditional tribal African cultures. Ancestor worship in Africa is often related to the rebirth ritual of circumcision (Vorbichler, 1980), in which the young are sworn in by their ancestors. Thus initiation and rebirth are connected with reference to traditional wisdom, represented by the ancestors.

An extended life course initiation model is found exhibited by the Senoufo and the Peul peoples in West Africa, to give just two examples. An elite of elders furnishes the interpretation of tribal history, particularly where they are connected with the veneration of ancestors and the orientation towards "the Beyond." It is easy to see that when the old become the carriers of tradition the historical value of tradition becomes an additional supporting factor for the status of the aged in nonliterate civilizations. The African sage, Amadou Hampaté Bâ, who originated from the partially nomadic Peul people, coined the saying, "An old man who dies is like a library which burns down."

AGING AND THE FAMILY UNDER CONDITIONS OF ANCESTOR WORSHIP

One might hold that such topics are extremely remote from present day practices which determine the position of older people in society. Yet in Japan ancestor worship, even under conditions of otherwise dramatic secularization, continues to be an important part of ritual as well as every day life. With strong roots in Hinduism ancestor worship is also alive in Thailand and Burma (Cowgill, 1972). Although we are relatively well informed about continuing familialism which has survived the Cultural Revolution and Maoism in the People's Republic of China, it is difficult to empirically substantiate in detail the statement, "The Chinese worship their ancestors for reasons of filial piety, clan unity, and social approval" (Rohlen, 1971). Wherever certain animistic mediation between human life and the unknown beyond is considered important, and where this mediation is firmly rooted and institutionalized in a society, certain traits of ancestor worship continue to be important. The cult of cemeteries, of caring for graves and worshipping at them, even in cultures which developed under Christian influence, bears traits of ancestor worship. There are even differences between societies according to Christian denominations: in Catholic societies the cult of the dead is generally stronger than in Protestant ones. The Catholic concept of the "saint" is not unrelated to such ideas of mediation.

The original model for the worship of ancestors and the *respect of the elders is the father–son relationship* (Fortes, 1965; Grindal, 1972). But all elders are neither equal in importance and status nor eligible to become ancestors. Although ancestors and elders have a common responsibility for their descent group and although, according to many tribal traditions, both have wisdom, the "dead elders" (ancestors) have a certain power not given to the living elders. The elders have custodial functions in connection with shrines. In the mythological European tradition that parallels the African cosmological-magical way of life, the pious old couple Philemon and Baucis find their ultimate fulfillment in becoming guardians of the temple, yet guardianship is not only ritualistic in nature but contains jural elements. A high status is attributed to those elderly who have a special jural function in balancing and resolving internal strife. This function may qualify them to become guardians of ancestor shrines.

In many traditional African societies we find an *"eldership complex"* (Kopytoff, 1971; Vorbichler, 1980) which includes both living and dead ancestors. A specific animistic perspective (Kossodo, 1978) attributes the souls of deceased family members to objects, particularly masks, as a special kind of magic life. Ancestors are believed to have a certain existence behind masks kept as treasured objects within the family (Schweeger-Hefel, 1980). In Japan masks are revered in pictures and in special corners of the house. This animism creates a strong bond between the family and the ancestry wherein the living elders serve a special "linkage" function between the "Here" and the "Beyond."

Ancestor worship and respect for the old is related to the kinship system; thus it brings about definite forms of the ritualization of filial piety (Fortes, 1959; Hsu, 1971). Elders take important positions in the council of clans and village communities. Tribal societies that are age-grade structured, like many nomadic or semi-nomadic tribes of East Africa (Eisenstadt, 1974; Fosbrooke, 1978; Rosenmayr, 1978a), follow an organization of cohorts rather than of intergenerational and clan relations. Therefore, tribal societies more explicitly downgrade the very old and clearly differentiate between various subgroups of "young old" and "old old". (The two or three oldest cohorts gradually move out of the central sphere of power and prestige, and although they may retain some religious and particularly ritual functions, they lose power and influence within the tribe and its age group system.) In societies based on family and kinship systems downgrading of the elderly is much less the case, if it occurs at all. The kinship system tends to perpetuate the power of the weak old person on account of authority definitions and sacred powers, and also because of the (magically sanctioned) control over property.

There are important distinctions between "ancestors" and the living old which can be proven by linguistic analysis. As far as the living old are concerned, age alone does not qualify one for the valued position of "elder." Even a relatively young member of the family who was important enough to the tribe may become an "elder" and an "ancestor" after death. In some societies an old bachelor—on account of familialism and the prominence of the fertility principle—cannot become an ancestor. Apart from these specifications the status of an ancestor is irreversible, once ascribed after death.

A final note of caution should be added: The status of older people in traditional societies is generally high. It is based on the seniority principle which secures a high position to old people. The old obtain and prolong their status by performing definite functions such as interpretation of dreams, counseling, the extinguishing of the flames of beginning social conflict, the re-establishment of peace, and, as we have seen, the worship of ancestors. Special knowledge of how to heal wounds may raise older women to the top of a clan (Kossodo, 1978); their role as midwives or for the initiation of young girls is also important.

Poor and isolated elderly do not generally receive high status, as African social researchers report from recent field studies (Ssenkoloto, 1981). In reviewing available literature on the topic of the position of older people we are faced with a particular dilemma: while anthropologists who focus on traditional tribal culture emphasize a structural preference and priority for the elderly, empirical social researchers who have recently discovered the topic for themselves tend to underline status deficiencies of the elderly. Social researchers often focus on regions where migration and social change toward modernization have occurred. Anthropologists, on the other hand, aim at isolated and relatively integrated communities which follow traditional norms and life styles. Research on the same populations by different methods might help to clarify the discrepancies which characterize present findings.

VARIOUS TYPES OF SOCIAL EXCLUSION AND RITUAL AMBIVALENCE VIS-À-VIS THE ELDERLY IN TRADITIONAL SOCIETIES

If we study the position of the elderly in an anthropological and historical comparative perspective we must not overlook certain minority forms of traditional and radical social exclusion of the elderly, which, in very ambivalent ways, were sometimes connected with their magical and religious reintegration. For this reason we will have to look into an often neglected or carefully avoided and tabooed topic, namely, the copiously yet not systematically documented phenomenon of radical exclusion by various forms of direct or indirect senilicide. Even in historical societies, senilicide has not completely been restricted to acts of a purely criminal character (Stearns, 1977). In some medieval Western societies the exposition of various instruments used for senilicide in prominent public places demonstrates traces of this institution.

We have gained little knowledge from animal societies of the practice of annihilation of the elderly by members of the same species. Dying or weak old elks or elephants become easy prey for predatory animals like leopards and wolves, which have the best chances of feeding on the old and weakening individuals of a species. Killing of the old by members of the same species does occur in the battle for succession as a unit or troop leader, and there is also killing ("murder") of weaker individuals in some primate societies. As far as we know, no special protection exists for the old against environmental hardship or enemies. There is, however, a furious protection of the brood; mother individuals use suicidal devices such as the display of helpless vulnerable behavior to distract threatening predators in order to rescue their young. Yet in animal societies there is no special protection of old congeners.

In perpetuating culture, and in order to find magical and spiritual protection, man has defined ways to "use" older congeners, including their physical destruction. Although the extension and frequency of senilicide in anthropological and historical societies is still debated, there is a plethora of unsystematic testimony which states that for a minority killing of the old and frail was an important way to end relatives' lives (Koty, 1934).

Such practices were reported in early Indian, Siberian, Western Asiatic, Slavic, Nordic, Mediterranean, and other societies (Gutmann, 1977). No testimony has been given on Middle Eastern cultures, and the practice is conspicuously absent from Judaism. Interpretations of the sociocultural phenomenon of senilicide differ widely. Some authors feel that ritualization was necessary to frame and render acceptable a revulsive practice of social egoism (Koty, 1934). Others make it plausible that senilicide may be interpreted as a remnant of more general ritual killing for magical purposes, including the sacred eating of human flesh. According to some magical belief systems selected aged individuals were killed so that their powers might transgress to others of the same group. The phenomenon of senilicide must not be reduced to perspectives of sheer economic utilitarianism. When senilicide occurred, the old were certainly not killed because they could no longer be fed. Whereas such measures of "population policy" seem to have played a more significant part in infanticide, other aspects were more relevant in senilicide. The elders' resource of power—their control of both existing social and economic relations, and spiritual forces—always mattered, particularly in pre-modern human societies.

Senilicide could have facilitated both the liberation of a clan or group from the exertion of power by a tyrannical old member, and the "profiting" from his spiritual resources after his death. It may be significant to note that all senilicide reported by anthropologists involved killing old men, never women! Some theories uphold that the death of an older man is necessary in order to allow his forces to pass through the soil, so that they can be received by other members of his group. Expulsion of an old man from the living in this sense did not include spiritual annihilation; on the contrary, it might well have meant his incorporation into the group on a higher level. We may well apply the notion of ambiguity or ambivalence to the apparent contradiction between veneration and destruction.

In some African tribes decorated skullcaps were worshipped and partly used as sacred drinking vessels. From the skulls of famous ancestors comes the vital strength of experience. Some aged persons were killed for their wisdom. We can only understand such ideas of soul and strength on the basis of a cosmologic magical belief system, and the priority of clan or tribal unity over individual well-being or personal integrity. In this connection it is important to understand that to exile the old in Vedic times in Indian tradition meant their social and finally physical death. After relinquishing their property to their sons in complete renouncement, Vedic elderly had no right to return, not even to pick a fruit from one of the fields over which they had had command the day before. All that remained was to become a "Sanyasin" in the forest and feed on what they found there, and later to go begging practically unclothed. Some saintly old people practiced complete nudity as a form of radical exposure to death.

The Indian example shows that on account of the special legal rules that defined the passage of property from one generation to the other, and the resulting dispossession of the old generation, the exile of Vedic elderly became a sort of institutionalized exclusion. The elderly were sent into a social nowhere leading to their physical weakenning and death (Sprockhoff, 1979). The social forms derived therefrom served as important foundations for Indian asceticism and mysticism that flourished in Buddhism.

ORIGINS OF THE EVALUATION OF HIGHER AGE IN WESTERN CULTURE

Early European history allows us to understand how we outgrew the veneration of our ancestors. Aristotle's life stage theory and Cicero's dialogue "On Old Age" emphasize that the human individual is capable of lifelong learning, and endurance and perseverance in old age. Therefore, man ought to prepare himself for aging with life styles that combine modesty and activity. This shows an important shift from an other-worldly to a this-worldly attitude. Instead of looking to ancestors, man was oriented toward himself.

We must also study Jewish and Christian religious and social concepts in order to fully understand Western attitudes toward old age. First we should note that to worship a dominant God like Yahweh, who provides social and political leadership, gives powerful personal protection, and demands as well as grants a covenant, leaves little room for the veneration of ancestors. Old people, however, often accompany religious and political leaders and heroes, as the Jewish sacred books of the Bible show. In the messianic future of the eschatological "New Jerusalem" gerontocratic assistance will be necessary for the "reign of fulfillment" (Zach. 8,4). Judaism of the 2nd century B.C. developed a rising sensitivity for the uniqueness and integrity of the individual (Flusser, 1968), and a conviction of personal continuity and resurrection after death. Long life and the survival of the chosen people were no longer the only means for continuity. During the last two centuries B.C., trends of a general eschatological egalitarianism spread; consequently, a long life became less important and the status of the old diminished.

The basic Christian message sprang up as a hope for individual human development and as a theory of fulfillment, emphasizing spiritual and psychological openness and the principle of "rebirth." The Christian tradition underlines a dynamic age-egalitarianism and therefore a neglect of biological age and seniority. This radicalism, however, could not stand on its own and had to be supplemented by a social support concept. For pastoral reasons the young Christian community adopted elements of the traditional Jewish "veneration" of the old. After the eschatological expectations of the imminent end of the world and the reappearance of Christ were not fulfilled, the Christian community had to base itself more and more on traditional family solidarity. "Do not rebuke an older man but exhort him as you would a father; treat younger men like brothers, older women like mothers" (1 Tim. 5, 1). This family model gave an element of order to the community, which in spite of its moral and spiritual radicalism reaching beyond family interest, had to cope with daily life. The pastoral letters attributed to Saint Paul clearly established or reaffirmed the "filial" duty of compensation. Under common household conditions the repayment idea of the Mosaic Law was re-institutionalized; the need for special consideration and assistance to older members of the community was emphasized (1 Tim. 5, 8). Social work done for the old was seen to be an aspect of personal and moral repayment or "exchange." If one behaved in an obliging manner toward the family and community in earlier phases of the life cycle, the chances of being integrated into the community during phases of weakness and old age were much better. The community was supposed to maintain a collective consciousness of standards of integrated moral "exchange."

"EXCHANGE" AND "OVERBALANCE" AS KEY CONCEPTS IN SOCIAL GERONTOLOGY

Modern secularized society has tried to explore exchange as a general framework for the evaluation of its relation to older people. In this search, the sociological concepts of the exchange and balance of benefits became a construction within which to think, both politically and morally. Recent developments in postaffluent or postmodern society spurred by value changes have underlined the need for radically new and more positive evaluations of the biographic and psychological "heritage" of older people. In this new vision of culture the elderly may be able to transmit to the young guidelines for orientation. Although there are certain important levelling tendencies at work toward a society where age will be less relevant, interage group exchange will remain a significant economic, political, and social issue. We will therefore briefly review some examples of the exchange frame of thought (Maddox, 1976; Rosenmayr, 1974a), in which actors are involved and definitions of society must transcend concepts of functionality (Dowd, 1978).

We discussed biological agents and sociobiological aspects involved in a social concept of aging earlier in this chapter. If, however, we want to adequately analyze human acts, we will have to widen the study of compensation, exchange, and the "principle of self-interest" to include social affection and "overbalancing," which take us beyond self-preservation and mutually balanced interests. "Overbalancing" is marked by a purposeful and processed disequilibrium in psychosocial exchange, where more is given or yielded than taken or assimilated. Acts of overbalancing are necessary to constitute social solidarity. In such a system ideally everyone gives more than he expects to receive. There are noncontractual elements in a "contract of solidarity" (Durkheim, 1893). Solidarity support for dependent elderly must go beyond a contractual balance not only in expressive but also in instrumental support. The direction of overbalancing in age relations is both up and down the generations. Overbalancing is necessary to enable aging persons to change their views and to accept assistance, as well as to "open up" society to the aged so that support for the necessary and desired functions is provided (Rosenmayr, 1978c).

The norm of reciprocity (Gouldner, 1960) contributes to the stability of social systems if their functions are intact, but reciprocity is insufficient to balance off dysfunctions. Support to social groups in a particular need of help cannot be conceptualized only in retributive terms of reciprocity.

Those theorists who refer to exchange concepts have not realized the limitations of the applicability of the norm of reciprocity. The aged as a general group, were seen, for example, to be in a power deficit, or in a disequilibrium of power, thought to result in unilateral exchange action (Dowd, 1978). The result of theorization on the power deficit recently was hardly more than a general social criticism that the more powerful exchange partners, namely the power centers of society and state, dictate the conditions of the relationship and that such one-sided distributive justice lowers the level of satisfaction. The weaker strive for access to resources, and can do so only with compliance. Child-parent support (in the form of social and emotional aid) may be seen as repayment for the benefits received during the time the child was dependent on the parent, and also as a strategy to gain recognition in the social environment. With the increase in longevity overbalancing becomes a structural necessity for the younger generations. The reciprocity obligation felt by children decreases as parents' age increases. Children are therefore challenged to "overbalance" if they want to continue their support (Schneider, 1974; Guillemard & Lenoir, 1974).

The exchange principle is insufficient for the family; the benefits can neither be objectively evaluated nor clearly remembered because they are always transformed by interpretation. Modern society lacks continuity in social reference which increases tendencies of ingratitude. Social mobility between generations, differences in religious or ideological attitudes (i.e., a pluralism of values even within the family), the decline of the family as an institution, discontinuities such as divorce and remarriage are all exemplary factors which contribute to the insufficiency of reciprocity as a source of solidarity. While the lifelong face-to-face-exchange in the frame of the extended family (Morioka, 1972; Aoi, 1975) and other chances for exchange shrink, the social and psychological demands of the old rise. In order to support, rehabilitate, and care for older people, society cannot base distribution only on the former contributions and achievements of the old. Repayment must be replaced by social and cultural acknowledgement of life chances as well as organized social and empathic interpersonal support for the legitimized needs of the elderly. The fulfillment of "life chances," although a general goal of society, will require an increased amount of solidarity and self-organization of those concerned who desire acknowledgement and support of such chances. Self-induced support for the elderly is on the rise and in the future we will have to employ different paths in this upward direction (Attias-Donfut, 1975).

SELF-THEORY AS AN APPROACH TO SOCIAL GERONTOLOGY AND GERIATRICS

For the modern notion of the self, emphasis on the unity of the individual with culture and society is typical. In the spirit of the systems theory approach developed earlier in this chapter, the self may be seen in an aura of autonomy, characterized by its relation to and dialectical unity with culture (Riegel, 1976). A revised and strengthened self furnishes a complex set of criteria for decision making which creates the potential for decisive change in the image of oneself. Such a vision of change is crucial for the improvement of expectations and decisions in the mid-life or preretirement phases. Insecurity and neurotic prohibitions block, through compulsive ideas and emotional fixations, the ability to change one's orientation. The formation of self-image, however, is a decisive pivotal point for the subjective regulation of one's basic orientation and is very important for behavioral modification. A strengthened actual self and the resulting increase in flexibility for renewal of the self-image are conditions for a change in the "aspiration framework" (Rosenmayr, 1974b). Changes in this framework are necessary for the successful approach to new emotional, social, and intellectual learning fields. These areas may be of high importance for new sexual or erotic choices, for compensation of a loss, or for recovery after an illness in mid-life or later. A change in one's aspiration framework has important consequences for motivation, and perseverance in taking on and realizing tasks. However, modification of the self-image is necessary for such change and requires the incentive of strong emotional experiences. These could include the involvement and subsequent detachment in a "separation of the lovers" (Caruso, 1968), or a certain inner radicalness resulting from meditation or religious acts. Purposeful detachment is necessary for inner self-criticism and acceptance of change.

Significant changes in the self-image require a paradoxical mixture of security and risk during (late) middle age—sufficient security to revise present evaluations, and sufficient desire for, and attachment to, the "early dream" which is part of the ideal self. Thus, later middle age is the phase of withdrawal and must be regarded as perhaps the key phase for gerontology in its classical sense. To be able to question oneself or one's behaviorally decisive principles means the ability to overcome one's own defensiveness and regressiveness. Chances for self-questioning rate much higher when the relation to one's own body is not substantially threatened or made insecure, which is more likely to happen at an older age. With advancing age, solutions are more likely sought in an already acquired psychological repertory than in attempts at working out novel solutions (Birren, 1964).

The connections between philosophical concepts of the self and psychotherapeutic treatment and theory have been strongly developed during the last decade (Stein, 1979). This opening offers as an advantage that a special therapeutic and pedagogic framework for the mass phenomena of aging may be drafted. Scientific reorientations have to be sought. It is no longer possible to accommodate central phenomena such as defensiveness, incapacity to change, lack of assimilation, and conviction within the framework of a science which looks upon the mind as an apparatus that processes biological drives (Kohut, 1979). Instead, personality ought to be seen as a self, capable of relating historical and autobiographical insight to the reformulation of life plans and life strategies (Fisher & Fisher, 1979).

"Self-expression" has to be seen as a particularly central problem area. Low education, lack of self-confidence, and depressive character structures hamper bodily or esthetic self-expression. Unresolved conflicts between superego structures and drives tend to block self-expression.

Particular emphasis needs to be given to self-acceptance and self-defense. Present societal conditions and trends hardly permit the high valuation of continuity, the capacity to wait, the self-determination of behavioral rhythms, leisure for "existential" reflection, and life revisions. Subjective experiences of chaos and disorientation may accompany these cultural trends. The search for security in the aging self therefore is a particularly important activity in post-modern society.

SUMMARY

The sociobiological sections emphasize two aspects: (a) The social organization of a species and group have decisive impact on task allocation and thereby set age standards and norms (biological age is shaped by social organization and is by no means to be considered as an immutable predetermination). (b) Information sharing in early humankind increasingly tended to move away from seniority and age-order principles, in a process where, first, genetic transfer dominated, second, generational initiation and knowledge control became powerful, and third, the system gave way to a much more generalized and less age-relevant exchange of information. The flexibility of a multitude of information universes was the decisive element in the devaluation of the old.

Any present day attempt to fight the devaluation of older people has to accept this irreversible devaluation principle and look for areas of knowledge and competence which are not affected by renewable information. In addition, fundamental attitudinal changes can be achieved only on the basis of sociostructural changes, such as the division of labor or the division of activity between work and leisure (Rosenmayr, 1982) and changes in the modes and evaluation of information and communication. A culturally now possible higher esteem for personal and biographic or autobiographic communication will contribute to raise the esteem for older human individuals.

The evaluation of old age is profoundly connected with the social system, and with status hierarchies related to magical or religious fundaments, such as those in our discussion of African cosmological cycles.

Monotheistic religion and new leadership principles in nonsedentary societies counteracted and finally destroyed traditional animistic ancestor cults and thereby devaluated the old who were the main partners of the dead ancestors.

Religions that emphasize human egalitarianism and the equal right of all individuals to participate in redemption (i.e., Christianity) were crucial in levelling the age statuses long before modern forms of production arose to devalue the traditional knowledge accumulated in higher age.

Exchange notions supporting an ideal of justice belong to the early philosophical foundations of Western culture and rightly serve as an orientation for modern gerontology. However, with the increased impact of state and other highly organized forms of social care, a mutual consensus on life chances is necessary which can no longer be achieved exclusively on the basis of exchange notions (Rosenmayr, 1978b). Reduction to exchange would mean weakening a growing proportion of old people who require assistance. Such an exchange system is neither morally nor politically adequate to respond to the proliferation of cultural, educational, psychological, and medical needs (Rosenmayr, 1984). Solidarity will have to rest on interindividual overbalancing and on the sociopolitical acknowledgement of enhanced quantitative and qualitative life chances of larger segments of the older population. The above cannot be argued from the point of view of "social order" or correcting "disorder," but may be seen as a strategy to satisfy needs within a hypothetical, step by step achievement of conflictual "distributive justice" (Rosenmayr, 1983a).

The last section of the chapter shows that all social intervention requires a corresponding notion of a self ready to assume responsibility for his/her own life conditions and chances for change. While indicating particular areas of deficiency and conflict, the section offers some means to conceptualizing social work, care, or psychiatric treatment as an attempt to strengthen the individual as a potential *actor* rather than treating him or her as an *object* of intervention.

REFERENCES

Aoi, K. (1975). *The elderly people and the return to childhood.* 10th International Congress of Gerontology, Jerusalem, June 22–27, 1975. *Congress Abstract,* Vol. II, p. 340.

Attias-Donfut, C. M. (1975). *Etudes et recherches. Etude sur le maintien à domicile des personnes âgées.* Enquête exploratoire: Les personnes âgées et leurs aides ménagères. Paris: C.N.A.V.T.S.

Bengtson, V. L. (1973). *The social psychology of aging.* The Bobbs-Merrill studies in sociology. New York: Bobbs-Merrill Comp.

Bengtson, V. L. (1975). Value socialization in three generations: Cohort and lineage effects. *American Sociological Review, 33,* 224–239.

Birren, J. E. (1964). *The psychology of aging.* Englewood Cliffs, NJ: Prentice-Hall.

Birren, J. E., & Schaie, K. W. (Eds.). (1984). *Handbook of the psychology of aging* (2nd ed.). New York: Van Nostrand Reinhold.

Campbell, B. G. (1976). *Human evolution, an introduction to man's adaptations.* Chicago: Aldine Publishing Company.

Caruso, I. (1968). *Trennung der Liebenden. Ein Phänomen des Todes.* Bern, Stuttgart: Huber.

Comfort, A. (1964). *The process of aging.* New York: Signet Science Library.

Cowgill, D. O. (1972). The role and status of the aged in Thailand. In D. O. Cowgill & L. D. Holmes (Eds.), *Aging and modernization* (pp. 91–102). New York: Appleton-Century-Crofts.

Dowd, J. J. (1978). Aging as exchange: A test of the distributive justice proposition. *Pacific Sociological Review, 21,* 351–375.

Durkheim, E. (1969). *The division of labor in society,* (G. Simpson, Trans.). New York: The Free Press.

Eisenstadt, S. N. (1974). *Tradition, change, and modernity.* New York, London: John Wiley & Sons.

Fischer, B., & Fischer, U. (1979). Konzeption einer frühgeriatrischen Klinik. In Bernd Fischer (Ed.) *Frühgeriatrie. Diagnostische und therapeutische Aspekte.* Frankfurt: Cassella Riedl-Pharma.

Flusser, D. (1968). A new sensitivity in Judaism and the Christian message. *Harvard Theological Review, 61,* 107–127.

Fortes, M. (1959). *Oedipus and Job in West African religion.* Cambridge: University Press.

Fortes, M. (1965). Some reflections on ancestor worship in Africa. In: M. Fortes & G. Dieterlen (Eds.), *African systems of thoughts,* (pp. 122–142). London: Oxford University Press.

Fosbrooke, H. (1978). Die Altersgliederung als gesellschaftliches Grundprinzip— Eine Untersuchung am Beispiel des Hirtenvolkes der Maasai in Ostafrika. In: Leopold Rosenmayr (Ed.), *Die menschlichen Lebensalter. Kontinuität und Krisen,* (pp. 80–104). Munich: Piper.

Fox, R. 1980. *The red lamp of incest.* London: Hutchinson & Co.

Freud, S. (1913). *Totem and Tabu.* In: Gesammelte Werke, Vol. IX, 1968. Frankfurt: S. Fischer.

Gouldner, A. W. (1960). The norm of reciprocity. *American Sociological Review, 25,* 161–178.

Grindal, B. T. (1972). *Growing up in two worlds: Education and transition among the Sisala of northern Ghana.* New York: Holt, Rinehart, & Winston.

Guillemard, A. M., & Lenoir, R. (1974). *Retraite et échange social. Tentative d'explication des systèmes de relations sociales en situation de retraite.* Paris: Centre d'étude des mouvements sociaux.

Gutmann, D. (1977). The cross-cultural perspective: Notes toward a comparative psychology of aging. In J. E. Birren & K. W. Schaie (Eds.), *Handbook of the psychology of aging*, (pp. 302–326). New York: Van Nostrand Reinhold.
Hsu, F. L. K. (1971). *Kinship and culture*. Chicago: Aldine Publishing Company.
Kabwasa, Nsang-O'Khan (1982). *La Personne Âgée dans la Cosmogonie Africaine: Concept, Place, Rôle et Problèmes de Vieillesse et du Troisième Âge en Afrique*. Communication Présentée au IV^c Congrès de la Fondation van Clé, Brussells.
Kohut, H. (1979). *The restoration of the self*. New York: International Universities Press.
Kopytoff, I. (1971). Ancestors as elders in Africa. *Africa*, (2), 129–142.
Kossodo, B. L. (1978). *Die Frau in Afrika. Zwischen Tradition und Befreiung*. Munich: List.
Koty, J. (1934) *Die Behandlung der Alten und Kranken bei den Naturvölkern*. Stuttgart: Hirschfeld.
Kummer, H. (1968). *Social organization of Hamadryas baboons. A field study*. Basel, New York: Karger.
Lévi-Strauss, C. (1949). *Les formes élémentaires de la parenté*. Paris: Presses Universitaires de France.
Lorenz, K. (1977) Die Stellung der Alten bei sozialen Tieren. In: Österreichisches Bundesinstitut für Gesundheitswesen (Ed.), *Der alternde Mensch* (pp. 137–152). Vienna: Österreichisches Bundesinstitut für Gesundheitswesen.
Maddox, G. L., & Wiley, J. (1976) Concepts and methods in the study of aging. In: R. H. Binstock & E. Shanas (Eds.), *Handbook of aging and the social sciences*, (pp. 3–34). New York: Van Nostrand Reinhold.
Mendonsa, E. L. (1976). Elders, office-holders, and ancestors among the Sisala of northern Ghana. *Africa*, 46, 57–65.
Morioka, K. (1972). Kazoku shûkiron kara mita sôjin. In Nasu and Masuda (Eds.), *Rôjin to kazoku no shakaigaku* Koza Nihon no sôjin, p. 3, Tokyo.
Portmann, A. (1976). *An den Grenzen des Wissens. Vom Beitrag der Biologie zu einem neuen Weltbild*. Frankfurt: Suhrkamp.
Riegel, K. (1976). Toward a dialectical theory of development. *American Psychologist*, 31, 689–700.
Rohlen, T. P. (1971). Father-son dominance: Tikopia and China. In F. L. K. Hsu (Ed.), *Kinship and culture*. Chicago: Aldine Publishing Company.
Rosenmayr, L. (1974a). *Elements of an assimilation-yield theory*. Paper presented at the 8th World Congress of Sociology, Toronto.
Rosenmayr, L. (1974b). Die Revision der These vom generellen Leistungsverfall im Alternsprozeß. In Karl Fellinger (Ed.), *Aktivitätsprobleme des Alternden*, (pp. 101–123). Basle: Editions Roche.
Rosenmayr, L. (1978a). Die menschlichen Lebensalter in Deutungsversuchen der europäischen Kulturgeschichte. In Leopold Rosenmayr (Ed.), *Die menschlichen Lebensalter. Kontinuität und Krisen*, (pp. 23–79). Munich: Piper.
Rosenmayr, L. (1978b). Elemente einer allgemeinen Alter(n)stheorie. In Leopold and Hilde Rosenmayr (Eds.), *Der alte Mensch in der Gesellschaft*, (pp. 46–70). Reinbek/Hamburg: Rowohlt.
Rosenmayr, L. (1978c, August). *Achievements, doubts, and prospects of the sociology of aging*, Paper prepared for the XIth International Congress of Gerontology, Tokyo.
Rosenmayr, L. (1982). Biography and identity. In T. K. Hareven (Ed.), *Aging and life course transitions: An interdisciplinary perspective*, (pp. 27–53). New York, London: Guilford Press.
Rosenmayr, L. (1983a). Reduced pragmatic solidarity: Multigenerational relations with the extended family in view of the social policy measures. In J. E. Birren, J.

Munnichs, H. Thomae, & M. Marois (Eds.), *Aging: A challenge to science and society*. Vol. 3. Behavioural Sciences and Conclusions. (pp. 134–155). London: Oxford University Press.

Rosenmayr, L. (1983b).

Rosenmayr, L. (1984). Changing values and positions of aging in western culture (A comparative analysis of the age status under different socio-structural conditions). In J. E. Birren & K. W. Schaie (Eds.), *Handbook of the psychology of aging* (2nd ed.). New York: Van Nostrand Reinhold.

Schneider, Hans-Dieter (1974). *Aspekte des Alterns. Ergebnisse sozialpsychologischer Forschung.* Frankfurt: Athenäum Fischer.

Schweeger-Hefel, A. (1980). *Masken und Mythen. Sozialstrukturen der Nyonyosi und Sikonse in Obervolta.* Vienna: Schendl.

Sprockhoff, J. F. (1979). Die Alten im alten Indien. Ein Versuch nach brahmanischen Quellen. *Saeculum, 30,* 374–433.

Ssenkoloto, G. M. (1981). *Social development and aging in developing and developed countries: A background document for policy makers.* Buea, Cameroon: Panafrican Institute.

Stearns, P. N. (1977). *Old age in European Society.* London: Croom Helm.

Stein, H. (1979). *Psychoanalytische Selbstpsychologie und die Philosophie des Selbst.* Meisenheim am Glan: Anton Hain.

Vorbichler, A. (1980). Das Leben im Rhythmus von Tod und Wiedergeburt in der Vorstellung der schwarzafrikanischen Völker. *Zeitschrift für Missionswissenschaft und Religionswissenschaft, 2,* 93–109.

Wilson, E. O. (1975). *Sociobiology. The New Synthesis.* Cambridge, Mass: The Belknap Press.

4
Psychological Aspects and Disorders Associated with Aging

Lawrence W. Lazarus

In this chapter, a review of the normal psychology of late life will be followed by a discussion of some typical neurotic disorders of old age and finally suggestions regarding future research. Emphasis will be placed on conceptualizing the aging process from a developmental life cycle perspective in which the last phase of the life cycle is viewed as having developmental challenges, tasks, and goals, as well as losses and depletions.

Attempts to define normal aging are complicated by the diversity of the aging experience, the changing nature of late life resulting from the dramatic increase in longevity, limitations of our knowledge about the biologic underpinnings of the aging process, and controversies regarding which empirical model is best suited for investigating this phase of the life cycle.

There is more diversity among people over age 65 than within any other age group. They demonstrate more within-group performance variability on physiological, cognitive, and personality measures than any other age group. One factor that contributes to this intragroup diversity is the broad age range incorporated in what is considered late life. Neugarten (1974) captured this distinction in her classification of the "young-old" (ages 65 to 75) and the "old-old" (over age 75). People in the 65- to 75-year-old age group are more similar to those in the 55- to 65-year-old age group with regard to health, socioeconomic status, and cognitive, personality, and

This chapter was supported, in part, by the Geriatric Mental Health Academic Award, 1K07 MH00445-01A1, from the National Institute of Mental Health, Center for Studies of the Mental Health of the Aging.

developmental issues than they are to people over age 75. In contrast, a significantly greater percentage of people over age 75 live in long-term care facilities and experience debilitating physical illness. In the United States, for example, only 2% of people between the ages of 65 and 74 live in long-term care institutions compared to about 8% of people 75 years of age and older (Busse, 1981). The unique manner in which each older person has attempted to resolve the developmental tasks and challenges during earlier phases of the life cycle, and the values, attitudes, and personality characteristics they have developed through personal development and interaction with others also contribute to the marked diversity among people over 65.

Another difficulty in studying normal aging is to define an appropriate empirical model for this period of life. The traditional assumption has been that the changes that accompany aging are quantitative in nature. Cross-sectional research designs that assume differences between the performance of young and old subjects reflect the impact of age have been the predominant models for studying these quantitative changes. Measures used in much of this research were generally developed for use with younger adults and thus are more relevant to their experience than to the experience of older people. Evidence that older subjects perform more poorly than younger subjects on many psychological measures has provided support for the belief that generalized decline occurs in late life. This research methodology has tended to contaminate age and cohort variables without elucidating the unique aspects of late life.

An alternative model for studying normal aging has grown out of the developmental framework used to study various phases of the life-span. This model assumes that the changes that occur in each phase of the life cycle, including those of late life, are qualitative rather than quantitative in nature. The belief is that old age is a stage of the life cycle in its own right with unique developmental tasks and potentials, as well as losses and depletions (Gutmann, 1980). Therefore, the relevant issues at each phase of the life cycle, as well as the methods of investigating these issues, are presumed to change across the life-span. This approach places less emphasis on age-group comparisons. Instead, direct observation and understanding of each life period is seen as the basis for the development of age-specific empirical measures and theories.

The following section addresses psychological developments that shape the lives of "normal" people over age 65 and focuses on empirical studies of the vast majority of elderly people who have adjusted to the challenges of late life without incapacitation due to psychological and physical problems. An understanding of the normal psychology of aging will provide a framework for a discussion of some typical neurotic disorders that afflict the elderly.

NORMAL PSYCHOLOGY OF LATE LIFE

There is considerable evidence from both cross-sectional and longitudinal research that many aspects of personality remain stable as one ages. Life satisfaction and morale remain consistent across the life-span (Palmore, 1970; Thomae, 1976). Income, self-rated health, and to a lesser extent, number of relationships, and access to means of achieving goals show a much stronger correlation to a person's general outlook on life, as defined by morale and life satisfaction, than to a person's age (Adams, 1971; Neugarten, 1977; Palmore & Kivett, 1977). One's individual perception of oneself as reflected in self-concept or self-image also remains stable with age. Contrary to previous beliefs, there is no evidence that the self-concept becomes negative with age (Monge, 1975; Trimakas & Nicolay, 1974). In interviews of 87 middle-aged and elderly men, Reichard, Livson, and Petersen (1962) found that self-acceptance is likely to become greater with age. Stability or similarity in personality traits as measured by objective means across age groups (Botwinick, 1981; Thomae, 1980) yields more impressive findings than the commonly believed personality traits usually associated with aging, such as increased cautiousness, increased introversion, and increased attention to practical needs.

Personality style also appears to be consistent from middle age into late life. No one particular personality style is predictive of adjustment in late life, although for many older people satisfactory adjustment is associated with continued activity and social involvement. Several investigators (Havighurst, 1968; Reichard, Livson, & Petersen, 1962) have found that equally important as the activity level in predicting adjustment in later life is the individual's ability to integrate the emotional and rational aspects of his or her personality, to come to terms with role changes, and to establish a sense of continuity with his past.

Although personality styles and traits do not appear to change with age, there does appear to be a shift in focus of the aging adult's inner life. This is reflected in the older person's view of himself in relation to the environment, in his preoccupations and values, and, to some extent, in the type of internal coping mechanisms used. Both cross-sectional and longitudinal research indicate that in late life there is a movement away from a preoccupation with the outer world and a movement toward an inner-world orientation. With aging, there is a greater preoccupation with inner life, decreased emotional cathexes toward environmental objects and persons, constriction in the ability to integrate complex impinging stimuli, and greater concern about satisfaction of one's own needs (Neugarten, 1964). Jung (1960) believed that this trend toward greater introversion begins as early as middle age and continues throughout late life. One aspect of this increased focus on the self in late life is a reorganization of values. Ryff and Baltes (1976) found a transition in middle to old age from emphasis on instrumental values, such as ambition, achievement, and work, to more philosophical concerns such as freedom and happiness. Increasing importance is placed on humanitarianism (Thomae, 1980), as well as on a reestablishing of personal priorities in light of greater awareness of both decreasing energy and the finitude of life.

This reorganization of values also includes greater emphasis on the establishment and maintenance of interpersonal affectional bonds. For example, in describing intergenerational relationships, adult children tend to emphasize the assistance-giving aspect of these relationships whereas their aging parents tend to emphasize the affectional components (Sussman, 1976). Similarly, in his study of long-married couples, Roberts (1979–1980) found that with increasing age more attention was given to the spouse's expressive affectional roles than to his or her instrumental functions.

Cath (1976) suggests that aging brings with it an accentuation of the role of the enteroceptive apparatus, so that messages or stimuli from within the organism are more quickly perceived, thought about, and responded to. This process is set in motion by an increased investment in the self because of somatic depletion, illness, or pain. Cath found the term "depletion anxiety" particularly attractive because the middle and later years can emerge as an age-specific crisis, a balance between factors of depletion and sources of restitution. The outcome between depletion and restitution depends increasingly upon the availability of a supportive environment. As the amount of psychological energy becomes more limited with aging, this increased narrowing of psychic focus to the self acquires some adaptive value in that it ensures survival by utilizing the available energy to meet one's essential needs. According to Cath, all these challenges of late life can be mastered.

Weinberg (1975) believes that one way the elderly focus their energy and ego functions on essential needs is exemplified by the phenomenon of "exclusion of stimuli." Because aging curtails one's capacity to deal with a complex multitude of stimuli, superfluous details of everyday life are no longer attended to while attention is given to information that is most pertinent and psychologically relevant to the individual. "Exclusion of stimuli" is reflected in the tendency of many older people who do not hear well to hear "what they should not hear" when issues pertaining to their well-being are discussed.

Aging individuals become less oriented toward coping with stress by changing the environment or the stressful situation itself, and more likely to accommodate themselves to the environment. As a result, adjustment is achieved in older people through changed attitudes and self-perceptions as well as through modified views of the world. This process was identified and examined by Neugarten et al. (1964) in the Kansas City Studies of Adult Life, a study of the personality changes that take place in the second half of life. The majority of men aged 40 to 49 assumed a stance of active mastery (Gutmann, 1964). That is, these men viewed their environment as one that rewards boldness and risk taking and themselves as capable of meeting those opportunities. They looked to the external world for justification, challenge, and stimulation. In contrast, men in older age groups tended to view the world as complex and dangerous and themselves as accommodating and conforming to outer world demands. As a result, these older men withdrew from active engagement with the external world and disengaged themselves from feelings and excitement. These men reshaped themselves to conform to external demands or their own superego strictures.

From the perspective of cognitive personality theory, Thomae (1970) believes that cognitive revisions of the way one views the self and the self in an environmental context are essential to an individual's maintenance of a stable self-concept, despite the multiple and varied narcissistic insults of late life. The elderly use "cognitive restructuration" to maintain a balance between motivational needs and cognitions of the world and of oneself. This process does not involve perceptual distortion. Instead, beliefs, attitudes, and ways of thinking about stressful situations change so that meaning and relevance are given to failure and loss.

DEVELOPMENTAL TASKS OF LATE LIFE

A number of researchers have speculated about developmental tasks of late life. The most widely known theories are those of Erikson (1963). He identifies late-life tasks as involving issues of generativity versus stagnation and ego integrity versus despair. Generativity is the capacity to become invested in establishing and guiding the next generation. The achievement of ego integrity involves emotional integration of life experiences and acceptance of life as it has been lived. This process involves the reconciliation of earlier goals and dreams to achievements actually accomplished, reevaluation and reconceptualization of earlier life experiences in light of later ones, and the revision of one's sense of self in a way that is compatible with those experiences.

Many theorists agree with Erikson that putting one's life into perspective is a major task of late life and suggest that reminiscence and self-reflection are key mechanisms for achieving this goal. Butler and Lewis (1977) believe that reminiscence occurs in all people in the final years of life, and is characterized by the "progressive return to consciousness of past experiences and particularly the resurgence of unresolved conflicts which can be looked at again and reintegrated" (p. 43).

PSYCHOLOGY OF AGING FROM THE PERSPECTIVE OF SELF-PSYCHOLOGY

The psychology of the self, as theorized by psychoanalyst Heinz Kohut (1966, 1971, 1977) and others (Cath, 1976; Meissner, 1976) adds another dimension to our understanding of personality development across the life cycle that has particular relevance to aging. The self may be defined as a developmental psychological structure responsible for the maintenance of one's self-image, self-esteem, feelings, and affects associated with bodily and psychological integrity, and relative need for others to idealize and to regulate self-esteem. Kohut believes that personality development in the course of life can be viewed not only from the traditional perspective of the progression from infantile autoeroticism to object love, but also from a second line of development, one that begins with what he terms the "archaic nuclear self," progresses to the "cohesive self," and finally attains, in varying degrees, higher forms of the self including potential transformation of the self across the second half of life.

According to Kohut, during normal childhood development of the self sector of the personality, the child's tendency toward self-centeredness and grandiosity is responded to more or less empathically by the parenting objects who serve as self-objects. The parents serve partly as self-objects for the child in that they respond empathically to the child's normal, age-appropriate exhibitionistic behavior and to the child's wish for the parents' mirroring or confirmation of the child's essential goodness. The child experiences these attributes of the parenting objects as functions of the self or self-objects. The parents' age-specific empathic and mirroring responses lead to the child's budding sense of confidence and sense of self, leading eventually and in varying degrees to feelings of cohesiveness and relative stability of self-esteem, as well as to the capacity to seek others in a sustaining and satisfying way during times of need.

In addition to the gradual transformation of grandiosity into self-integrated ambitions and goals, childhood idealizations of what the child perceives to be all-powerful and perfect parents (idealized parent images) gradually become modulated, internalized, and transformed into the ideals to which one aspires, as healthy admiration of others, and the wish to be associated with those one admires. During childhood and the later phases of life, the self may be expressed through such developmental achievements as wisdom, creativity, humor, and an acceptance of life's finitude (Fig. 4.1). Across adulthood, based on the more or less successful development of an integrated cohesive self, persons vary in their sense of cohesiveness and integration, from sustained feelings of vitality, spontaneity, and vigor, to feelings of enfeeblement, depletion, and, where functioning is seriously disrupted, a sense of inner fragmentation (Kohut & Wolf, 1978).

In the late 1970s Kohut made a slight but significant shift in conceptualizing the self, not in isolation but as a lifelong sequence of changing self-selfobject relationships. Psychopathology in general and self-pathology in particular are therefore defined in terms not of this or that defect in the self but in terms of a disturbance of the self-selfobject relationship during a particu-

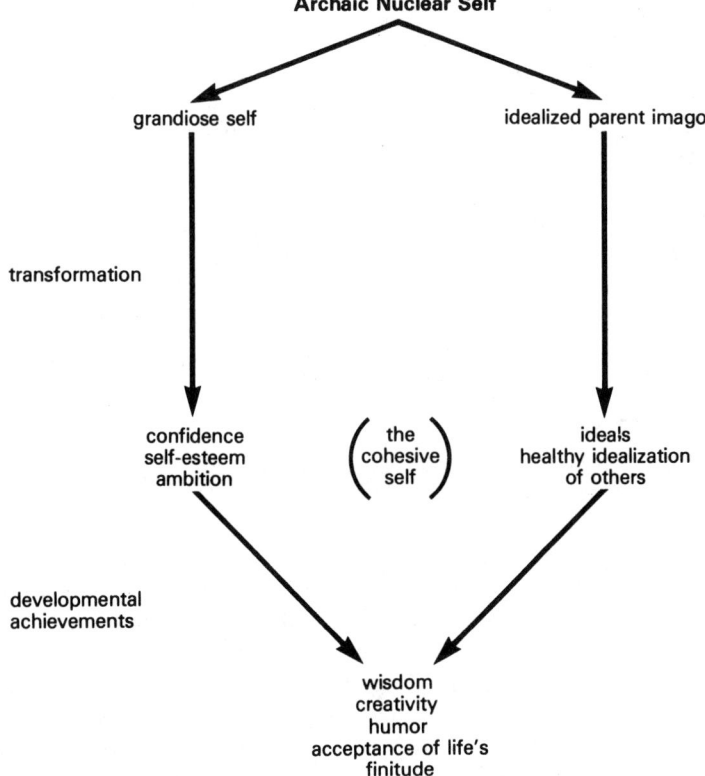

FIGURE 4.1 The development of the self.
From Newton, N., Lazarus, L. W., and Weinberg, J. Aging: Biopsychosocial Perspectives. In D. Offer & M. Sabshin (Eds.), *Normality*, pp. 230–285. New York: Basic Books, 1984. © 1984 Basic Books. Reprinted by permission.

lar stage of development. Applying these concepts to the psychopathology of the elderly, Kohut (personal communication, 1980) suggests "focusing on the old and his environment as a unit rather than focusing only on the failures of the aged and on the defects of the self." In his summary statement at the 1978 Chicago Conference on Self Psychology, Kohut explained:

> In the view of self psychology man lives in a matrix of selfobjects from birth to death. He needs selfobjects for his psychological survival, just as he needs oxygen in his environment throughout his life for physiological survival. . . . Self psychology does not see the essence of man's development as a move from dependence to independence, from merger to autonomy, and, yes, not even as a move from no-self to self. . . . What we have begun to study, therefore . . . is the sequence of self-selfobject relationships throughout man's life. How accurately in tune with the small baby's various, specific needs were the responses of the selfobject at the beginning of extrauterine life, we will ask. Did the selfobject respond with proud mirroring to the first strivings for a move away, will be another question. How, we will ask, does the selfobject milieu respond to a person's dying? With pride in him for being an example of courage in pain and decline? Or by withdrawing their mirroring from him at this ultimate point in the curve of life?

According to Meissner (1976), the basic problem of aging is that of narcissistic loss. Referring to Rochlin's (1965) discussion of the issue:

> The greatest test of narcissism is aging or old age. All that has come to represent value and with which narcissism has long been associated is jeopardized by growing old. The skills, mastery, and powers, all painfully acquired, which provided gratifications as they functioned to effect adaptation wane in the last phase of life. One's resources, energies, adaptability, and function, the intimacies of relationships upon which one depended, family and friends, are continually being depleted and lost. (pp. 377–378)

From the viewpoint of self psychology, the magnitude of an elderly person's reactions to a loss is dependent, to some degree, on the amount of narcissistic investment in the lost function or object. For example, for aged persons whose intellectual achievements accounted for much of their pride and self-esteem, reminders of failing memory may provoke anger, rage, and depression. Kohut (1972) cites the example of the aging person who, because of brain injury, is unable to solve simple problems. He becomes enraged over the fact that "he is not in control of his own thought processes, of a function which people consider to be most intimately their own, i.e., as a part of the self" (p. 383).

Self psychology provides a useful theoretical model for understanding the older person's attempt to cope and to find restitution for the biopsychosocial losses and stresses that occur in late life. From the point of view of self psychology, regression within the self sector of the personality may serve adaptive functions by preserving one's self-esteem and warding off feelings of emptiness and fragmentation. For example, the retired industrialist whose self-esteem rests upon financial successes may brag exhibitionistically about past accomplishments as a way of compensating for current feelings of loss of self-esteem. The tendency of older persons to reminisce about the past may serve not only to stave off depression and to preserve a sense of continuity with the past, but also to remind them of a time when they felt worthwhile, vital, and competent.

Self psychology also provides a useful conceptualization of normality in the self sector of the personality in late life (Lazarus, 1980). Elderly persons with a healthy reservoir of self-esteem and confidence have achieved, to varying degrees, such developmental goals as the acquisition of wisdom, creativity, acceptance of the finitude of life, and a sense of humor. They enjoy sharing with those younger than themselves the knowledge and wisdom accumulated from a lifetime of experience. Rather than dreading and despairing the inevitability of death, they approach this and other existential matters philosophically.

If illness restricts activities that previously contributed to feelings of pride and self-esteem, the elderly can mourn and work through the loss and eventually depend more on those physical and mental capabilities they still posess. Having related to others throughout life primarily as objects separate from the self rather than solely and psychopathologically as selfobjects, they can mourn the loss of loved ones. By a realistic appraisal of current abilities and impairments elderly persons with a healthy, integrated self in later life can gradually modify the cherished ideals and goals of their youth. In doing so, they are better protected from the depression that may ensue if they expected to perform as they once did. As Kohut and Wolf (1978) note: "If our self is firmly established, we shall neither be afraid of the dejection that may follow a failure nor of the expansive fantasies that may follow a success— reactions that would endanger those with a more precariously established self" (p. 415). Cath (1976) has noted that psychologically healthy older people have the capacity to tolerate loss, to grieve, and to be depressed without losing basic self-respect or suffering irreparable damage to self-esteem.

Although the majority of persons aged 65 and older adjust to the later years in a psychologically healthy manner, the biopsychosocial stresses of this period render certain older persons particularly vulnerable to the development of psychological problems for the first time in late life, or to a reactivation of unresolved neurotic problems from earlier phases of the life cycle.

PSYCHOLOGICAL DISORDERS IN LATE LIFE— ETIOLOGIC FACTORS

Older people of certain personality types may be predisposed to psychological disorders in late life, especially when compensatory external sources of support are not available. For example, elderly people who were excessively dependent throughout their lives may be more vulnerable to depressive disorders when their supports, such as family and friends, have moved away or died. Elderly people with narcissistic personality disorders may decompensate into depression, paranoid disorders, or withdrawal when they can no longer depend on physical or occupational successes to bolster a chronically insecure sense of self and self-esteem (Lazarus, 1980).

Certain stresses and losses that are ubiquitous in later life may contribute to neurotic symptom formation. In later life, the magnitude and rapidity of external stresses and losses may occur at a time when the physical and psychological apparatus may be least equipped to adapt to the stresses. In addition, the availability of compensations and substitutions for the losses are diminished. As Weinberg (1975) has noted:

> Each loss necessitates a rearrangement of the equilibrium that one had set up for comfortable functioning. Each loss, too, releases the energy that was previously invested but that now needs a new object to be attached to. One searches for a substitute, but there are no takers. There may be no replacement of family, and there are no bidders for the friendship of the aged. When the aging person attempts to re-establish equilibrium by attempting to reinvest the freed libido into objects in the environment, he sometimes meets a wall of resistance. (p. 2407)

Psychodynamic factors play an important role in the development of neurotic disorders in late life. Neurotic disorders may be considered as arising from the individual's attempts to cope with the anxiety aroused by psychological problems and stresses. The neurotic symptoms may reveal the anxiety directly or may represent the person's defenses against anxiety, for example, conversion, compulsive, or phobic manifestations. In a neurosis, there is both a feeling of anxiety and the formation of repetitive unconscious defense mechanisms to control the anxiety. The form of the neurosis is determined by the type of defensive measure the patient uses to control anxiety.

The same general mechanisms that contribute to the development of neurotic patterns earlier in life operate in old age as well, although in late life the mechanisms are usually modified by biologic aging, the extent of the socioeconomic support systems, lifelong personality traits, and the individual's capacity to cope with the stresses of aging.

Simon (1980) believes that decline in physical strength and the occurrence of chronic illness is particularly stressful for the elderly. Physical decline may precipitate efforts at adaptation that become expressed in real or imagined somatic complaints. There may be complaints of easy fatigability, weakness, or pain or overcompensatory (counterphobic) efforts to prove to oneself or others that one is as good as ever. Should these fail, anxiety, depression, and hypochondriasis may develop.

PRESENTATION OF NEUROSIS IN LATE LIFE

In understanding the etiology and natural history of the neuroses of late life, an important issue is whether these disorders began in earlier phases of the life cycle, such as in adolescence or adulthood, or whether these disorders make their appearance for the first time in late life. Bergmann (1971) reported that 11% of his community sample of 300 persons age 65 and over had developed a neurosis for the first time after the age of 60. Kay and Bergmann (1966) found a higher than expected mortality rate in elderly neurotic patients, which they attributed to the higher prevalence of physical illness and disability among them compared to normal subjects.

According to Bergmann (1975), elderly people who present with a neurosis for the first time in late life have some of the following characteristics: (a) greater association of late life neurosis with impaired physical health, especially cardiovascular disease, (b) more acute suffering from loneliness and lack of recreational activities, (c) the neurosis concealed, manifesting itself mainly in social disabilities and a decline in the quality of life, and (d) a history of fairly good premorbid functioning. In comparison, the neurotic individual who has had lifelong difficulties appears to suffer comparatively less from the neurosis in late life, even when symptoms are florid. Perhaps the lifelong neurotic has made necessary adjustments and accommodations to the neurotic symptoms and is less bothered by them than the person whose neurosis develops for the first time in late life. According to Ciompi (1969), previously existing neurotic disorders tend to improve later in life, although they are often replaced by minor affective disorders and residual states.

Perhaps the most common symptoms of late life psychological dysfunction are those of depression. Bergmann (1971) found that depression accounted for 75% of elderly people with late onset neurotic disorders. Simon (1980) believes that older people who develop a neurosis late in life do not usually present with classic signs and symptoms, but rather a mixture of psychiatric symptoms that are modified by a complex array of physical, social, psychological, and cultural factors. For example, neurotic depression in older people often presents atypically, with complaints of memory loss, loneliness, and rejection, somatic or hypochondriacal preoccupations, irritability, withdrawal, and apathy.

The presentation of neurotic disorders in late life is additionally complicated by the occurrence of concomitant mental and behavioral disorders associated with organic brain disease, such as Alzheimer's disease or other dementing illnesses. The development of neurologic signs may, in and of themselves, lead to neurotic symptoms as the cognitively impaired older person attempts to cope with catastrophic assaults on his self-image and self-esteem.

Unfortunately, neurotic disorders often go undetected by the family physician (Williamson et al., 1964), are sometimes misdiagnosed as organic mental disorders, or are dismissed altogether as being expected concomitants of "old age." Because of the complex interplay of medical, psychological, sociocultural, and other factors influencing the clinical picture of neurosis in late life, a comprehensive psychiatric and medical assessment is crucial in order to arrive at an accurate diagnosis. For example, a psychiatric symptom such as anxiety or depression may be the first manifestation of an undiagnosed medical illness, a side effect of medication, an early manifestation of an organic mental disorder, an expression of family conflict, or other factors. In addition to several diagnostic interviews of the identified patient, the diagnostic process often requires a review of pertinent medical records and discussion with family members.

Epidemiologic Considerations

Epidemiological studies that indicate psychiatric morbidity in the aged have been carried out mostly in Great Britain and Scandinavia. A comparison of the results of the various studies is difficult because of differences in the cultural and social characteristics of the populations studied, the methods and diagnostic categories used, the aims of the investigators, and the form in which the results are presented (Simon, 1980).

In the northern European countries where numerous studies were conducted, the tendency is for the aged to remain at home rather than to move to institutional settings. Consequently the populations studied live, for the most part, in the community. Most populations studied are from well-defined groups such as inhabitants of an island or a small town. In these surveys of general populations, the neuroses are by far the most common category of psychiatric disorder (Kay, Beamish, & Roth, 1964). From 5 to 10% of the aged population are found to be suffering from fairly definite neurosis. When less clear-cut conditions related to personality factors are included, the percentage rises from 8 to 17. Almost half of these neurotic illnesses are believed to have begun after the age of 60. The most frequent neurotic diagnoses were anxiety neurosis, neurotic depression, or a mixture of both. Other studies have suggested a similar prevalence of neurotic disorders in the aged (Gurland, 1976; Kessel & Shepherd, 1962; Nielsen, Homma, & Biorn-Henriksen, 1977).

A recent U.S. large-scale epidemiologic study by Robins, Helzer, Weissman et al. (1984) tested the lifetime prevalence (the proportion of persons who have ever experienced that disorder up to the date of assessment) of 15 major DSM-III psychiatric diagnoses using the Diagnostic Interview Schedule (American Psychiatric Association, 1980). It was found that from 29 to 38% of the sample had experienced at least one of the 15 disorders in their lifetime. The two most common diagnoses were alcohol abuse or dependence (accounting for between 11 and 16%) and phobic disorder (accounting for between 8 and 23% of the sample). The third most prevalent diagnosis was major depressive disorder (experienced by about 5% of the population). Dysthymic disorder affected about 3%. When different age groups were compared with regard to the rate of specific diagnoses, the 25- to 44-year-old age group had the highest rates for most disorders. It was expected that the older age groups (i.e., over age 65), having passed through more years of life and hence, more years of risk than younger groups, should have lifetime rates as high or higher than the young. Instead, lifetime prevalence was generally lowest in those over age 65 (except for cognitive impairment). Possible explanations for this unexpected low prevalence among the elderly included the elderly's hesitation to disclose their psychiatric symptoms, a tendency to attribute psychogenic symptoms to physical illnesses, difficulty in recall, and disorder-associated mortality before age 65.

Psychiatric Diagnosis

Neurotic conditions that afflict adult and elderly people have been classified by the 1980 Diagnostic and Statistical Manual-III (DSM-III) of the American Psychiatric Association as disorders, such as affective, anxiety, somatoform, dissociative, and psychosexual disorders. To facilitate the identification of these DSM-III categories, which in the former DSM-II nomenclature and in the International Classification of Diseases-9-CM are grouped together as the neuroses, the term neurosis may be included separately in parentheses after the corresponding "disorder." For example, a phobic disorder in DSM-III may also be referred to as a phobic neurosis. The DSM-III classification system, compared to the DSM-II, places greater emphasis on the phenomenology of psychiatric disorders, providing specific diagnostic criteria for specific diagnoses. In other words, the DSM-III emphasizes the descriptive symptoms that may be used to make the diagnosis and classifies them into operational criteria. However, as Simon (1980) has noted, it is not very common for the elderly person to present with pure or classic symptoms of a specific neurosis. Instead, the neuroses present as a mixture or complex array of signs and symptoms influenced by biopsychosocial changes and stresses of late life. The following section focuses on three common neurotic disorders that afflict the elderly—dysthymic, anxiety, and somatoform disorder—as well as the ubiquitous adjustment disorders.

Dysthymic Disorder (Depressive Neurosis)

Compared with many other psychiatric classification systems that are based on such dichotomous distinctions as endogenous versus reactive depression or neurotic versus psychotic depression, the Affective Disorders are divided in the DSM-III into three major groups. The first major category is Major Affective Disorders, which include bipolar manic depressive disorder and major depression; the second major category is Other Specific Affective Disorders, which include cyclothymic disorder and dysthymic disorder; and the third is the Atypical Affective Disorders for affective disorders that cannot be classified in the other two major groups.

Dysthymic disorder is closest to the previous DSM-II diagnosis neurotic depression. According to the DSM-III, the essential feature of a dysthymic disorder is a chronic disturbance of mood involving either depressed mood or loss of interest or pleasure in all, or almost all, activities and pastimes. Psychotic features are not present and symptoms are not of sufficient severity and duration to meet criteria for a major depression. The depressed mood can be either persistent or intermittent, but periods of normal mood generally last less than a few weeks. Another criteria for dysthymic disorder is that the depressed mood and associated symptoms are present for at least two-year duration; the disorder usually begins early in adult life. In some instances, it occurs following a more severe depression, such as a major depression. Dysthymic disorder is particularly common in individuals with borderline, histrionic, and dependent personality disorders.

According to Simon (1980), classical presentations of dysthymic disorder (neurotic depression) are not often seen as mixtures of anxiety, depression and hypochondriasis. The symptoms of a dysthymic disorder may include insomnia, fatigue, loss of self-esteem, social withdrawal, irritability, pessimism, tearfulness, and complaints of impaired memory. Kahn et al. (1975) noted that depressed elderly people often complain of poor memory, which is not substantiated by cognitive testing, suggesting that these complaints may be indicative of a depression.

Depression in the elderly is likely to occur in association with real or symbolic losses. Reactions to these losses may be understood in terms of threats to the patient's self-esteem and security. Among those elderly patients who have trouble coping with loss are those with a chronically impaired sense of self and self-esteem.

Anxiety Disorders (Anxiety Neurosis)

According to the DSM-III, in this group of disorders anxiety is either the predominant disturbance, as in panic disorder and generalized anxiety disorder, or anxiety is experienced if the individual attempts to master the symptoms, as in confronting the feared situation in a phobic disorder or resisting the obsessions and compulsions in an obsessive-compulsive disorder. One common type of anxiety disorder in the elderly is generalized anxiety disorder, the essential feature of which is generalized persistent anxiety of at least one month's duration without the specific symptoms that would characterize either phobic, panic, or obsessive-compulsive disorder. In generalized anxiety disorder, there are signs of motor tension, such as jitteriness and trembling, autonomic hyperactivity, such as sweating and tachycardia, and apprehensiveness, vigilance, irritability, and distractibility. Mild depressive symptoms are also common. The diagnosis generalized anxiety disorder is not used if the anxiety is due to another physical or mental disorder.

Seeking relief for these unpleasant states, some elderly people resort to abuse of alcohol and antianxiety medication. Since anxiety in the elderly may be the first manifestation of a medical illness or drug toxicity, a thorough medical assessment is carried out before considering antianxiety medication and/or psychotherapy, environmental manipulation or another treatment approach. Some of the etiologies of anxiety in the elderly are listed below.

- Major depressive disorder
- Neurotic depression or adjustment disorder
- Medical illness, either known or occult (angina, cerebral arterial disease, endocrine disorders, hypoglycemia, paroxysmal tachycardia, pulmonary embolus, gastrointestinal bleeding, or carcinoma are common causes)
- Late-life neurotic disorder
- The continuation of lifelong recurrent anxiety such as chronic phobic disorder
- Late-onset acute phobic disorder, sometimes in response to acute illness or surgery
- Late-onset hypochondriasis which may be a new problem in late life or simply the continuation of lifelong hypochondriasis in association with a personality disorder

The first sign of a dementia
A manifestation of underlying paranoid disorder
An early symptom of acute organic confusional state (delirium)
Caffeinism or from sympathomimetic drugs such as ephedrine, and occasionally antidepressants—over-the-counter drugs also may cause confusion and anxiety
Withdrawal from alcohol or barbiturates
Obsessional disorders

SOMATOFORM DISORDERS

Pfeiffer and Busse (1973) believe that somatoform disorders are particularly important among the neuroses of old age. According to the DSM-III, the essential features in this group of disorders are physical symptoms suggesting physical disorders for which there are no demonstrable medical findings, and for which there is evidence, or a strong presumption, that the symptoms are linked to psychologic factors or conflicts. The most common of the four subtypes of somatoform disorders seen in the elderly is hypochondriasis (or hypochondriacal neurosis) in which the predominant disturbance is an unrealistic interpretation that vague physical signs or sensations are abnormal and the fear or belief that these signs indicate the presence of a serious disease.

Some investigators suggest that hypochondriasis is closely related to depression (Jacobs, Foselson, & Charles, 1968; Kay & Bergmann, 1966; Earley & Von Mering, 1969). Bergmann (1978) cautions that when hypochondriacal complaints arise for the first time late in life they may be indicative of depression and increased risk of suicide as well as signalling an underlying physical illness, unbeknownst to patient and physician, Although a physical disorder may coexist with hypochondriasis, medical evaluations do not reveal a diagnosis that can account for the patient's physical complaints or interpretation of them. The patient's fear persists, despite reassurance, and causes impairment in functioning.

In hypochondriasis, the belief of having a disease does not include the fixed quality of a true somatic delusion. The feared disease or diseases may involve several body systems simultaneously or at different times. These patients commonly have some associated anxiety and depression and often go from physician to physician, expressing dissatisfaction with the previous one. The disorder frequently begins in people in their thirties or forties and is commonly seen in medical practice. Because these patients are offended at the suggestion that psychological problems play a role, they often are either not seen by mental health professionals or, when seen, are unfortunately considered unsuitable for treatment. Important differential diagnostic considerations, especially in the elderly hypochondriacal patient, include affective disorders, such as a major depression, or a previously undiagnosed medical illness.

Weinberg (1975) provides an intuitive understanding of hypochondriasis in the elderly. The loss of family and friends that the elderly experience necessitates the establishment of a new equilibrium. The elderly search for a substitute for their lost loved ones, but unfortunately there are sometimes no takers. Having no person to become emotionally invested in, the older person's attention is turned inwardly and invested in organs or organ systems, becoming expressed as somatic complaints, pain, and/or ruminatory recapitulations of the past.

ADJUSTMENT DISORDERS

Although adjustment disorders (formerly termed transient situational disturbances in the DSM-II) are not neurotic disorders, their prevalence in the elderly warrants their inclusion in this chapter. These disorders are especially seen in reaction to the stress of medical illness, hospitalization, or of relocation to new surroundings. The stressors may be single or multiple, may be recurrent, may occur in a family setting or be limited to the patient, or may occur in a group or community setting where the stressor involves many other people. According to the DSM-III, the use of coping styles judged to be maladaptive is characteristic of an adjustment disorder. The maladaptive nature of the response is indicated by impairment in social or occupational functioning or symptoms that are in excess of a normal and expectable reaction. The presenting symptoms in an adjustment disorder are not sufficient in number or severity to qualify for a diagnosis of a major mental disorder. Features of depression, anxiety, hypochondriasis, and paranoia are common, with frequent use of relatively simple defense mechanisms such as withdrawal, somatization, projection, and denial. It is assumed that the disturbance will eventually remit after the stressor ceases or when a new level of adaptation is achieved. The particular subtype of an adjustment disorder depends on the major clinical manifestations; therefore, descriptive phrases such as "with depressed mood," "with withdrawal," etc., are used.

In late life, losses are frequent stressors. Verwoerdt (1976) believes that the capacity to develop or use adaptive mechanisms diminishes as one grows older. Psychologic decompensation may occur in predisposed older people as stress states hasten a process of withdrawal and regression. These tendencies are magnified if brain disease diminishes brain function.

Gaitz and Varner (1980) believe that adjustment disorders in late life are not diagnosed as often as they should be. Early recognition and intervention to neutralize (or at least to minimize) the effects of stressors carries with it the promise of modifying the course of adjustment disorders in late life, thereby preventing the development of a more serious, irreversible, or less treatable psychiatric disorder.

CONCLUSION

Epidemiological studies indicate a high prevalence among the elderly of neurotic disorders and almost half of these begin in late life. Neurotic disorders in the elderly continue to go undetected by the family physician because of inadequate training in geriatric medicine and psychiatry, lack of recognition that somatic complaints may be the first manifestation of a treatable neurosis or adjustment disorder, or the tendency to attribute psychiatric symptoms and behavioral changes in the elderly to "old age."

Research directed at understanding these neuroses has received comparatively less attention than investigations conducted on other psychiatric disorders of the elderly, such as depression and the dementias. Clinical investigations are needed in a number of areas. Although more recent classification systems, such as the DSM-III, have some distinct advantages over previous systems, there needs to be a diagnostic system specifically developed for psychiatric disorders of late life (just as there are specific classification systems for children) that can be used universally by clinical investigators and clinicians.

Despite the many etiological factors contributing to the high prevalence of neurotic symptoms in late life, according to Lowenthal, Berkman, and associates (1964) we still know too little about the causal and other relationships that may exist among hereditary factors, lifelong personality characteristics, and psychogenic or functional and biologic disorders which occur during the early, middle, and later years. Whether neurotic illness arises primarily as a reaction to the aging process or as the culmination of lifelong conflicts in particularly vulnerable individuals, or as a combination of these, still remains an open question.

Research needs to be done into the natural history of somatoform disorders of the elderly, particularly hypochondriasis, and in how frequent these disorders are part of the symptom complex of a depressive disorder and/or an unrecognized physical illness. Studies also need to be conducted into the relationship, prevalence, and natural history of adjustment and dysthymic (neurotic depressive) disorders that occur in acute and chronically ill older people. Investigations into the efficacy of various treatment approaches, both psychopharmacological and psychotherapeutic, are also needed to guide clinicians in providing effective treatment for this group of treatable, reversible disorders in the elderly.

REFERENCES

Adams, D. L. (1971). Correlates of satisfaction among the elderly. *Gerontologist, 2,* 64–68.
American Psychiatric Association. (1980). *Diagnostic and statistical manual of mental disorders* (3rd ed.). Washington, DC: Author.
Bergmann, K. (1971). The neuroses of old age. In D. W. K. Kay & A. Walk (Eds.), *Recent developments in psychogeriatrics, A symposium* (pp. 39–50). British Journal of Psychiatry Special Publication No. 6.
Bergmann, K. (1975). Nosology. In J. G. Howells (Ed.), *Modern perspectives in the psychiatry of old age* (pp. 170–187). New York: Brunner/Mazel, 1975.
Bergmann, K. (1978). Neurosis and personality disorder in old age. In A. D. Isaacs & F. Post (Eds.), *Studies in geriatric psychiatry* (pp. 41–75). Chichester, UK, New York, Brisbane, Toronto: Wiley.
Botwinick, J. (1981). Neuropsychology of aging. In S. B. Filskov & T. J. Boll (Eds.), *Handbook of clinical neuropsychology* (pp. 135–171). New York: Wiley.
Busse, E. W. (1981). Old age. In S. I. Greenspan & G. H. Pollock (Eds.), *The course of life: Psychoanalytic contributions toward understanding personality development* (pp. 519–544). Washington, DC: U.S. Government Printing Office.
Butler, R., & Lewis, M. (1977). *Aging and mental health: Positive psychological approaches* (2nd ed.). St. Louis, MO: C. V. Mosby.
Cath, S. H. (1976). Functional disorders: An organismic view and attempt at reclassification. In L. Bellak & T. B. Karasu (Eds.), *Geriatric psychiatry: A handbook for psychiatry and primary care physicians* (pp. 141–172). New York: Grune & Stratton.
Ciompi, L. (1969). Follow-up studies on the evolution of former neurotic and depressive states in old age. *Journal of Geriatric Psychiatry, 3,* 90–106.
Earley, L. W. & Von Mering, O. (1969). Growing old the outpatient way. *American Journal of Psychiatry, 125,* 964–967.
Erikson, E. H. (1963). Childhood and society. New York: W. W. Norton.
Gaitz, C. M., & Varner, R. V. (1980). Adjustment disorders of late life: Stress disorders. In Busse, E. W. & Blazer, D. G. (Eds.), *Handbook of geriatric psychiatry* (pp. 381–388). New York: Van Nostrand Reinhold.
Gurland, B. J. (1976). The comparative frequency of depression in various adult age groups. *Journal of Gerontology 31,* 283–292.
Gutmann, D. L. (1980). Observations on culture and mental health in later life. In: J. Birren & R. B. Sloane (Eds.), *Handbook of Mental Health and Aging,* (pp. 429–447). Englewood Cliffs, NJ: Prentice-Hall.
Gutmann, D. L. (1964). An exploration of ego configurations in middle and later life. In B. L. Neugarten (Ed.), *Personality in middle and late life: Empirical studies* (pp. 114–148). New York: Atherton Press.
Havighurst, R. J. (1968). Personality and patterns of aging. *Gerontologist, 8,* 20–23.
Jacobs, T. J., Fogelson, S., & Charles, E. (1968). Depression ratings in hypochondria. *New York State Journal of Medicine,* December 15, 3119–3122.
Jung, C. G. (1960). The stages of life. In H. Read, M. Fordham, & G. Adler (Eds.), *The collected works of C. G. Jung.* (Vol. 8). *The structure and dynamics of the psyche* (pp. 384–403). New York: Pantheon.
Kay, D. W. K., Beamish, P., & Roth, M. (1964). Old age mental disorder in Newcastle-upon-Tyne. (Part I) A study of prevalence. *British Journal of Psychiatry, 110,* 146–158.

Kay, D. W. K., & Bergmann, K. (1966). Physical disability and mental health in old age. *Journal of Psychosomatic Research* (London), *10*, 3–12.

Kahn, R. L., Zarit, S. H., Hilbert, N. M., & Niederehe, G. (1975). Memory complaint and impairment in the aged: The effect of depression and altered brain function. *Archives of General Psychiatry, 32*, 1569–1573.

Kessel, N., & Shepherd, M. (1962). Neurosis in hospital and general practice. *Journal of Mental Science, 108*, 159–166.

Kohut, H. (1966). Forms and transformations of narcissism. *Journal of the American Psychoanalytic Association, 14*, 243–272.

Kohut, H. (1971). *The analysis of the self*. New York: International Universities Press.

Kohut, H. (1977). *The restoration of the self*. New York: International Universities Press.

Kohut, H. (1972). Thoughts on narcissism and narcissistic rage. *Psychoanalytic Study of the Child, 27*, 360–400.

Kohut, H., & Wolf, E. (1978). The disorders of the self and their treatment: An outline. *International Journal of Psycho-Analysis, 59*, 413–425.

Lazarus, L. W. (1980). Self psychology and psychotherapy with the elderly: Theory and practice. *Journal of Geriatric Psychiatry, 13*, 69–88.

Lazarus, L. W., & Weinberg, J. (1980). Treatment in the ambulatory care setting. In E. Busse & D. G. Blazer (Eds.), *The handbook of geriatric psychiatry* (pp. 427–452). New York: Van Nostrand Reinhold.

Lowenthal, M. F., Berkman, P., et al. (1964). *Aging and mental disorder in San Francisco*. San Francisco: Jossey-Bass.

Meissner, W. W. (1976). Normal psychology of the aging process revisited—1:Discussion. *Journal of Geriatric Psychiatry, 9*, 151–159.

Monge, R. H. (1975). Structure of the self-concept from adolescence through old age. *Experimental Aging Research 1*, 281–291.

Neugarten, B. L. (1974, September). Age groups in American society and the rise of the young–old. *Annals of American Academy*, (pp. 187–189).

Neugarten, B. L. (1977). Personality and aging. In J. E. Birren & K. W. Schaie (Eds.), *Handbook of the psychology of aging* (pp. 626–649). New York: Van Nostrand Reinhold.

Neugarten, B. L. (1964). *Personality in middle and late life: Empirical studies*. New York: Atherton Press.

Nielsen, J., Homma, A., & Biorn-Henriksen, T. (1977). Follow-up 15 years after a geronto-psychiatric prevalence study. *Journal of Gerontology, 32*, 554–561.

Palmore, E., (Ed.). (1970). *Normal aging, Reports from the Duke Longitudinal Study* (pp. 1955–1969). Durham, NC: Duke University Press.

Palmore, E., & Kivett, V. (1977). Changes in life satisfaction: A longitudinal study of persons aged 46–70. *Journal of Gerontology, 32*, 311–316.

Pfeiffer, E., & Busse, E. W. (1973). Affective disorders. In E. W. Busse & E. Pfeiffer (Eds.), *Mental illness in later life* (pp. 199–232). Washington, DC: American Psychiatric Press.

Reichard, S., Livson, F., & Petersen, P. G. (1962). *Aging and personality: A study of eighty-seven older men*. New York: Wiley.

Roberts, W. L. (1979–1980). Significant elements in the relationship of long-married couples. *International Journal of Aging and Human Development, 10*, 165–172.

Robins, L. N., Helzer, J. E., Weissman, M. M., et al. (1984). Lifetime prevalence of specific psychiatric disorders in three sites. *Archives of General Psychiatry, 41*, 949–958.

Ryff, C. D., & Baltes, P. B. (1976). Value transition and adult development in women. The instrumentality–terminality sequence hypothesis. *Developmental Psychology, 12,* 567–568.

Simon, A. (1980). The neuroses, personality disorders, alcoholism, drug use and misuse, and crime in the aged. In J. Birren & R. B. Sloane, (Eds.), *Handbook of mental health and aging,* (pp. 653–670). Englewood Cliffs, NJ: Prentice-Hall.

Sussman, M. (1976). The family life of old people. In R. H. Binstock & E. Shanas, (Eds.), *Handbook of aging and the social sciences* (pp. 218–43). New York: Van Nostrand Reinhold.

Thomae, H. (1976). Patterns of successful aging. In H. Thomae (Ed.), *Patterns of aging: Findings from the Bonn longitudinal studies of aging* (pp. 147–161). Basel: S. Karger.

Thomae, H. (1980). Personality and adjustment to aging. In J. Birren & R. B. Sloane, (Eds.), *Handbook of mental health and aging* (pp. 285–309). Englewood Cliffs, NJ: Prentice-Hall.

Thomae, H. (1970). Theory of aging and cognitive theory of personality. *Human Development, 13,* 1–16.

Trimakas, K. A., & Nicolay, R. C. (1974). Self-concept and altruism in old age. *Journal of Gerontology, 29,* 434–439.

Verwoerdt, A. (1976). *Clinical Geropsychiatry.* Baltimore: Williams and Wilkins.

Weinberg, J. (1975). Geriatric psychiatry. In A. M. Freedman, H. L. Kaplan, & B. J. Sadock (Eds.), *Comprehensive textbook of psychiatry* Vol. 2 (2nd ed., pp. 2405–2420). Baltimore, MD: Williams & Wilkins.

Weinberg, J., & Lazarus, L. W. (1980). Treatment in the ambulatory care setting. In E. W. Busse, & D. G. Blazer, (Eds.). New York: Van Nostrand Reinhold.

Williamson, J., Stokoe, I. H., Gray, S., Fisher, M., Smith, A., McGhea, A., & Stephenson, E. (1964). Old people at home—Their unreported needs. *Lancet, 1,* 117–120.

5
Psychosomatic Problems in Geriatrics

Joep M. A. Munnichs

This comprehensive theme evokes varying associations and expectations. First, the relationship between psychosomatics and geriatrics will be discussed, followed by a description of the relationship between morbidity and life-span, which may also shed light on the different perspectives of psychosomatics. The latest views are those of Ursin. The central concepts he uses will be expanded, including the use of empirical data. Society's attitude toward people with psychosomatic symptoms will be discussed along with a possible therapeutic approaches.

PSYCHOSOMATICS AND GERIATRICS

The principle of classical psychosomatics is that emotional experiences not only can influence health and bodily functions but can also trigger psychosomatic diseases. The idea that only physical causes can change the body has been discarded. Psychosomatics, hence, is a movement opposing the dualistic view of man, which began with Descartes, who regarded man as "res cogitans" on the one hand and "res extensa" on the other hand. The latter concept considered the body an autonomous organism. The idea expressed in psychosomatics is akin to that of geriatrics, although not everybody employed in geriatrics will or would like to recognize this. The field of gerontology attempts to present the old and very old individual as a compartmentalized whole. A person's state of health is associated not only with their physical condition but with the whole person, which contributes to a person's well-being to an important degree. This holistic point of view in geriatrics can be traced to the discourses on psychosomatics.

A second common characteristic between geriatrics and psychosomatics is that the geriatrician, as the medical doctor involved with psychosomatic symptoms, looks for the long-term effects in a patient's life. Psychosomatic symptoms are usually not an expression of a suddenly appearing disease. A significant period of time usually elapses before the effect of a particular emotional response has had the chance to influence the body. The same can be said of the usually multiple ailments of the elderly. When treating the elderly it is often very enlightening to know how they learned to cope with a chronic complaint. Only once this is known should an interpretation—both diagnostic and therapeutic—be made.

A third common characteristic can be seen as an extension of the second, that is, in order to obtain a true view of a patient's emotional state, an accurate view of his/her life-span is required. The geriatrician needs this because man, in the course of his life, becomes more and more his body, contrary to his youth when he rather owns his body. It is quite true therefore to say that the body becomes more individualized with aging, more like the person whose body it is.

Another reason for the kinship between geriatrics and psychosomatics is that the geriatrician is used to multicausal thinking. He knows that not only somatic but also other factors are involved in diagnostics and in understanding the body messages.

These four, mainly formal, points characterize the relationship between geriatrics and psychosomatics. However, there is no denying the fact that there are fewer new instances of psychosomatic disorders in old age than in the years preceding. As Hunter et al. (1982) stated: "Fresh cases of classical psychosomatic disease are reduced in frequency after 65 and often show a somewhat different clinical picture than those occurring in the younger age groups" (p. 364). Others even state that psychosomatics changes during the aging process into normal somatic pathology, i.e., psychosomatic ailments slowly become normal somatic ailments. This point of view may be too radical and may contradict some of the formal characteristics mentioned above. But if, for a moment, we would accept this point of view, we could be faced in our old age with mainly psychosomatic patients who have grown old, e.g., patients with stomach complaints or those who have to be careful because of them; patients who are aware of their high blood pressure and have learned to live with it.

These simple examples already show a probably very strong "body-preoccupation" (Peck, 1968)—a strong involvement on the part of the patient with his or her body, resulting undoubtedly in psychosomatic effects. There is another reason to question the thesis that psychosomatics is a rare phenomenon in old age. It is well known that many people approaching retirement have to take it easy. And although retirement entails new stress for some, the small amount of research on this topic (Wasylenski et al., 1981) shows that most people respond positively to retirement. Taking it easy indeed has a mental effect on the body, and there are certain positive psychosomatic effects of retirement as well. It remains to be seen, however, whether the concept of psychosomatics has been taken too broadly. Adler et al. (1980) also warned about this. They stated that by recognizing the drastic effects of stress on the body, psychosomatic medicine presumes that all diseases have mental components and that medicine as a whole is contained in psychosomatic medicine. If this concept is extended, it will be difficult to distinguish psychosomatics from the newly rising discipline of "behavioral medicine" (p. 580).

MORBIDITY AND LIFE-SPAN

A relationship between the appearance of psychosomatic diseases and certain periods of life was mentioned. This can be expanded on. It is obvious that, apart from the symptoms caused by the body itself or by an unambiguous influence of the physical environment, all the remaining symptoms are influenced by the interaction between the whole human being and his environment. To that extent, the life course of a human being largely determines his health. It would be wonderful if we could present an overview of the morbidity and the changes in the pattern for various personality types or organizations. However, this is not yet possible. Nor can we present such an overview for those still alive. We can, however, present an overview of the most frequent causes of death for various age categories. These are American data from 1976, applicable, in our opinion, to most countries of the Western world. (See Table 5.1.)

The table shows the eleven most important causes of death for seven successive life-span periods. These periods extend from the age of 25 to 85 and beyond. The change in order is particularly interesting. In the youngest age group (25–34) "accidents" constitute the most important cause of death. But this cause moves to third place in the 35–44 age group, to fourth in 55 to 64-year olds, ending as the sixth cause in those 85 and over.

Diseases that increase with age are, as is known, diseases of the heart and malignant neoplasms. Heart diseases initially rank third among the young, those between 25 and 34 years old, moving to first place in people between 45 and 55, and keeping that place to the end, age 85 and above. Cerebrovascular disease shows a similar pattern, with arteriosclerosis following at a distance.

When one compares this schema with the classic psychosomatic symptoms, one realizes that these are missing. Does this mean that psychosomatic

TABLE 5.1 Order of Ten Leading Causes of Death, by Death Rate[a] for Seven Age Groups, 1976

Total	Age: 25–34	35–44	45–54	55–64	65–74	75–84	85+
Diseases of the heart (337.2)	Accidents	Malignant neoplasm	Diseases of the heart	Diseases of the heart	Diseases of the heart	Diseases of the heart	Diseases of the heart
Malignant neoplasm (175.8)	Suicide	Diseases of the heart	Malignant neoplasms	Malignant neoplasms	Malignant neoplasms	Malignant neoplasms	Malignant neoplasms
Cerebrovascular disease (87.9)	Malignant neoplasm	Cerebrovascular disease	Cerebrovascular disease	Cerebrovascular disease	Cerebrovascular disease	Cerebrovascular disease	Cerebrovascular disease
Accidents (46.9)	Diseases of the heart	Accidents	Accidents	Accidents	Influenza and pneumonia	Influenza and pneumonia	Influenza and pneumonia
Influenza and pneumonia (28.8)	Cirrhosis	Cirrhosis	Cirrhosis	Cirrhosis	Accidents	Arteriosclerosis	Arteriosclerosis
Diabetes (16.1)	Cerebrovascular disease	Suicide	Cerebrovascular disease	Influenza and pneumonia	Diabetes	Diabetes	Accidents
Cirrhosis (14.7)	Influenza and pneumonia	Influenza and pneumonia	Suicide	Diabetes	Bronchitis, emphysema, and asthma	Accidents	Diabetes
Arteriosclerosis (13.7)	Diabetes	Diabetes	Influenza and pneumonia	Bronchitis, emphysema, and asthma	Cirrhosis	Bronchitis, emphysema, and asthma	Bronchitis, emphysema, and asthma
Suicide (12.5)	Bronchitis, emphysema, and asthma	Bronchitis, emphysema, and asthma	Diabetes	Suicide	Arteriosclerosis	Cirrhosis	Suicide
Bronchitis, emphysema, and asthma (11.4)	Arteriosclerosis	Arteriosclerosis	Bronchitis, emphysema, and asthma	Arteriosclerosis	Suicide	Suicide	Cirrhosis

[a]Death rate per 100,000 estimated population per age group.

Source: U.S. Department of Health, Education, and Welfare, Monthly Vital Statistics Report, Final Mortality Statistics, 1976. Washington, D.C.: U.S. Government Printing Office, March 30, 1978, pp. 20–21.

diseases cannot be lethal? It certainly does not mean that they cannot be tremendously troublesome to the individual person. However, using a different classification, for example, one from the WHO (1968), we find that cardiovascular and endocrine diseases are mentioned as psychosomatic disorders too. Diabetes is explicitly included in the latter. Both—diabetes and cardiovascular diseases—appear in the schema just presented. What does this mean? The achievements of medicine after Alexander's publications on psychosomatics (1968) have increased our knowledge about the background of the two conditions mentioned above: cardiovascular diseases and diabetes. We will expand on the former.

It seems superfluous to describe in detail Rosenman and Friedman's (1970) discovery of the so-called A and B typology which they distinguished in their respondents. The A-type was twice as likely to get a heart attack as type B. Type A behavior may be characterized by an excessively competitive mentality and an enormous drive toward achievement. Type A displays aggressive, restless and impatient behavior. He/she is short-tempered, uses explosive language and tends to struggle continuously with the environment in his/her feelings.

Type B is mostly characterized by the absence of these traits. From an objective point of view it is obvious that type A has organized his/her life and personality in a less healthy way than type B. The question remains, however, how a physical response that may be called a cardiovascular disease can be evoked from this behavior. Only when this can be shown can the psychosomatic nature of the disease be proven.

The afore-mentioned typology also points out that such behavior does not develop overnight. For psychologists the question then remains how such behavior does develop. It probably received its stimuli in childhood, with the environmental factors in the first professional years being of fundamental importance. Does one have to prove oneself and to whom? What does one want to achieve and why? If other stress situations, like family illness, a child's accident or the death of one of the parents to whom it is attached, are added to such a typology, exhaustion may result, with that state becoming the last decisive factor in a myocardial infarct.

It is evident that this disease, and probably the majority of the other diseases, reflects the personality's approach to life and his/her life style. The infarct is not the result of a suddenly developed situation but of a pattern developed over time and leading to cardiovascular disease. Once the disease is there, the question arises of how it developed. The answer to this and the consequences a person draws from it determine the way in which he/she organizes the remaining years.

The crucial question then is: Does one wish to change or not? From a psychological viewpoint it would be interesting to ask: Can one still change?

VIEWS ON PSYCHOSOMATICS

Warwick-Evens (1983) provides some examples that are of interest to us. As an illustration of psychological factors that coincide with different actions, she mentions that peeling onions and reading poetry may both lead to tears. Only the latter, however, is a psychological factor. If an asthmatic patient inhales pollen to which he is allergic, he may have breathing problems. This may also happen when he sees a photograph of pollen. Again, only in the latter case is the cause internal and psychological. We may therefore conclude that the personal interpretation or "appraisal" is the central psychological core in question. This conclusion can be found in various theories on psychosomatics.

In Alexander's psychodynamic theory three conditions for psychosomatics are named: (1) a "psychodynamic constellation," or a specific attitude; (2) a provoking situation (e.g., an important life event); and (3) factor X, being the vulnerability of a particular organ or organic system (1968). The first condition resembles what we called "personal appraisal." Moreover we should mention that until now Alexander's theory has not been supported by unambiguous empirical data. Warwick-Evens, presenting an up-to-date overview of various theoretical starting points, gives us some interesting statements in the commentary.

She suggests that while psychosomatic ailments should be distinguished from other complaints, we should check every complaint to see whether it is psychosomatic or not. Not all heart complaints are psychosomatic. We may conclude, however, that psychological factors cause a number of *physiological* complaints. Here we could use the following reference points:

- in the course of evolution, reflex mechanisms have been inextricably attached to subject-dependent mental events like emotions, memories and expectations;
- these act in accordance with the laws of operant and classic conditioning;
- there are crucial biochemical, physiological and psychic differences between individuals (p. 182).

The crucial psychic factors have to do with emotions and expectations, and undoubtedly with memories associated with emotions. "Being moved," as one may initially describe emotions, is therefore the beginning. The way in which this "being moved" is interpreted follows. Lazarus uses the concept "appraisal," this also being a cognitive act by which whatever moves one is interpreted as something pleasant, or something demanding careful attention, or something within one's power, not something that leaves one indifferent. After interpretation Lazarus lists action which, depending on the nature of the interpretation, he calls "coping." We would say that one deals with one's experience in a particular way. If you have been mistreated and you can respond to it, counterattack is an adequate response. If, however, such response only worsens the situation, action may be postponed. In that case the emotional tension may continue—you feel frustrated.

Frustration and stress are necessary concepts in this context. Ursin (1980), also engaging in theories of psychosomatics, holds a different view. What is more important to him than stress is the response to what is called stress, and he distinguishes between two categories: the "defense mechanisms" and "the coping mechanisms." What does he mean by this?

The response is related to the defense mechanism in the Freudian sense. In less threatening circumstances the response style could be harmless, but not so in serious circumstances. The defense mechanism tries to reduce the influence of particular stimuli and in that way is related to denial. The coping response, however, tries to deal with the stimulus by an effective way of handling the environment. It contributes to a successful mastering of the situation. Contrary to the defense mechanism, which unfolds automatically, coping is a conscious process. By using the coping mechanism dramatic, even threatening events cannot lead to continuous activation. Coping reduces the arousal that arises in the physiology. Further research has shown that it is plausible that certain mechanisms coincide with different hormones. Prolonged arousal could be the most important mediator of frequently occurring psychosomatic illness in man. And the extent of experienced and unresolved conflicts is responsible for it. There is no balance between tension and relaxation in these persons. The attention paid by professionals to stressful, important life events is as important as the knowledge of the individual biography. Through a description of past experiences, it is possible to learn how a person has interpreted different experiences and responded to them. Hence we may suggest a possible correlation between behavior and symptoms.

EMPIRICAL FOUNDATION

After this mainly theoretical discourse we ask ourselves whether empirical research supports the typology suggested in the literature. We already mentioned the type A and B division with respect to patients with cardiovascular disease. And if there was ever any question that prolonged tension leads to this disease, especially in addition to a long period of physiological strain, that question no longer exists. But is there any support for this hypothesis in other studies? We would prefer to look for it in longitudinal research where the long-term effects are best shown. Cross-sectional research is therefore of less value.

Our question then is: Does research show that there is a differentiation, e.g., in personality organization, to the effect that one type of person shows characteristics that suggest a psychosomatic disease whereas the other does not?

We are acquainted with the results of two longitudinal American studies that followed respondents (totaling 136) from their birth onward—the Oakland Growth Study (OGS) and the Guidance Study (GS). The former started in 1921, the latter in 1928. In 1968 (cf. the overview) these respondents were 47 and 40 years old, respectively.

This is not the occasion to describe these two very complex studies. (For details see the recent study "Present and past in middle life," Eichorn, Mussen, Clausen, Haan, & Honzik, 1981.) We would like to expand, however, on one important aspect: the personality organization of these respondents. This should tell us something about personality style. Haan (1985), who has dealt with this, presents nine personality organizations in the schema shown below. We only list one dimension for the sake of convenience. The schema also indicates whether the personality organization in question may be regarded as efficient (+) or inefficient (−).

1. Self-confident/cognitively invested +
2. Open to self/cognitively invested +
3. Overcontrolled heterosexual/closed to self −
4. Closed to self/emotionally overcontrolled −
5. Hostile/not cognitively invested −
6. Closed to self/not cognitively invested −
7. Undercontrolled heterosexual −
8. Nurturant/cognitively invested +
9. Mixed.

Haan was also in a position to observe the stability of certain personality organizations over time. This analysis could only be done on a limited number of patients, i.e., the type, labeled "open to self" and "closed to self." The difference was highly significant ($p < 0.001$). The "open-to-self" type changed far more often over time. The problematic "closed-to-self" type appeared to remain stable over time and to possess a less efficient personality organization. Since a less efficient personality organization was found only in men, with few exceptions, it appears that women have more of a coping style, to speak in Ursin terms, and men more of a defending style. This difference may also explain the greater number of cardiovascular complaints in men—in whom type A is also more often found than in women.

What can we conclude from these data? Apparently a certain fixed personality organization is developed in early adulthood, characterized by a particular coping style, this style is probably not physically neutral, i.e., apart from the so-called objective health condition, it leaves its traces in the body.

Persons who are able to deal with their experiences, who are open to them, seem to have a better adaptation capacity than those who evade them. The consequences, however, may appear only after a long time. They also depend on the amount and kind of strain. If the strain increases all of a sudden as a result of one or more important events, then the negative process of falling ill may be accelerated. If this is not the case, it may lie dormant during normal strain and only surface at an advanced aged. This empirical research suggests the same direction as does our own rather more theoretical discourse.

EPILOGUE

When restating our question about the link between psychosomatics and geriatrics, we arrive at the following provisional conclusions: It is difficult at present to tell where psychosomatics starts and where it ends. This is due to the fact that as Ursin only recently showed, physiological reactions may be aroused in a person that may influence various systems. The question still remains if any other complaints by a patient should be included, apart from those associated with psychosomatics from the early days. Pseudodementia and depression may be candidates for inclusion, but that is still debatable.

It is not the disease that is indicative of psychosomatics, but rather the person's physiological reaction to a given event. Stated otherwise: the physiological response is organ-neutral. It depends on the individual whether he/she responds with a stomach ulcer or a heart complaint. The determinants remain unknown. Also important is the fact that by the time geriatrics usually starts, i.e., in early old age—for many this is retirement age—the individual and his body have either achieved health or have been victimized by morbidity. (The geriatrician may study the person's morbidity history—and his health history for that matter—and try to understand it; he may explain to the person in question his situation, because there is not much more left to do.) The choice the person made during adulthood in favor of a particular coping style cannot be undone. If it was an unhealthy coping style, the effects will be visible. If it was not, the geriatrician has an unexpected chance to discuss his patient's life pattern, indicating which behavior style bears the fewest risks. Usually this means that the geriatrician, faced with numerous complaints, cannot boast of spectacular results—

as can the pediatrician—but that he must develop a therapy and a daily pattern for the patient that will preserve his/her life and continue to make it meaningful.

REFERENCES

Adler, N. E., Cohen, F., & Stone, G. C. (1980). Themes and professional prospects in health psychology. In G. C. Stone, F. Cohen, & N. E. Adler (Eds.), *Health psychology, a handbook*. San Francisco: Jossey-Bass.

Alexander, F., French, T. M., & Ollock, G. H. (Eds.). (1968). *Psychosomatic specificity*. Chicago: University of Chicago Press.

Eichorn, D. H., Mussen, P. H., Clausen, J., Haan, N. & Honzik, M. (Eds.). (1981). *Present and past in middle life*. New York: Academic Press.

Haan, N. (1985). Common personality dimensions or common organizations across the life span? In J. M. A. Munnichs et al. (Eds.), *Life span and change in a gerontological perspective* (pp. 17–44). New York: Academic Press.

Hunter, R. C. A., & Cleghorn, R. A. (1982). Psychosomatic disorders in the elderly. *Canadian Journal of Psychiatry, 27,* 362–365.

Lazarus, R. S., & Cohen, F. (1980). Coping with the stresses of illness. In G. C. Stone, F. Cohen, & N. E. Adler (Eds.) *Health psychology, a handbook* (pp. 217–254). San Francisco: Jossey-Bass.

Peck, R. C. (1968). Psychological developments in the second half of life. In B. L. Neugarten (Ed.) *Middle age and aging* (pp. 88–92). Chicago: University of Chicago Press.

Rosenman, R. H., Friedman, M., et al. (1970). Coronary heart disease in the western collaborative group study: A follow-up experience of four-and-one-half years. *Journal of Chronic Diseases, 23,* 173–190.

Stein, S. & Shamoian, C. (1981). Psychosomatic disorders in the middle-aged. In J. G. Howells (Ed.), *Modern perspectives in the psychiatry of middle age* (pp. 266–278). New York: Brunner/Mazel.

Stevens-Long, J., (1979). *Adult life, developmental processes*. Palo Alto, CA: Mayfield.

Ursin, H. (1980). Personality, activation and somatic health, a new psychosomatic theory, (pp. 259–279). In S. Levine & H. Ursin (Eds.), *Coping and health*. New York: Plenum.

Warwick-Evens, L. A. (1983). Psychosomatic disorders: theories and evidence. In A. Fale, & J. A. Edwards (Eds.) *Physiological correlates of human behavior, Vol. III Individual differences and psychopathology* (pp. 169–185). London: Academic Press.

Wasylenski, D., & MacBride, A. (1981). Retirement. In J. G. Howells (Ed.), *Modern perspectives in the psychiatry of middle age* (pp. 144–166). New York: Brunner/Mazel.

PART II
Diagnostics

6
New Perspectives in the Classification and Diagnosis of Psychiatric Disorders in Late Life

Sir Martin Roth

The rapid growth of clinical and scientific interest in the mental disorders of the aged has been intensified during the past decade by the advances achieved in knowledge of the neurobiologic basis of Alzheimer's disease and related forms of dementia. Social concern over the growing burden created within aging societies by the mental disorders of late life increased over many decades. Half a century ago most of these disorders were considered to cause infirmity and dependence on others. This view began to be modified by clinical observations first published about 30 years ago that showed mental illness in senescence to comprise a number of distinct disorders which differed in their courses and outcomes.

The unitary etiological theories of the past that had attributed all forms of psychiatric disease in the elderly to cerebral degeneration began to be increasingly called into question. As in other branches of psychiatry the burgeoning of scientific interest and achievement had probably begun with advances in classification and clinical diagnosis. In the intervening years progress has been achieved through not only the validation of the clinical distinctions initially made, but also through modifications and refutations of some of the hypotheses initially advanced.

COMPARISON OF THE RESULTS OF RECENT AND EARLY STUDIES OF CLASSIFICATION

Two recent investigations into the natural history of mental disorders in old age (Blessed & Wilson, 1982) have attempted to ascertain the extent to which the patterns of outcome of the initial inquiries were still in evidence among elderly psychiatric patients admitted to a hospital. The new observations are timely for a number of reasons. These may have been secular changes during a period of more than 30 years in the character and course of mental disorders in the elderly. There have been important developments in the area of diagnosis and classification of psychiatric disorders in general. They include new systems of classification such as DSM III which have substituted strict operational definitions of all psychiatric disorders for open textbook descriptions upon which diagnosis and classification had been based until 10 to 15 years ago. The ninth version of the International Classification of Disease with its accompanying glossary has been published (WHO, 1977) and proposals for the tenth version are available in preliminary form. A number of the novel features of DSM III have a special relevance for the mental disorders of the elderly. In old age, disorders diagnosed as "organic" both on the strength of etiological and phenomenological criteria are to be found in greater prevalence than in earlier stages of adult life. But a number of the new categories introduced in DSM III, and adumbrated for ICD 10, reflect abandonment or radical revision of the concepts of "organic" and "functional" mental illness, and the implication for psychogeriatric clinical practice and inquiry needs to be assessed.

An Earlier Classification

The five broad groups of conditions into which the disorders of the aged were classified with the aid of definitions of a descriptive and phenomenological character were "affective disorder," "senile dementia," "late paraphrenia," "acute confusion," and "arteriosclerotic dementia" (Roth, 1955). Although the existence of overlap was recognized, hybrid diagnoses were not allowed. Independent validation for the sharp distinctions was sought from several lines of inquiry. The outcome of the disorders was formed to differ in terms of the proportion of discharged in-patients and those patients dead at 6 months, 2 years and 6–7 years after admission (Roth & Kay, 1962). The results at 2 years and 6 to 7 years are shown in Figures 6.1 and 6.2. At 2 years following admission more than three-fourths of patients with senile and multiinfarct dementia were dead; three-fourths of those with depressive illness and late schizophrenia were alive; while those with "acute confusion" (clouded and delirious states) occupied an intermediate position. After 6 to 7 years the differences, although partly blurred by the high

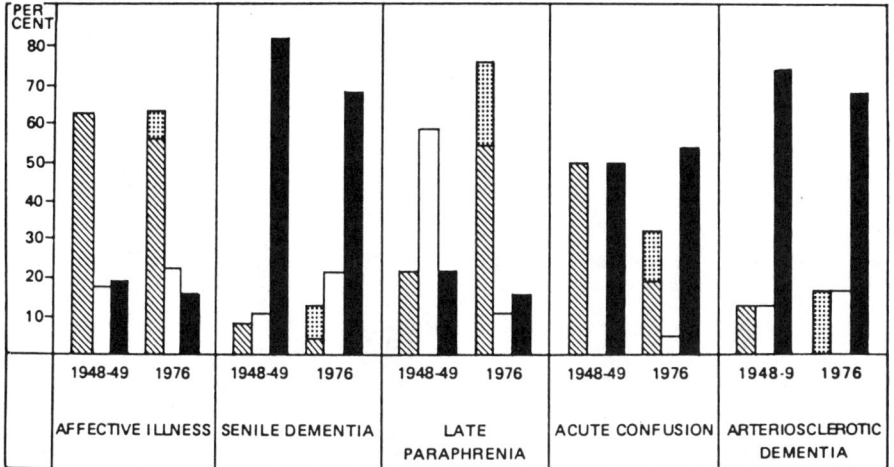

FIGURE 6.1 The contemporary natural history of mental disorder in old age. Status of elderly mentally ill patients two years after admission in 1948 and 1949 (318 patients), and 1976 (287 patients): discharged (*hatched* column), residential care (*dotted* column), inpatient (*white* column), dead (*black* column). (From Blessed & Wilson 1982. Reprinted by permission.)

mortality in all clinical groups in a sample of aged subjects, were still in evidence (Figure 6.2). The differences in mortality rate and distinctive patterns of outcome defined in the different groups were shown to be independent to a considerable extent, from the differences in mean age between them.

The groups differed significantly from each other with respect to performance on standardized psychological tests (Roth & Hopkins, 1953; Hopkins & Roth, 1953), the prevalence of physical illness, postmortem findings (Kay & Roth, 1955; Roth & Kay, 1956), and life expectation in comparison with normal population samples (Kay, 1962). It was found that for depressions that made their first appearance in later life, hereditary factors proved less important and exogenous influences more important in causation than in the comparable affective disorders of later life (Kay, 1962; Kay & Roth 1961; Roth & Kay, 1956).

With regard to the recent controversy over the validity of the distinction between "functional" and "organic" disorders in a phenomenological sense, it is perhaps pertinent that their mortalities showed such a marked disparity in these early inquiries in comparison with life expectation in comparable normal population samples. Patients with late paraphrenia proved to have a normal life expectation and affective disorders to enjoy about three-quarters of the life duration of general population samples of comparable age. But the senile and arteriosclerotic dementias taken together had a life expectancy of approximately 25% of the normal (Kay, 1962).

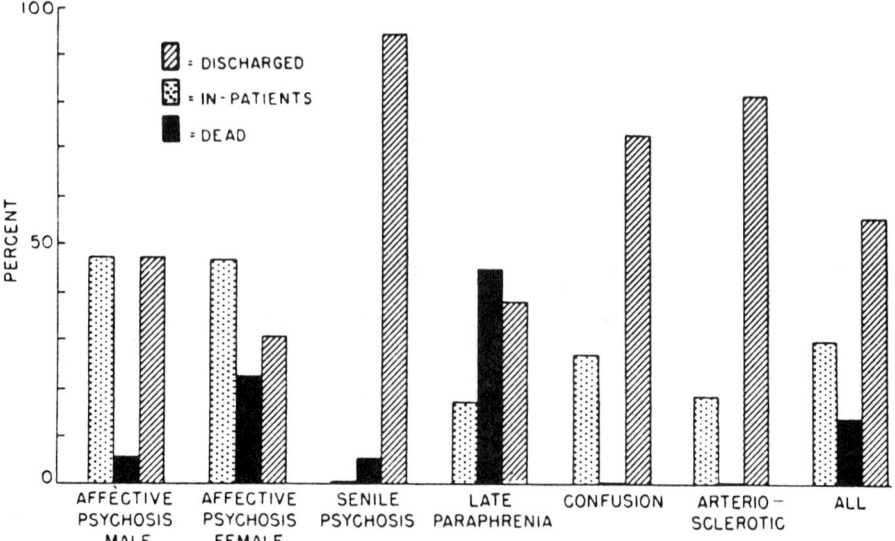

FIGURE 6.2 Pattern of outcome in 1955 of 322 cases admitted at 60 years of age and over with mental disease in 1948 and 1949. The status of the patients is shown in terms of discharged (*hatched* column), inpatients (*dotted* column), and dead (*black* column).

The body of the validating evidence derived from brain pathology posed a number of fresh questions in relation to the neurobiologic basis of senile and multi-infarct dementia. Until 30 years ago, the conclusion that generally emerged from investigations into the pathology of the dementias was that the clinical picture and the course of mental disorders in late life and their brain pathology were related to one another only in loose and ill-defined ways. The effects of brain pathology upon mental functioning during life were influenced among other factors by resources at the disposal of the personality to compensate for cerebral damage (Rothschild, 1956). With the aid of the new classification which drew sharp clinical distinctions between senile and arteriosclorotic disorders and "functional" syndromes, it was shown that a strict and orderly relationship obtained between clinical diagnosis and measures of dementia on the one hand, and the extent of neuropathological change on the other (Roth et al., 1967; Blessed et al., 1968; Corsellis, 1962; Tomlinson et al., 1968; Tomlinson et al., 1970).

Recent Enquiries into Classification

Two recent enquiries into classification have made it possible to compare and contrast the current course and outcome of different forms of mental disorder in late life with that obtained 30 or more years ago (Blessed &

Wilson 1982; Christie, 1982), as well as to assess how the classification, first suggested more than 30 years ago, has stood the test of time and thus shed light on its validity. A number of fresh questions have also been posed for further enquiry.

In the investigation by Blessed and Wilson, conducted similarly to the earlier study in Newcastle, it proved possible to allocate 90% of the 320 patients investigated into one of the five categories originally established. Of the remainder, 12 cases were classified as "other neurotic: personality disorder." These 12 cases had been classified in the group "affective psychoses" in the earlier investigation. The term "psychosis" was loosely used at that time particularly in relation to disorders of affect which first appeared in late life and were therefore presumed to be of endogenous aetiology. However, even in the second study only 27 cases out of a total of 87 received a diagnosis of "neurotic depression," and 60 of "affective psychosis" of monopolar or bipolar type. It is of interest that the majority of aged patients with affective illness admitted to a modern mental hospital are, as they were more than 30 years ago, psychotic or endogenous in character. The four cases of schizo-affective illness would have been probably diagnosed as "late paraphrenia" in the previous enquiry.

There were 97 cases of senile dementia and 25 of arteriosclerotic (multiinfarct) dementia. Only 14 of the total of 136 patients with dementia, a little over 10%, were diagnosed as having neither of these conditions and classified with "other dementias." The proportion of patients with dementia unclassifiable either on clinical or pathological criteria or both would be regarded as substantially higher by some authorities. This defines an area of crucial importance for clinical and neurobiologic research. The phenomenology of these indeterminate disorders requires definition to prevent their inclusion with the main classes of dementia, in clinical trials and other enquiries. Their pathology needs to be investigated lest there be conditions more susceptible to treatment or prevention than the senile or multiinfarct dementias have proven to be, for the present time.

As far as the outcome and mortality rates are concerned, both the similarities and the differences between the results of the earlier and the later studies are of interest (Fig. 6.1). Patterns of outcome and differences between the groups are broadly similar in the three studies despite the fact that the patients in the studies by Christie and Blessed had been admitted almost three decades later than those in the earlier inquiry. Cases now diagnosed as "functional" continue to have a markedly higher discharge rate and a lower rate of mortality than those which fall into the demented groups. Acute confusional states (or "clouded and delirious states") occupy an intermediate position.

The proportion of those with affective disorder who remain discharged at two years is similar in Blessed's study to that in the earlier inquiry by Roth (1955). There has been a slight increase in those under residential care in the

1976 inquiries, which possibly reflects the view of Post (1978) that in about a third of all cases, the depressive and related disorders of old age have the character of chronic and disabling disorders. But Christie (1982) found the outcome of affective psychosis to have improved since 1955. The most striking change in the functional group is to be found with respect to late paraphrenia, where most cases were predominantly in the inpatient group in the earlier study, well over half are now discharged in both recent inquiries, although a minority in Blessed's study are now in residential homes (Fig. 6.1). The transformation of outlook is attributed to the efficacy of neuroleptic drugs in the treatment of the schizophrenic group of disorders.

In the study by Blessed and Wilson, mortality in senile dementia had declined six months after admission and the difference from the 1955 study was statistically significant. Similar observations were recorded in the Christie study. Moreover, after two years 35% of Christie's patients, and 28% of Blessed's were found to be long-term residents in institutions. Two years after admission mortalities among the two dementia groups were only slightly lower but they were an older cohort than the earlier cases, those aged 60 to 64 years having been omitted. This evidence regarding changes in rate of survival accords with the findings of Hagnell, which suggest a steep decline in mortality rate for senile dementia. These observations are given further credence by the more recent studies conducted by Hagnell and his colleagues (Hagnell et al. 1981, 1983) indicating a decline in the prevalence and incidence of the dementias of late life. They suggest that improved socioeconomic conditions may have diminished the severity and prevalence of the disease.

As far as the disparity in mortality rates between the patients with senile dementia in the recent studies, as compared with earlier ones is concerned, other explanations than those advanced by the Swedish groups merit consideration. With an increase in the rate of employment of women as well as other changes in the domestic scene, it is more difficult to care for patients with senile and other dementias of late life at home. They may therefore have to be admitted to hospitals at an earlier stage of their illness than was the case some decades ago. If this proves to be the case the higher survival rate will be shown to be more apparent than real. However, the epidemiological findings of Hagnell and his colleagues urgently need replication in other communities.

Both the Scottish and the Newcastle recent studies record a greater mortality among cases in the group "Acute Confusion" at two years than did the 1955 investigation. The difference in mortality between 1955 and 1976 does not declare itself in either study until two years have elapsed. It is difficult to interpret the findings without more detailed information. To make valid comparisons between the outcome of the confusional states in the three studies a breakdown according to underlying aetiology would be needed. Differences in diagnostic practice might also be responsible for the changes recorded. In the presence of early, doubtful dementia together with a superimposed and indubitable confusional state, priority in diagnosis would have been given to the former in the 1955 study. Where "confusion" or "delirious" or "clouded state" is diagnosed in all cases in which this syndrome is the most conspicuous component of the presenting clinical picture, the group of clouded and confused states will inevitably contain a proportion of progressive dementias. The mortality rate is bound to be raised above that of pure and primary "clouded" cases since the outcome will in the long term be that of the underlying degenerative disorder in such states.

DEVELOPMENTS IN THE MAIN INDIVIDUAL GROUPS OF MENTAL DISORDER IN LATE LIFE

The revised classification of the mental disorder discussed in the previous section paved the way for fresh inquiries into each of the different disorders. The results that emerged and the new questions posed will be described in the present section.

Depressions of Late Life

The view implicit in classifications employed in all three follow-up studies reviewed, that the depressions that became manifest in old age were essentially similar in etiology to those of earlier life and only exceptional harbingers of later cerebral degeneration, was in conflict with authoritative opinion. Diagnostic terms such as "senile dementia of depressive type" implied that the contrary was the case. In his influential textbook of psychiatry Bleuler (1916) had said, "I should not like to class 'senile melancholias' with mild organic features or organic confusions and deliria because on closer examination it is always found that after the disappearance of the striking symptoms the patient is, in the sense of dementia senilis, a weakened individual. Therefore, I conceive such storms as intercurrent manifestations of a senile brain degeneration, . . ."

The issue could be settled only by detailed follow-up investigations. (Kay, 1962) studied the outcome in 52 manic-depressive subjects and in 45 patients with affective disorder of late onset; the patients in both groups were more than 60 years of age at the onset of the current illness. The follow-up period ranged from 16 to 25 years in the course of which only one case of senile dementia was recorded in each of the groups. Among manic-depressive patients who had also had attacks of affective disorder before the age of 60 years, there was physical evidence of cerebrovascular disease in four patients at the time of admission. But similar evidence was found in only one of the patients in the later affective group. The findings showed that dementia did not evolve in the course of depressive disorders with a frequency beyond chance expectation, and also that it was rare for cerebral disease to contribute to the development of an ordinary depressive illness. Coexistence of the two conditions probably resulted from the fortuitous association of two common types of illness. A depressive coloring is found in a minority of early cases of multiinfarct dementia, but evidence of cognitive impairment and/or personality change is nearly always manifested so that the diagnosis of an organic syndrome is not in question.

Although cerebral disease was shown to play little or no part in the causation of depressive illness, the hypothesis that the association of affective disorder with somatic disease was also due to chance has not been upheld. Studies of hospitalized patients have shown an excessive prevalence of a variety of chronic physical diseases among the aged with depression (Kay & Roth 1955; Roth & Kay 1956; Stenstedt, 1959). In studies of a community sample, Kay and Bergmann (1966) found the same increased prevalence of chronic somatic disease among men (but not women) with affective disorder, and also a significantly increased mortality among depressed men. In a 2½- to 4-year follow-up study, 50% of the men aged 65 and over were found to have died, almost twice the expected number in a normal population sample. This showed that the common combination of physical disease with depression was neither a sampling artifact nor the result of hypochrondrical exaggeration of minor ailments.

Somatic disease has therefore been shown to play some part in the genesis of affective disorder in late and also middle life (Kerr et al. 1969), partly through its metabolic affects, and in some measure through the implications carried by somatic disease and disability for men in particular (Roth, 1984). But it does no more than contribute to a limited and variable extent. Most patients, even in old age, do not have significant somatic disease, and the mental and physical disease may pursue quite different courses. The association has not therefore provided insight into the fundamental causation of depressive, manic, and other affective disorders. In addition, the overlap found in old age has not erased the line of demarcation between "functional" and "organic" disorders either in a phenomenological or an aetiological sense.

Depressive Pseudodementia

Kiloh (1961) first pointed out that depressed patients can present with a picture comprising failure of concentration and attention, loss of memory, disorientation, poor appetite, and weight loss. This picture may simulate dementia. Post (1965) and Hemsi (1968) have drawn attention to the Ganser-like responses that are given by some patients. Where a history is available of recent onset and previous family history of depression the presence of depressive ideation and perceptual disturbance provide clues to the diagnosis. Moreover, observation of behavior over a period will often reveal the presence of cognitive and other skills which may have appeared absent or impaired in the course of a formal testing. Only a limited range of the developmental and presenting features of true dementia are simulated by these disorders.

The following description, although set down 25 years ago, still delineates the clinical lines of the demarcation from senile dementia (Roth & Myers, 1962):

> The onset of an endogenous depression is usually recent and acute, in dementia it is insidious, and at the time of presentation, distant. The endogenously depressed patient will often communicate a sense of distress whereas, in dementia, the emotions are usually shallow. He can sometimes be distracted from his morbid and self-critical ruminations for long enough to establish both that his cognitive impairment is not as gross as initial impression suggests, and that it is inconsistent: he may do badly on some simple tests of memory and intellect but unexpectedly well on others, and his performance varies considerably from day to day. In depression there is frequently a family history of depressive illness and, in the cases which most resemble dementia, the family pattern of depression is also atypical. Finally, the whole picture in depression including the defects of memory, grasp and reasoning, will generally respond dramatically to electroconvulsive treatment.

A substantial proportion of cases are now known to respond to antidepressant drugs which are usually given as the first treatment.

Late Paraphrenia

This group of disorders may now be regarded, on the grounds of a number of lines of evidence, as having a close kinship with schizophrenic illness of early life (Roth, 1955; Kay & Roth, 1961; Kay, 1963). The morbid risk for schizophrenia in first degree relatives is significantly beyond normal expectation although smaller than in schizophrenic subjects of earlier life. Similarities in clinical picture, premorbid personality, sexual adaptation, fertility, and treatment response of these disorders are testimony to their kinship with schizophrenic illness.

The interesting question as to why manifestation of the disorder is postponed to late life in these patients is presently unanswered. The clinical focus brought to bear on late paraphrenia after it was differentiated from other mental disorders of late life, has helped to define some contributory aetiologic factors of the condition. Deafness of a kind different from that found in patients with affective disorder is present in some 35 to 40% of cases (Kay & Roth, 1961; Cooper et al., 1974). Visual defects are found in a smaller proportion. The fact that paraphrenics without sensory defects prove to be more abnormal in premorbid personality as assessed by reliable measures than those in whom there is concomitant deafness, confirms the contribution to aetiology made by sensory defect (Kay et al., 1976). In a minority of patients evidence suggesting circumscribed nonprogressive cerebral disease has been found (Kay & Roth, 1961; Post, 1966). In Blessed's recent investigations, only 3 of 28 patients developed dementia; 2 from Alzheimer's disease, and 1 as the result of a succession of strokes. However, at postmortem examination, plaque and tangle counts were rarely found to be at above threshold levels in paraphrenic cases (Roth, 1971).

The finding of sensory deficit has adduced a piece of new knowledge about the etiology of late onset schizophrenia, the significance of which for the early life forms of the disease is presently unclear. The limited overlap with cerebral disease represents the old age counterpart of the schizophreniform psychoses associated with cerebral diseases such as Huntington's chorea and general paralysis in their early stages, cerebral tumours in certain sites, and toxic agents such as amphetamine, alcohol, and chronic L.S.D. ingestion. These subjects have been extensively reviewed in the papers of Davison and his colleagues (Davison & Bagley, 1969; Davison, 1976).

The contribution of cerebral disease and drug intoxication to the paraphrenias is therefore limited. Even if the dopaminergic or some other neurochemical hypothesis is substantiated in schizophrenia, it will have been shown to be a cerebral disease in a quite different sense from syndromes such as dementia or delirium. Such advances are not within sight and for the present, paraphrenias have to be set apart from the organic syndromes of late life. This view of its nosological status is confirmed by the normal life expectation of those who suffer from this disease in contrast with the marked abridgement found to obtain among those with organic mental disorder proper. The partition advanced here applies a fortiori to schizophrenia in early life and the evidence calls into question the recommendations in some recent classifications which seek to eliminate the "functional-organic" concept.

Alzheimer's Disease

There have been some noteworthy changes of opinion regarding the unity or heterogeneity of this disorder since it was first described by Alzheimer (1907). He considered that the pathological changes that he described were confined to the presenile dementias, and believed that plaques, tangles, and granulovacuolar change were absent from the primary forms of mental deterioration of the aged as well as from the brains of well-preserved old people. When later investigators established that the changes described by

Alzheimer were to be found to some extent in the brains of well-preserved aged people (Gruntahl, 1927; Gellerstedt, 1933), these changes were for a time regarded as unimportant epiphenomena. It was not until a quantitative relationship was shown to obtain between the intensity of plaque formation on the one hand, and clinical diagnosis and dementia scores registered during life on the other, that the finding of Alzheimer changes in well preserved elderly people was reconciled with their presence in patients with Alzheimer's disease of early and late onset (Roth et al., 1967; Blessed et al. 1968; Tomlinson et al., 1970; Roth, 1971).

Finally, in quite recent years, diversity and heterogeneity have been demonstrated within this unitary concept. A large body of evidence testifies to the more extensive and severe nature of the morphologic and neurochemical lesions in Alzheimer's disease of early life than in Alzheimer's disease of later life (Rossor et al., 1984; Roth et al., 1985). In the light of recent inquiries, the early and late groups are separated also, by some clinical features. Selzer and Sherwin (1983) found a higher prevalence of language deficits, more common gait disturbances, and selective vulnerability of the left hemisphere. A study by Evans et al. (1985) has confirmed the difference with respect to gait and also found echolalia and differential performance on cognitive tests and scales for dementia. There is both a continuity and discontinuity between the early life and late life forms of Alzheimer's disease. Account has to be taken of both of these findings with regard to classification when inquiries are being made into aetiology or new methods of treatment.

Multiinfarct Dementia

The differential diagnosis between multiinfarct and primary forms of dementia, as well as clouded and confusional states is important in everyday clinical practice as well as scientific inquiry. This section will be largely devoted to the differentiation between primary and multiinfarct dementia.

From the point of view of clinical management it is germane that a substantial proportion of multiinfarct cases are hypertensive. Early treatment of hypertension can be expected to make some impression on the prevalence of this form of dementia. The decline in the prevalence of morbidity and mortality from strokes in the United States, among other affluent countries, in the past two to three decades may well have been due to the prophylactic measures in relation to cardiovascular disease widely recommended in these societies and followed by some sections of the population (National Center for Health Statistics, 1975). A further point is that in a substantial proportion of multiinfarct dements the syndrome arises from multiple emboli that emanate from atheromatous plaques in cerebral or extracerebral artery. In these cases also prophylactic treatment will on occasion be indicated, although the case for intervention has to be weighed with care.

As far as diagnostic criteria are concerned, those recommended for differentiating between senile and multiinfarct dementia in the past (Roth, 1955; Slater & Roth, 1969) have received a measure of validation from postmortem findings (Corsellis, 1962; Tomlinson, et al. 1968, 1970). Problems in discrimination are presented by the "mixed cases" combining Alzheimer change with cerebral infarct. They have been estimated by different authors as constituting between 15–25% of the total number of dementias presenting in clinical practice. There are no generally accepted criteria for identifying mixed cases, either in clinical practice or on neuropathological examination. One common pattern is the commencement of dementia in the absence of evidence of cerebral infarct. A continually progressive course will then be complicated by infarction or a solitary episode of cerebral ischemia, which leaves behind physical signs and is followed by a stepwise change in the rate of progression of intellectual and personality deterioration. Such cases may have begun with the features of Alzheimer's disease complicated and accelerated in progression after some years by cerebral infarction. At postmortem they prove to be "mixed" cases (predominantly Alzheimer in pathology when there have been only 1 or 2 transient ischemic episodes) and not examples of pure multiinfarct dementia (a diagnosis which is often made).

Hachinski et al. (1975) have adapted established criteria into a scale that makes it possible to compute an "ischemic" score that assists discrimination between multiinfarct and Alzheimer cases.

Loeb (1980) applied the 13 features of the scale to 49 demented subjects with a mean age of 64.7±2.5 years. Twenty of the cases were judged on clinical grounds to suffer from definite multiinfarct dementia. Loeb concluded that the scale enabled him to identify about 50% of the ischemic cases. But the independent diagnostic criteria that had been used in clinical diagnosis were not specified. There were indications that the success rate achieved with the scale would have been higher had a discriminant function or analytic technique been used to assign differential quantitative weights to the various clinical features. For example, abrupt onset, fluctuating course, history of a stroke, focal symptoms, and focal signs were all entirely confined to the multiinfarct cases and absent from all patients with senile dementia. Further highly significant differences were observed with respect to the presence of depression, and emotional lability. Some of these features probably have earned higher ratings than the narrow one–two range of scores allowed in the Hachinski scores.

In atypical cases features such as epileptic fits, the presence of mild Parkinsonism, and subtle degrees of emotional lability provide the hint that the underlying process arises from multiple infarcts.

Concomitant depression, at times accompanied by psychotic features, is more common in multiinfarct than in senile or presenile dementia. This kind of overlap (and there is a more limited one with respect to paranoid features) has also been construed as invalidating the "functional-organic" distinction. However, the affective disorder is distinctive in its fragmented features with depressive ideation or delusions that may be in sharp contrast to the sustained background of wooden unchanging affect. The blend of clouded consciousness and depression sometimes culminates in serious and violent attempts at self-destruction.

However, the diagnosis is rarely in doubt because cognitive and other manifestations of multiinfarct dementia are present and thus have to be given priority in diagnosis. Here again the etiological association between the two components is loose; the depression will often respond to antidepressant treatment while the dementia proceeds on its course. At a later stage depressive and other forms of emotional disturbance are submerged by the affective impoverishment that results from the dementing process.

The hypothesis that multiinfarct (and other) dementias, on the one hand, and "functional" disorders such as affective and paranoid psychoses and neurotic states, on the other, requires modification to take account of these new facts, although the character of the overlap is such that a clear allocation to dementia with depression or functional disorder can still be made in the great majority of patients. The new findings merely enlarge the picture of this form of dementia and also create fresh opportunities for treatment. Further, a fresh scientific question is posed. What factors in terms of heredity or cerebral lesion of the underlying disorder differentiate those patients who develop a conspicuous and lasting depression or paranoid coloring to their multiinfarct dementia from the 70–75% of patients who do not manifest such a coloring? The general point that arises here in relation to the functional-organic dichotomy is taken up again at a later stage.

IMPLICATIONS OF DSM III AND RELATED SYSTEMS OF CLASSIFICATION AND DIAGNOSIS FOR PROBLEMS OF GERIATRIC PSYCHIATRY

The advances in knowledge regarding the character and origins of the mental disorders of the aged have posed certain conundrums for the classification of mental illness. Some of these arise in relation to geriatric psychiatry alone. Others are of more general significance for taxonomic problems in psychiatry. Somatic disease has been shown to contribute to the causation of affective disorders, particularly in aged and middle aged men. In the schizophrenias of late life, cerebral disease and perceptual defects have been shown to be responsible for at least a small part of causation. Would these conditions not be more appropriately described as "organic" or "symptomatic" psychoses, rather than "functional" disorders?

To make these changes in terminology would be to perpetuate the errors of the past. The use of terms such as "alcoholic hallucinosis" probably helped to obscure the close similarity of some of the psychoses associated with chronic alcoholism to schizophrenia. This has emerged with particular clarity from Cutting's study of 114 patients with alcoholic psychosis (Cutting, 1978), in which 40% were given a "Catego" diagnosis (a computerized diagnostic system associated with the Present State Examination of Wing et al.) of schizophrenia, and a further 18% of paranoid or "possible" paranoid psychosis. The hallucinatory experience often had Schneiderian features. The term "senile paranoid psychosis" falsely imputes an organic aetiology to the schizophrenias of late life. Even terms such as "arteriosclerotic psychosis" have been misconceived. Evidence of peripheral or retinal atheroma was until 25 years ago erroneously presumed to be correlated with cerebrovascular disease and the explanation of associated psychiatric disorder of many kinds. Such findings are now known to be irrelevant. Cerebral infarction is the only lesion that matters and it has to be sufficiently extensive to give rise to dementia.

One source of these ambiguities was identified some years ago in the following manner, "A major disadvantage of the many classifications that derive from the Kraepelinian system is that they reify incompletely worked out aetiologies in diagnostic terms principles of classification" (Roth, 1971). For obvious reasons alcoholism and senescent cerebral change cannot be the whole cause of alcoholic paranoid states and paraphrenia respectively. We deal here with that important minority of cases in which a psychiatric syndrome that satisfies the criteria for "functional" disorder is associated with concomitant cerebral or somatic disease. Such disease plays a limited part in causation. The strength of this contribution and the manner in which it interacts with genetical and personality factors remain to be defined by scientific investigation.

Such problems are familiar to those engaged in the treatment and investigation of mental diseases of late life when cerebral or somatic diseases of some degree are found to be highly prevalent. This was one type of dilemma in psychiatric diagnosis and classification that led Essen-Möller (1961) to suggest a new system of diagnostic procedure which entailed setting down both a descriptive and an etiological diagnosis and later a statement about personality setting in every case. This multiaxial system is a prominent feature of a number of recently introduced systems of diagnosis.

The most widely known and influential of these is the third version of the Diagnostic and Statistical Manual of Mental Disorders adopted by the American Psychiatric Association or "DSM III." The bearing of this new scheme upon the problems of psychogeriatric diagnosis and taxonomy will now be considered.

The Multiaxial System

The multiaxial system is a central feature of DSM III and will therefore be considered first. Under Axis I all forms of mental disorder, with the exception of personality disorder in adults, and specific developmental disorder in children are included. Personality and developmental disorders are recorded in Axis II. Axis III provides for denotation associated physical disorders, whether judged to contribute to causation or thought relevant for other reasons. Under Axis IV, psychosocial stress factors judged to have contributed to the genesis of current illness can be recorded on a 7-point scale. Axis V was intended for to record the highest level of adaptive functioning achieved during the preceding year. Although Axes IV and V are intended for research and special purposes they are already being employed in the course of comprehensive clinical assessment in ordinary practice. However, only the first three axes are intended to constitute the "official diagnostic assessment."

DSM-III invites comments under two main headings. The first relates to the character and the utilization of information to be recorded under the individual axes, the second to the problems posed by the concept of multiaxial classification.

Individual Axes

The additional information that will be yielded through use of the axes will fulfill one of the objectives which Essen-Möller envisaged when he first made the case for a diagnostic system which entailed the recording of information regarding descriptive and etiologic diagnosis, as well as other relevant clinical items under separate headings. The concept of a multiaxial system essentially as a starting point for clinical research in psychiatry, was also outlined by other workers (Slater & Roth, 1969; Roth, 1971).

Problems of definition, however, are posed by each of the subsidiary axes. In relation to mental disorders of late life, chronic physical disability and disease are so common that there is bound to be a certain amount of fortuitous association between psychiatric and physical disorder. No rules are set down to enable clinician or investigator to assess the relevance or importance to be attached to concomitant cerebral or somatic disease as a possible or definite factor in causation. A robust, vigorous 69-year-old man may have received a diagnosis of hypertension made six months previously with equanimity and have taken the prescribed medication with care and consistency. His blood pressure may now be within normal limits, but it may be the emotional implications of the diagnosis for a successful, dynamic body proud man suffering his first serious disability, rather than the physical effects that help to generate the depression which develops 14 months later. There would be wide variation among psychiatrists regarding the role to be ascribed to physical disease in such a case. Is an attack of pneumonia successfully treated a fortnight ago, or diverticulitis causing intermittent discomfort diagnosed 2 years ago to be recorded? Unless there is further specification there will be wide variation in the relevance and aetiologic significance of types of physical disorder done in Axis III.

The problem of specification is even more important in relation to Axis II. The personality dimension is important in the commonest forms of depression as it is in other emotional disorders observed in the community. Those with neurotic affective disorder presenting in late life have proved in a high proportion of cases to have had difficulties in personal relationships during their entire lives (Kay et al., 1964a, b; Garside et al., 1965; Lowenthal, 1964).

Although they complain, often with bitterness, of loneliness investigations have shown such "lonely" individuals not to be socially isolated. In contrast, those isolated have chosen this mode of existence as the life style that gives them greatest satisfaction. Such personality data are relevant for purposes of clinical managements and scientific investigation. However, the problem of developing reliable and valid measures of such personality traits and profiles awaits solution. Unless the manner in which such information is elicited and the interpretations made standardized, measures are unlikely to prove of value.

Axis IV has its own difficulties as life events research has shown in recent years. Whether it is used for research or in clinical practice, more guidance will be necessary regarding criteria for evaluating potentially relevant information. Moreover, it cannot be assumed that data on Axes II and IV are independent. Those who suffer from lifelong personality disorder may be the passive victims of sudden bereavement or loss. But they are also liable to generate stressful circumstances in their lives as a result of the manner in which they interact with others. Axis V is vague in meaning unless a more clear definition can be given of the spheres of existence in which adaptation requires assessment. A 74-year-old distinguished composer of music was highly successful and admired by a large public for her artistic achievements, but her personal relationships were in a chaotic state. She was happy, fulfilled in mind, full of creative enthusiasm in her artistic life, but in her family circle there was constant strife and tension which engulfed her at times.

The multiaxial system of DSM III and other classifications such as ICD 10 in which a set of subsidiary axes are to be included, can make a valuable contribution to clinical practice, for they encourage psychiatrists to attend consistently to a wider range of physical psychosocial and personality variables than can be subsumed within a descriptive diagnosis. This enrichment of the body of systematically recorded information is indispensable for improvement of standards in treatment and rehabilitation. The practice of exploring these areas has yet to be assimilated into psychogeriatric and general psychiatric practice. However, the multiaxial system will not advance knowledge unless the associations between the main diagnosis and the variables recorded under other axes can be investigated in a rigorous manner. In their present form the data that will be assembled in relation to the Axes in the course of ordinary practice are unlikely to prove of value for scientific purposes.

As far as ICD 10 is concerned, preliminary notice has been given that in its final form it will incorporate a multiaxial system essentially similar to DSM-III.

The Concept of Multiaxial "Classification"

There is an implicit assumption in some of the literature describing features of DSM-III that the addition of subsidiary axes and the expanded body of information that will be provided alongside the diagnosis of the main psychiatric disorder will pave the way for more clear replicable and useful classifications of psychiatric disorder than older systems such as ICD 9 (Spitzer et al., Appendix II, pp. 93–95). The term "multiaxial classification" has been used in connection with the multiaxial system devised for diagnostic purposes in the field of child psychiatry (Rutter et al., 1968).

There can be little doubt that the additional information recorded under the Axes will encourage more comprehensive clinical assessment. However, multiaxial classification is unlikely to improve on the system of rubrics to be found at the present time within ICD 9 or comparable classifications.

To take first the example of mental disorder in old age, it is hoped that when information regarding physical illness, personality, and life events is added to clinical diagnoses such as "affective disorder," "acute confusion" or "delirium" and "senile dementia," these disorders will be more sharply delineated and separated from each other than they can be with the aid of the criteria employed to arrive at the main diagnosis. Such facts as are available suggest that the outcome of any attempt to build a classification on such a basis will be the direct opposite of what is anticipated. For there is likely to be considerable overlap between the syndromes on Axes I and II and the data on each of the subsidiary axes, and consequently greater blurring of the lines of demarcation between them. If so the disorders recorded under Axis I, DSM-III will become more confluent rather than more distinct.

Among the aged suffering from mental disorder, for example, physical disease or disability is found to be of relatively high prevalence in all groups and stressful circumstances of different kinds are ubiquitous. Depressive illness, Alzheimer's disease, and paranoid states would not likely be clearly differentiated from each other in terms of concomitant somatic disease. The data recorded on the subsidiary axes will probably prove valuable for the purpose of drawing upon all available methods of treatment and social support that might ameliorate or cure the presenting disorder, and should also be helpful in the mitigation of current personal and social difficulties.

The term "multiaxial diagnosis" is therefore of dubious validity. Diagnosis should be decided on the basis of clear and reliable operational criteria that command a wide consensus. It would not be possible to incorporate such criteria from the subsidiary axes for the purpose of formulating a revised diagnosis of Alzheimer's disease that had an acceptable measure of clarity or validity. It would be equally difficult to succeed in this task in the case of affective disorder or even in relation to an indubitably clouded or delirous state where over 90% of the patients can be expected to have a concomitant and specific physical disease. For it would defeat the central purpose of arriving at a psychiatric diagnosis if one were not permitted to make a diagnosis of confusion or delirium until a physical disease had been identified.

It follows, therefore, that multiple axes may prove useful adjuncts for the delineation of a global picture and/or the possibility of a rich and informative *clinical formulation* in everyday practice. No classification of psychiatric disorders could be developed from such axes for purposes of record keeping, national or international morbidity statistics, or operational definition for scientific inquiry. With more stringently defined criteria for the axes, valuable scientific investigations could be undertaken into the strength of the relationship of each subsidiary axis to the main descriptive syndromes of psychiatry. The correlations that obtain between the different axes and the clinical disorders within the "core classification" of ICD 10 and related systems would also prove of considerable interest, as would a comparison of the results obtained in inquiries into different systems of classification.

COMMENT ON SPECIFIC CATEGORIES AND OPERATIONAL DEFINITIONS IN DSM III

Operational criteria for a number of specific categories within DSM III require critical scrutiny from the point of view of mental disorders of the aged.

SCHIZOPHRENIA

The criterion that signs of illness be continuous for at least 6 months during an individual's life to qualify for a diagnosis of schizophrenia has already been submitted to a great deal of criticism. The criterion has only limited relevance for schizophrenias of late life which pursue a chronic course in large part and rarely present in the form of acute, transient disorder. However, occasional acute cases of brief duration are seen. To separate those in whom schizophrenic features have been manifest for less than 6 months into a separate class of "schizophreniform disorder" assumes what is in need of proof. Some cases of severe and chronic schizophrenic illness are first manifest as an acute psychotic episode which remits only to recur in the form of a more enduring illness refractory to treatment. Moreover, termination of the psychosis in a period of less than 6 months is commonly achieved today through the administration of neuroleptic drugs. Termination may occur even in seemingly malignant forms of hebephrenic or paranoid illness in a proportion of cases. To class these cases under a rubric such as "schizophreniform disorder," which continues to carry connotations of a benign illness, may encourage premature or false optimism and inadequate management.

A more important defect from the point of view of geriatric psychiatry is the exclusion criterion which prohibits the diagnosis of schizophrenia in those over the age of 45 years. This is an arbitrary demarcation line and fails to take account of the advances achieved in diagnosis and aetiologic basis of the paranoid-hallucinatory psychoses of late life, shown in the last few decades to meet the criteria for the diagnosis of schizophrenia in DSM III and related systems. (Kay & Roth, 1961; Roth, 1985). As already indicated in an earlier section, these disorders have been shown to be genetically and in other respects homologous to schizophrenia (Kay, 1963).

The division into separate categories of schizophrenias in different parts of the life-span makes the attempt to extract lessons from a comparison between manifestations of one and the same disorder at different stages of the life-span inadmissible. At the present time there is no theory available to explain the ability of some individuals shown to be predisposed to schizophrenia by genetic and a range of other criteria, to postpone breakdown until the last phase of life. But certain lines of enquiry can be developed in an attempt to answer the questions posed. If postponement of the manifestation of schizophrenia could be achieved for the majority of those predisposed, mental hospitals could be emptied in all parts of the world of about 40 to 50% of their beds.

THE ORGANIC GROUP OF DISORDERS

The account of the main syndromes and the operational criteria for the diagnoses of the main groups of disorders are clear and authoritative. The comments will be confined here to the rubrics.

Organic Mental Disorder

A number of the new categories included in DSM III under this heading have important implications for clinical diagnosis, and scientific work in each category merits critical scrutiny.

Until 35 to 40 years ago, diagnoses such as "organic delusional state," "senile paranoid psychosis," and "senile depressive psychosis" were commonplace as reflected in the quotation from Bleuler in an earlier section. The causation of such conditions was regarded as stemming from progressive, primary cerebral degeneration or cerebral arteriosclerosis. Such disorders were expected to pursue a course marked by progressive deterioration. These predictions were fulfilled in a proportion of cases for a number of reasons. As pointed out by Post (1971), a proportion of patients with depressive illness commencing in late life are liable to frequent relapse or to a chronic course. This derives in part from the high prevalence of concomitant physical disease. It is a chronic rather than an acute somatic disease that is specially associated with the depressions of late life (Roth & Kay, 1956). To some extent this outcome was the result of a self-fulfilling prophecy because many such patients suffered the effects of long-term institutional care in chronic wards as well as inadequate medical care. As the histograms in Figure 6.1 indicate, inpatient status was the commonest fate of patients with paraphrenia at 2 years, and even 7 to 8 years, after admission. Those with depressive psychoses fared better since electroconvulsive treatment was introduced for some depressive illnesses diagnosed in patients of advanced age in the 1940s (Mayer-Gross, 1945).

The observations relating to the natural history of mental disorders of the aged published in the 1950s reflected a vigorous and positive approach toward the treatment and resocialization of patients with depressive and related affective disorders, paranoid psychotic states, and severe neuroses. Large numbers of patients were relieved of mental suffering and enabled to return home and to the community. These successes were achieved despite the presence of concomitant somatic disease often of a chronic character in a substantial minority of cases.

If implemented in clinical practice, the proposals in DSM III and similar classifications are likely to set the clock back. Under the heading of Organic Mental Disorders the rubrics "organic delusional syndrome," "organic hallucinosis," "organic affective syndrome," and "organic personality syndrome" are to be found. In each case, the diagnostic criteria stipulate that there must be neither clouding of consciousness nor a significant loss of intellectual abilities as in delirium and dementia. Another criterion states that there has to be evidence, "of a specific organic factor that is judged to be etiologically related to the disturbance." But instructions are nebulous as to how the etiologic relevance of concomitant physical somatic disease is to be determined.

All these conditions differ in fundamental ways from "organic mental disorder" in the strict sense of the term. In "dementia" as well as "confusional states and deliria," a cerebral lesion or some somatic disease is invariably present. Somatic diseases are therefore necessary causes of associated psychiatric syndromes. Further, where such diseases can be eradicated as in a proportion of confusional states those who are psychiatrically disordered can be restored to their erstwhile state of mental well-being. This is not true of the delusional, depressive, and personality syndromes listed in this section of DSM III. For example, under "organic delusional syndrome," reference is made to "schizophrenia or paranoid disorders" among the conditions from which differential diagnosis has to be established. It is difficult to see how this can be accomplished because they do not differ in their phenomenological counterparts from syndromes to be found in DSM-III, if under rubrics such as "affective disorders," "schizophrenic disorders," and "paranoid disorders." It is plain, also, that the associated organic disease can be neither the necessary nor a sufficient cause of associated psychiatric disorder. The great majority of those in depressive and paranoid states do not suffer from associated or relevant somatic disease. It is a delirious, amnestic, or demented state that usually complicates cerebral and somatic disease, although functional syndromes of complex etiology are formed in a minority. If there is evidence drawn from scientific inquiry to contravert such views, it has nowhere been presented.

A further reason that invalidates the grouping of purely affective or paranoid syndromes with organic disorders is the fact that the former have a different course and outcome. The manner of their response to treatment is also far removed from the other organic syndromes with which they have been grouped in DSM-III. Organic depressive, manic, and paranoid states will often respond to antidepressant drugs, Lithium, and neuroleptics, respectively, even where there is concomitant physical disability or disease.

A further argument against the incorporation of these new conditions under the heading "Organic Mental Disorder" is that doubt is cast upon the purpose and relevance of the multiaxial system. The association of typical, depressive or paranoid syndromes with physical disorder can be most logically and empirically handled by listing the psychiatric syndrome under Axis I, and concomitant somatic disease under Axis III. The strength of the correlation between the two phenomena could then be subjected to empirical investigation.

Hence, the whole area of "organic" syndromes without organic phenomenology should be thrown open to scientific inquiry. This would be preferable to the closure likely to result if controversial and conjectural theories are given premature authority.

THE RELATIONSHIP BETWEEN CLINICAL DIAGNOSIS AND REFERENCE DIAGNOSES IN SCIENTIFIC INQUIRY AND CLINICAL PRACTICE

A great deal of effort has been devoted during the last thirty years to the development of operational criteria for arriving at psychiatric diagnoses that have an acceptable level of reliability. The Feighner criteria (Feighner et al., 1972), the Research Diagnostic Criteria (Spitzer et al., 1978), and DSM III, respectively were all fruits of this endeavor. The development of standardized methods of examining the present mental state such as the PSE (Wing et al., 1984), represents another result of the quest to achieve more stringent standards and replicable results in clinical examination for purposes of scientific inquiry. Wing's "Catego" diagnostic system codifies the main concepts of the classifications that derive from Kraepelin and the ninth version of The International Classification of Diseases. With the aid of advances in statistical methodology such as the statistic "kappa" for quantifying agreement in psychiatric diagnosis reached by a group of observers (Fleiss et al., 1972), it has been demonstrated that diagnoses made with the aid of strict operational criteria show a high measure of interobserver reliability. This holds for the diagnostic criteria formulated in DSM III as demonstrated in the course of extensive field trials.

In relation to treatment, it is now accepted that randomized controlled clinical trials are the only means to arrive at a verdict regarding the efficacy of new treatments. This agreement is reflected in the editorial policy of leading psychiatric journals which confine publications in the field of treatment to studies that have used clearly defined criteria in the selection of patients, and double-blind controlled techniques in the evaluation of therapy.

There are, however, important limitations to the diagnostic procedures that have been described in this section. Diagnoses arrived at with the aid of rigid operational criteria are, for the large part, cross-sectional; the main diagnosis is made on a basis of features elicited from examination of the patient's presenting mental state. The addition of Axes has helped to incorporate data regarding personality, adjustment, and possibly relevant psychosocial factors. But the range of information recorded and the manner in which decisions are made to reach a diagnosis differs in important respects from the assembly of data and the manner in which inferences are drawn in the course of clinical evaluation and diagnosis. The question arises as to whether reference diagnoses, such as those made with the aid of DSM III or the PSE examination aided by the "Catego" program, have replaced and rendered obsolete the more subjective, but flexible, procedures followed in clinical practice.

It is doubtful whether the claim often made in recent years in the form of a positive answer given to this question, can be justified. Only a limited part of the interview and examination employed in clinical practice has been standardized in interview and diagnostic techniques such as those set down in DSM-III. The findings elicited during ordinary clinical examination are interpreted and often reinterpreted in the light of a wide range of observations relating to developmental history, adaptation in social and familial settings, the pattern of interpersonal relationships, and recent personal vicissitudes that have been suffered (or are conspicuous in their absence). A tentative diagnosis made in the course of examination may need revision or total reformulation in light of observations conducted over a period of time in a psychiatric ward or information obtained from relatives and a succession of further interviews. Clinical diagnosis entails a comparison of patterns of conduct manifest since the onset of symptoms, the ability to conduct an independent life, and other features of adjustment and interpersonal relationships, with the manner in which the patient acquitted himself in his premorbid state in all these circumstances.

In relation to geriatric psychiatry, the diagnosis of dementia made in the course of interview even when aided by psychometric investigation may have to be rejected in light of an observation of the patient's behavior and the intellectual assets, skills, and capacities for problem solving as manifest over a period in a psychiatric ward during which relevant data are systematically recorded. Conversely, an interview that suggests no organic deficit may need revision in the light of reports from a relative who observes the patient's failure to find his way in familiar surroundings, the deterioration of personal habits, the parody of his premorbid traits or the total chaos into which his affairs and home environment have degenerated.

Despite the evidence that the use of DSM III has improved reliability of psychiatric diagnosis even in clinical practice, the advantages of open and flexible clinical examination and diagnosis should not be jettisoned.

Diagnoses made with the aid of standardized examination techniques and strict operational definitions will prove a valuable aid in the course of arriving at a categorical diagnosis and formulation, but should not be allowed to supplant it.

DSM III evolved from a set of operational definitions derived from the published clinical literature for the purpose of achieving reliability and replicability in the course of scientific research in psychiatry. The Feighner definitions (Feighner et al., 1972) and the Research Diagnostic Criteria from which DSM III has evolved were both intended for this purpose. The new methods of diagnosis and classification have an important part to play in the course of multicenter investigations into specific problems in the course of clinical trials, and for the purpose of comparing systems of classification in different countries and cultural settings. But even in such exercises, it would be a mistake to regard the diagnostic verdict reached after comprehensive clinical evaluation of the traditional open kind as redundant. The findings and results obtained with the aid of the two different methods should be compared and contrasted with each other. This would be to the mutual benefit of each and would be bound to enrich the total body of information available for scientific investigation. And ample room remains for more comparisons of the results achieved by the two techniques in clinical practice so that they can be refined by an incorporation of the best features of each into one technique. The mental disorders of the aged are in particular need of such endeavors.

REFERENCES

Alzheimer, A. (1907). On a peculiar disease of the cerebral cortex. *Allg. Z. Psychiat., 64,* 177–179.

Blessed, G., Tomlinson, B. E., & Roth, M. (1968). The association between quantitative measures of dementia and senile changes in the cerebral grey matter of elderly subjects. *Br. J. Psychiatry, 114,* 797–811.

Blessed, G., & Wilson, I. D. (1982). The contemporary natural history of mental disorder in old age. *Br. J. Psychiatry, 141,* 59–67.

Bleuler, E. (1916). *Lehrbuch der Psychiatrie.* Berlin: Springer.

Christie, A. B. (1982). Changing patterns in mental illness in the elderly. *Br. J. Psychiatry, 140,* 154–159.

Cooper, A. (1974). Hearing loss in paranoid and affective psychoses of the elderly. *Lancet, II,* 851–854.

Corsellis, J. A. N. (1962). *Mental illness and the aging brain.* Maudsley Monographs Number Nine. London: Oxford University Press.

Davison, K. (1976). Drug induced psychoses and their relationship to schizophrenia. In D. Kemali, G. Bartolini, & D. Richter (Eds.), *Schizophrenia today* (pp. 105–133). Oxford, New York: Pergamon Press.

Davison, K., & Bagley, C. R. (1969). Schizophrenia-like psychoses associated with organic disorders of the CNS: A Review of the Literature. In Herrington, *Current problems in neuropsychiatry. Br. J. Psychiatry, Special Pub.* No. 4, 113–184.

Essen-Möller, E. (1961). On classification of mental disorders. *Acta Psychiat. Scand., 37,* 119–126.

Evans, N. J. R., Roth, M., & Mountjoy, C. Q. (in preparation). Similarities and differences in clinical findings between pre-Senile and senile dementias.

Feighner, J. P., Robins, E., Guze, S. B., et al. (1972). Diagnostic criteria for use in psychiatric research. *Arch. Gen. Psychiatry, 26,* 57–63.

Fleiss J. L., Spitzer R. L., Endicott J., et al. (1972). Quantification of agreement in multiple psychiatric diagnosis. *Arch. Gen. Psych., 26,* 168–171

Garside, R. F., Kay, D. W. K., & Roth, M. (1965). Old age mental disorders in Newcastle upon Tyne. Part III. A factorial study of medical, psychiatric and social characteristics. *Br. J. Psychiatry,* 939–943.

Gellerstedt, N. (1933). Zur Keutins der Hirnveranderung bei der Normalen Altersunvolution. *Uppsala Lakareforenings Forhandlingar, 38,* 193.

Grünthal, E. (1927). Klinisch-Anatomisch Vergleichende Untersuchungen uber den Greisenblodsinn. *Zeitschrift fur die Gesamte Neurologie und Psychiatrie* (Berlin), *111,* 763–818.

Hachinski V. C., Iliff L. D., Du Boulay G. H., McAllister V. L., Marshall J., Ross Russell, R. W., & Symon, L. (1975). Cerebral blood flow in dementia. *Arch. Neurol., 32,* 632–637

Hagnell, O., Lanke, J., Rorsman, B., & Ojesjo, L. (1981). Does the incidence of age psychosis decrease? A prospective longitudinal study of a complete population investigated during the 25-year period 1947–1972: The Lundy Study. *Neuropsychobiology, 7,* 201–11.

Hagnell, O., Lanke, J., Rorsman, B., Ohman, T., & Ojesjo, L. (1983). Current trends in the incidence of senile and multi-infarct dementia. *Arch. Psych. and Neurol. Sci.,* 423–438.

Hemsi, L. K., Whitehead, A., & Post, F. (1968). Cognitive functioning and cerebral arousal in elderly depressives and dements. *J. Psychosom. Res., 12,* 145–156.

Hopkins, B., & Roth, M. (1953). Psychological test performance in patients over sixty. II. Paraphrenia, arteriosclerotic psychosis and acute confusion. *J. Ment. Sci., 99,* 451–463.

Kay, D. W. K., & Roth, M. (1955). Physical accompaniments of mental disorder in old age. *Lancet, ii,* 740–745.

Kay, D. W. K., & Roth, M. (1961). Physical illness and social factors in the psychiatric disorders of old age. *Proceedings of the Third World Congress of Psychiatry,* (pp. 303–308). Montreal.

Kay, D. W. K. (1962). Outcome and cause of death in mental disorders of old age: A long-term follow up of functional and organic psychoses. *Acta Psych. Scand., 38,* 249–276.

Kay, D. W. K. (1963). Late paraphrenia and its bearing on the aetiology of schizophrenia. *Acta Psychiat. Scand., 39,* 159–169.

Kay, D. W. K., & Bergmann, K. (1966). *J. Psychosom. Res., 10,* 3–12.

Kay D. W. K., Cooper A. F., Garside R. F., & Roth M. (1976). The differentiation of paranoid from affective psychoses by patients' premorbid characteristics. *Br. J. Psych., 129,* 207–215.

Kerr, T. A., Schapira, K., & Roth, M. (1969). The relationship between premature death and affective disorders. *Br. J. Psychiatry, 115,* 1277–1282.

Kiloh, L. G. (1961). Pseudo-dementia. *Acta Psychiat. Scand., 37,* 336–351.

Loeb, C. (1980). Clinical diagnosis of multi-infarct dementia. In L. Amaducci, A. N., Davison, P. Antuono (Eds.), *Aging of the Brain and Dementia* (pp. 251–260). New York: Raven Press.

Lowenthal, M. F. (1964). *Lives in distress.* New York: Basic Books.

Mayer-Gross, W. (1945). Electric convulsive treatment in patients over sixty. *J. Ment. Sci., 91,* 101–105.

National Center for Health Statistics (1975). *United States life tables by cause of death: 1969–71.* Vol. 1, No. 5 (DHEW Pub. No. HRA), 75–1150.

Post, F. (1965). *The clinical psychiatry of late life.* Oxford: Pergamon Press.

Post, F. (1966). *Persistent persecutory states of the elderly.* London: Pergamon Press.

Post, F. (1975). Dementia, depression and pseudo-dementia. In D. F. Benson & D. Blumer (Eds.), *Psychiatric aspects of neurologic disease.* New York: Grune & Stratton.

Post, F. (1978). The functional psychoses. In *Studies in geriatric psychiatry.* Chichester: John Wiley & Sons.

Rossor, M. N., Iversen, L. L., Reynolds, G. P., Mountjoy, C. Q., & Roth, M. (1984). Neurochemical characteristics of early and late onset types of alzheimer's disease, *Br. Med. J., 288,* 361–364.

Roth, M. (1955). The natural history of mental disorder in old age. *J. Ment. Sci., 101,* 281–301.

Roth, M., & Hopkins, B. (1953). Psychological test performance in patients over 60. I. Senile psychosis, and the affective disorders of old age. *J. Ment. Sci., 99,* 439–450.

Roth, M., & Kay, D. W. K. (1956). Affective disorders arising in the senium. II. Physical disability as an aetiological factor. *J. Ment. Sci., 102,* 141–150.

Roth, M., & Kay, D. W. K. (1962). Psychoses among the aged. In H. T. Blumenthal (Ed.), *Medical and clinical aspects of aging* (pp. 74–96). Aging Around the World, Proceedings of the Fifth Congress of the International Association of Gerontology. New York: Columbia University Press.

Roth, M., Tomlinson, B. E., & Blessed, G. (1967). The relationship between quantitative measures of dementia and of degenerative changes in the cerebral grey matter of elderly subjects. *Proc. R. Soc. Med., 60,* 254–260.

Roth, M. (1971). Classification and aetiology in mental disorders of old age: Some recent developments. In D. W. K. Kay & A. Walk (Eds.), *Recent developments in psychogeriatrics. Br. J. Psychiatry,* Special Pub. No. 6.

Roth, M. (1984). Senile dementia and related disorders. In J. Wertheimer, & M. Marois (Eds.), *Senile dementia: Outlook for the future.* (pp. 493–515).

Roth, M., Wischik, C. M., Evans, N., & Mountjoy, C. Q. (1985). Convergence and cohesion of recent neurobiological findings in relation to Alzheimer's Disease and their bearing on its aetiological basis. In *Thresholds in aging, The 1984 Sandoz Lectures in gerontology.* London: Academic Press.

Rothschild, D. (1956). Senile psychoses and psychoses with arteriosclerosis. In D. J. Kaplan (Ed.), *Mental disorders in late life.* Stanford, CA: Stanford University Press.

Rutter, M., Shaffer, D., & Shepherd, M. (1973). An evaluation of the proposal for a multi-axial classification of child psychiatric disorders. *Psychol. Med., 3,* 244–250.

Selzer, B., & Sherwin, I. (1983). A comparison of clinical features in early and late onset primary degenerative dementia. *Arch. Neurol. 40,* 143–146.

Slater, E., & Roth, M. (1969). *Clinical psychiatry* (3rd ed.). London: Bailliere Tindall.

Spitzer, R. L., Endicott, J., & Robins, E. (1978). Research diagnostic criteria: Rationale and reliability. *Arch. Gen. Psychiatry, 35,* 773–782.

Stenstedt, A. (1959). Involutional melancholia. *Acta Psychiat. Scand.* (Suppl. 127).

Tomlinson, B. E., Blessed, G. & Roth, M. (1968). Observations on the brains of non-demented old people. *J. Neurol. Sci., 7,* 331–356.

Tomlinson, B. E., Blessed, G. & Roth, M. (1970). Observations on the brains of non-demented old people. *J. Neurol. Sci., 11,* 205–242.

Tomlinson, B. E. (1977). The pathology of dementia. In C. E. Wells (Ed.), *Dementia* (2nd ed.). Contemporary Neurology Series. Philadelphia: F. A. Davis.

World Health Organization (WHO) (1977). ICD-9. Classification of mental disorders. *Manual of the international statistical classification of diseases, injuries, and causes of death.* Vol. 1. Geneva.

Wing, J. K., Cooper, J. E., & Sartorius, N. (1974). *The measurement and classification of psychiatric symptoms.* London: Cambridge University Press.

7
Multidimensional Assessment in Geriatric Psychiatry

M. Robin Eastwood and Sandra Corbin

The team approach has long been a part of medical practice. Traditionally, this took the form of the professor and his entourage, with a clear hierarchy of authority, sweeping magnificently around the hospital. There was no doubt who was in charge, who took responsibility, and who received the glory. As health care has increased in complexity, however, the team has changed and the approach has become more egalitarian. The problems presented in the assessment and treatment of geriatric psychiatry patients may be best solved by a team composed of members with diverse professional training, meeting frequently to plan investigations, discuss findings and formulate coherent and comprehensive treatment plans. Such a group must function with little overlap of tasks, few interdisciplinary jealousies, be problem oriented, and exercise communication skills in order to be effective and efficient. Although the physician typically chairs team meetings and takes medical and legal responsibility, each member of the team must make a definite contribution, either in direct patient care or with technical and backup services.

Since geriatric psychiatry units may be in a variety of settings, the assessment and treatment team varies with type of care and availability of staff. Bearing in mind that the majority of geriatric psychiatrists practice in a consultant capacity, the model described here is based on the service which can be provided in acute or chronic care hospitals with a discrete geriatric psychiatry unit. Such units may provide a range of services, from short term assessment and treatment to management of chronic patients.

The ideal setting for a geriatric psychiatry unit has been much discussed. Some health care workers stress the importance of maintaining the elderly in the community and avoiding hospitalization at all costs. Others argue that detailed observation and medical investigations cannot be properly conducted on an outpatient basis, and require at least short-term admission to a hospital. There are also geriatric psychiatry patients with chronic disorders who require continuous care, supervised by a physician with access to acute psychiatry services. To meet these various demands, the optimal geriatric psychiatry unit would be able to provide home visits and linkage with other medical and social services in the community, outpatient and day care services, some inpatient beds for short to intermediate stay admissions, and access to chronic care facilities for longer term placements. Most units will have some, but few will have all of these features. Whatever the level of sophistication, a geriatric psychiatry unit should be able to provide an holistic and eclectic approach to assessment of the patient. In addition to the psychiatrist, who acts as chief of service, it also may be advisable to have available the services of another staff psychiatrist, one or more residents in psychiatry, and the consulting services of specialists in internal medicine, cardiology, neurology, ophthalmology, and otolaryngology. In addition, other team members, nurses, social workers, occupational and physiotherapists, psychometrists, dieticians, audiologists, and pharmacists, play critical roles in the assessment and treatment of geriatric psychiatry patients. The following account of a multidisciplinary approach describes protocols which are desirable, but with the caveat that they may not be available in settings outside an active treatment facility.

PREADMISSION ASSESSMENT AND HOME VISITS

Despite differences of opinion regarding the optimal setting for assessment, there can be little doubt that observation of the patient in the home environment provides valuable information. Not only does the home visit facilitate functional assessment, and provide a basis for predicting the necessary level of function in that environment, but it also permits a determination, prior to admission, of the necessary level of care and support during the process of assessment. In some cases inappropriate referrals, or patients requiring immediate medical attention, may be identified in the preadmission home visit. Where home visits by the physician are not feasible, due to economic or time constraints, another representative of the team can gather information to be presented and reviewed by the team. The preadmission assessment should be standardized, ensuring adequate information is gathered in a uniform manner to facilitate review. Some areas for assessment prior to admission are summarized in Table 7.1.

TABLE 7.1 Preadmission Assessment

Nature of presenting problem
Source and reason for referral
Medical history—including past and present medical problems, medications, general practitioner contact information
Psychiatric history—including family history, previous illness, and current mental state
Behavioral and physical assessment—including observation of disabilities, family interaction, and environment
Interviewer's comments

Review of this information will enable the team to decide whether admission to the unit is required or whether referral elsewhere or placement recommendations would be more appropriate. If the patient is to be admitted, the type of admission (i.e., inpatient, day-care or outpatient), purpose of admission, and investigation strategy can be planned. Most admissions can be elective; however, some must bypass this procedure and be admitted directly, or on referral, due to a crisis situation.

ADMISSION

Cases should be admitted to a geriatric psychiatry unit for a definite purpose. In an active treatment setting, the purpose will usually be to investigate and diagnose or, more infrequently, to determine appropriate level of placement. Such units may be small, in the 10- to 15-bed range, and intended for short stays of a month or less. In a chronic care setting, cases may be more mixed, with some admitted for short stays from other units within the same setting for psychiatric investigation, and others admitted for longer courses of rehabilitation or management of behavior problems. In either the active treatment or chronic setting, a standard assessment protocol can be implemented on admission which will provide both diagnostic information and baseline measures. In addition to a careful mental state examination, preferably using a standardized interview schedule linked to a recognized diagnostic system e.g., the Present State Examination, PSE, Wing et al., 1974) or the Diagnostic Interview Schedule, DIS (Robins et al., 1981) a full medical history should be obtained and a physical examination conducted. Given the prevalence of sensory deficits in geriatric populations, and the implications these may have for psychosocial assessment, all cases should be referred for ophthalmological and otological consultation. Internists, neurologists, cardiologists, and other specialists should be available for consultation on request, although major health problems in these areas may result in transfer to another unit or setting. As an adjunct to the medical examination procedures, certain laboratory investigations are imperative to identify or rule out physical health problems. A suggested list of these procedures is presented in Table 7.2. Although not exhaustive, this list represents a survey of systems in which problems are commonly found in geriatric psychiatry patients and is practicable on units in both active and chronic settings.

In addition to the medical admission protocol, all cases admitted to the unit should be assessed by the members of the team involved in direct patient care. In the active treatment setting, these should include a member of the nursing team, the social worker, and the occupational therapist. In the chronic care setting, a physiotherapist may also be a member of the direct care team. Technical support, from individuals trained in the disciplines of psychology, pharmacy, audiology, and nutrition, may be available in either setting. Examples of admission protocols for each of these disciplines are described below.

Nursing

In many settings a primary model of nursing care has been implemented, allowing each patient to have one nurse who is responsible for the nursing care plan, and for the coordination of patient care. This model, which

TABLE 7.2 Medical Admission Protocol

Examination:	Full medical history. Physical examination by resident
	Examination by internist and neurologist optional
	Examination by ophthalmologist and ENT physician
Tests:	ECG
	Chest x-ray
	EEG
	Complete blood count (CBC) and differential, hematocrit and smear, platelet count
	Serum electrolytes: potassium, chloride, sodium
	Fasting blood sugar
	Thyroid indices: T4 T3 uptake. TSH
	Renal function tests: serum creatinine
	Liver function tests: SGOT and alkaline phosphates
	FT AB-BS
	Urinalysis
	Serum digoxin—inpatients suspected of taking digoxin during past month

appears to be particularly suitable for geriatric patients who may become easily confused or distressed, allows for greater continuity of care. Where nursing staff are responsible for preadmission assessments, it should be possible to arrange for the patient to have the same primary nurse from initial contact to discharge and follow-up.

Initial assessments by nursing staff following admission to a geriatric psychiatry unit should include questioning and observation of the patient and relatives to determine presence of immediate safety or security risks (e.g., suicide, aggression or elopement) and necessary or advisable prostheses (e.g., dentures, eye glasses, hearing aid). A nursing history should be taken to record nature and expression of the presenting problems, daily activity patterns (e.g., nutrition, sleep, hygiene, elimination, physical activity), drug or food sensitivities, culture and religion, and social relationships. From an initial problem list, immediate nursing interventions can be planned. As nursing staff represent the closest and most continuous contact with inpatients, they generally provide direct observation of patient behavior and monitor fluctuation or changes in medical and psychological status, social interaction patterns, and requirements for support or assistance with activities of daily living. In addition to narrative form-written and oral communication of observations, nursing staff may utilize a variety of cognitive state, e.g., the Mini Mental State Examination, MMSE (Folstein et al., 1975), the Mental State Questionnaire, MSQ (Kahn et al., 1960), and ward behavior scales, e.g., Multidimensional Observation Scale for Elderly Subjects, MOSES (Short & Csapo, 1979), and London Psychogeriatric Scale, LPGS (Hersch et al., 1978), as repeated measures to document treatment response or change in status.

Social Work

Where a clinical social worker is attached to the geriatric psychiatry unit, it may be advisable for this member of the team to accompany the nurse or physician in making the domicilliary visit for preadmission assessment of the patient. In addition to providing assistance in gathering information regarding the nature of the presenting problem, reason for referral, and history of present illness, the social worker will be trained in the formulation of social history and social relationships. If potential placement problems can be foreseen, the social worker can also advise and begin preparations for discharge planning even prior to admission.

If it is not feasible for the social worker to participate directly in preadmission assessments, sufficient information should be gathered to permit access to present and potential sources of social support (e.g., family, friends, neighbors, community agencies). On admission the social worker can assess the strengths and weaknesses of the patient's current social network and evaluate the potential for benefit from relationship or individual counselling and supportive psychotherapy.

Occupational Therapy

Through team review of cases presented prior to admission, admission assessments documented by the physician, nursing and social work, and by direct patient interview, the occupational therapist can evaluate the patient's needs in relation to the goals of the ward program and connections with community agencies. Taking into account the patient's physical and psychosocial state, education, and work and social history, the occupational therapist can assess the patient's current ability to plan and occupy time with meaningful activities. Over the course of admission the occupational therapist can also assess the patient's response to social, physical, and intellectual stimulation, and evaluate both direct and instrumental activities of daily life (e.g., self-care, money management, use of telephone and transportation). The results of the occupational therapist's assessments should be useful in providing a specific positive focus for intervention, such as individual hobbies and interests. Occupational and leisure needs can also be assessed over the course of admission with a view of assisting linkages with community agencies on discharge.

Psychology

The psychologist can provide assessment of global intellectual and specific task performance on a variety of standardized psychometric and neuropsychological tests. In addition to assisting in the determination of presence or extent of cognitive deficits, repeated measures may provide a baseline and index of the course in fluctuating or degenerative organic disorders. Careful psychological assessment of the geriatric psychiatry patient, comparing timed versus untimed performance and testing over several sessions, may reveal the relative contributions of fatigue, anxiety, and dysfunction due to cognitive impairment. The psychologist may also provide consultant services or direct patient care in the assessment or management of behavior modification and relaxation therapy programs.

Pharmacy

The pharmacist may provide consultation on drug dosage levels, potential interactions, reactions, and contradictions. This function may be of particular value in the treatment of geriatric psychiatry patients in chronic care settings, where many patients have multiple medical conditions and a variety of medications.

Nutrition

The nutritionist or dietician may provide specialist assessment of nutritional deficiencies and need for nutrition counseling. In an active treatment setting, the focus should be on determining food preferences and intolerances, diet history, attitudes toward diet, and usual food intake on admission. In a chronic care setting, assessment should focus on diet and activity level required to attain and maintain ideal weight and nutritional status and to avoid drug reactions. Prior to discharge, the dietician may collaborate with nursing and occupational therapy to assess patient independence in obtaining and preparing nutritional foods.

Physiotherapy

The physiotherapist may be either a consultant on an active treatment unit, or a member of the direct care team in chronic care settings. Initial assessment should focus on the extent of physical functional disability and potential for rehabilitation. Over the course of rehabilitation therapy, or following training with prostheses, aided functions and necessary support systems can be evaluated.

Audiology

A clinical audiologist, either as a consultant or on staff in an active treatment or chronic care facility, can provide assessment of hearing and evaluation of rehabilitation potential. Following otological examination to ensure removal of cerumen and clearance of acute ear disease, the audiologist can test thresholds for sound across frequencies, and ability to hear and understand speech. If warranted on the basis of audiometry, the audiologist can also evaluate the potential for benefit from a hearing aid, or other aural rehabilitation procedures, and institute a hearing aid trial. As many elderly psychiatric patients are unable or unwilling to comply with aural rehabilitation recommendations, the audiologist may provide inservice training for other staff in communication with the hearing impaired.

In summary, although the above general admission protocols focused on the specialist skills of each member, in practice, patient assessment on a geriatric psychiatry unit must be a team effort. Conjoint assessment and effective communication are essential in order to achieve an holistic approach which acknowledges the contribution of psychological and physical states, individual and interpersonal function.

ADDITIONAL DIAGNOSTIC PROTOCOLS

Frequently patients are admitted with presumptive or provisional diagnoses, or the results of the initial investigations suggest a diagnostic category which demands a more specific investigation of dementia or confusional states, affective disorders, paraphrenia or paranoid psychoses, neuroses or personality disorders, and alcohol or other substance abuse.

Dementia Protocol

In addition to the general admission medical protocol, patients with evidence of cognitive impairment should receive a complete neurological assessment by a consulting neurologist, and be referred for CT brain scan and neuropsychological assessment. Because there are one hundred purported causes of secondary dementia, the majority obscure, the several admission laboratory investigations listed in Table 7.2 should be supplemented if a specific disorder is suspected. Cognitive state and ward function scales should be completed more frequently (i.e., daily or weekly) in order to monitor closely for fluctuations. If reliable informants are available, a careful history of the dementing disorder should be taken including nature and onset of first signs of subsequent course.

Affective Disorders

As accurate diagnosis of affective disorder may have important implications for both immediate and long-term treatment plans, and careful documentation of symptoms and signs is critical. In addition to determining the nature and duration of the current episode, it is important to establish whether there is family history of either. Current and previous medications should be evaluated both for potential deleterious effects on mood, and for history of benefit in prior episodes. The Dexamethasone Suppression Test, DST (Carroll, 1983) and the Ritalin Challenge Test (Sabelli et al., 1983), although still in experimental stages, may be useful as biological markers or to assist treatment choice. Repeated mental state examinations should be conducted over the course of treatment to monitor for changes in symptoms and severity.

Paraphrenia or Paranoid Psychoses

Suspected cases of paranoid disorders require careful documentation of symptoms and symptom severity. Frequency, form, and content of hallucinations and delusions should be documented. As there does appear to be an association between paraphrenia and sensory deficits (Cooper, 1976), and some degree of congruence between modality of sensory deficit and type of hallucination (Eastwood & Corbin, 1983), suspected cases should be examined for both hearing and vision impairment. Either medication or remediation of sensory deficits may provide symptom control, but assessment of patient compliance may indicate needs for continuous support and assistance.

Neuroses, Personality Disorders, Psychosocial Crises

An essential component of specific assessment for patients with suspected neuroses and personality disorders is the determination of onset of functional disturbance and examination for possible precipitants (e.g., significant losses or other major life events). Even disorders of long duration may be amenable to appropriate therapy; therefore, careful assessment of the patient's strengths and responses to various treatments, and linkage with appropriate services on discharge may have beneficial effects.

Alcohol or Drug Dependency or Abuse

Evidence of substance dependency or abuse, based on observation, patient self-report or informant report can be assessed using standardized instruments such as the Alcohol Dependence Scale, Lifetime Drinking History, and Drug Abuse Screening Test (Skinner, 1984). In evaluating alcohol and drug problems in the elderly population, however, it should be kept in mind that changes in tolerance and potential drug interactions may result in exaggerated reactions at relatively low intake levels. Although treatment with medication and psychotherapy can be started during admission to a geriatric psychiatry unit, evidence that geriatric clients may be particularly responsive to support group therapy (Brody, 1982) suggests the benefit of linkage with community agencies.

TREATMENT AND MANAGEMENT

Observation and assessment for all diagnoses is continuous. Each team member may be called upon to present a synopsis of findings prior to formulation of the case by the physician, and to provide information specific to the assessment of treatment and management of the case through the course of stay. In addition to general measures, specific diagnostic categories require specific treatment assessment protocols. These are outlined below.

Affective Disorders

Depending upon urgency, severity, chronicity, or previous treatment response, affective disorders may be treated with tri- or tetracyclic antidepressants, MAOI antidepressants, lithium carbonate or electroconvulsive therapy. Each of these treatments requires careful monitoring in geriatric psychiatry. The antidepressants require monitoring for anticholinergic side effects, symptom change and regular checks on ECG, serum drug levels and blood pressure. Electroconvulsive therapy also requires monitoring for signs of headache or confusion. Although most patients with affective disorders can be discharged home, they frequently are at risk of repeated episodes and require follow-up at discharge. These patients may be seen in outpatient clinics or day hospital, and may benefit from telephone contact or occasional home visits by any member of the team.

Dementia

Since there is no treatment specific for dementia, attention is directed to achieving and maintaining the maximum functional ability. Management of behavior secondary to the confusional state, such as wandering, incontinence, and aggression, are problematic. Wandering requires skilled redirection and can be difficult to handle without restraint in settings with few staff. Incontinence may often be a result of both reduced control and poor communication, and may be best dealt with by frequent toileting. Aggression may be reduced by neuroleptic medications; however, this requires monitoring for evidence of excessive sedation, hypotension, extrapyramidal signs or further confusion. Prognosis is generally poor for primary dementia, and most cases will ultimately require skilled custodial care, but some patients can be maintained at home for a long while if their families obtain sufficient support in the form of respite care and home help. Placement for the severely disabled, who can no longer be maintained at home, is frequently difficult and often inadequate. Follow-up for these patients may focus on monitoring the adequacy of level of care and family counselling to assist with a common pattern of grief, guilt, and concern.

Paraphrenia

The psychotic features of this illness may respond to neuroleptic medication; however, the patient will require monitoring for signs of sedation, extrapyramidal signs, hypotension and confusion. If hearing is impaired, the evaluation of potential for benefit from a hearing aid or other aural rehabilitation is warranted. Since compliance with hearing aids is frequently poor among elderly patients, support and assistance in learning the appropriate use and care of the aid is essential in the early stages of adjustment, and some support may always be necessary for continuous use.

Neuroses, Personality Disorder, and Psychological Crises

Although antidepressant, anxiolytic or mild sedative medications may be beneficial for short-term intervention, the mainstays of treatment are counseling, psychotherapy and linkage with support services in the community.

DISCHARGE AND FOLLOW-UP

Depending upon the psychiatric and physical diagnoses, functional level, family and community supports, and even income, patients will eventually be discharged to home or to appropriate care facilities. This task of discharge, which often starts on admission, is both complex and delicate and the final decision is the result of many observations and determinations. The social worker, primary therapist, nurse, and occupational therapist are particularly involved. The discharge requires careful preparation and planning beforehand and consolidation afterward. Because, for example, the affective disorders are associated with a high relapse rate, monitoring at follow-up is imperative. The medical aspect may be done in the outpatient clinic or day hospital. Home visits, again done by any member of the team, are particularly useful in determining function in the community.

EFFICIENCY AND EFFICACY

The hospital team is only a part of the large array of health workers serving the needs of the elderly. The multiple problems of the aged have become very familiar to us, and in most western countries health, education, and research solutions are being sought. Only a few of the elderly ever need psychiatric hospital care, but those who do seem to require much expert assessment. Inpatient care is expensive and should be used judiciously. It has been argued that dementia, although common, is largely idiopathic and would be best assessed by general practitioners (Eastwood & Corbin, 1981). There are, however, frequent occasions when the diagnosis is in doubt, emergencies develop at home, or families need a rest from home care.

In these cases, admission is critical. The functional psychiatric disorders of old age also deserve proper investigation and close attention to treatment effects. The well practiced team can manage fine observation in a quick turnover setting, with minimal upset to the patient and a reduction in the risk of institutionalization.

REFERENCES

Brody, J. A. (1982). Aging and alcohol abuse. *J. Am. Geriatr. Soc., 30*(2), 123.
Carroll, B. J. (1983) Biologic markers and treatment response. *J. Clin. Psychiatry, 44*(8, Sec. 2), 30.
Cooper, A. F. (1976). Deafness and psychiatric illness. *Br. J. Psychiatry, 129,* 216.
Eastwood, M. R., Corbin S. (1981). Investigation of subject dementia. *Lancet, i,* 1261.
Eastwood, M. R., Corbin, S. (1983). Hallucinations in patients admitted to a geriatric psychiatry service: Review of 42 cases. *J. Am. Geriat. Soc., 31*(10), 593.
Folstein, M. F., Folstein, S. E., McHugh, P. R. (1975). "Mini-Mental State." A practical method for grading the cognitive state of patients for the clinician. *J. Psychiatr. Res., 12,* 189.
Hersch, E. L., Csapo, K. G., Palmer, R. B. (1978). Development of the London Psychogeriatric Rating Scale. *London Psychiatr. Hosp. Res. Bull., 1,* 3.
Kahn, R. L., Goldfarb A. I., Pollack M., Peck A. (1960). Brief objective measures for the determination of mental status in the aged. *Am. J. Psychiatry, 117,* 326.
Robins, L. N., Helzer, J. E., Croughan, J., Ratcliff, K. S. (1981). National Institute of Mental Health Diagnostic Interview Schedule: Its history, characteristics and validity. *Arch. Gen. Psychiatry, 38,* 381.
Sabelli, H. C., Fawcett, J., Javaid, J. I., Bagri, S. (1983). The Methylphenidate Test for differentiating desipramine responsive from nortriptyline responsive depression. *Am. J. Psychiatry, 140,* 212.
Short, J., Csapo, K. G. (1979). Multidimensional Observation Scale for Elderly Subjects: A research scale designed for assessing the behaviour of the institutionalized elderly. *London Psychiatr. Hosp., Res. Bull., 2,* 15.
Skinner, H. A. (1984). Instruments for assessing alcohol and drug problems. *Bull. Soc. Psychol. Addict. Behav., 3,* 21.
Wing, J. K., Cooper, J. E., Sartorius, N. (1974). *The measurement and classification of psychiatric symptoms.* London: Cambridge University Press.

8
Brain Hemodynamic and Metabolic Approaches in Senile Cerebral Impairment Related to Dementia

Willy J. Dekoninck

The central nervous system is one of the ideal tools for the study of the phenomenon of aging. Indeed, as a largely postmitotic tissue subject to the attrition in structure-function that affects all incompletely replenishing physical entities, the nervous system provides a model that can be analyzed at all levels of complexity, from changes at the molecular-genetic level to subjective reports on the results of its own activities mainly including classic human psychological research. The other organs of the body usually cannot report directly on their functional integrity; the brain can and does.

It is still a common belief that normal aging as well as many types of abnormal aging are due to an insufficient blood supply to the brain. The main cause of the reduction of the flow is generally assumed to be atherosclerosis of the vessels leading to the brain and/or arteriosclerosis of cerebral vessels. According to this view, the reduced function of the central nervous system, including signs of failing intellectual functions frequently observed in elderly people during senility, would be due to cerebral ischemia which leads to a successive reduction of brain metabolism and a decrease in the number of brain neurons. As Lassen and Ingvar have recently written (1980), this concept also implies that aging of the brain might be counteracted if the blood flow or oxygen delivery to the brain is increased by cerebral vasodilatation or by hyperbaric oxygen, respectively. However, clinical experience often yields unexpected or poor results in using such treatments.

We will try to give a general view of the most important studies done on cerebral flow and metabolism in order to get a better understanding of different types of senile chronic brain impairment. But, whatever the results of these studies, and whatever the importance of an altered cerebral circulation, the question still remains whether in senile chronic states, this eventual altered cerebral circulation chronologically precedes a metabolic impairment or whether it is simply an adaptative phenomenon (autoregulation), and also whether endogenous changes observed within the brain parenchyma are not really the primary events.

CLASSICAL CEREBRAL BLOOD FLOW AND METABOLIC STUDIES IN NORMAL AND ABNORMAL BRAIN AGING

Definition of Cerebral Aging

It is unquestionable that the brains of elderly subjects, particularly those with significant cognitive impairment, undergo two major forms of anatomical changes: (1) neuronal loss, senile plaques, neurofibrillary tangles, modification of the dendritic tree, and granulovacuolar degeneration, all of which are considered to be the manifestation of cellular degeneration; and (2) focal cerebral softening or multiple lacunar infarcts, considered to be the manifestation of vascular disorders (Tomlinson, 1973). A relationship between these structural brain changes and cognitive decline surely seems to exist, but it is still unresolved whether the difference among normal aging, senile dementia, and presenile dementia is an intensity, extensity, locational or subtle qualitative ultrastructural difference.

Another controversial issue is whether the severity of cognitive impairments is correlated with the severity of brain changes (Lenzi & Jones, 1980). All these observations are biased by several factors, namely that ordinary patients were studied only when they present with clear-cut clinical conditions, the natural history of the brain during aging is not well established, and morphology does not directly reflect function. Therefore the new atraumatic and repetitive techniques now available to measure in vivo regional cerebral blood flow and metabolic oxygen-glucose consumptions may provide in the future better approaches, on the one hand, to early discovery of the real causes of functional changes related to regional impairments of the brain's metabolism occuring during cognitive decline and, on the other, to following them during a sufficient period of life. Actually, in abnormal brain aging, we may be facing patients with dementia who present with similar clinical conditions, but the differential diagnosis often remains uncertain and complicated for the clinician. It is assumed, in organic brain syndrome, that senile dementia of the Alzheimer type (SDAT) accounts for 50% of the cases, multiinfarct dementia (SDMI) for 12%, and a combination of the two, 8%. Another 16% are probably related to the former two types. Nearly 14% remain unclassifiable (Tomlinson, 1973). Moreover, biochemical studies on brain tissue ex vivo and in vivo reveal with increasing frequency instances of specific neurotransmitter deficiency as the basis for dementia (Bowen et al., 1977, 1982). How many of these are specifically treatable cases is unknown. Therefore, one approach that may be fruitful is the study of the cerebral distribution of flow and metabolic activity in young and healthy, in normal elderly, in slightly demented, and in severely demented people.

Results of Superficial Cortical Flow and Global Metabolic Measurements

The nitrous oxide technique introduced by Kety and Schmidt (1945) enabled measurement of the total mean cerebral blood flow (CBF) and a calculation of the total cerebral oxygen and glucose consumptions (CMR_{O_2} and CMR_{glc}) from the arteriovenous oxygen and glucose differences. Regional, but always superficial, CBF techniques were then introduced based on intracarotid injection of freely diffusible isotopes like ^{85}Kr and ^{133}Xe with multiple cranial probes detectors (Lassen, 1959; Lassen & Ingvar, 1972). For biophysical reasons related to properties of the tracers and of the external probes, cerebral flow measurements are applied only to superficial regions of the brain (mainly cortex) and are thus unable to detect flow lower in the cerebral nervous system. Using a 254-channel intracarotid regional CBF method (gamma camera system) Lassen and colleagues have shown colored maps of human cerebral functions during resting and during sensorimotor activations (Lassen et al., 1977) (Fig. 8.1).

Normal Aging

Numerous studies in man have demonstrated that aging is generally associated with a reduction in average CBF and energy metabolism of the brain as a whole (measured by CMR_{O_2} and CMR_{glc} because aerobic glycolytic is the most important energy pathway for cerebral work) (Kety, 1956). In some of the studies surveyed by Kety, age-related systemic and vascular disease may have contributed to the changes in cerebral flow and energy metabolism. In order to minimize the effects of disease and to identify the effects of chronological aging per se, the National Institute of Mental Health in Bethesda, Maryland, carried out a broad multidisciplinary study in aged subjects rigorously selected for normal performance in the community and as great a freedom from disease as possible (Dastur et al., 1963). Although in this very select group CBF and CMR_{O_2} remained quite unchanged from the levels in normal subjects fifty years younger, CMR_{glc} was significantly reduced.

Diagnostics 151

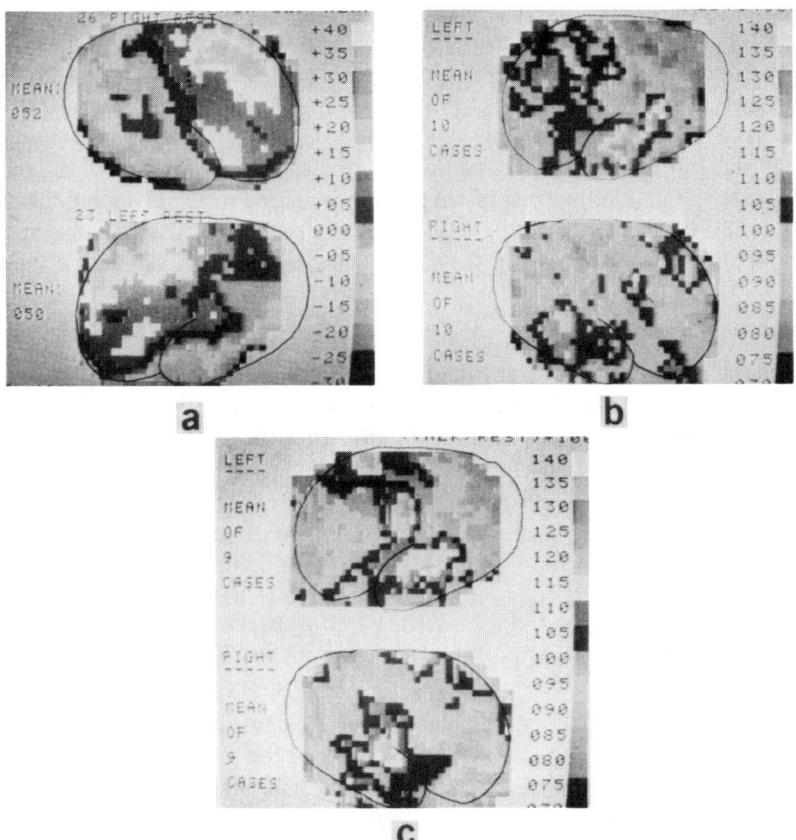

FIGURE 8.1 Normal regional CBF patterns with lateral views of the left and right hemispheres in resting state where (a) frontal hyperaemia is noted by a colored scale representing CBF as a percentage above or below the mean hemispheric flow. CBF increases in both temporal auditory areas as well as in Broca's and Wernicke's speech areas in the left hemisphere during a listening test (b). During automatic speech (c), increases are seen in both temporal auditory and rolandic face areas and in the left supplementary motor areas (Lassen et al., 1977). (Reprinted by permission.)

The dissociation between oxygen-glucose cerebral consumptions may possibly have been due in part to ketosis with consequent cerebral utilization of ketone bodies as substrates for oxidative metabolism (Sokoloff, 1975) or for transamination to form amino acids (Dekoninck et al., 1980a). Another explanation for the decrease of cerebral glucose consumption may be found in the modification of the activity of two key enzymes of the glycolytic pathway occurring during normal aging and observed in human frontal cortex and putamen: increase in hexokinase and decrease in phosphofructokinase activities (Fig. 8.2). The reduction in fructokinase activity may impair glucose splitting capacity of the glycolytic pathway with loss of energy formation by decreased synthesis of the ATP carrier (Iwangoff et al., 1979). But normal appearing elderly subjects may exhibit impairments of cognitive and psychomotor functions during special examinations (Birren et al., 1963). These impairments are probably related to the observed CMR_{glc} reduction and to the decrease in the EEG dominant rhythm, indicating abnormalities somewhere in the brain (Obrist, 1963).

Abnormal Aging

Patients with signs of arteriosclerosis of vessels leading to the brain but without clinically intellectual deficits or symptoms of "chronic brain syndrome" show only a moderate reduction of CBF and energy metabolism (Lassen, 1959). Such patients also show a normal cerebrovascular reactivity to CO_2 and a normal autoregulatory response to changes of the systemic pressure (Strandgaard et al., 1974). In patients with arteriosclerotic changes of brain vessels who show signs of intellectual impairment and/or a history of one or several cerebrovascular lesions, some authors find a reduction of CBF and of energy metabolism grossly proportional to the clinical neurologic and psychiatric symptomatology (Lassen & Ingvar, 1980). Others (Dekoninck et al., 1975; 1977 a,b) report a lack of close correlation between brain function and CBF-energy metabolism as measured as a whole, but this is probably due to both the weak sensitivity of the techniques used and the heterogeneity of the patients studied. In those demented subjects (SDMI), regional CBF measurements show diffuse areas of flow reduction while global metabolism is decreased (Dekoninck et al., 1977a; Hachinski et al., 1975).

The regional CBF pattern seems quite different in SDAT (compared to SDMI) where global CBF is decreased with the most important reduction in frontal and postcentral-temporal areas in advanced cases with severe mental deterioration. It has been established that subsymptoms of dementia such as memory disturbances, disorientation, speech impairment, gnostic deficits, and apraxia show regional CBF decreases which correlate surprisingly well to the distribution of the neuronal degeneration: temporal regions for memory deficit, occipito-parieto-temporal regions for agnostic symptoms, and disorientation (Gustafson, 1975; Hagberg & Ingvar, 1976).

What has been said about Alzheimer's disease (presenile or senile forms) also holds for patients suffering from other types of dementia, for example Pick's and Jakob-Creutzfeldt's disease. In both groups, CBF is reduced and the distribution of the reduction relates to the morphologic changes (Lassen & Ingvar, 1980). One very important finding is that in patients with any type of dementia, activation stimuli, whether sensorimotor activity or men-

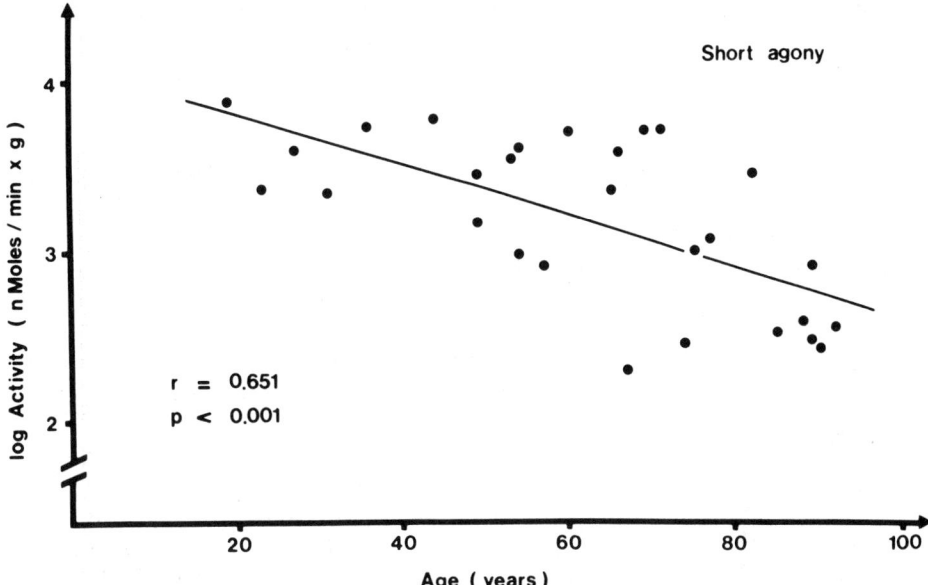

FIGURE 8.2 Age-induced decrease of phosphofructokinase (PFK) activity in human brain cortex ($n = 28$) from cases with sudden death (Iwangoff et al., 1979).

tal effort, do not result in the expected flow increases seen in normal subjects (Ingvar et al., 1975).

Concerning global metabolism of the brain, most of the studies confirm the decrease of CMR_{O_2} and CMR_{glc} in senile dementia compared to adults and healthy elderly people. However the SDMI type seems to present the largest metabolic decreases (Dekoninck et al., 1977a). Some senile demented patients (mainly SDAT) paradoxically may conserve an excellent CBF and glycolytic metabolism with a possibility of concomitant utilization of intermediate glucose pathways (Hoyer, 1969; Hachinski et al., 1975; Dekoninck et al., 1980). But this utilization of such intermediate metabolic pathways instead of, or together with, the usual glycolytic pathway does not generate much energy and seems rather to preserve vegetative life or nerve cells in senile patients.

NEW NONINVASIVE APPROACHES

Regional Superficial or Cortical CBF Studies

Noninvasive CBF measurements after ^{133}Xe intravenous injection or inhalation are now usually performed with specially designed multidetector equipment (Obrist & Wilkinson, 1980). The most important clinical application of the method in psychiatry is the early diagnosis of the different types of organic dementias, and also the differentiation between organic dementia and pseudodementia caused by systemic organic diseases or psychiatric illness, such as depressive psychosis.

The principal interest of such a method of regional CBF measurement is, first, its total atraumatic approach, allowing repetitive measures of both hemispheres in awake subjects and, second, the high validity and reliability of the method with good correlations with the intraarterial technique (Reivich et al., 1975). It becomes possible to study large groups of normal, healthy and very old elderly yielding approximately the same conclusions as the intraarterial technique, except for a small but significant progressive decline of the mean resting CBF from age 24 through age 82, with a persistent but decreased vasodilator response to hypercapnia during aging (Fig. 8.3) (Meyer, 1980; Dekoninck et al., 1980b). The progressive decline of CBF observed in normal aging may have an explanation other than the fact that it is an expression of incipient senile organic-atrophic brain disease. Young subjects, especially children, are more readily aroused than are elderly people. Arousal and psychologic tension increase CBF and metabolism, as does pain, all conditions which cannot always be avoided in studying awaked subjects. If pain is often absent with the inhalation technique (compared to the intraarterial one), individual anxiety and nervous tension may be present and give false results in some cases (Lassen & Ingvar, 1980). With the intraarterial method, this is also true if a supplementary factor such as pain is added. Complete steady states are difficult to obtain in this type of examination. Inhalation is a better approach and new complete atraumatic approaches now begin to afford more information on physiopathological processes occuring in advancing age without a series of usual artefacts.

As with the intracarotid method, hemispheric CBF is significantly reduced in demented patients compared to normal elderly and to age-matched patients with depression who have generally normal CBF results (Risberg, 1980, 1983). In SDAT subjects there are focal flow decreases of at least 20% below the hemispheric mean in postcentral regions, predominantly in the parietal area (Fig. 8.4). For Pick's disease, focal flow abnormalities are found in the frontal region in addition to a global flow decrease, whereas SDMI patients show diffuse regional and/or global hemispheric right–left asymmetries (Fig. 8.4). Thus the results indicate that a differential diagnosis of organic dementia and depression is possible by this easy method of CBF measurement. Moreover, the degenerative dementias are more easily recognizable than the cerebrovascular ones—such an examination is also useful in the evaluation of the effects of drug therapy and in the study of the progression of the disease. Several other applications in psychiatry have been investigated, including alcohol withdrawal, senile paranoia (flow de-

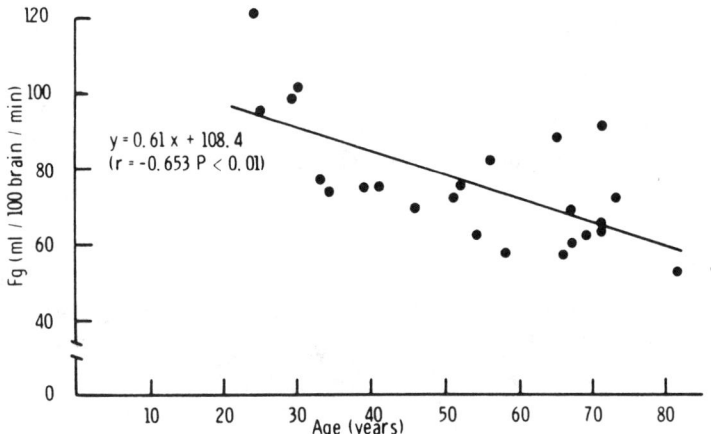

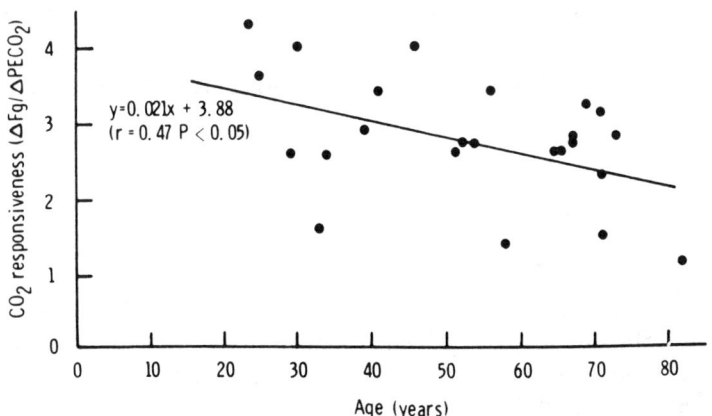

FIGURE 8.3 Correlation between mean hemispheric steady state CBF values (Fg = gray matter flow) and advancing age in normal healthy volunteers ($n = 24$) with absolute cerebral vasodilation response to hypercapnia expressed as CBF per mmHg PE_{CO_2} (end-tidal carbon dioxide pression) correlating with age (Meyer, 1980).

creases especially in frontotemporal regions), and drug intoxications demonstrating the clinical and experimental neuropsychological potential of the method (Risberg, 1980; Zemcov et al., 1983). In both dementia groups (AT and MI), cerebral autoregulation and vascular response during CO_2 inhalation seem to be maintained but are less normal in the MI type of dementia (Miyazaki et al., 1983).

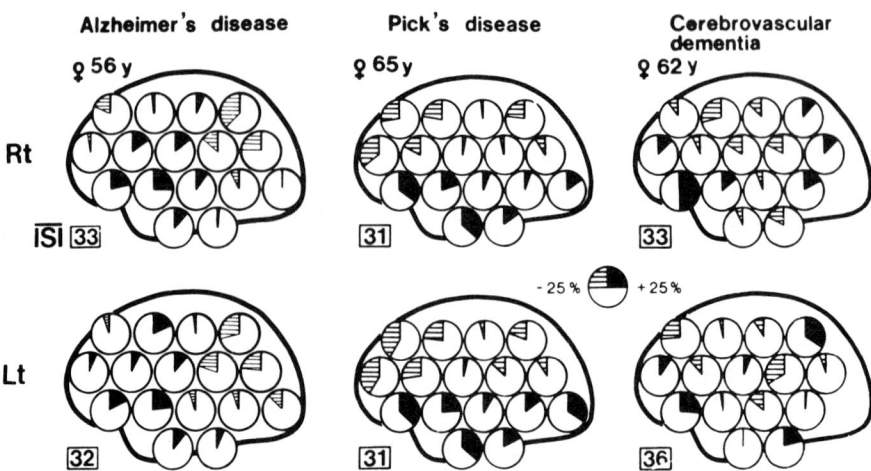

FIGURE 8.4 Regional CBF patterns (Xenon-133 inhalation method) in three typical cases of Alzheimer's disease, Pick's disease, and multiinfarct dementia. "Clock symbols" show percentage deviation from hemispheric mean □ for right (Rt) and left (Lt) hemispheres (Risberg, 1980).

Regional Cortical Subcortical Flow and Metabolism Studies

Measurement of Regional CBF Using Computed Tomography and Stable Xenon

The inhalation of nonradioactive or stable xenon provides adequate contrast enhancement for quantitative computed tomography measurements of regional CBF within regions of interest using the Kety's formula for the autoradiographic method. Cortical and subcortical areas (basal ganglia, putamen, caudate nucleus, thalamus, centrum semiovale, internal capsule, optic radiation) are so defined in a hemodynamic way (Rottenberg et al., 1981; Sakai et al., 1981).

This method was recently employed to differentiate dementias from normal aging and to make a distinction between SDAT and SDMI (Meyer et al., 1983). In normal aging, this method shows reductions of mean cortical gray matter (mainly in frontal lobes), basal ganglia, thalamic and white matter flow values. In SDAT, cortical and thalamic grey matter flows are diffusely reduced compared to age-matched normals. In SDMI, the coefficient of variation is greater than in SDAT and normals whereas cortical flow declines from 85 to 65 ml/100 g brain/min between 35 and 80 years with similar declines in basal ganglia and thalamic flow. No great difference is observed between SDAT and MI but reductions of CBF correlate well with severity of dementia (Meyer et al., 1983).

Use of Positron Emission Tomography for Regional Flow and Metabolism Determinations

Positron emission tomography (PET) is a noninvasive scanning method that can provide a cross-sectional image of brain radioactivity. The process resembles x-ray CT but, unlike studies that can only show static qualities such as anatomic structure or cerebrovascular membrane permeability, PET can illustrate dynamic actions such as blood flow, metabolism, and other physiologic cerebral functions, depending on the labeled compound chosen as a tracer.

For PET studies, a cyclotron prepares compounds labeled with short-lived isotopes of carbon, oxygen, nitrogen, or fluorine (Phelps et al., 1978). During radioactive decay, these isotopes emit positrons that rapidly annihilate with electrons, producing two photons diverging at 180°; the photons can be detected by electronic coincidence counting (Phelps et al., 1975). The improvement of temporal resolution in the recent PET devices (from a few seconds to a few nanoseconds) raises the possibility of passage from static or slow variance with time studies to very fast dynamic ones (Ter-Pogossian et al., 1981).

Among the most usual labeled compounds employed in PET studies for regional CBF and CMR_{O_2} measurements let us point out the ^{15}O inhalation technique (Lammertsma et al., 1981), whereas for regional CMR_{glc} determination the fluorodeoxyglucose labeled with ^{18}F intravenous method seems mostly to be used (Phelps et al., 1979; Huang et al., 1980). Beside glycolytic pathway studies in normal and abnormal conditions, PET makes possible the in vivo study of brain protein synthesis in some diseases where abnormalities of amino acids are suspected, such as phenylketonuria, schizophrenia, Parkinson's disease, and senility (Bustany et al., 1981, 1983). Local coupling among CBF, oxygen consumption, and glucose utilization now becomes possible in humans with PET combination of the ^{15}O steady-state technique followed by intravenous injection of ^{18}F deoxyglucose in order to obtain brain tomographic images of regional CBF, CMR_{O_2}, oxygen extraction fraction, and CMR_{glc} (Baron et al., 1983).

Because size and shape of heads vary among individuals, PET scans at identical levels above an externally defined inferior orbitomeatal line do not always include corresponding brain regions. In order to evaluate corresponding regions among brains of different subjects, each scan is compared with anatomical sections of a single human brain at specified levels above the inferior orbitomeatal line for that brain, and the "intrinsic" height for each scan from the comparable brain section is defined. Regions of interest are identified by comparing the scan with the section, and are outlined with the computer program of the used positron tomography (Fig. 8.5).

In *normal aging,* some PET studies have shown no correlation between age and cerebral metabolic rate for glucose or any difference between left

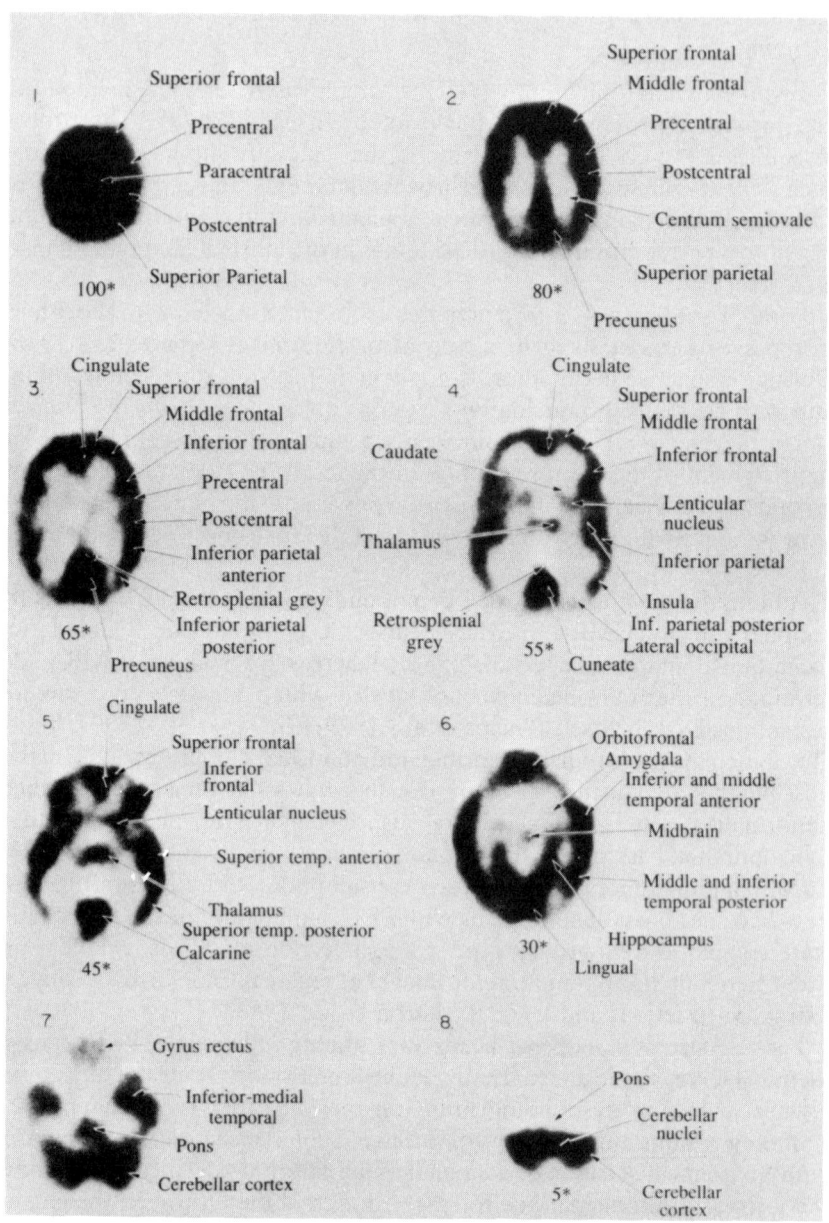

FIGURE 8.5 PET scans and regions of interest at different levels (mm) above the inferior orbitomeatal line (Duara et al., 1983).

and right hemispheres (total hemispheric and local rates of 31 different brain structures) (Duara et al., 1983) (Fig. 8.6). However, other studies using PET have found a mild decrease of hemispheric as well as regional CMR_{glc} in gray and white matter regions in healthy elderly (Frackowiak et al., 1980; Kuhl et al., 1982). These apparent differences may be due to inclusion of subjects with asymptomatic cerebrovascular disease or to methodological reasons, depending principally on unregulated sensory stimulation during measurements (eyes and ears open or not) (Duara et al., 1983). Changes in local CMR_{glc} reflect what occurs in given brain regions, but do not indicate how regions work together as a neurofunctional unit. Regional brain function does not exist in isolation, but depends on interactions with other regions. Thus, if metabolism changes across subjects in one region, corresponding changes should occur in other regions where some interdependence exists (Metter et al., 1983). These authors have found differences in regional metabolic relationships between young and old nor-

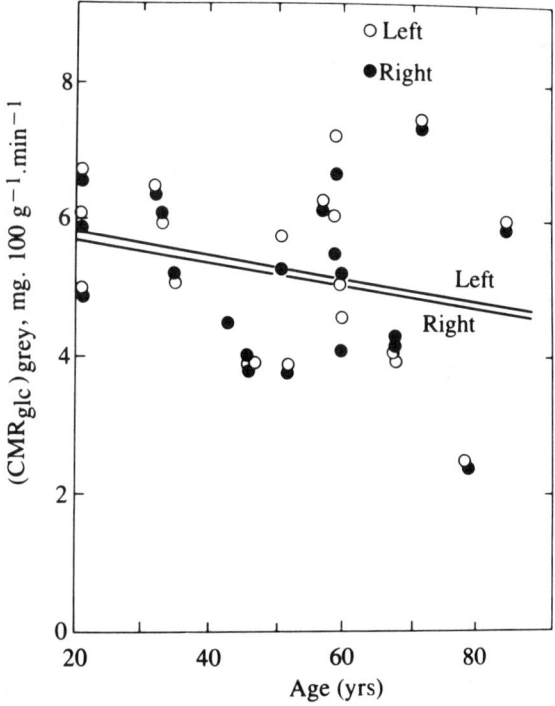

FIGURE 8.6 Absence of significant decrease of cerebral metabolism rate for glucose in gray matter of the hemispheres in relation to age in 21 healthy subjects ($p > 0.05$) (Duara et al., 1983).

mal subjects; relationships were more focused in the elderly, with most intercorrelations between the superior frontal parietal and occipital regions.

This functional system has been shown to correlate with memory recognition and decision criteria, and in fact may represent an attentional system. These metabolic cortical interrelations may reflect a better ability of the older brain to focus regional interactions in response to functional demands, with a more selective arousal pattern. By relying on these more limited relationships, the older brain may compensate for dwindling brain reserves demonstrated by measures of atrophy and decreasing CMR_{glc}. Alternatively, it may relate to decreased sensory or cognitive awareness during PET deoxyglucose procedure (resting state with eyes and ears not occluded).

The constancy of glucose metabolic rates with age, despite morphological and functional decrements, might reflect the fact that the metabolic rates are intensive per gram of tissue. If the net volume of a brain region, such as the thalamus, were reduced in the elderly, then metabolism for the region as a whole might be reduced even though metabolism per gram of region was not. The fact that the subjects were examined under resting conditions (eyes covered and ears plugged with cotton) may also explain the stability of CMR_{glc} with age. But age deficits might become evident if the brain were subjected to pharmacological or physiological stimulation (Rapoport et al., 1983).

In *abnormal aging,* and particularly in demented patients, PET data reveal decreasing values ($\pm$ 30%) for regional CBF and CMR_{O_2} with no significant modification of oxygen extraction fraction (oxygen-15 steady state technique) as compared with the values obtained in age-matched, normal, healthy volunteers (Frackowiak et al., 1981). A correlation between severity of dementia and decline in CBF and CMR_{O_2} is also observed with an absence of difference between type of dementia (degenerative or vascular). The relative stability of the regional oxygen extraction fraction suggests that chronic ischaemia does not play a significant pathogenic role in any of the types of dementia (Tables 8.1 and 8.2).

By always using PET, but with the 18-fluorodeoxyglucose technique, the results obtained in demented patients reveal progressive decreased cerebral glucose utilization from young to old age and a further decline from old age to the demented state; however the only significant metabolic mean changes are between young controls and dementias. This can be partially explained by the relatively poor resolution of the system used (Alavi et al., 1982). These authors do not find a correlation between the mean cortical metabolic rates for glucose and the global mental function in either old controls or demented patients; a possibility may exist for brain to utilize other substrates than glucose in aging and/or dementia.

TABLE 8.1 PET ^{15}O Results Obtained in the Temporal/Insula Region and in the Centrum Semiovale in Demented Patients Compared to the Normal Age-Matched Subjects

	rCBF (ml/100 ml/min)	rOER	rCMR$_{O_2}$ (ml O$_2$/100 ml/min)
Gray matter			
Normal ($n = 14$)	50.08±8.7^a	0.53±0.07	4.69±0.64
Demented	35.6±9.0^b	0.54±0.08	3.31±0.47^b
% Change	−30%	+20%	−29%
White matter			
Normal ($n = 14$)	21.5±2.6	0.49±0.07	1.81±0.21
Demented	15.4±4.9^b	0.51±0.10	1.33±0.32^b
% Change	−28%	+4%	−27%

^{a} ± SD. ^{b} $p = <0.001$.
rCBF: regional cerebral blood flow; rOER: regional oxygen extraction fraction; rCMR$_{O_2}$: regional cerebral oxygen utilization.
From Frackowiak et al. (1981). Reprinted by permission.

With a better spatial resolution, PET has shown lower glucose utilization mainly in regions such as the temporal-parietal cortex of patients with Alzheimer's disease (mean age = 65 years), compared to healthy subjects of the same age (Friedland et al., 1983). Concerning differences between unipolar depression, multiple infarct dementia, and Alzheimer's disease (with a mean age for all patients of 64 years), it is worth pointing to the recent study of Kuhl and colleagues who used a PET with middle spatial resolution (12 mm). These authors found a normal global CMR$_{glc}$ in depression, a decrease of 17% in vascular dementia, and a reduction of 33% in Alzheimer's disease, with the lowest results in the most severely demented patients. Regional CMR$_{glc}$ patterns were different in vascular and degenerative dementias: metabolic defects in cortex, caudate, thalamus, white matter, and cerebellum were observed for vascular types of dementia whereas, for degenerative ones, the most important abnormalities were observed in association cortex (Fig. 8.7). The values of the ratio of parietal cortex to caudate-thalamus CMR$_{glc}$ clearly separated Alzheimer's patients from normal, depressed, and multiple-infarct demented subjects (Kuhl et al., 1983).

Initial studies performed with the PET method (deoxyglucose technique) in other dementing processes seem to suggest several important metabolic differences. Pick's disease shows striking hypometabolism in the frontal and temporal areas, with lesser alteration of subcortical structures. In contrast,

TABLE 8.2 Gray Matter rCBF, rOER, and rCMRo₂ According to Severity and Type of Dementia, Compared to Normals

	rCBF (ml/100 ml/min)	rOER	rCMRo$_2$ (ml O$_2$/100 ml/min)
Mild dements ($n = 11$)	40.2±9.9^a	0.51±0.06	3.60±0.35
	−21%^{bc}	− 4%	−23%^{d}
Severe dements ($n = 11$)	31.1.±5.0	0.57±0.08	3.02±0.40
	−39%^{d}	+ 8%	−36%^{d}
Degenerative ($n = 13$)	35.0±6.9	0.54±0.06	3.32±0.43
	−31%^{c}	+ 2%	−29%^{c}
Vascular ($n = 9$)	36.5±11.8	0.53±0.11	3.29±0.56
	−28%^{d}	0	−30%^{c}

^{a} ±SD. ^{b} Change from normal. ^{c} $p = < 0.01$. ^{d} $p = < 0.001$.
Abbreviations as in Table 8.1.
From Frackowiak et al. (1983).

Huntington's disease with well-advanced dementia indicates total hypometabolism of the caudate region with well-preserved cortical metabolism. Similarly, individuals with dementia based on normal pressure hydrocephalus, Wilson's disease, suggest relative retention of cortical metabolic activity, at least in comparison to the patients with Alzheimer's disease. Finally, patients with relatively early Jakob-Creutzfeldt's disease seem to reveal a pattern characterized by mottled areas of hyper- and hypometabolism scattered in both cortical and subcortical regions (Benson et al., 1982). Table 8.3 gives a summary of the main regional metabolic differences observed with the PET technique in different varieties of demented patients (compared to normal and depressed elderly), offering a useful index of focal cerebral function, both cortical and subcortical, in living patients in order to make a better clinical distinction and diagnosis in elderly subjects. If global CMR$_{glc}$ is always reduced in abnormal brain aging with a relationship to severity of clinical mental impairment, Table 8.3 shows the cortical and subcortical regions where the CMR$_{glc}$ reduction is principally located with occasional (Jakob-Creutzfeldt's disease) areas of hyper- and hypometabolism. Besides in vivo studies concerning the metabolic glycolytic pathway in abnormal brain aging, there is also a postmortem "compositional" approach of brain modifications in senile dementia: decrease of RNA, total brain protein, proteolipid, enzyme activities in some regions (choline acetyltransferase, ATP-ases . . .), gangliosides,

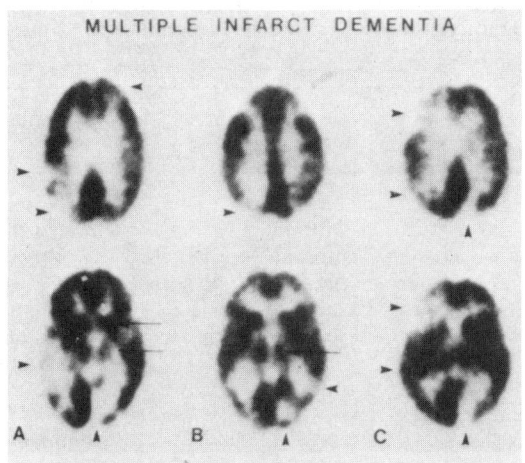
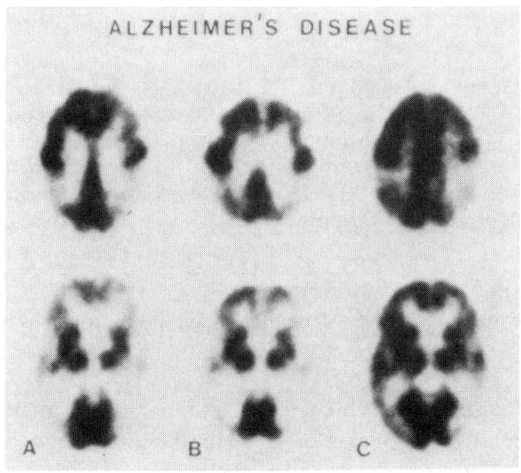

FIGURE 8.7 Deoxyglucose PET scans in three patients with multiinfarct dementia *(top)*: global metabolic rates are depressed and there are multiple focal metabolic defects scattered throughout the brain *(arrows)*. Three patients with Alzheimer's disease *(bottom)* with global CMR$_{glc}$ decrease particularly in the parietal cortex (Kuhl et al., 1983).

neuropeptides (somatostatin in cortex), neurohormones (vasopressin). But it appears that the approach of "compositional neurochemistry" which was so very fruitful in giving us insight into various lipidoses of childhood, has not been productive of more than baseline information in neurological aging. More interesting in the field of neurochemistry is the "structural or

TABLE 8.3. Regional Metabolic Patterns (CMR$_{glc}$ Reductions) Observed with the PET Deoxyglucose Method in Normal and Abnormal Brain Aging [a]

Patients with	Cortical area defects	Subcortical area defects
Normal aging	± Normal	± Normal
Unipolar depression	± Normal	± Normal
Alzheimer's disease	Temporal Parietal External occipital	
SDAT	Association cortex	Basal ganglia Thalamus
Multiple infarct dementia (senile or not)	Diffuse	White matter Caudate Thalamus Cerebellum
Pick's disease	Frontal Temporal	
Huntington's disease	Minor	White matter Caudate
NPH	Minor	
Wilson's disease	Diffuse	Putamen Lentiforme nuclei
Jakob-Creutzfeldt disease	Minor	Diffuse

[a] See also Figure 8.7.
SDAT: senile dementia of the Alzheimer type; NPH: normal pressure hydrocephalus.

cell-biological" approach, which leads to the modern neurobiology with synaptic molecular biology and bioelectric phenomenon using enzyme histochemical and immunocytochemical methods.

CONCLUSION

One consistent problem disturbing both clinical and research approaches to abnormal brain aging is the establishment of the diagnosis during the patient's life. That many widely different disorders can underly dementia is well established (Haase, 1977; Yesavage, 1979) but it is also apparent that the features distinguishing the varieties of dementia in vivo are not all clear. Several mental tests exist in order to quantify the degree of mental deterioration and to measure clinical changes during drug therapy, but the psychometric tests are so numerous that it seems difficult to make the best choice for universal and standardized utilization. Reisberg, however, using a global cognitive deterioration scale, seems to have succeeded in making a clinical distinction among the different stages of SDAT with a prediction (risk factors) for each of the seven degrees of the disease, taking into account borderline cases between normal and abnormal brain aging. The seven stages quantified by Reisberg in SDAT seem to relate to neuroradiologic and neurometabolic examinations (Reisberg et al., 1982, 1983; de Leon et al., 1983). The metabolism of aged controls (the two first stages of the global deterioration scale) was comparable to that of young normal subjects. Thus, for Reisberg the metabolism decrement observed from stage 3 of his scale appears to represent the first neurophysiologic evidence of a discontinuity between normal brain aging and Alzheimer's disease (Reisberg, 1984).

Recent technical advances (nuclear magnetic resonance, positron emission tomography) have improved the situation to obtain a correct in vivo diagnosis, but the widespread cerebral abnormality of many causes of dementia leads to poor definition until the disease is well advanced. The new techniques developed in this chapter are often complicated to carry out because, for example, in the case of PET, a cyclotron is necessary near the hospital (short-lived isotopes) where a specialized full-time staff has to attend to expensive machinery. Therefore, we think that these techniques are presently necessary for clinical research to obtain a better understanding of the brain vs physiopathological processes occuring during life. Regional cerebral blood flow determinations are now more easy to obtain and they give a credible reflection of metabolic disturbances either in cortical regions (^{133}Xe inhalation technique) or in subcortical areas (stable xenon with CT scan).

Finally, as Professor Exton Smith (University College of London) has said in a recent symposium, the only certain way to diagnose Alzheimer's disease is by brain biopsy. Histological examination reveals characteristic senile plaques and neurofibrillary tangles whereas histochemical procedures allow the examiner to reveal biochemical change like reduction of choline acetyltransferase activity which has been shown to correlate both with the degree of histopathological damage and with the mental test score of the patient (Bowen et al., 1982). Most clinicians at present do not think that brain biopsy is ethically justified for the diagnosis of dementia. However, if any agent became available that could specifically affect the progression of the dementing process, a precise diagnosis, with evaluation of the biochemical disturbance, would be necessary. But one must consider several obstacles that impede research relating to senile dementia, including the ethical and legal issue of informed consent. Therefore the National Institute on Aging (USA) has plans to convene a major workshop and invite philosophers, lawyers, and scientists to explore this difficult subject (Butler, 1982).

For all these reasons, our knowledge of the chemical changes in the aging brain is still limited and our understanding of the functional implications of these alterations is always slight indeed. Concerning the influence of age per se on cerebral metabolism, one school of thought emphasizes a breakdown of delivery systems providing essential substances as a primary feature whereas another argues that endogenous change within brain tissue marks the primary event.

Evidence supporting both points of view is apparent in the literature reviewed and would serve to remind us that the end-point, namely, an eventual decline in metabolism and concomitant intellectual changes, may result from multiple causes. Between these causes cerebral arteriosclerosis and cerebral ischemia do not seem to play a primary role in brain aging. However, sclerosis of the vessels leading to the brain may enhance symptoms of aging and produce, in some cases, dementia. In such cases, the reactivity of the cerebral vessels to CO_2 and to variations of blood pressure (autoregulation) appears to be retained in unaffected parts of the brain. It has been demonstrated that induced brain work, be it sensorimotor activity or pure mental effort, gives rise to both localized and generalized augmentations of CBF (Ingvar et al., 1975). It is not yet known whether a reduction or a complete absence of cerebral activation of this type may lead to a secondary loss of neurons and/or modifications of neurotransmitters released with reduction of synapses and loss of dendritic spines eventually inducing decreases in metabolism reflected by CBF defects. The semistatic in vivo measurements of regional cerebral metabolism based on PET now make it possible to obtain changes that occur in given brain regions, but do not indicate how regions work together as a neurofunctional unit. Present PET studies (Metter et al., 1983) have already tried to give an answer by studying the intercorrelations between brain areas in healthy young and elderly but not yet in the mentally disturbed. These findings seem to demonstrate changes with age in the functional interactions of the brain which go beyond local CMR_{glc} and include the interrelationships of regional metabolism.

REFERENCES

Alavi, A., Reivich, M., Ferris, S., Christman, D., Fowler, J., MacGregor, R., Farkas, T., Greenberg, J., Dann, R., & Wolf, A. (1982). Regional cerebral glucose metabolism in aging and senile dementia as determined by 18-deoxyglucose and positron emission tomography. In S. Hoyer (Ed.), *The aging brain: Physiological and pathophysiological aspects* (pp. 187–195). Berlin, Heidelberg, New York: Springer-Verlag.

Baron, J. C., Rougemont, D., Soussaline, F., Crowzel, C., Bousser, M. G., & Comar, D. (1983). Positron tomography investigation in humans of the local coupling among CBF, oxygen consumption, and glucose utilization. In A. Bès, E. T. MacKenzie, & J. Seylaz (Eds.), *Journal of Cerebral Blood Flow and Metabolism, 3* (Suppl. 1), S242–S243.

Benson, D. F. (1982). The use of positron emission scanning techniques in the diagnosis of Alzheimer's disease. In S. Corkin, K. L. Davis, J. H. Growdon, E. Usdin, & R. J. Wurtman (Eds.), *Alzheimer's disease: A report of progress in research* (*Aging*, Vol. 19) (pp. 79–82). New York: Raven Press.

Birren, J. E., Botwinick, J., Weiss, A. D., & Morrisson, D. F. (1963). Interrelations of mental and perceptual tests given to healthy men. In J. E. Birren (Ed.), *Human aging* (pp. 143–156). Washington, DC: U.S. Dept. of Health, Education and Welfare.

Bowen, D. M., Smith, C. B., White, P., Goodhardt, M. J., Spillane, J. A., Fluck, R. H., & Davison, A. N. (1977). Chemical pathology of the organic dementias. I. Validity of biochemical measurements on human postmorten brain specimens. *Brain, 100,* 397–426.

Bowen, D. M., Sims, N. R., Benton, S., Hean, E. A., Smith, C. C. T., Neary, D., Thomas, D. J., & Davison, A. N. (1982). Biochemical changes in cortical brain biopsies from demented patients in relation to morphological findings and pathogenesis. In S. Corkin, K. L. Davis, J. H. Growdon, E. Usdin, & R. J. Wurtman (Eds.), *Alzheimer's disease: A report of progress in research* (*Aging,* Vol. 19) (pp. 1–8). New York: Raven Press.

Bustany, P., Sargent, T., Saudubray, J. M., Henry, J. F., & Comar, D. (1981). Regional human brain uptake and protein incorporation of 11-c-1-methionine studied in vivo with PET. In M. E. Raichle, R. L Grubb, Jr., & M. M. TerPogossian (Eds.), *Journal of Cerebral Blood Flow and Metabolism, 1* (Suppl. 1), S17–S18.

Butler, R. N. (1982). *Alzheimer's disease: Priorities for the future.* In S. Corkin, K. L. Davis, J. H. Growdon, E. Usdin, & R. J. Wurtman (Eds.), *Alzheimer's disease: A report of progress in research* (*Aging,* Vol. 19) (Foreword). New York: Raven Press.

Dastur, D. K., Lane, M. H., Hansen, D. B., Kety, S. S., Butler, R. N., Perlin, S., & Sokoloff, L. (1963). Effects of aging on cerebral circulation and metabolism in man. In J. E. Birren (Ed.), *Human aging* (pp. 59–78). Washington, DC: U.S. Dept. of Health, Education and Welfare.

Dekoninck, W. J., Collard, M., & Jacquy, J. (1975). Comparative study of cerebral vasoactivity in vascular sclerosis of the brain in elderly men. *Stroke, 6,* 673–677.

Dekoninck, W. J., Jacquy, J., Jocquet, Ph., & Noel, G. (1977a). Cerebral blood flow and metabolism in senile dementia. In J. S. Meyer, H. Lechman, & M. Reivich (Eds.), *Cerebral vascular disease* (pp. 29–32). Amsterdam, Oxford: Excerpta Medica.

Dekoninck, W. J., Calay, R., & Hongne, J. C. (1977b). Cerebral blood flow in elderly with chronic cerebral involvement. *Acta Neurol. Scand., 56*(Suppl. 64), 412.

Dekoninck, W. J., Jacquy, J., Jocquet, Ph., Gerebtzoff, A., & Noel, G. (1980a). Uptake and release of amino acids in the senile brain. In D. G. Stein (Ed.), *The psychobiology of aging: Problems and perspectives* (pp. 319–329). New York, Oxford, Amsterdam: Elsevier North Holland.

Dekoninck, W. J., Jacquy, J., Gerebtzoff, A., & Collard, M. (1980b). Le débit sanguin cérébral régional chez le vieillard normal âgé de 80 ans et plus. In A. Bès & G. Géraud (Eds.), *Circulation Cérébrale* (pp. 263–265). Ann. Congrès International de Circulation Cérébrale de Toulouse, Septembre, 1979.

de Leon, M. J., Ferris, S. H., George, A. E., et al. (1983). Regional correlation of PET and CT in senile dementia of the Alzheimer's type. *Am. J. Neuroradiol., 4,* 553–556.

Duara, R., Sokoloff, L., Weingartner, H., Kessler, R. M., & Rapoport, S. I. (1983). Cerebral glucose utilization as measured with positron emission tomography in 21 resting healthy men between the ages of 21 and 83 years. *Brain, 106,* 761–775.

Frackowiak, R. S. J., Lenzi, G. L., Jones, T., H. & Heather, J. D. (1980). Quantitative measurement of regional cerebral blood flow and oxygen metabolism in man using 0–15 and positron emission tomography: theory, procedure and normal values. *J. Comput. Assist. Tomogr., 4,* 727–736.

Frackowiak, R. S. J., Pozzilli, C., Legg, N. J., DuBoulay, G. H., Marshall, J., Lenzi, G. L., & Jones, T. (1981). A prospective study of regional cerebral blood flow and oxygen utilization in dementia using positron emission tomography and oxygen-15. In M. E. Raichle, R. L. Grubb, Jr., & M. M. Ter-Pogossian (Eds.), *Journal of Cerebral Blood Flow and Metabolism, 1* (Suppl. 1), S453–S454.

Friedland, R. P., Budinger, T. F., Yano, Y., Huesman, R. H., Knittel, B., Derenzo, S. E., Koss, B., & Ober, B. A. (1983). Regional cerebral metabolic alterations in Alzheimer-type dementia: kinetic studies with 18-flourodeoxyglucose. In A. Bès, E. T. MacKenzie, & J. Seylaz (Eds.), *Journal of Cerebral Blood Flow and Metabolism, 3* (Suppl. 1), S510–S511.

Gustafson, L. (1975). Psychiatric symptoms in dementia with onset in the presenile period. *Acta Psychiatr. Scand.* (Suppl. 257), 9–35.

Haas, G. R. (1977). Diseases presenting as dementia. In C. E. Wells (Ed.), *Dementia* (2nd ed.) (pp. 27–67).

Hachinski, V. C., Yliff, D., Zilhka, E., DuBoulay, G. H., MacAllister, V. L., Marshall, J., Russel, R. W. R., & Symon, L. (1975). Cerebral blood flow in dementia. *Arch. Neurol., 32,* 632–637.

Hagber, B., & Ingvar, D. H. (1976). Cognitive reduction in presenile dementia related to regional abnormalities of the cerebral blood flow. *Br. J. Psychiatry, 128,* 219–222.

Hoyer, S. (1969). Cerebral blood flow and metabolism in senile dementia. In M. Brock, C. Fieschi, D. H. Ingvar, N. A. Lassen, & K. Schürmann (Eds.), *Cerebral blood flow* (pp. 235–236). Berlin, Heidelberg, New York: Springer-Verlag.

Huang, S. C., Phelps, M. E., Hoffman, E. J., Sideris, K., Selin, C., & Kuhl, D. E. (1980). Noninvasive determination of local cerebral metabolic rate of glucose in man. *Am. J. Physiol., 238,* E69–E82.

Ingvar, D. H., Risberg, J., & Schwartz, M. S. (1975). Evidence of subnormal function of association cortex in presenile dementia. *Neurology, 10,* 964–974.

Iwangoff, P., Reichlmeier, K., Enz, A., & Meier-Ruge, W. (1979). Neurochemical findings in physiological aging of the brain. In W. Meier-Ruge (Ed.), *Central nervous system aging and its neuropharmacology* (pp. 13–33). Basel, New York: Karger.

Kety, S. S., & Schmidt, C. F. (1945). The determination of cerebral blood flow in man by use of nitrous oxide in low concentrations. *Am. J. Physiol., 143,* 53–66.

Kety, S. S. (1956). Human cerebral blood flow and oxygen consumption as related to aging. *Res. Publ. Assoc. Res. Nerv. Ment. Dis., 35,* 31–45.

Kuhl, D. E., Metter, E. J., Riegl, W. H., & Phelps, M. E. (1982). Effects of human aging on patterns of local cerebral glucose utilization determined by 18-F-fluorodeoxyglucose method. *Journal of Cerebral Blood Flow and Metabolism, 2,* 163–171.

Kuhl, D. E., Metter, E. J., Riegl, W. H., Hawkins, R. A., Mazziotta, J. C., Phelps, M. E., & Kling, A. S. (1983). Local cerebral glucose utilization in elderly patients with depression, multiple infarct dementia, and Alzheimer's disease. In A. Bès, E. T. MacKenzie, & J. Seylaz (Eds.), *Journal of Cerebral Blood Flow and Metabolism, 3* (Suppl. 1), S494–S495.

Lammertsma, R. S., Frackowiak, R. S. J., Lenzi, G. L., Heather, J. D., Pozzili, C., & Jones, T. (1981). Accuracy of the oxygen-15 steady state technique for measuring rCBF and rCMRO$_2$: tracer modelling, statistics and special sampling. In M. E. Reichle, R. L. Grubb, Jr., & M. M. Ter-Pogossian (Eds.), *Journal of Cerebral Blood Flow and Metabolism, 1* (Suppl. 1), S3–S4.

Lassen, N. A. (1959). Cerebral blood flow and oxygen consumption in man. *Physiol. Rev., 39,* 183–238.

Lassen, N. A., & Ingvar, D. H. (1972). Radioisotopic assessment of regional cerebral blood flow. *Prog. Nucl. Med., 1,* 376–409.

Lassen, N. A., Roland, P. E., Larsen, B., Metamed, E., & Soh, K. (1977). Mapping of human cerebral functions: A study of the regional CBF pattern during rest, its reproducibility and the activations seen during basic sensory and motor functions. In D. H. Ingvar & N. A. Lassen (Eds.), *Cerebral function, metabolism and circulation* (pp. 262–263). [*Acta Neurol. Scand.* 56, (Suppl. 64).] Copenhagen: Munksgaard.

Lassen, N. A., & Ingvar, D. H. (1980). Blood flow studies in the aging normal brain and in senile dementia. In L. Amaducci, A. N. Davison, & P. Antuono (Eds.), *Aging of the brain and dementia (Aging,* Vol. 13) (pp. 91–98). New York: Raven Press.

Lenzi, G. L., & Jones, T. (1980). Cerebral metabolism-to-blood flow relationships with respect to aging and dementia. In L. Amaducci, A. N. Davison, & P. Antuono (Eds.), *Aging of the brain and dementia (Aging,* Vol. 13) (pp. 99–102). New York: Raven Press.

Metter, E. J., Riege, W. H., Kuhl, D. E., & Phelps, P. E. (1983). Differences in regional glucose metabolic intercorrelations with aging. In A. Bès, E. T. MacKenzie, & J. Seylaz (Eds.), *Journal of Cerebral Blood Flow and Metabolism, 3* (Suppl. 1), S482–S483.

Meyer, J. S. (1980). Effects of normal aging versus disease on cerebral vasomotor responsiveness. In A. Bès & G. Géraud (Eds.), *Cerebral circulation and neurotransmitters* (pp. 133–138). Amsterdam, Oxford, Princeton: Excerpta Medica.

Meyer, J. S., Shaw, T. G., Okayasu, H., & Tachibana, H. (1983). Multi-infarcts and Alzheimer dementias differentiated from normal aging by Xenon contrast CT-CBF measurements. In A. Bès, E. T. McKenzie, & J. Seylaz (Eds.), *Journal of Cerebral Blood Flow and Metabolism, 3* (Suppl. 1), S506–S507.

Miyazaki, T., Tezuka, H., Kasahara, N., Kitamura, S., Goto, T., Miura, T., Ujike, T., Kato, T., Imazu, O., Kuroki, S., Chiba, T., & Terashi, A. (1983). Cerebral blood flow and mental function in dementia. In A. Bès, E. T. McKenzie, & J. Seylaz (Eds.), *Journal of Cerebral Blood Flow and Metabolism, 3* (Suppl. 1), S514–S515.

Obrist, W. D. (1963). The electroencephalogram of healthy aged males. In J. E. Birren (Ed.), *Human aging* (pp. 79–96). Washington, DC: U.S. Dept. of Health, Education and Welfare.

Obrist, W. D., & Wilkinson, W. E. (1980). The non-invasive Xenon-133 method: Evaluation of CBF indices. In A. Bès & G. Géraud (Eds.), *Cerebral circulation and neurotransmitters* (pp. 119–124). Amsterdam, Oxford, Princeton: Excerpta Medica.

Phelps, M. E., Hoffman, E. J., Mullani, N. A., & Ter-Pogossian, M. M. (1975). Application of annihilation coincidence detection to transaxial reconstruction tomography. *J. Nucl. Med., 16,* 210–224.
Phelps, M. E., Hoffman, E. J., Huang, S. C., & Kuhl, D. E. (1978). A new computerized tomographic imaging system for positron-emitting radiopharmaceuticals. *J. Nucl. Med., 19,* 635–647.
Phelps, M. E., Huang, S. C., Hoffman, E. J., Selin, C., Sokoloff, L., & Kuhl, D. E. (1979). Tomographic measurement of local cerebral glucose metabolic rate in humans with (F-18) 2-fluoro-2-deoxy-D-glucose: Validation of method. *Ann. Neurol., 6,* 371–388.
Rapoport, S. I., Duara, R., London, E. D., Margolin, R. A., Schwartz, M., Cutler, N. R., Partanen, M., & Shinowara, N. (1983). Glucose metabolism of the aging nervous system. In D. Samuel, S. Algeri, S. Gershon, V. E. Grimm, & S. Toffano (Eds.), *Aging of the brain (Aging,* Vol. 22) (pp. 111–121). New York: Raven Press.
Reisberg, B., Ferris, S. H., de Leon, M. J., et al. (1982). The global deterioration scale (GDS): An instrument for the assessment of primary degenerative dementia. *Am. J. Psychiatry, 139,* 1136–1139.
Reisberg, B., Ferris, S., deLeon, M. J., & Crook, T. (1985). Age-associated cognitive decline and Alzheimer's disease: Implications for assessment and treatment. In M. Bergener, M. Ermini, and H. B. Stähelin (Eds.), *Thresholds in aging: The 1984 Sandoz lectures in gerontology* (pp. 255–292). London: Academic Press.
Reisberg, B., Schulman, E., Ferris, S. H., et al. (1983). Clinical assessments of age-associated cognitive decline and primary degenerative dementia: Prognostic concomitant. *Psychopharmacol. Bull., 19,* 734–739.
Reivich, M., Obrist, W., Slater, R., Greenberg, J., & Goldberg, H. I. (1975). A comparison of the Xenon-133 intracarotid injection and inhalation techniques for measuring regional cerebral blood flow. In A. M. Harper, W. B. Jennett, J. D. Miller, & J. O. Rowan (Eds.), *Blood flow and metabolism in the brain* (pp. 8.3–8.6). Edinburgh, London, New York: Churchill Livingstone.
Risberg, J. (1980). Cerebral blood flow measurement by Xenon-133 inhalation. Validity and clinical applications in psychiatry. In A. Bès & G. Géraud (Eds.), *Cerebral circulation and neurotransmitters* (pp. 125–131). Amsterdam, Oxford, Princeton: Excerpta Medica.
Risberg, J., Johanson, M., Gustafson, L., & Brun, A. (1983). Differential diagnosis of dementia by rCBF and psychometric methods. In A. Bès, E. T. McKenzie, & J. Seylaz (Eds.), *Journal of Cerebral Blood Flow and Metabolism, 3* (Suppl. 1), S496–S497.
Rottenberg, D. A., Lu, H. C., Thaler, H. T., & Kearfott, K. (1981). The measurement of regional CBF using CT and stable Xenon. In M. E. Raichle, R. L. Grubb, Jr., & M. M. Ter-Pogossian (Eds.), *Journal of Cerebral Blood Flow and Metabolism, 1* (Suppl. 1), S27–S28.
Sakai, F., Gotoh, F., Ebihara, S., Kitagawa, Y., Hata, T., Takagi, Y., & Komagamine, M. (1981). Xenon enhanced CT method for the measurement of local CBF in man. In M. E. Raichle, R. L. Grubb, Jr., & M. M. Ter-Pogossian (Eds.), *Journal of Cerebral Blood Flow and Metabolism, 1* (Suppl. 1), S29–S30.
Sokoloff, L. (1975). Cerebral circulation and metabolism in the aged. In S. Gershon & A. Raskin (Eds.), *Genesis and treatment of psychological disorders in the elderly (Aging,* Vol. 2) (pp. 45–54). New York: Raven Press.
Strandgaard, S., MacKenzie, E. T., Sengupta, D., Rowan, J. O., Lassen, N. A., & Harper, A. M. (1974). Upper limit of autoregulation of CBF in the baboon. *Circ. Res., 34,* 435–440.

Ter-Pogossian, M. M., Raichle, M. E., & Ficke, D. C. (1981). Dynamic positron emission tomography of the brain. In M. E. Raichle, R. L. Grubb, Jr., & M. M. Ter-Pogossian (Eds.), *Journal of Cerebral Blood Flow and Metabolism, 1* (Suppl. 1), S1–S2.

Tomlinson, B. E. (1973). Morphological changes and dementia in old age. In W. L. Smith & N. Kinsbourne (Eds.), *Aging and dementia* (pp. 25–26). New York: Spectrum.

Yesavage, J. (1979). Dementia: Differential diagnosis and treatment. *Geriatrics, 34,* 51–59.

Zemcov, A., Barclay, L., Vitale, V., & Blass, J. (1983). Measurement of CBF in the diagnosis of dementias. In A. Bès, E. T. McKenzie, & J. Seylaz (Eds.), *Journal of Cerebral Blood Flow and Metabolism, 3* (Suppl. 1), S512–S513.

9
Noninvasive Diagnostic Techniques to Study Age-Related Cerebral Disorders

Steven B. Waller and Edythe D. London

Human senescence is characterized by a progressive and cumulative deterioration in the vitality of body tissues and their associated functions. Although some age-related physiological and biochemical changes are considered normal, senescence is associated with an increased frequency of certain pathological conditions, including Parkinson's disease and senile dementia of the Alzheimer type (Alzheimer's disease).

Traditionally, the study of human brain aging has focused on cataloging structural and biochemical changes, which have been assessed postmortem. These studies have demonstrated that senescence of the human brain is associated with decrements in brain weight and volume (Blinkov & Glezer, 1968), a tendency for increased variability in ventricular size (Last & Tompsett, 1953; Blinkov & Glezer, 1968), accumulation of pigments such as lipofuscin (Riese, 1946), neuronal loss (Brody, 1955), and dendritic atrophy (Brizzee, 1981). However, these findings need not have a direct bearing on cerebral function prior to death.

Because a critical review and commentary on each approach used to study human brain aging is beyond the scope of this chapter, this review has been limited to noninvasive investigative approaches used in living subjects to provide information regarding cerebral function as related to senescence or pathology. These techniques include the assay of chemical markers in samples of cerebrospinal fluid (CSF) and blood, and cerebral imaging techniques.

PROBLEMS IN DIAGNOSIS OF AGE-RELATED CEREBRAL DISORDERS

An increasing mass of data indicates that specific neurochemical changes in the aging brain may adversely affect performance. The associations between neurochemistry and performance largely reflect correlations between premortem clinical evaluations and postmortem neurochemical studies. For example, the role of nigrostriatal dopaminergic deficits in the pathophysiology and extrapyramidal symptoms in parkinsonism (Bernheimer et al., 1973) has been established largely by the postmortem findings of a major loss of nigrostriatal dopamine neurons (Hornykiewicz, 1966; Lloyd et al., 1975), associated with striatal decreases in dopamine, its major metabolite homovanillic acid, and its synthetic enzyme L-dopa decarboxylase (Bernheimer et al., 1973; Lloyd et al., 1975). The brains of subjects who died with Alzheimer's disease, manifested mainly by progressive dementia, have marked reductions of choline acetyltransferase, the enzyme which catalyzes acetylcholine biosynthesis, in the neocortex and hippocampus (Bowen et al., 1976; Davies & Maloney, 1976; Perry et al., 1977; White et al., 1977; Davies, 1979; Rossor et al., 1980).

However, despite knowledge about the changes in brain chemistry that occur in age-related diseases, means of accurate and reliable diagnosis are often lacking. This situation is quite evident in the case of Alzheimer's disease, where a definitive diagnosis requires direct examination of brain tissue, obtained during brain biopsy or autopsy, and demonstration of the characteristic pathologic findings (i.e., neurofibrillary tangles, neuritic plaques, and granulovacuolar degeneration) (McKhann et al., 1984). The clinical diagnosis of Alzheimer's disease is made by exclusion of other syndromes that exhibit some similar symptoms. This exclusion procedure often entails extensive review of the patient's history, an exhaustive physical examination, and a thorough psychological evaluation of the patient. Syndromes easily confused with Alzheimer's dementia include delirium, simple memory loss, multiinfarct dementia, focal neurological disease, depression, normal pressure hydrocephalus, and Creutzfeldt-Jakob disease (Kerzner, 1984). The need for better and more specific diagnostic procedures is apparent, as 20% or more of cases with a clinical diagnosis of Alzheimer's disease are found at autopsy to have been misdiagnosed (McKhann et al., 1984). These cases might have benefited from appropriate therapeutic measures, had the correct diagnosis been made.

NEUROCHEMICAL MARKERS IN CSF AND BLOOD AS INDICES OF ALTERED BRAIN FUNCTION

Considerable attention recently has been directed at determining the diagnostic value of the CSF and blood in indexing the physiological, biochemical, and functional status of the brain. These body fluids have been used because they are obtained easily and come in very close contact with the tissues of the central nervous system. As such, substances carried within these fluids may reflect the cerebral environment and serve as markers for disturbed brain function. CSF is the more suitable of the fluids, as it bathes the central nervous system continually and is not likely to be contaminated with substances of peripheral origin; whereas, blood is circulated throughout the body, with each peripheral site a potential source of contamination.

Recent research that relates CSF- and blood-borne substances to central nervous system neurotransmission has involved patients diagnosed as having Alzheimer's disease. Presumably, these studies were initiated to duplicate the success of CSF studies in Parkinson's disease. The motor impairments of Parkinson's disease are related to dopaminergic deficiencies in the nigrostriatal system. This deficiency is reflected by low CSF levels of homovanillic acid (Bernheimer et al., 1966), negatively correlated with the akinesia of Parkinson's disease (Rinne & Soininen, 1972; Korf et al., 1974). What follows is an overview on research directed at identifying markers in CSF and blood elements which can be related to the disturbed brain function of Alzheimer's disease.

The most consistent neurochemical finding in Alzheimer's disease has been a reduction in the specific activity of choline acetyltransferase in various brain regions (Bowen et al., 1976; Davies & Maloney, 1976; Perry et al., 1977; Davies, 1979). Choline acetyltransferase is found exclusively in cholinergic neurons (Kuhar, 1976), and its loss is thought to reflect a decrease in cholinergic innervation (Whitehouse et al., 1981). In contrast, cholinesterase catalyzes the enzymatic degradation of acetylcholine and, unlike choline acetyltransferase, it is not a reliable marker of cholinergic neurons, as it is found in regions relatively devoid of cholinergic innervation (Silver, 1974). Nonetheless, abnormalities in cerebral specific activities of cholinesterase follow closely the changes in choline acetyltransferase activity (Davies & Maloney, 1976; Op den Velde & Stam, 1976; Perry et al., 1978; Davies, 1979; Henke & Lange, 1983). Two isozymes of cholinesterase are present in the body, and can be distinguished on the basis of substrate preference for acetylcholine ("true" acetylcholinesterase) or other substrates ("pseudo" or butyrylcholinesterase). Significant reductions in acetylcholinesterase activity and increases in butyrylcholinesterases have been observed in samples of the hippocampus and temporal cortex from patients who died with Alzheimer's disease, as compared with samples from control brains.

In the blood, acetylcholinesterase is the predominant cholinesterase isozyme found in red blood cells, and pseudocholinesterase the predominant isozyme in the plasma (Garry & Routh, 1965). Several studies have dealt with the activities of cholinesterase isozymes in the blood of patients with Alzheimer's disease. All reports to date have noted decreased red blood cell acetylcholinesterase activity in Alzheimer's disease (Chipperfield et al., 1981; Perry et al., 1982; Smith et al., 1982). While this finding approximates the previously reported change in brain acetylcholinesterase activity, the utility of blood acetylcholinesterase activity as a screen for Alzheimer's disease is limited, as similar changes in red blood cell acetylcholinesterase activity have been reported in other disorders such as depression, which are often misdiagnosed as Alzheimer's dementia (Milstoc et al., 1975; Perry et al., 1982). However, Perry et al. (1982) reported that plasma acetylcholinesterase activity is reduced in Alzheimer's disease, but is unchanged in plasma from depressed patients. This finding suggests that measurements of both red blood cell and plasma acetylcholinesterase activity may be of value as markers for Alzheimer's disease. Reports of plasma pseudocholinesterase activity have been less consistent, as Perry et al. (1982) reported no change, and Smith et al. (1982) reported a 101% greater activity in the plasma of Alzheimer's patients compared to controls.

In human CSF, acetylcholinesterase is the predominant cholinesterase isozyme (Johnson & Domino, 1971; Davies, 1979; Scarsella et al., 1979; Deutsch et al., 1983) and is thought to derive exclusively from within the central nervous system (Yaksh et al., 1975; Bareggi & Giacobini, 1978). Moreover, the secretion of cholinesterases into the CSF reflects the functional activity of discrete populations of central neurons. For example, Greenfield and co-workers (1979, 1980) reported that electrical stimulation of brain regions such as the caudate nucleus, substantia nigra or lateral hypothalamus resulted in higher CSF acetylcholinesterase activity. Therefore, there seems to be a justification for measuring CSF acetylcholinesterase activity as a marker for disturbed cholinergic neuronal activity.

Davies (1979) and Wood et al. (1982) observed no differences in the activities of cholinesterases, expressed per CSF volume, in samples taken from patients with Alzheimer's dementia, as compared with samples from age-matched control subjects. In contrast, Deutsch et al. (1983) and Soininen et al. (1981a, 1984) found that acetylcholinesterase activity, expressed per CSF volume, was significantly lower in the Alzheimer's group compared to the control group. Furthermore, Soininen et al. (1984) determined that acetylcholinesterase activity, expressed per CSF volume was positively correlated with a battery of psychological test scores used to measure the severity of the dementia. However, when cholinesterase activity was expressed per mg CSF protein, the differences between the Alzheimer's and control groups became nonsignificant (Soininen et al., 1981a; Deutsch et al., 1983); and age was positively correlated with CSF protein and acetylcholinesterase activity (expressed per CSF volume) and not with diagnosis (Deutsch et al., 1983). Considered together, these findings suggest that CSF acetylcholinesterase activity may not be a specific or useful biochemical marker of disturbed central cholinergic neurotransmission in Alzheimer's disease.

Davis et al. (1982) measured the acetylcholine and choline content of CSF from patients with Alzheimer's disease, and related these levels to the severity of dementia. Although the reported levels of these substances approximated those reported by Welch et al. (1976) for normal individuals, CSF acetylcholine levels in the dements were correlated significantly with scores on a memory impairment test, such that a low acetylcholine concentration correlated with a severe dementia score. Choline levels were not related significantly with dementia scores.

While the decline in choline acetyltransferase in Alzheimer's diseased brains supports a cholinergic defect, numerous less striking changes have been noted in other neurotransmitter systems; these include decrements in L-glutamic acid decarboxylase, which catalyzes γ-aminobutyric acid (GABA) biosynthesis, and L-dopa-decarboxylase in various brain regions (Bowen et al., 1974; Davies, 1979), and reduced cortical levels of norepinephrine, GABA, and somatostatin (Rossor et al., 1984). As was the case with the cholinergic system, extensive research has been performed to determine if peripheral markers of these systems might be used as diagnostic indices for Alzheimer's disease.

Dopamine-β-hydroxylase, the enzyme that catalyzes the conversion of dopamine to norepinephrine, is released from noradrenergic nerve endings together with norepinephrine during neurotransmission. As such, its presence in serum and CSF may reflect levels of noradrenergic neurotransmission in the peripheral and central nervous systems, respectively (North & Mulrow, 1976; Miyata et al., 1984). Miyata et al. (1984) reported that serum dopamine-β-hydroxylase activity increased between the third and eighth decade, but decreased thereafter; and no age difference was noted in CSF dopamine-β-hydroxylase activity. They also noted that dopamine-β-hydroxylase activity was significantly lower in serum samples from patients diagnosed as having Alzheimer's disease compared with the activity measured in samples from multiinfarct dementia or control subjects. Dopamine-β-hydroxylase activity also was significantly lower in the CSF of patients with Alzheimer's dementia than in samples from age-matched controls, whereas in samples from multiinfarct dementia patients, it was not significantly different from either Alzheimer's dementia or control values.

These findings support central and peripheral involvements of noradrenergic neurons in the neuropathology of Alzheimer's dementia.

The decrease in serum and CSF dopamine-β-hydroxylase activities in Alzheimer's disease patients compared to age-matched controls would suggest reduced levels of norepinephrine synthesis and, perhaps, neurotransmission. This conclusion opposes the one reached by Raskind et al. (1984), who reported higher norepinephrine and 3-methoxy-4- hydroxy-phenylglycol levels in the plasma and CSF of patients with severe Alzheimer's dementia compared with the values in moderate Alzheimer's dementia and control subjects, which did not differ significantly from one another. As 3-methoxy-4-hydroxyphenylglycol is the major metabolite of central norepinephrine, this finding suggests enhanced central and peripheral noradrenergic neurotransmission in patients with severe Alzheimer's disease. Earlier studies measuring 3-methoxy-4- hydroxy-phenylglycol in the CSF of patients with Alzheimer's disease and nondemented controls revealed no significant differences between the two groups (Mann et al., 1981; Wood et al., 1982). According to Raskind et al. (1984), discrepancies between their study and earlier work may reflect differences in the severity of Alzheimer's dementia. Nonetheless, further studies are needed to delineate the role of noradrenergic neuronal systems in Alzheimer's disease.

Homovanillic acid, the principal metabolite of dopamine, and 5-hydroxyindoleacetic acid, the principal serotonin metabolite, also have been studied in the CSF of Alzheimer's patients, with greatly conflicting results. In general, studies with moderately severe Alzheimer's dementia patients yielded little or no change in the CSF levels of either metabolite compared to age-matched normal subjects (Parkes et al., 1974; Mann et al., 1981; Bowen et al., 1982; Direnfeld, 1983). Davis et al. (1982) found no relation between CSF levels of either metabolite and the severity of dementia in Alzheimer's patients. Although this study included no normal volunteers, the CSF levels of both metabolites in demented patients approximated previously reported control values. However, studies that included a severely demented Alzheimer's group reported a significant reduction in homovanillic acid and/or 5-hydroxyindoleacetic acid levels in CSF samples from the severely demented group compared to levels in samples from less demented or normal patients (Gottfries et al., 1969; Soininen et al., 1981b; Bucht et al., 1984). As changes in homovanillic acid and 5-hydroxyindoleacetic acid reflect altered dopaminergic and serotonergic neurotransmission, respectively, these findings are consistent with the hypothesis that patients with advanced Alzheimer's dementia, in which dopaminergic or serotonergic lesions are not part of the primary pathological process, have additional neurochemical pathology. In this regard, dementia often accompanies Parkinson's disease (Pollock, 1966), although it does not represent the primary disorder.

Taking into account the normal age-related decrease (Hare et al., 1982), CSF GABA levels are significantly reduced in samples obtained from Alzheimer's dementia patients (Enna et al., 1977; Manyam et al., 1980). While this finding may suggest a central defect of GABA systems, it is not characteristic of Alzheimer's dementia; similar changes also have been reported in Huntington's chorea (Enna et al., 1977), Parkinson's disease (Lakke & Teelken, 1976; Manyam et al., 1980), and other disease processes characterized by local atrophy (Lakke & Teelken, 1976; Manyam et al., 1980). Further studies are needed to determine what the decrements in CSF GABA levels represent in Alzheimer's disease and how they relate to the clinical state.

Oram et al. (1981) and Wood et al. (1982) found reduced levels of somatostatin in CSF from a small group of Alzheimer's dementia and mixed dementia patients compared to age-matched, nondemented subjects. Soininen et al. (1984) confirmed these findings in a larger sample and determined that CSF somatostatin-like immunoreactivity was correlated with the severity of dementia, as measured by a battery of psychological tests. The correlation was such that the lowest CSF somatostatin-like immunoreactivity was associated with the most severe dementia. However, as the authors pointed out, reduced CSF somatostatin levels are not specific to Alzheimer's dementia. They have been reported in Parkinson's disease (Dupont et al., 1982), multiple sclerosis (Sorenson et al., 1980), and Huntington's chorea (Cramer et al., 1981). Levels of other neuropeptides such as hypothalamic thyrotropin-releasing hormone and gonadotropin-releasing hormone, were significantly lower in the CSF of patients with Alzheimer's disease than in age-matched control subjects (Wood et al., 1982). However, the lack of knowledge regarding the role of these neuropeptidergic systems in brain function leaves the significance of this finding as yet to be determined.

Serum somatomedins—hormones that are thought to act as growth and maintenance factors for nervous tissue (Sara et al., 1981) and for which receptors are found throughout the brain (Sara et al., 1980)—decline with age in normal subjects, but are elevated in patients diagnosed as having Alzheimer's disease (Sara et al., 1982). Preliminary evidence suggests that CSF levels of somatomedins also are elevated in Alzheimer's disease compared to those of normal subjects (Sara et al., 1982). In light of the postulated anabolic role of somatomedins, the elevated serum and CSF levels of these substances in patients with Alzheimer's disease may represent an ineffective compensatory mechanism to overcome the degenerative processes characteristic of Alzheimer's disease.

There also is considerable evidence for disturbed immunological function in Alzheimer's disease. Nandy (1978) reported significantly elevated levels of brain-reactive antibodies in serum taken from Alzheimer's disease patients compared to age-matched control subjects. In normal individuals, serum IgG levels decrease with age until the sixth or seventh decade of life, after which they tend to increase (Buckley & Dorsey, 1971). However, unlike normal aging, dementia is associated with serum IgG levels that decrease with age (Cohen et al., 1980). The decline in disease-elevated serum levels of IgG also is correlated positively with scores on tests of cognitive status (Cohen et al., 1980). The early elevation of IgG levels in the serum of patients diagnosed as having Alzheimer's disease was interpreted as evidence of a heightened immune response to accelerated somatic changes, whereas, the subsequent decline in IgG levels was thought to represent progressive immunoincompetence, often observed in the latter stages of Alzheimer's disease. However, the elevation of IgG levels with the subsequent decline is not a consistent finding in all Alzheimer's patients (Matsuyama & Fu, 1983), and probably is characteristic of a subpopulation of patients with the disease.

Experiments by Matsuyama and co-workers (Jarvik et al., 1982; Matsuyama & Fu, 1983) demonstrated that the philothermal response of polymorphonuclear leukocytes (the tendency of polymorphonuclear leukocytes to migrate along a temperature gradient to a warmer environment) was dramatically different in patients diagnosed as having Alzheimer's disease as compared to age- and sex-matched normal individuals. Although the number of polymorphonuclear leukocytes that migrated was not different, polymorphonuclear leukocytes from patients with Alzheimer's disease did not migrate as far as those of normal subjects. The philothermal response of polymorphonuclear leukocytes also was determined in three patients diagnosed as having multi-infarct dementia and seven individuals suffering from depression (Jarvik et al., 1982). With the exception of one depressed patient, all multiinfarct and depressed patients demonstrated a normal philothermal response profile. The one exception had a profile similar to that observed in Alzheimer's disease. The disturbed philothermal response profile of polymorphonuclear leukocytes from Alzheimer's disease patients appears to result from a serum-borne factor (Matsuyama & Fu, 1983). This conclusion is supported by the finding of a disturbed migratory response profile exhibited by polymorphonuclear leukocytes obtained from normal individuals, but incubated in sera from Alzheimer's disease patients (Matsuyama & Fu, 1983). Although all Alzheimer's patients in these studies were receiving medication at the time of the test, it seems unlikely that the altered polymorphonuclear leukocyte philothermal response reflected a drug effect, as no single class or type of drug was common to the test subjects (Matsuyama & Fu, 1983). Nonetheless, a generalized drug effect cannot be discounted; and additional tests are warranted to verify the specificity of the altered philothermal response for Alzheimer's disease and to relate this abnormal response profile to the pathogenesis of the disease.

DIRECT STUDY OF THE BRAIN THROUGH CEREBRAL IMAGING TECHNIQUES

Although substances in CSF, blood, and even urine have been used as valuable indicators of cerebral function, they are far removed and diluted from the primary area of interest. Recent developments in tomographic technology have allowed noninvasive study of the living brain in various normal and pathological states. X-ray transmission tomography (computed tomography, CT) scans have provided measures of ventricular size and sulcal atrophy, which have been studied in relation to the major psychoses as well as aging and dementia. Nuclear magnetic resonance (NMR) images provide higher structural resolution without exposure to x-rays, and can be used for similar analyses.

Positron emission tomography (PET) is a computer-assisted nuclear medicine approach that utilizes the mathematics of CT scanning to produce tomographs of radioisotope location. Positron emitting isotopes, such as ^{11}C and ^{18}F have been attached to glucose, amino acids, and specific receptor ligands to produce cerebral metabolic and receptor maps *in vivo*.

This portion of the chapter deals with how cerebral imaging techniques have been used to reveal structural and functional alterations in normal aging and dementia. In some cases, correlations with performance in neuropsychological tests may reveal anatomical sites important in age-related functional impairments.

CT and NMR Studies of Normal Aging and Dementia

Pathological studies of the human brain have suggested that age per se induces cerebral atrophy (Brizzee, 1981). Gross pathological evaluations of patients with Alzheimer's disease have demonstrated shrinkage of the cerebral convolutions, widened cerebral sulci, and ventricular dilatation (Tomlinson et al., 1970; Corsellis, 1976). Although the brains of patients with dementia show more atrophy than tissue from nondemented age-matched persons, there is substantial overlap (Tomlinson et al., 1970). This overlap predicts that studies of brain structure would not be useful in the diagnosis of dementia. However, since the clinical introduction of CT (Ambrose, 1973), numerous investigators have applied CT to the study of normal aging and dementia. Initially, the studies mainly involved measures of ventricular size and sulcal width. More recently, they were extended to brain parenchyma (see review by de Leon & George, 1983).

Generally, CT studies of people in different age groups have shown ventricular dilatation with age, although the magnitude of the measured differences range from striking (Barron et al., 1976) to nonsignificant tendency (Haug, 1977). Glydensted and Kosteljanetz (1976) found significant age correlations for linear measures of the lateral ventricles and the third ventricle, which increased in size with advancing age. In another study using linear measures, the transverse diameter of the frontal horns and the bicaudate diameter increased with age (Hahn & Rim, 1976). In still another study, the area of the lateral ventricles and linear measures of the transverse diameter of the frontal horns, the bicaudate diameter and the width of the bodies of the lateral ventricles were positively correlated with age, but these measures were not significantly related to cognitive performance (Earnest et al., 1979). Using an automated method to estimate intracranial CSF, Zatz et al. (1982) studied 123 normal subjects of various ages (23 to 88 years). Their results indicated that ventricular size remained relatively constant until 60 years of age, and then increased. This finding was consistent with results of an earlier study by Yamamura et al. (1980) on 228 hospitalized patients between the ages of 2 and 89 years, and free of severe brain disease. In this study, a measure of the brain volume was divided by the cranial cavity measure for each CT slice. These ratios were summed across all slices to yield a quantity reflecting all intracranial CSF. This quantity was found to increase during the sixth decade. Takeda and Matsuzawa (1984) measured CSF space volume above the level of the tentorium cerebelli in 483 men and 497 women ranging in age from 10 to 88 years. They reported that CSF space volume increase significantly in an exponential manner in both sexes after the third decade.

Most of the CT studies concerned with age effects on cortical sulcal width during senescence revealed increases with advancing age. Glydensted and Kosteljanetz (1976) reported a nonsignificant trend towards increased width of cortical sulci with age. In contrast, Earnest et al. (1979) found that the average width of the four largest sulci was significantly greater in a group of senescent normals (80 to 99 years) as compared with a younger elderly group (60 to 79 years). Using a four-point rating scale in subjective evaluation of the degree of sulcal prominence, Jacoby and Levy (1980) showed a significant correlation between cortical atrophy and age. Takeda and Matsuzawa (1984) used a CT-derived brain atrophy index, and noted that in Japanese men and women, brain atrophy increased exponentially after the third decade. Their results suggested that the male brain is especially susceptible to atrophy during the fourth decade, as compared with the female brain.

CT studies have demonstrated an association between cerebral atrophy and advanced age in normal persons as well as those with dementia. Jacoby (1981) noted that groups of demented patients had significantly more atrophy than controls; however, dementia occurred without atrophy, and atrophy without dementia, indicating that primary neuronal dementia cannot be diagnosed on the basis of CT alone. Nonetheless, CT as a diagnostic tool has been tested in studies correlating CT and performance measures.

Roberts and Caird (1976) found a high negative correlation between maximum ventricular area and performance on a simple test of cognitive function. Whereas de Leon et al. (1980) reported significant correlations between ventricular as well as sulcal rankings and various measures of dementia, Ford and Winter (1980) found significant correlations between dementia measures and ventricular rankings only. Jacoby and Levy (1980), who provided data that support these findings, observed a negative correlation between ventricular area and a test of cognitive function in an amalgamated group of healthy controls, depressed patients, and dements. Within the group of dements, there were only weakly significant relationships or nonsignificant trends between psychological impairment and measures of ventricular enlargement, but not of cortical atrophy. More recently, Gado et al. (1983) reported on another study suggesting that ventricular dilation might be a more useful diagnostic index than atrophy. Using normal control and age-matched subjects diagnosed as having Alzheimer's disease but living in the community, they assigned a clinical dementia rating to each subject, and rank-ordered them according to subjective impressions of ventricular or sulcal size. The CT scans from the subjects also were analyzed with linear measurements, and a ventricular score was derived as a percentage of the maximum width of the cranial cavity. The correlation between the subjective ventricular rankings and the dementia rating was highly significant ($p = 0.0001$), but the correlation between the sulcal rankings and the dementia score was less significant ($p < 0.05$). The authors suggested that better correlations were obtained with ventricles than with sulci because it is easier for the observer to correctly compare sizes of ventricular systems than to compare sulci. In comparing sulci, the observer must consider the size of each sulcus as well as the number of sulci. Nonetheless, the same group (Gado et al., 1982) reported that controlling for age, both ventricular and sulcal size correlate strongly with mild dementia (presumptive Alzheimer's disease) using volumetric measures of brain atrophy. They indicated that linear measures were not as sensitive to the presence of dementia as volumetric ones.

Despite overlapping CT findings in control and demented subjects (Jacoby & Levy, 1980; Jacoby, 1981), the study by Gado et al. (1983) suggests some diagnostic value in ventricular CT measures. Because the subjects in their study were living in the community and exhibited either no dementia or mild dementia, it appears that brain atrophy may be demonstrated by CT very early in the course of Alzheimer's disease. Another study which supports a diagnostic role for CT is that of Soininen et al. (1982). In this report, ventricular dilatation was greater in patients with Alzheimer's disease than those with multiinfarct dementia or in control subjects. The dilatation also was greater with more severe dementia. Nonetheless, one of the major limitations in the use of CT for diagnosis of dementia is the lack of diagnostic criteria (de Leon & George, 1983).

Most recently, imaging studies of dementia have involved proton NMR imaging. Besson et al. (1983) reported that spin-lattice relaxation times and proton density values permit differentiation of demented from nondemented subjects. They classed demented patients as having Alzheimer's disease or multiinfarct dementia on the basis of their scores on the Hachinski rating scale. Spin-lattice relaxation times for all white matter areas were significantly greater in both dementia groups than in controls, but there was no significant difference between Alzheimer's disease and multiinfarct dementia. Proton density values were significantly greater in Alzheimer's disease patients than in controls or those with multiinfarct dementia, although there was significant overlap. As NMR technology becomes more available, it may provide a diagnostic advantage over CT.

PET Studies of Aging and Dementia

PET requires the introduction into the body of radiopharmaceuticals labeled with positron-emitting radionuclides (i.e., ^{11}C, ^{15}O, ^{18}F). Such compounds have been used as radiotracers for regional metabolic processes, including oxygen and glucose consumption and protein synthesis, in studies of normal aging and dementia.

The development by Kety and Schmidt (1945) of the nitrous oxide technique allowed *in vivo* measurements of global cerebral blood flow and oxidative metabolism in human volunteers. Since then, numerous studies have measured these parameters as a function of age and dementia. Cerebral blood flow, usually coupled with oxidative metabolism (Kety, 1956), was reduced with age in some studies (Fazekas et al., 1952; Scheinberg et al., 1953), but not in others (Shenkin et al., 1953). Similar discrepancies were observed in studies of the cerebral metabolic rate for oxygen (CMR_{O_2}). While some studies suggested age-dependent declines (Fazekas et al., 1952; Lassen et al., 1960), others did not (Shenkin et al., 1953; Scheinberg et al., 1953).

More recently, cerebral blood flow and CMR_{O_2} have been studied using PET in combination with $C^{15}O_2$ and $^{15}O_2$ (Frackowiak et al., 1980). The methodological basis of the procedure depends upon creating a "steady-state" tracer concentration within the tissues by the continuous inhalation of $C^{15}O_2$ and $^{15}O_2$. The theoretical concepts underlying the measurements have been discussed in papers by Jones et al. (1976), Subramanyam et al. (1978), and Lenzi et al. (1978).

Using the ^{15}O steady-state technique, Frackowiak and Gibbs (1983) found that gray matter cerebral blood flow was significantly correlated with age, whereas, CMR_{O_2} was not reduced with age in white matter, and an age-related decline in gray matter barely reached statistical significance. Indeed, when two exceedingly high values were excluded, there was no relationship between cortical oxygen consumption and age. Regional analysis showed the parietal and frontal cortices to be the regions with the lowest impairment of metabolism. The authors concluded that the lack of a change in CMR_{O_2} reflected a compensatory increase in oxygen extraction during aging.

In the same study (Frackowiak & Gibbs, 1983), cerebral blood flow and CMR_{O_2} were reduced simultaneously in demented subjects. Generally, oxygen consumption fell with increased functional ability. Furthermore, there was a selective decline in CMR_{O_2} in the parietal and frontal cortices, suggesting that the pathogenic process in Alzheimer's disease affects neuronal populations unique to these areas.

Another index of cerebral oxidative metabolism is the cerebral metabolic rate for glucose (CMR_{glc}). The results of animal and human experiments have indicated that glucose is the main substrate for cerebral metabolism in adults, and that most of the glucose extracted by the brain is oxidized (Sokoloff, 1972; Siesjö, 1978). Glucose oxidation is coupled to ATP formation and is stoichiometrically related to CMR_{O_2} under physiologic conditions. Measurements of CMR_{glc}, therefore, provide information on CMR_{O_2} and on cerebral energy metabolism in general.

The regional cerebral metabolic rate for glucose ($rCMR_{glc}$) has been studied in human volunteers as a function of age and dementia using PET and ^{18}F-2-deoxy-D-glucose (FDG), which serves as a tracer for the exchange of glucose between plasma and brain and its phosphorylation by hexokinase in the tissue (Reivich et al., 1979). In one of these investigations, Kuhl et al. (1982) reported that overall CMR_{glc} in forty normal resting volunteers between the ages of 18 and 78 years demonstrated a gradual decline, when plotted as a function of age. At age 78, whole brain mean CMR_{glc} was 26% less than at age 18. However, this alteration was of the same order as the variance among subjects at any age, and no statement was made about the statistical significance of this decline or of other results in the study. A study by de Leon et al. (1984) showed age-related ventricular and cortical sulcal dilation by CT examination, but no metabolic decrement, as measured with FDG. Using similar methods to measure $rCMR_{glc}$, Duara et al. (1983) found that in twenty-one subjects between the ages of 21 and 83 years, neither mean hemispheric CMR_{glc} nor $rCMR_{glc}$ in thirty-one brain regions was correlated significantly with age. The lack of decline in resting $rCMR_{glc}$ with age, despite performance decrements (Arenberg, 1978), suggests an insensitivity of resting $rCMR_{glc}$ measurements to functional decline in normal aging. Greater benefit might be derived from $rCMR_{glc}$ studies during functional challenge of the brain. Thus, metabolic measures might elucidate the anatomical loci associated with performance deficits in aging (London, 1984).

In contrast to the negative results in FDG studies of normal aging, applications of the PET-FDG technique to localize neuronal dysfunction in

Alzheimer's disease suggest a potential diagnostic use for the procedure, and may help direct future studies. Benson et al. (1983) reported that in a group of eight patients diagnosed as having Alzheimer's disease or three subjects with multiinfarct dementia, global CMR_{glc} was reduced as compared with metabolism in sixteen age-matched controls. However, patients with Alzheimer's dementia showed sparing of the primary motor and sensory cortices. The pattern differed in the brains of patients with multiinfarct dementia, where areas of hypometabolism were focal and asymmetric. Thus, in this study of few subjects, Alzheimer's disease could be distinguished from multiinfarct dementia.

Although Benson et al. (1983) reported equally severe changes in the frontal and temporal cortices, Friedland et al. (1983) presented evidence that the metabolic effects of Alzheimer's disease were most concentrated in the temporoparietal cortex. In ten subjects with the clinical diagnosis of Alzheimer's disease, the frontal to temporoparietal ratio of $rCMR_{glc}$ exceeded 1.10 in both hemispheres. In contrast, none of six control subjects had a frontal to temporoparietal ratio greater than 1.08. The anteroposterior differences seen in $rCMR_{glc}$ in the Alzheimer's disease group were not observed on CT, suggesting a diagnostic advantage of FDG-PET studies over CT.

Correlative studies of $rCMR_{glc}$ and neuropsychological test results may provide information on the importance of different brain regions in various aspects of functional performance. In this regard, Friedland et al. (1983) found strong negative correlations of both the Mattis Dementia Rating score and the verbal IQ with the right frontal/left frontal ratio, suggesting that these tests may reflect left frontal impairment. A high correlation between the performance IQ and the right temporoparietal/left temporoparietal ratio indicated the sensitivity of this measure to right posterior hemisphere impairment (Friedland et al., 1983). These results agreed with those of Foster et al. (1983), who studied thirteen patients with clinically diagnosed Alzheimer's disease. Three of the subjects had predominant language deficits, four had a major failure of visuoconstructive function, and the other six presented primarily with memory loss. Those patients who showed a disproportionate failure of language function had markedly reduced $rCMR_{glc}$ in the left frontal, temporal, and parietal regions, as compared with corresponding areas of the right hemisphere. Patients with predominant constructional apraxia showed hypometabolism in the right temporal and parietal regions. Furthermore, scores on tests of verbal competency generally correlated with $rCMR_{glc}$ in the left frontal and temporal lobes, whereas scores on tests of the ability to deal with two-dimensional designs and three-dimensional objects correlated with right parietal $rCMR_{glc}$. Furthermore, the cortical localization of regions with a high correlation between $rCMR_{glc}$ and performance on visuoconstructive tests was in the posterior right hemisphere.

Another index of local cerebral function that can be assessed with PET is amino acid incorporation into protein. Bustany et al. (1983) have developed a dynamic three-compartment model to measure methionine incorporation. This method uses an intravenous bolus injection of ^{11}C-L-methionine as a radiotracer for the incorporation of methionine into cerebral proteins. The procedure has been validated in rats and baboons for quantitative autoradiographic studies of protein synthesis in animals, and has been applied in forty-eight patients diagnosed as having Alzheimer's dementia. Compared with twenty normal volunteers of about the same age, the Alzheimer's disease group showed a net decrease in frontal metabolism. This effect was seen dramatically in occipital-to-frontal ratios of protein incorporation rates. Decrements of greater than 65% were measured in patients with the most severe condition. The authors reported that preliminary results of psychometric tests correlated with protein synthesis. These results indicated that like FDG-PET studies, measures of local cerebral protein synthesis ultimately may provide a means to evaluate and study dementia in the living brain.

CONCLUSION

Since the discovery of neurodegenerative diseases associated with senescence, investigative tools for the study of these conditions mainly have consisted of analytic techniques and pathological studies applied to postmortem material. Although these studies have provided valuable information, in vivo monitoring techniques for various neurochemical processes in biological fluids or the living brain allow measurements which can be related to the clinical and functional status of the patient. Because of the difficulty in distinguishing Alzheimer's disease from other dementing disorders, diagnostic advances in this area would be particularly helpful. Advances in neuroradiology and the development of specific probes with appropriate mathematical models for regional cerebral metabolism will facilitate the diagnosis of neurodegenerative disorders and the study of their underlying pathogenic processes.

REFERENCES

Ambrose, J. (1973). Computerized transverse axial scanning (tomography): Part 2. Clinical application. *Br. J. Radiol.*, 46, 1023–1047.

Arenberg, D. (1978). Differences and changes with age in the Benton Visual Rentention Test. *J. Gerontol.*, 33, 534–540.

Bareggi, S., & Giacobini, E. (1978). Acetylcholinesterase activity in ventricular and cisternal CSF of dogs: Effect of chlorpromazine. *Neurosci. Res.*, 3, 335–339.

Barron, S. A., Jacobs, L., & Kinkel, W. R. (1976). Changes in size of normal lateral ventricles during aging determined by computerized tomography. *Neurology, 26,* 1011–1013.

Benson, D. F., Kuhl, D. E., Hawkins, R. A., Phelps, M. E., Cummings, J. L., & Tsai, S. Y. (1983). The fluorodeoxyglucose ^{18}F scan in Alzheimer's disease and multi-infarct dementia. *Arch. Neurol., 40,* 711–714.

Bernheimer, H., Birkmayer, W., & Hornykiewicz, O. (1966). Homovanillic acid in the cerebrospinal fluid. *Experientia, 22,* 609–610.

Bernheimer, H., Birkmayer, W., Hornykiewicz, O., Jellinger, K., & Seitelberger, F. (1973). Brain dopamine and the syndromes of Parkinson and Huntington. *J. Neurol. Sci., 20,* 415–455.

Besson, J. A. O., Corrigan, F. M., Foreman, E. I., Ashcroft, G. W., Eastwood, L. M., & Smith, F. W. (1983). Differentiating senile dementia of Alzheimer type and multi-infarct dementia by proton NMR imaging. *Lancet, ii,* 789–790.

Blinkov, S. M., & Glezer, I. I. (1968). *The human brain in figures and tables.* New York: Plenum.

Bowen, D. M., White, P., Smith, C. B., & Davison, A. N. (1974). Brain-decarboxylase activities as indices of pathological change in senile dementia. *Lancet, i,* 1247–1249.

Bowen, D. M., Smith, C. B., White, P., & Davison, A. N. (1976). Neurotransmitter-related enzymes and indices of hypoxia in senile dementia and other abiotrophies. *Brain, 94,* 459–496.

Bowen, D. M., Sims, N. R., Benton, S., Hahn, E., Smith, C., Neary, D., Thomas, D., & Davison, A. (1982). Biochemical changes in cortical brain biopsies from demented patients in relation to morphological findings and pathogenesis. In S. Corkin, K. Davis, J. Growdon, E. Usdin, & R. Wurtman (Eds.), *Alzheimer's disease: A report of progress (Aging,* Vol. 19). (pp. 1–7). New York: Raven Press.

Brizzee, K. (1981). Structural correlates of the aging process in the brain. *Psychopharmacol. Bull., 17,* 43–52.

Brody, H. (1955). Organization of the cerebral cortex. *J. Comp. Neurol., 102,* 517–557.

Bucht, G., Adolfsson, R., & Winblad, B. (1984). Dementia of the Alzheimer type: A clinical description and diagnostics problem. *J. Am. Geriatr. Soc., 32,* 491–498.

Buckley, C., & Dorsey, F (1971). Serum immunoglobulin levels throughout the life-span of healthy man. *Ann. Intern Med., 75,* 673–683.

Bustany, P., Henry, J. F., Soussaline, F., & Comar, D. (1983). Brain protein synthesis in normal and demented patients—a study by positron emission tomography with ^{11}C-L-methionine. In P. L. Magistretti (Ed.), *Functional radionuclide imaging of the brain.* (pp. 319–326). New York: Raven Press.

Chipperfield, B., Newman, P., & Moyes, I. (1981). Decreased erythrocyte cholinesterase activity in dementia. *Lancet, ii,* 199.

Cohen, D., Eisdorfer, C., Prinz, P., Leverenz, J., & Davis, M. (1980). Immunoglobulins, cognitive status, and duration of illness in Alzheimer's disease. *Neurobiol. Aging, 1,* 165–168.

Corsellis, J. A. N. (1976). Aging and the dementias. In W. Blackwood, & J. A. N. Corsellis (Eds.), *Greenfield's neuropathology* (3rd ed.) (pp. 796–848). Chicago: Year Book Medical Publishers.

Cramer, H., Kohler, J., Oepen, G., Schomburg, G., & Schroter, E. (1981). Huntington's chorea—measurements of somatostatin, substance P and cyclic nucleotides in the cerebrospinal fluid. *J. Neurol., 225,* 183–187.

Davies, P., & Maloney, A. J. F. (1976). Selective loss of central cholinergic neurons in Alzheimer's disease. *Lancet, ii,* 1403.

Davies, P. (1979). Neurotransmitter-related enzymes in senile dementia of the Alzheimer's type. *Brain Res., 171,* 319–327.

Davis, K., Hsieh, J., Levy, M., Horvath, T., Davis, B., & Mohs, R. (1982). Cerebrospinal fluid acetylcholine, choline, and senile dementia of the Alzheimer's type. *Psychopharmacol. Bull., 18,* 193–195.

de Leon, M. J., & George, A. E. (1983). Computed tomography in aging and senile dementia of the Alzheimer type. In R. Mayeux, W. G. Rosen (Eds.), *The dementias* (pp. 103–122) New York: Raven Press.

de Leon, M. J., Ferris, S. N., George, A. E., Reisberg, B., Kricheff, I. I., & Gershon, S. (1980). Computed tomography evaluations of brain–behavior relationships in senile dementia of the Alzheimer type. *Neurobiol. Aging, 1,* 69–79.

de Leon, M. J., George, A. E., Ferris, S. H., Christman, D. R., Fowler, J. S., Gentes, C. I., Brodie, J., Reisberg, B., & Wolf, A. P. (1984). Positron emission tomography and computed tomography assessments of the aging human brain. *J. Comput. Assist. Tomogr., 8,* 88–94.

Deutsch, S., Mohs, R., Levy, M., Rothpearl, A., Stockton, D., Horvath, T., Coco, A., & Davis, K. (1983). Acetylcholinesterase activity in CSF in schizophrenia, depression, Alzheimer's disease and normals. *Biol. Psychiatry, 18,* 1363–1373.

Direnfeld, L., Albert, M., Volicer, L., Langlais, P., Marquis, J., & Kaplan, E. (1983). Parkinson's disease: The possible relationship of laterality to dementia and neurochemical findings. *Arch. Neurol., 41,* 935–941.

Duara, R., Margolin, R. A., Robertson-Tschabo, E. A., London, E. D., Schwartz, M., Renfrew, J. W., Koziarz, B. J., Sundaram, M., Grady, C., Moore, A. M., Ingvar, D. H., Sokoloff, L., Weingartner, H., Kessler, R. M., Manning, R. G., Channing, M. A., Cutler, N. R., & Rapoport, S. I. (1983). Cerebral glucose utilization, as measured with positron emission tomography in 21 resting healthy men between the ages of 21 and 83 years. *Brain, 106,* 761–775.

Dupont, E., Christensen, S. E., Hansen, A. P., Olivarius, B. F., & Orskov, H. (1982). Low cerebrospinal fluid somatostatin in Parkinson's disease: An irreversible abnormality. *Neurology* (NY), *32,* 312–314.

Earnest, M. P., Heaton, B. K., Wilkinson, W. E., & Manke, W. F. (1979). Cortical atrophy, ventricular enlargement and intellectual impairment in the aged. *Neurology, 29,* 1138–1143.

Enna, S. J., Stern, L. Z., Wastek, G. J., & Yamamura, H. I. (1977). Cerebrospinal fluid γ-aminobutyric acid variations in neurological disorders. *Arch. Neurol.* (Chicago), *34,* 683–685.

Fazekas, J. K., Alman, R. W., & Bessman, A. N. (1952). Cerebral physiology of the aged. *Am. J. Med. Sci., 223,* 245–257.

Ford, C. V., & Winter, J. (1980). Computerized axial tomograms and dementia in elderly patients. *J. Gerontol., 36,* 164–169.

Foster, N. L., Chase, T. N., Fedio, P., Patronas, N. J., Brooks, R. A., & Di Chiro, G. (1983). Alzheimer's disease: Focal cortical changes shown by positron emission tomography. *Neurology, 33,* 961–965.

Frackowiak, R. S. J., Lenzi, G-L, Jones, T., & Heather, J. D. (1980). Quantitative measurement of regional cerebral blood blow and oxygen metabolism in man using ^{15}O and positron emission tomography: Theory, procedure, and normal values. *J. Comput. Assist. Tomogr., 4,* 727–736.

Frackowiak, R. S. J., & Gibbs, J. M. (1983). The pathophysiology of Alzheimer's disease studied with positron emission tomography (pp. 317–327). Banbury Report 15: Biological Aspects of Alzheimer's Disease. Cold Spring Harbor, New York: Cold Spring Harbor Laboratory.

Friedland, R. P., Budinger, T. F., Ganz, E., Yano, Y., Mathis, C. A., Koss, B., Ober, B. A., Huesman, R. H., & Derenzo, S. E. (1983). Regional cerebral metabolic alterations in dementia of the Alzheimer type: Positron emission tomography with [^{18}F]fluorodeoxyglucose. *J. Comput. Assist. Tomogr., 7,* 590–598.

Gado, M., Hughes, C. P., Danziger, W., Chi, D., Jost, G., & Berg, L. (1982). Volumetric measurement of the cerebrospinal fluid spaces in demented subjects and controls. *Radiology, 144,* 535–538.

Gado, M., Patel, J., Hughes, C.P., Danzinger, W., & Berg, L. (1983). Brain atrophy in dementia judged by CT scan ranking. *Am. J. Neuroradiol., 4* 499–500.

Garry, P., & Routh, J. (1965). A micro method for serum cholinesterase. *Clin. Chem., 11,* 91–96.

Glydensted, C., & Kosteljanetz, M. (1976). Measurements of the normal ventricular system with computed tomography. *Neuroradiology, 10,* 20S–21S.

Gottfries, C. G., Gottfries, I., & Roos, B. E. (1969). Homovanillic acid and 5-hydroxyindoleacetic acid in the cerebrospinal fluid of patients with senile dementia, presenile dementia and Parkinsonism. *J. Neurochem., 16,* 1341–1345.

Greenfield, S., & Smith, A. (1979). The influence of electrical stimulation of certain brain regions on the concentration of acetylcholinesterase in rabbit cerebrospinal fluid. *Brain Res., 177,* 445–459.

Greenfield, S., Chubb, I., & Smith, A. (1979). The effects of chlorpromazine on the concentration of acetylcholinesterase in the cerebrospinal fluid of rabbits. *Neuropharmacology, 18,* 127–132.

Greenfield, S., Cheramy, A., Leviel, V., & Glowinski, G. (1980). In vivo release of acetylcholinesterases in cat substantia nigra and caudate nucleus. *Nature, 284,* 355–357.

Hahn, F. J. Y., & Rim, K. (1976). Frontal ventricular dimensions on normal computed tomography. *Am. J. Roent., 126,* 593–596.

Hare, T., Wood, J., Manyam, B., Gerner, R., Ballenger, J., & Post, R. (1982). Central nervous system gamma-aminobutyric acid activity in man: Relationship to age and sex as reflected in CSF. *Arch. Neurol., 39,* 247–249.

Haug, G. (1977). Age and sex dependence of the size of normal ventricles on computed tomography. *Neuroradiology, 14,* 201–204.

Henke, H., & Lang, W. (1983). Cholinergic enzymes in neocortex, hippocampus and basal forebrain of non-neurological and senile dementia of Alzheimer-type patients. *Brain Res., 267,* 281–291.

Hornykiewicz, O. (1966). Dopamine (3-hydroxytyramine) and brain function. *Pharmacol. Rev., 18,* 925–964.

Jacoby, R. (1981). Dementia, depression and the CT scan. *Psychological Medicine, 11,* 673–676.

Jacoby, R. J., & Levy, R. (1980). Computed tomography in the elderly: 2. Senile dementia: Diagnosis and functional impairment. *Br. J. Psychiatry, 136,* 256–269.

Jarvik, L., Matsuyama, S. S., Kessler, J., Fu, T., Tsai, S., & Clark, E. (1982). Philothermal response of polymorphonuclear leukocytes in dementia of the Alzheimer type. *Neurobiol. Aging, 3,* 93–99.

Johnson, S., & Domino, E. (1971). Cholinergic enzymatic activity of cerebrospinal fluid of patients with various neurologic diseases. *Clin. Chim. Acta, 35,* 421–428.

Jones, T., Chesler, D. A., & Ter-Pogossian, M. M. (1976). The continuous inhalation of oxygen-15 for assessing regional oxygen extraction in the brain of man. *Br. J. Radiol., 49,* 339–343.

Kerzner, L. (1984). Diagnosis and treatment of Alzheimer's disease. In G. Stollerman (Ed.), *Advances in internal medicine* (Vol. 29) (pp. 447–470). Chicago: Year Book Medical Publishers.

Kety, S. S. (1956). Human cerebral blood flow and oxygen consumption as related to aging. *Research Publications of the Association for Research in Nervous and Mental Disease, 35,* 31–45.

Kety, S. S., & Schmidt, C. F. (1945). The determination of cerebral blood flow in man by the use of nitrous oxide in low concentrations. *Am. J. Physiol., 143,* 53–66.

Korf, J., Van Pragg, H., & Schut, D. (1974). Parkinson's disease and amine metabolites in cerebrospinal fluid. *Eur. Neurol., 12,* 340–350.

Kuhar, M. J. (1976). The anatomy of cholinergic neurons. In A. M. Goldberg & I. Hanin (Eds.), *Biology of Cholinergic Function* (pp. 3–27). New York: Raven Press.

Kuhl, D. E., Metter, E. J., Reige, W. H., & Phelps, M. E. (1982). Effects of human aging on patterns of local cerebral glucose utilization determined by the [^{18}F]flurodeoxyglucose method. *J. Cereb. Blood Flow Metab., 2,* 163–171.

Lakke, J., & Teelken, A. (1976). Amino acid abnormalities in cerebrospinal fluid in patients with Parkinsonism and extrapyramidal disorders. *Neurology, 26,* 489–493.

Lassen, N. A., Feinberg, I., & Lane, M. H. (1960). Bilateral studies of cerebral oxygen uptake in aged normal subjects and in patients with organic dementia. *J. Clin. Invest., 39,* 491–500.

Last, R. J., & Tompsett, D. H. (1953). Casts of cerebral ventricles. *Br. J. Surg., 40,* 525–543.

Lenzi, G. L., Jones, T., McKenzie, C. G., Buckingham, P. D., Clark, J. C., & Moss, S. (1978). Study of regional cerebral metabolism and blood flow relationships in man using the method of continuously inhaling oxygen-15 and oxygen-15-labelled carbon dioxide. *J. Neurol. Neurosurg. Psychiatry, 41,* 1–10.

Lloyd, K. G., Davidson, L., & Hornykiewicz, O. (1975). The neurochemistry of Parkinson's disease: Effect of L-dopa therapy. *J. Pharmacol. Exp. Ther., 195,* 453–464.

London, E. D. (1984). Metabolism of the brain: A measure of cerebral function in aging. In J. E. Johnson (Ed.), *Aging and Cell Function* (pp. 187–210). New York: Plenum.

Mann, J., Stanley, M., Neophytides, A., de Leon, M., Ferris, S., & Gershon, S. (1981). Central amine metabolism in Alzheimer's disease: *In vivo* relationship to cognitive deficits. *Neurobiol. Aging, 2,* 57–60.

Manyam, B., Katz, L., Hare, T., Gerber, J., & Grossman, M. (1980). Levels of gamma-aminobutyric acid in cerebrospinal fluid in various neurologic disorders. *Arch. Neurol., 37,* 352–355.

Matsuyama, S., & Fu, T. (1983). Inhibition of normal polymorphonuclear leukocyte philothermal response by serum from dementia of the Alzheimer-type patients. *Age, 6,* 72–75.

McKhann, G., Drachman, D., Folstein, M., Katzman, R., Price, D., & Stadlam, E. (1984). Clinical diagnosis of Alzheimer's disease: Report of the NINCDS–ADRDA work group under the auspices of Department of Health and Human Services Task Force on Alzheimer's Disease. *Neurology, 34,* 939–944.

Milstoc, M., Teodoru, C., Fieve, R., & Kambaraci, T. (1975). Cholinesterase activity and the manic depressive patient. *Dis. Nerv. Syst., 36,* 197–199.

Miyata, S., Nagata, M. S., Yamao, S., Nakamura, S., & Kameyama, M. (1984). Dopamine-β-hydroxylase activities in serum and cerebrospinal fluid of aged and demented patients. *J. Neurol. Sci., 63,* 403–409.

Nandy, K. (1978) Brain-reactive antibodies in aging and senile dementia. In R. Katzman, R. Terry, K. Bick (Eds.), *Alzheimer's disease: Senile Dementia and Related Disorders* (pp. 503–512). New York: Raven Press.

North, R., & Mulrow, P. (1976). Serum dopamine-β-hydroxylase as an index of sympathetic nervous system activity in man. *Circ. Res., 38,* 2–5.

Op den Velde, W., & Stam, F. (1976). Some cerebral proteins and enzyme systems in Alzheimer's presenile and senile dementia. *J. Am. Geriatr. Soc., 24,* 12–16.

Oram, J., Edwardson, J., & Millard, P. (1981). Investigation of cerebrospinal fluid neuropeptides in idiopathic senile dementia. *Gerontology, 27,* 216–223.

Parkes, J., Marsden, C., Rees, J., Curzon, G., Kantamaneni, B., Knill-Jones, R., Akbar, A., Das, S., & Kataria, M. (1974). Parkinson's disease, cerebral arteriosclerosis and senile dementia. *Q. J. Med., 43,* 49–51.

Perry, E., Perry, R., Gibson, P., Blessed, G., & Tomlinson, B. (1977). A cholinergic connection between normal aging and senile dementia in human hippocampus. *Neorosci. Lett., 6,* 85–89.

Perry, E. K., Perry, R. H., Blessed, G., & Tomlinson, B. E. (1977). Necropsy evidence of central cholinergic deficits in senile dementia. *Lancet, i,* 189.

Perry, E., Perry, R., Blessed, G., & Tomlinson, B. (1978). Changes in brain cholinesterases in senile dementia of Alzheimer type. *Appl. Neurobiol., 4,* 273–277.

Perry, E., Tomlinson, B., Blessed, G., Bergmann, K., Gibson, P., & Perry, R. (1978). Correlation of cholinergic abnormalities with senile plaques and mental test scores in senile dementia. *Br. Med. J., 2,* 1457–1459.

Perry, R., Wilson, I., Bober, M., Atack, J., Blessed, G., Tomlinson, B., & Perry, E. (1982). Plasma and erythrocyte acetylcholinesterase in senile dementia of Alzheimer type. *Lancet, i,* 174–175.

Pollock, M., & Horbabrook, R. W. (1966). The prevalence, natural history and dementia of Parkinson's disease. *Brain, 89,* 429–448.

Raskind, M., Peskind, E., Halter, J., & Jimerson, D. (1984). Norepinephrine and MHPG levels in CSF and plasma in Alzheimer's disease. *Arch. Gen. Psychiatry, 41,* 343–346.

Reivich, M., Kuhl, D., Wolf, A., Greenberg, J., Phelps, M., Ido, T., Casella, V., Fowler, J., Hoffman, E., Alavi, A., Som, P., & Sokoloff, L. (1979). The ^{18}F-fluorodeoxyglucose method for the measurement of local cerebral glucose utilization in man. *Circ. Res., 44,* 127–137.

Riese, W. (1946). The cerebral cortex in the very old human brain. *J. Neuropathol. Exp. Neurol., 5,* 160–164.

Rinne, U., & Sonninen, V. (1972). Acid monoamine metabolites in the cerebrospinal fluid of patients with Parkinson's disease. *Neurology, 22,* 62–67.

Roberts, M. A., & Caird, F. I. (1976). Computerized tomography and intellectual impairment in the elderly. *J. Neurol. Neurosurg. Psychiatry, 39,* 986–989.

Rossor, M. N., Fahrenkrug, J., Emson, P., Mountjoy, C., Iversen, L., & Roth, M. (1980). Reduced cortical choline acetyltransferase activity in senile dementia of Alzheimer type is not accompanied by changes in vasoactive intestinal peptide. *Brain Res., 201,* 249–253.

Rossor, M. N., Iversen, L. L., Reynolds, G. P., Mountjoy, C. Q., & Roth, M. (1984). Neurochemical characteristics of early and late onset types of Alzheimer's disease. *Br. Med. J., 288,* 961–964

Sara, V., Hall, K., Ottosson-Seeberger, A., & Wetterberg, L. (1980). The role of somatomedins in fetal growth (pp. 453–456). In I. Cumming, J. Funder, F. Mendelson (Eds.), Endocrinology 80, (pp. 453–456). *The Role of Somatomedins in Fetal Growth.* Australian Academy of Science, Canberra, Australia.

Sara, V., Hall, K., Rodeck, C., & Wetterberg, L. (1981). Human embryonic somatomedin. *Proc. Natl. Acad. Sci. USA, 78,* 3175–3179.

Sara, V., Hall, K., Enzell, K., Gardner, A., Morawski, R., & Wetterberg, L. (1982). Somatomedins in aging and dementia disorders of the Alzheimer type. *Neurobiol. Aging, 3,* 117–120.

Scarsella, G., Toschi, G., Bareggi, S., & Giacobini, E. (1979). Molecular forms of cholinesterases in cerebrospinal fluid, blood plasma, and brain tissue of the Beagle dog. *J. Neurosci. Res., 4,* 19–24.

Scheinberg, P., Blackburn, I., Rich, M., & Saslaw, M. (1953). Effects of aging on cerebral circulation and metabolism. *Arch. Neurol. Psychiatry (Chicago), 70,* 77–85.

Shenkin, H. A., Novak, P., Goluboff, B., Soffe, A. M., & Bortin, L. (1953). The effects of aging, arteriosclerosis, and hypertension upon the cerebral circulation. *J. Clin. Invest., 32,* 459–465.

Siesjö, B. K. (1978). *Brain Energy Metabolism.* Chichester: John Wiley and Sons.

Silver, A. (1974). Acetylcholinesterase in the context of nervous transmission. In A. Silver (Ed.), *The Biology of Cholinesterases* (pp. 303–354). New York: Elsevier.

Smith, R., Ho, B., Hsu, L., Vroulis, G., Claghorn, J., & Schoolar, J. (1982). Cholinesterase enzymes in the blood of patients with Alzheimer's disease. *Life Sci., 30,* 543–546.

Soininen, H., Halonen, T., & Riekkinen, P. (1981a). Acetylcholinesterase activities in cerebrospinal fluid of patients with senile dementia of Alzheimer type. *Acta Neurol. Scand., 64,* 217–224.

Soininen, H., MacDonald, E., & Rekonen, M. (1981b). Homovanillic and 5-hydroxy-indole-acetic acid levels in cerebrospinal fluids of patients with senile dementia of Alzheimer type. *Acta Neurol. Scand., 64,* 101–107

Soininen, H., Puranen, M., & Reikkinen, P. J. (1982). Computed tomography findings in senile dementia and normal aging. *J. Neurol. Neurosurg. Psychiatry, 45,* 50–54.

Soininen, H., Jolkkonen, J., Reinikainen, K., Holonen, T., & Reikkinen, P. (1984). Reduced cholinesterase activity and somatostatin-like immunoreactivity in the cerebrospinal fluid of patients with dementia of the Alzheimer type. *J. Neurol. Sci., 63,* 167–172.

Sokoloff, L. (1972). Circulation and energy metabolism of the brain. In G. J. Siegel, R. W. Albers, R. Katzman, & B. W. Agranoff (Eds.), *Basic Neurochemistry* (2nd ed.) (pp. 338–413) Boston: Little Brown and Co.

Sorenson, K., Christensen, S., Dupont, E., Hansen, A., Pedersen, E., & Orskov, H. (1980). Low somatostatin content in cerebrospinal fluid in multiple sclerosis—An indicator of disease activity? *Acta Neurol. Scand., 61,* 186–191.

Subramanyam, R., Alpert, N. M., Hoop, B., Brownell, G., & Laveras, J. M. (1978). A model for regional cerebral oxygen distribution during continuous inhalation of $^{15}O_2$, and $C^{15}O$ and $C^{15}O_2$. *J. Nucl. Med., 19,* 48–53.

Takeda, S., & Matsuzawa, T. (1984). Brain atrophy during aging: A quantitative study using computed tomography. *J. Am. Geriatr. Soc., 32,* 520–524.

Tomlinson, B. E., Blessed, G., & Roth, M. (1970). Observations on the brains of demented old people. *J. Neurol. Sci., 11,* 205–242.

Welch, M., Markham, C., & Jenden, D. (1976). Acetylcholine and choline in cerebrospinal fluid of patients with Parkinson's disease and Huntington's chorea. *J. Neurol. Neurosurg. Psychiatry, 39,* 367–374.

White, P., Hiley, O. R., Goodhardt, M. J., Carrasco, L. H., Keet, J. P., Williams, I. E. I., & Bowen, D. M. (1977). Neocortical cholinergic neurons in elderly people. *Lancet, i,* 668–670.

Whitehouse, P., Price, D., Clark, A., Coyle, J., & De Long, M. (1981) Alzheimer's disease: Evidence for selective loss of cholinergic neurons in the nucleus basalis. *Ann. Neurol., 10,* 122–126.

Wood, P., Etienne, P., Lal, S., Gauthier, S., Cajal, S., & Nair, N. (1982). Reduced lumbar CSF somatostatin levels in Alzheimer's disease. *Life Sci., 31,* 2073–2079.

Yaksh, T., Filbert, M., Harris, L., & Yamamura, H. (1975). Acetylcholinesterase turnover in brain, cerebrospinal fluid and plasma. *J. Neurochem., 25,* 853–860.

Yamamura, H., Ito, M., Kubota, K., & Matsuzawa, T. (1980). Brain atrophy during aging: A quantitative study with computed tomography. *J. Gerontol., 4,* 492–498.

Zatz, I. M., Jernigan, T. L., & Ahumada, A. J. (1982). Changes on computed cranial tomography with aging: Intracranial fluid volume. *J. Neuroradiol, 3,* 1–11.

10
Electrophysiologic Methods for Assessing Sleep Disorders in the Elderly

Horst W. Ebeling

Disturbed sleep may considerably alter our physiological and psychological performance (Johnson et al., 1983). Insomnia is an extremly prevalent symptom associated with a variety of psychiatric and medical disorders, as well as situational disturbances. In studies of the general population, the prevalence of insomnia has been estimated at 14 to 35% (Balter & Bauer, 1974; Bixler et al., 1979; Karacan et al., 1976), while excessive daytime sleepiness is thought to be considerably less, 0.3 to 4% (Bixler et al., 1979; Coleman et al., 1980, Karacan et al., 1976). In a follow-up study of 8,000 patients (Coleman, 1983) the most prevalent disorder of initiating and maintaining sleep (DIMS) was diagnosed as insomnia associated with psychiatric disorders. The frequency was 34.9 and 34.8%, respectively, for two samples. Psychophysiological insomnia ranked as the second most frequent DIMS diagnosis (about 16%). Periodic movements in sleep, restless legs syndrome, and drug-dependency insomnia were the next most frequent diagnoses. The remaining categories had frequencies less than 10%. Related to age, insomnia is relatively uncommon under 20 years of age. It becomes more common in the age range 20 to 60 (about 12 to 14%) and increases at an age of 60 years and more (about 25 to 33%) (Lugaresi et al., 1983; Miles & Dement, 1980).

Objective methods in sleep research have existed since Loomis, Harvey, and Hobart in 1937 described the electrophysiology of sleep and classified specific stages of sleep (Loomis et al., 1937). Modern sleep research, as we know it today, began in the 1950s, when Aserinsky and Kleitman observed that clusters of conjugated, rapid eye movements (REM) occurred periodically during sleep (Aserinsky & Kleitman, 1953, 1955). With the discovery of REMs, researchers divided sleep stages into REM sleep and nonREM (NREM) sleep (stage 1, 2, 3, and 4), based on each stage's characteristic electroencephalogram (EEG), electrooculogram (EOG), and electromyogram (EMG) patterns. Specialized and standardized electrophysiologic recording techniques have enabled scientists to study sleep in subjects whose sleep was normal and those with sleep disorders. To be most effective in managing insomnia, clinicians must acquire a basic understanding of electrophysiological methods of sleep research. This chapter provides such information.

SLEEP POLYGRAPHY

Recording Techniques

The sleep laboratory provides an ideal setting for the evaluation and analysis of sleep, primarily because measurements are objective and experimental conditions can be rigorously controlled (Kales et al., 1975; Rechtschaffen & Kales, 1968). In sound-attenuated rooms, that are also temperature and humidity controlled, EEG, EOG, and EMG tracings are recorded continuously during the night by a polygraph machine. In recent years, mobile polygraphic recordings using telemetry or Holter recording technology (Holter & Gengerelli, 1949; Ives & Woods, 1975) have also been obtained. The standardized techniques of human sleep research are described in a manual edited by Rechtschaffen and Kales (1968). According to Rechtschaffen and Kales, the minimal technique records the EEG in 1 tracing, the EOG in 2 tracings, and the EMG in 1 tracing.

EEG Recording

For electrode placement the Ten-Twenty Electrode System of the International Federation (Jasper, 1958) is adopted (Fig. 10.1). When EEG information is limited to one derivation, the recommended derivation is C4/A1 or C3/A2. Either the right or left side may be used. To minimize artificial potentials the mastoid on the opposite side of the central electrode (C4/Cb1 or C3/Cb2) can be used for electrode placement. If multiple channels of EEG can be recorded, the results from the additional derivations should be compared with the results from C4/A1 or C3/A2. However, to maximize comparability and replicability, the EEG criteria for scoring sleep stages should always be based on tracings obtained from C4/A1 or C3/A2.

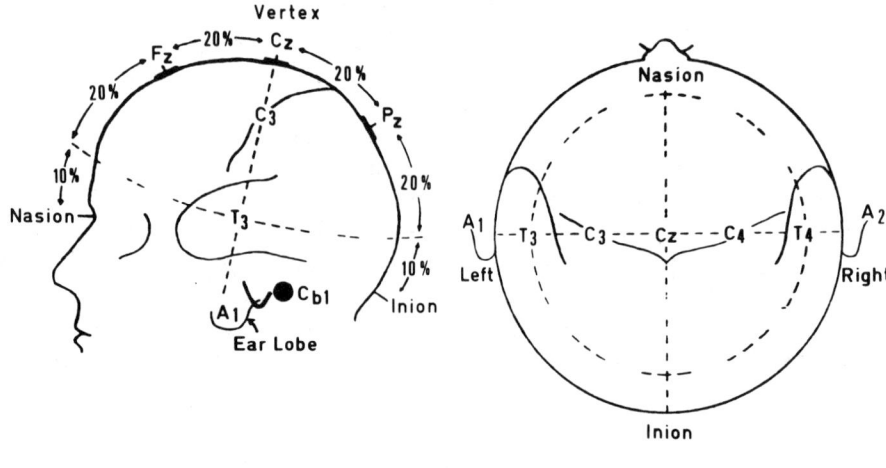

LEFT SIDE OF HEAD   **TOP OF HEAD**

FIGURE 10.1 Electrode placement adopted in the Ten-Twenty Electrode System of the International Federation (Jasper, 1958) to derive EEG tracings according to Rechtschaffen and Kales (1968).

Eye Movement Recording

To distinguish between eye movements and other signals that resemble them, two channels are necessary for recording the EOG. On the first EOG channel the potentials from an electrode 1 cm above and slightly lateral to the outer canthus of one eye, and a reference electrode on either the homolateral earlobe or mastoid are recorded. On the second EOG channel the potentials from an electrode 1 cm below and slightly lateral to the outer canthus of the other eye referred to the contralateral ear lobe or mastoid are recorded, i.e., both eyes are referred to the same reference electrode. This array does not permit differentiation between horizontal and vertical eye movements. With the use of a common supranasion reference such differentiation is possible (Fig. 10.2). However, the use of a supranasion reference could result in confusion because an EEG signal may also be recorded.

EMG Recording

The recording of EMG is derived from two electrodes attached to the mental or submental muscle areas on and beneath the chin (Fig. 10.2). High gains should be used, preferably 20 μV for 10 mm or higher. If there are additional channels for polygraphic recording, the ECG, breathing, the actogram, or the phallogram can be recorded.

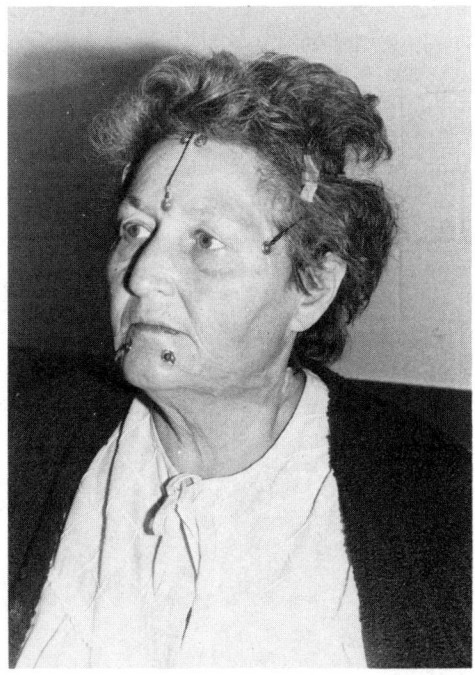

FIGURE 10.2 Electrode placement for derivation of the EOG in 2 channels (with the use of a supranasion reference) and the EMG in 1 channel (mental muscle areas).

Technical Conditions for Qualified Polygraphic Recordings

In order to produce qualified EEG, EOG, and EMG recordings, the biological signals have to be free of artifacts; there should be no frequency-dependent reduction of amplitude or alteration in phase. Silver–silverchloride electrodes produce a minimum of polarization voltage (Ferries, 1974); therefore they are relatively unsusceptible to movement artifacts (Irrgang, 1979). They also transfer the biological signal independently of the frequency (Cooper et al., 1974).

Holter Recording Technology

Following Dr. Norman J. Holter's interest in measuring the electrical activity of the brain in ambulatory humans in 1949, in the early 1970s telemetry techniques were developed (Porter et al., 1971; Ives et al., 1973) and similar to electrocardiographic techniques, a long-term 4-channel continuous Holter recorder (Medilog 4-24, Oxford Medical Systems Ltd., Oxfordshire,

England) has evolved (Ives & Woods, 1975). Quite recently, a 9-channel Holter recorder has appeared on the market (Medilog 9000, Oxford Medical Systems Ltd., Oxfordshire, England). Basically, the present recording equipment consists of three elements: (1) silver–silverchloride electrodes, (2) miniature multiparameter preamplifiers, and (3) a recording device, for example, a 4-channel portable 24-hour cassette recorder (Fig. 10.3). Electrode placement is performed as described above. The electrodes are attached to a miniature preamplifier which is mounted on the scalp between each pair of electrodes (Fig. 10.3). The lead wires are then passed down the back of the neck under the clothing to the Holter recorder.

Playback analysis is done by a page mode playback device (PMD-12 Replay and Visual System, Oxford Medical Systems Ltd., Oxfordshire,

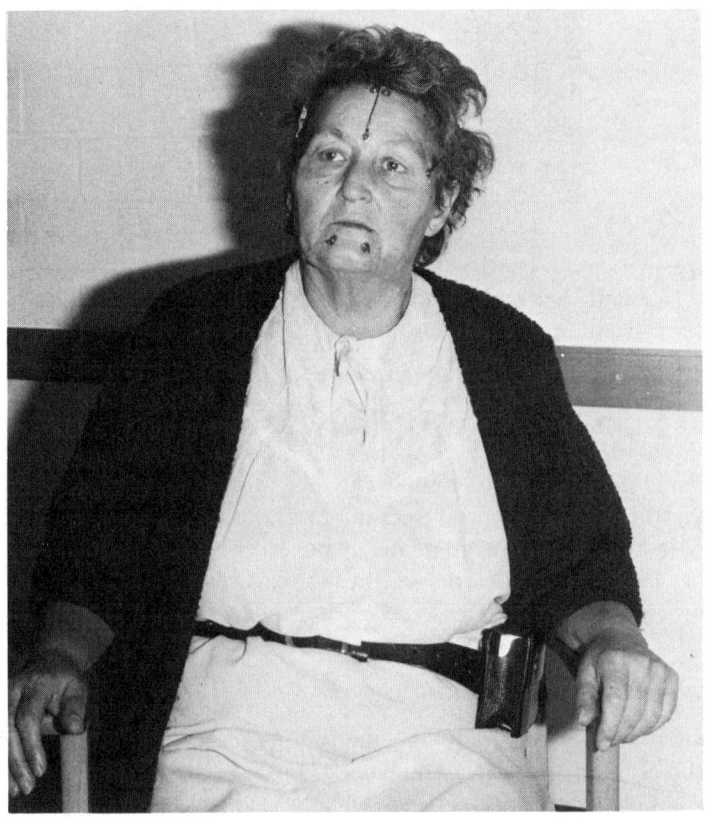

FIGURE 10.3 Polygraphic sleep recording unit using Holter technique (4-channel multiparameter cassette recorder, Medilog 4-24, Oxford Medical Systems Ltd., Oxford, England).

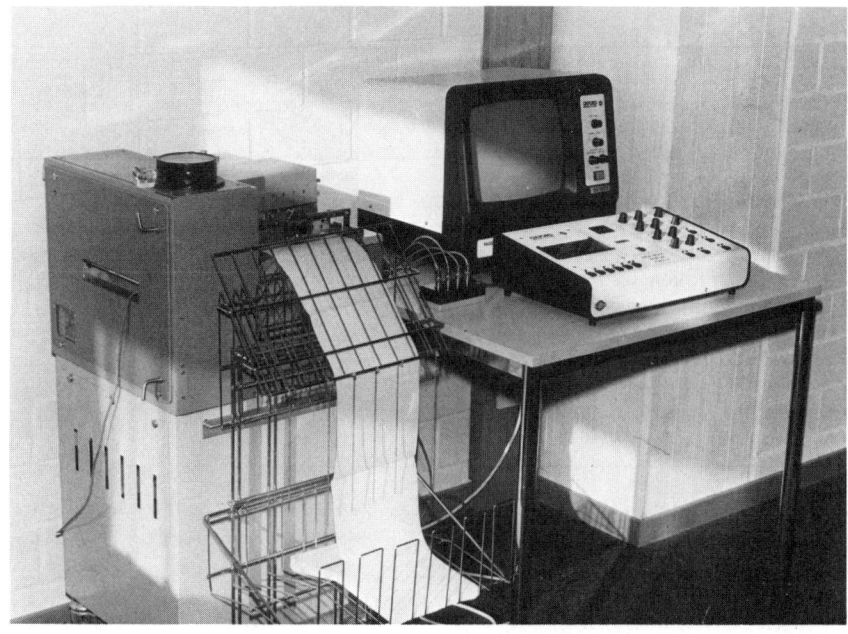

FIGURE 10.4 Playback analysis unit for transferring the EEG, EOG, and EMG signals from the 4-channel multiparameter cassette recorder Medilog 4-24 (Oxford Medical Systems Ltd., Oxfordshire, England) on paper. Right side: The page mode display (PMD 12, Oxford Medical Systems Ltd., Oxford, England). Left side: ECG writer Siemens Mingograph (Siemens, West Germany).

England) which displays 4 channels of recorded signals on a storage screen in 8- or 16-second pages at 20 or 60 times real time. For scoring sleep stages the recorded EOG, EEG, and EMG tracing has to be transferred to paper in a real time of 10 or 15 mm/s (Rechtscaffen & Kales, 1968). This is possible by using an EEG- or ECG-writer with a paper speed of 200 or 300 mm/s at 20 times real time playback (Fig. 10.4).

SCORING CRITERIA AND VISUALIZING SLEEP PARAMETERS

The scoring criteria below follow the Rechtschaffen und Kales Manual (Rechtschaffen & Kales, 1968). A convenient interval for most investigators would be a page record of 300 mm. This interval would result in epoch durations of 30 s at a paper speed of 10 mm/s or 20 s at a paper speed of 15 mm/s. If shorter or longer epochs should be used, it is suggested that investigators report them specifically. An epoch-by-epoch approach is

TABLE 10.1 Scoring Criteria for Sleep Stages of Human Subjects

Stage	EEG	EOG	EMG
W	Alpha activity and/or a low voltage, mixed frequency EEG	Frequent rapid eye movements (REM)	Relatively high tonic EMG level
1	Relatively low voltage, mixed frequency EEG with a prominence of activity in the 2–7 cps range. The faster frequencies are mostly of lower voltage than the 2–7 cps activity. The highest voltage 2–7 cps activity (about 50–75 μV) tends to occur in irregularly spaced bursts. Vertex sharp waves (as high as 200 μV) may appear	Slow eye movements. No REM	Tonic EMG levels are usually below those of relaxed wakefulness
2	Sleep spindles (12–14 cps) and/or K complexes. Absence of high amplitude, slow activity to define the presence of stages 3 and 4. Other polyphasic high voltage slow waves occurring paroxysmally which do not have the precise morphology of the K complex	No eye movements	Different tonic EMG levels
3	20–50% of the epoch consists of waves of 2 cps or slower (amplitudes greater than 75 μV peak to peak).	No eye movements	Different tonic EMG levels
4	More than 50% of the epoch consists of waves of 2 cps or slower (amplitudes greater than 75 μV peak to peak).	No eye movements	Different tonic EMG levels
REM	EEG pattern resembles the one described for stage 1, except that vertex sharp waves are not prominent, alpha activity is usually somewhat more prominent, the frequency is generally 1–2 cps slower than during stage W. "Saw-tooth" waves	Rapid conjugated eye movements	Tonic EMG level reaches its lowest level
MT	Epoches that immediately precede or follow sleep stages, but in which the EEG and EOG tracings are obscured in more than half the epoch by muscle tension and/or amplifier blocking artifacts	Eye movements	High tonic EMG level

From Rechtschaffen & Kales (1968).

strongly recommended in all scoring procedures. One single stage score is assigned to each epoch. When more than one stage is present in an epoch, the one that takes up the greatest portion of the epoch should be scored. The polygraphic characteristics are listed in Table 10.1. Examples of sleep stages according to these criteria are shown in Figure 10.5. The scored stages are then stored in a computer which calculates specific parameters and presents the sleep stage graphically. A simple home or personal computer is adequate. The sleep analysis shown in Figure 10.6 was calculated and drawn by a Commodore Personal Computer 8032 (Commodore Business Machines, Inc.) and an Epson FX 80 Printer (Epson Corporation, Japan). Definitions of frequently used sleep variables are given in Table 10.2.

TABLE 10.2 EEG Sleep Variables

Parameter		Definition
Average REM activity		RA/TSA
Awake	(A)	Time spent awake after sleep onset and before the final morning awakening
Awake/asleep ratio		A/TSA
Delta sleep		Sum of stage 3 and 4
Early morning awakening	(EMA)	Time spent awake from the final awakening until the patient gets out of bed
Percentage stage x	(%Sx)	Percentage of each stage of sleep expressed as a ratio to TSA
REM activity	(RA)	Each minute of REM sleep is scored on a 0–8 scale for REM patterns, the sum for the whole night providing RA
REM density	(RD)	RA/RT
REM latency	(RL)	Time from onset stage 2 to onset stage REM
Sleep efficiency	(SE)	(TSA/TRP) × 100
Sleep latency	(SL)	Time from light out until first stage 2
Sleep maintenance	(SM)	(TSA/(TRP-SL)) × 100
Total recording period	(TRP)	Minutes of total recording (time from lights out until the patient gets out of bed)
Time spent asleep	(TSA)	Time spent asleep less any awake (A) time during the night after sleep onset
Total stage x	(TSx)	Minutes of each stage of sleep

From Rechtschaffen and Kales (1968) and Ulrich et al. (1980).

METHODOLOGIC CONSIDERATIONS

Sleep measurements should reflect a typical nightly schedule in everyday life. It should thus be reproducible in single individuals and should allow comparisons between groups of subjects. It is well known that variations in methodologic considerations can markedly affect sleep variables (Dement et al., 1984). At the present time no widely accepted sleep recording standards have been specifically adopted by the sleep research community (Dement et al., 1984). It is therefore very important to define methodologic considerations in sleep research.

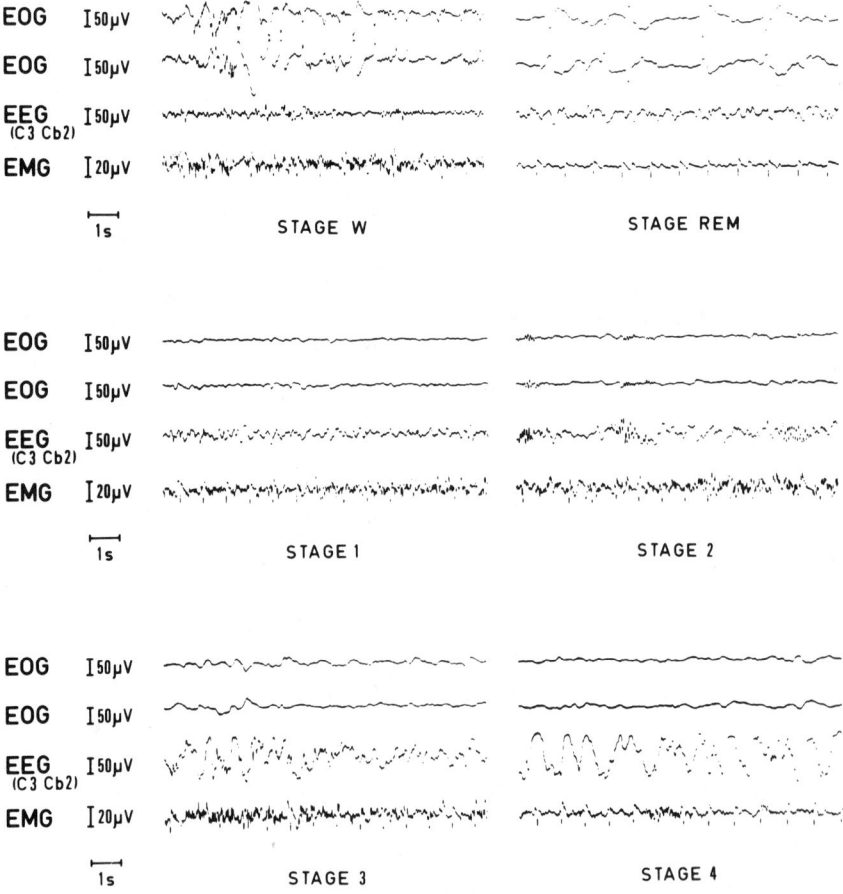

FIGURE 10.5 Polygraphic characteristics of sleep stages according to the Rechtschaffen and Kales criteria (Rechtschaffen & Kales, 1968).

```
Start of recording                     20.55  h
End                         600  min    6.55  h
Stage 1 onset                27  min   21.22  h
Final awakening             574  min    6.29  h
Sleep duration              542  min
Sleep latency                32  min
Early morning awakening      26  min
Awake                        13  min
Time spent asleep           530  min
Awake/asleep ratio          .02
Sleep efficiency             88    %
Sleep maintenance            93    %
Stage 1                     172  min   32.4  %
Stage 2                     176  min   33.1  %
Stage 3                      74  min   13.9  %
Stage 4                       3  min    .5   %
Delta sleep                  76  min   14.4  %
REM sleep                   107  min   20.1  %
REM latency                  99  min
REM activity                 96
Average REM activity        .18
REM density                  .9
```

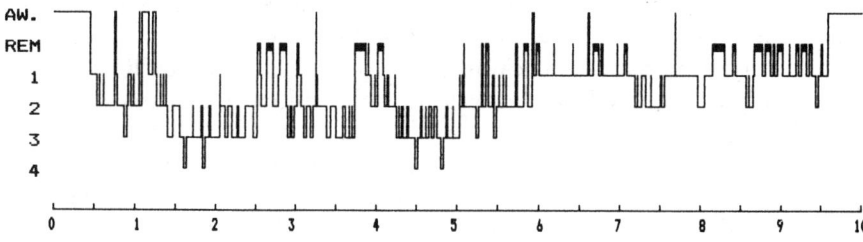

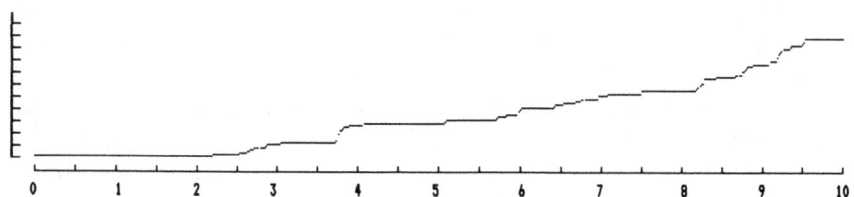

FIGURE 10.6 Sleep analysis of a depressive woman of 67 years of age (for explanation of terms see Table 10.2).

Length of the Recording Period

Two basic designs are used for sleep laboratory studies (Kales & Kales, 1984). One design uses an "ad-lib" protocol in which subjects are allowed to stay in bed as long as they wish (Feinberg, 1974; Webb, 1982; Williams et al., 1974). The other design is marked by a fixed recording period (Kales & Kales, 1984). The "ad-lib" design makes comparisons difficult between groups of subjects, as sleep onset, total waking time, and time spent asleep differ (Kales & Kales, 1984), but it reflects a more typical nightly schedule in an individual. The fixed recording period allows comparison between different groups of subjects, but reflects an artificial situation.

Influence of Environment and Recording Technique on Sleep Variables

Another exceedingly important issue in standardization is the number of nights required to yield an adequate characterization of sleep in a single individual. Most investigators agree that there is a First Night Effect (FNE) of adaptation to the sleep laboratory environment, characterized by more stage W and stage 2, less stage REM, an increased sleep latency and REM latency, more awakenings and stage shifts, and a decreased number of sleep cycles (Agnew et al., 1966; Mendel & Hawkins, 1967; Schmidt & Kaelbing, 1971). Therefore, one night is probably insufficient for investigations. Data from the first night are usually not included in the average values that represent baseline sleep patterns in a study protocol (Kales & Kales, 1984). But it has also been claimed that FNE is absent or minimal in insomniacs and elderly subjects (Webb & Campbell, 1979). Quite recently Reinertshofer et al. (1984) could demonstrate in eight normal males (mean age of 24.75) by using telemetry techniques that there was only a significant effect of adaptation to the sleep laboratory environment concerning the REM latency (increased in the first night and lasted several nights) compared to the fifth night. Other significant FNE existed for subjective parameters.

Concerning the use of different recording technology, Koerner et al. (1982) compared sleep stage patterns in a group of 11 normal subjects (mean of age 29.7) obtained both in a conventional sleep laboratory and mobile sleep recording at home by Holter technology. A significantly higher value for the evaluation of the sleep efficiency index (quotient of total sleep time and time spend in bed) was found with the mobile recording system. Furthermore, there was found to be a significant decrease of stage 1 in favor of REM sleep. Regarding the relation between the REM and NREM time, a distinct difference could also be shown. Studies concerning the FNE using Holter recording technology outside the sleep laboratory in age- and sex-matched groups consisting of normal subjects and those with sleep disorders are still inconclusive. Preliminary results of our running study in sleep research using Holter technology (Medilog 4-24, Oxford Medical System Ltd., Oxfordshire, England) outside a sleep laboratory suggest that there is no clear FNE in elderly normal subjects (older than 60, $n=6$) and in psychiatric patients requiring hospitalization (unselected, untreated, older than 60, $n=17$).

SLEEP AND AGING

Medical science knows little about the fundamental biology of aging. Changes in sleep appear to be one consistent sign of biological aging. But it has not always been obvious whether these findings are signs of maturation or of sleep pathology (Miles & Dement, 1980). Generally, the elderly do seem to be dissatisfied with their sleep. Methodologically heterogeneous surveys reported a clear consensus between increased age and increased time in bed, wake after sleep onset, and use of more sleeping pills (Ballinger, 1976; Bixler et al., 1979; Kales et al., 1974; McGhie & Russel, 1962).

Objective Sleep Parameters in Elderly Subjects

Because sleep patterns in normal subjects are influenced considerably by age, and to a lesser extent by sex, knowledge of sleep and its variations in normal subjects is essential for evaluation of the sleep of subjects with sleep disorders (Kales & Kales, 1984).

Time in Bed

The nocturnal time in bed is highest in childhood, lowest in adults, and rises in old age without reaching childhood levels (Williams et al., 1970). Feinberg et al. (1967) found an average nocturnal time in bed of 420.7 min (± 27 min) for young normal adults (19 to 36 years, $n=15$), and 468.9 min (± 38.3 min) for aged normal subjects (65 to 96 years, $n=15$). Prinz et al. (1975) found in polygraphic sleep studies in the homes of 12 healthy aged subjects (75 to 90 years) an average nocturnal time in bed of 475.6 min ($\pm$ 52 min).

Sleep Latency

Some studies have found normal sleep latency (Williams et al., 1970; Foret & Webb, 1974), some found increased sleep latency (Agnew & Webb 1971; Cavazzuti & Recaldin, 1975; Feinberg et al., 1967). In the Feinberg study (Feinberg et al., 1967) the average sleep latency of the elderly was 18.5 min ($\pm$ 11.1 min) versus 10.4 min ($\pm$ 7.2 min) in the young normal group. Hayashi et al. (1979) reported an average sleep latency of 39.8 min in the elderly (73 to 92 years, 5 males, 10 females) versus 11.5 min for young adults.

Total Sleep Time

Total sleep time seems to be reduced (Williams et al., 1970; Kahn & Fisher, 1969) or unchanged in the elderly (Feinberg et al., 1967; Prinz et al., 1975). Feinberg et al. (1967) reported a total sleep time of 384.4 ± 36.5 min; Prinz et al. (1975) showed a total sleep time of 390 to 420 min.

Wake After Sleep Onset

Waking time after sleep onset increases considerably with age (Agnew & Webb, 1968; Meyer, 1971; Kales & Kales, 1984; Webb, 1982; Williams, 1974), and men waken more often during the night than women. Older men also have been reported to have more wakefulness after sleep onset (Kales & Kales, 1984; Williams et al., 1974). Thus the increased wakefulness often experienced by the elderly is generally the result of more frequent and prolonged awakenings during the night (Feinberg et al., 1967; Feinberg & Carlson, 1968; Feinberg, 1974; Hayashi & Endo, 1982; Webb, 1982; Williams et al., 1974).

Sleep Stage Patterns

REM Sleep The absolute amount and percentage of REM sleep are inversely correlated with age (Roffwarg et al., 1966; Williams et al., 1964). This reduction in the percentage of REM sleep may be due to the fact that the elderly tend to be awake during the latter part of the night, when REM is usually most prevalent (Miles & Dement, 1980). Prinz et al. (1975) reported an average REM sleep time in elderly subjects of 75.8 ($\pm$ 13.5) min, representing 18.4% of total sleep time.

NREM Sleep Sleep stage patterns also change with age. Feinberg et al. (1967) report virtually no difference in the absolute amount of NREM sleep between the young normal (304.4 $\pm$ 28.9 min, $n=15$) and elderly normal subjects (303.4 $\pm$ 36.8 min, $n=15$).

Stage 1 sleep. Agnew et al. (1967) reported that an average of 10.91% ($\pm$ 5.67) of total sleep time was spent in stage 1. Men have a higher stage 1 percentage than women, from puberty onwards (Foret & Webb, 1974; Hursch et al., 1972). The mean percent of total sleep time spent in stage 1 increases steadily throughout life (Williams et al., 1970). An excessive total duration of stage 1 sleep and an increase in the number of shifts into stage 1 sleep are both considered to be indications of sleep disturbance (Miles & Dement, 1980).

Stage 2 sleep. Stage 2 sleep levels in old age are similar to those seen in early adult life (approximates an inverted U-curve throughout life) (Williams et al., 1970). Kales et al. (1967) reported an average of about 60% of total sleep time spent in stage 2 sleep in aged subjects with little night-to-night variation. Hayashi found that in the elderly an average of about 40.5% of total sleep time was spent in stage 2 sleep.

Slow wave sleep. Slow wave sleep decreases even more dramatically with age (Feinberg et al., 1967; Feinberg, 1974; Kales et al., 1967; Kleitman & Engelman, 1953; Roffwarg et al., 1966). Whereas children spent about 20–25% of their total sleep in slow wave sleep (Kleitman & Engelman, 1953), the elderly spent little or no time in slow wave sleep. There is an absolute and relative reduction in the time spent in stage 4 sleep in the elderly. Stage 3 sleep tends to be normal or even elevated in elderly females, and normal or reduced in males (Agnew et al., 1967; Kales et al., 1966; Meyer, 1971; Thompson & Marsh, 1973). Kales et al. (1967) found the percentage of stage 3 sleep with 10.6% of total sleep time to be very similar to that of younger subjects with 10.3%. Stage 4 sleep was reduced in the elderly subjects, accounting for 1.4% of sleep, compared with 11.2% in the younger subjects.

Distribution of Sleep Throughout 24 Hours

Webb and Swinburne (1971) reported an average of 558 min in men and 474 min in women spent sleeping throughout 24 hours ($n=19$, 66 to 96 years). Of this amount 92% occurred during the night; the number of daytime naps averaged 1.8 in males and 1.4 in females. The average time in bed over the 24-hour period was 716 min ($\pm$ 42 min) in men and 702 min ($\pm$ 30 min) in women.

Sleep Parameters in Pathological Aging

Feinberg et al. (1967) investigated 15 young normal (19 to 36 years of age), 15 aged normal (65 to 96 years of age), and 15 chronic brain syndrome subjects (64 to 92 years of age) by uninterrupted recording of sleep polygraphy for four or five nights. Their results indicate that normal aging is associated with a diminished ability to sustain sleep, decreased stage 4, and (less regularly) increased stage 3 activity, and a tendency toward decreased emergent stage 1 EEG and rapid eye-movement activity. Except for stage 3 and stage 4 EEG, each of these variables was correlated with both age and performance on psychometric tests over the range of 64 to 96 years. Pathological aging, as manifested in the chronic brain syndrome group, showed an accentuation of these changes. The authors suggested that the EEG of sleep may prove to be a diagnostic and research tool of special value to geriatric psychiatry. Other studies have directly assessed the relationship between intellect and sleep (Oliver-Martin et al., 1975; Prinz et al., 1975, 1978). REM sleep decrements appear to reflect normal age-related changes, as well as pathological changes, in the functional integrity of the brain; these decrements also change with stress and depression (Hartmann, 1966).

EVALUATION OF INSOMNIA

While electrophysiological methods for assessing sleep disorders could contribute basic data on insomnia that would be objective and precise, there is no definition of what constitutes disturbed sleep (Dement et al., 1984). A wide overlap exists between objective sleep parameters of normal sleepers and insomniacs (Carskadon et al., 1976; Monroe, 1967; Williams et al., 1972). Therefore, a multidimensional research assessment is necessary to identify those treatments that will produce a favorable outcome (Kales et al., 1974; Kales et al., 1976). By taking a complete sleep history in evaluating sleep disorders, the clinician obtains important information on the onset, progression, and clinical characteristics of the disorder, as well as its effect on the patient's life (Kales et al., 1980). Medical, psychological, and behavioral factors should be evaluated to complete the assessment of sleep disorders.

REFERENCES

Agnew, H. W., Webb, W. B., & Williams, R. L. (1966). The first night effect: an EEG study of sleep. *Psychophysiology, 2,* 263–266.

Agnew, H. Jr., Webb, W., & Williams, R. (1967). Sleep patterns in late middle aged males: an EEG study. *Electroencephalogr. Clin. Neurophysiol., 23,* 168–171.

Agnew, H. Jr., & Webb, W. (1968). Sleep patterns of healthy elderly. *Psychophysiol., 5,* 229.

Agnew, H., & Webb, W. (1971). Sleep latencies in human subjects-age, prior wakefulness, and reliability. *Psychosom. Sci., 24,* 253–254.

Aserinsky, E., & Kleitman, N. (1953). Regularly occurring periods of eye motility and concomitant phenomena during sleep. *Science, 118,* 273–274.

Aserinsky, E., & Kleitman, N. (1955). Two types of ocular motility occurring in sleep. *J. Appl. Physiol., 8,* 1–10.

Ballinger, C. (1976). Subjective sleep disturbance at menopause. *J. Psychosom. Res., 20,* 509–513.

Balter, M. B., & Bauer, M. L. (1974). Patterns of prescribing and use of hypnotic drugs in the United States. In A. D. Clift (Ed.), *Sleep Disturbances and Hypnotic Drug Dependence,* (pp. 261–194). New York: Exerpta Medica.

Bixler, E. O., Kales, A., Soldatos, C., Kales, J., & Healey, S. (1979). Prevalence of sleep disorders: A survey of the Los Angeles metropolitan area. *Am. J. Psychiatry, 136,* 1257–1262.

Carskadon, M. A., Dement, W. C., Mitler, M. M., Guilleminault, C., Zarcone, V. P., & Spiegel, R. (1976). Self-reports versus sleep laboratory findings in 122 drug-free subjects with the complaint of chronic insomnia. *Am. J. Psychiatry 133,* 1382–1388.

Cavazzuti, F., & Recaldin, E. (1975). Aspetti clinici dei disturbi del sonno nell' anziano e criteri di terapia (Clinical aspects of sleep disturbances in the elderly and treatment criteria). *Giornale Di Gerontologia (Firenze), 23,* 563–581.

Coleman, R. M., Zarcone, V. P., Redington, D., Miles, L. E., Dole, K. V., Perkins, W. C., Gananian, M., Moore, B. J., Stringer, J., & Dement, W. C. (1980). Sleep-wake disorders in a family practice clinic. In M. H. Chase, D. F. Kripke, & P. L. Walter (Eds), *Sleep Research, Vol. 9,* (p. 192). Los Angeles: University of California, UCLA Brain Information Service/Brain Research Institute.

Coleman, R. M. (1983). Diagnosis, treatment, and follow-up of about 8,000 sleep/wake disorder patients. In C. Guilleminault, & E. Lugaresi (Eds.), *Sleep/wake disorders: natural history, epidemiology, and long-term evolution* (pp. 87–97). New York: Raven Press.

Cooper, R., Osselton, J. W., & Shaw, J. C. (1974). *Elektroenzephalographie.* Stuttgart: Gustav Fischer Verlag.

Dement, W., Seidel, W., & Carskadon, M. (1984). Issues in the diagnosis and treatment of insomnia. In I. Hindmarch, H. Ott, & T. Roth (Eds.), *Sleep benzodiazepines and performance* (pp. 11–43). Berlin, Heidelberg, New York, Tokyo: Springer-Verlag.

Feinberg, I., Koresko, R. L., & Heller, N. (1967). EEG sleep patterns as a function of normal and pathological aging in man, *J. Psychiatr. Res., 5,* 107–144.

Feinberg, I., & Carlson, V. (1968). Sleep variables as a function of age in man. *Arch. Gen. Psychiatry, 18,* 239–250.

Feinberg, I. (1974). Changes in sleep cycle patterns with age. *J. Psychiatric. Res., 10,* 283–306.

Ferries, C. D. (1974). *Introduction to bioelectrodes.* New York: Plenum Press.

Foret, J., & Webb, W. (1974). The sleep of 50 year old people revisited. *Sleep Res., 3,* 71.

Hartmann, E. (1966). Dreaming sleep (the D-state) and the menstrual cycle. *J. Nerv. Ment. Dis., 10,* 406–416.

Hayashi, Y., Otomo, E., Endo, S., & Watanabe, H. (1979). The all-night polygraphies for healthy aged persons. *Sleep Res., 8,* 122.

Hayashi, Y., & Endo, S. (1982). All-night sleep polygraphic recordings of healthy aged persons: REM and slow-wave sleep. *Sleep Res., 5,* 239–250.

Holter, N. J., & Gengerelli, J. A. (1949). Remote recording of physiological data by radio. *Rocky Mtn. Med. J., 46,* 747.

Hursch, C., Karacan, I., & Williams, R. (1972). Stage 1-REM from infancy to old age. *Sleep Res., 1,* 87.

Irrgang, U. (1979). Technische Voraussetzungen fuer eine qualifizierte EEG-Ableitung. *Das EEG-Labor, 1,* 87–99.

Ives, J. R., Thompson, C. J., & Woods, J. F. (1973). Acquisition by telemetry and computer analysis of 4-channel, long term EEG recordings from patients subject to "petit-mal" absence attacks. *Electroencephalogr. Clin. Neurophysiol., 34,* 665.

Ives, J. R., & Woods, J. F. (1975). 4-channel 24 hour cassette recorder for long-term EEG monitoring of ambulatory patients. *Electroencephalogr. Clin. Neurophysiol., 39,* 88–92.

Jasper, H. H. (Committee Chairman). (1958). The ten twenty electrode system of the International Federation. *Electroencephalogr. Clin. Neurophysiol., 10,* 371–375.

Johnson, L. C., & Spinweber, C. L. (1983). Quality of sleep and performance in the navy: a longitudinal study of good and poor sleepers. In C. Guilleminault & E. Lugaresi (Eds.), *Sleep wake disorders: natural history, epidemiology, and long-term evolution* (pp. 13–28). New York: Raven Press

Kahn, E., & Fisher, C. (1969). The sleep characteristics of the normal aged male. *J. Nerv. Ment. Dis., 148,* 474–494.

Kales, A., Kales, J., Jacobson, A., Weissbach, R., Walter, R. D., & Wilson, T. (1966). All night EEG Studies: Children and elderly. *Electroencephalogr. Clin. Neurophysiol. 21,* 415.

Kales, A., Wilson, T., Kales, J. D., Jacobson, A., Paulson, M. J., Kollar, E., & Walter, R. D. (1967). Measurements of all-night sleep in normal elderly persons: effects of aging. *J. Am. Geriatr. Soc., 15,* 405–414.

Kales, A., Bixler, E. O., & Kales, J. D. (1974). Role of the sleep research and treatment facility: diagnosis, treatment and education, In E. D. Weitzman (Ed.), *Advances in sleep research,* Vol. 1. New York: Spectrum Publications.

Kales, A., Kales, J. D., Bixler, E. O., & Scharf, M. B. (1975). Methodology of sleep laboratory drug evaluations: further considerations. In F. Kagan, T. Harwood, K. Rickels, A. Rudzik, & H. Sorer (Eds.), *Hypnotics: methods of development and evaluation* (pp. 109–126) New York: Spectrum Publishers.

Kales, A., Caldwell, A., Preston, A., Healey, S., & Kales, J. (1976). Personality patterns in insomnia: Theoretical implications. *Arch. Gen. Psychiatry, 33,* 1128–1134.

Kales, A., Soldatos, C. R., & Kales, J. D. (1980). Taking a sleep history. *Am. Fam. Physicians, 22,* 101–108.

Kales, A., & Kales, J. D. (1984). Sleep laboratory studies of insomnia. In *Evaluation and treatment of insomnia* (pp. 61–86). New York, Oxford: Oxford University Press.

Karacan, I., Thornby, J., Anch, M., Holzer, C. E., Warheit, G. L., Schwabb, J. J., & Williams, R. L. (1976). Prevalence of sleep disturbance in a primarily urban Florida county. *Soc. Sci. Med., 10,* 239–244.

Kleitman, N., & Engelman, T. G. (1953). Sleep characteristics of infants. *J. Appl. Physiol., 6,* 269–282.

Koerner, E., Ladurner, G., Flooh, E., Reinhart, B., Wolf, R., & Lechner, H. (1982). Nachtschlafuntersuchungen: Mobile Registrierung im Vergleich mit Konventioneller Laborableitung. *Z EEG-EMG, 13,* 154–156.

Loomis, A. L., Harvey, E. N., & Hobart, G. A. (1937). Cerebral stages during sleep as studied by human brain potentials. *J. Exp. Psychol., 21,* 1217–144.

Lugaresi, E., Cirignotta, F., Zucconi, M., Mondini, S., Lenzi, P. L., & Coccagna, G. (1983). Good and poor sleepers: an epidemiological survey of the San Marino population. In C. Guilleminault & E. Lugaresi (Eds.), *Sleep/wake disorders: natural history, epidemiology, and long-term evolution.* New York: Raven Press.

McGhie, A., & Russel, S. (1962). The subjective assessment of normal sleep patterns. *J. Ment. Sci. 108,* 642–654.

Mendel, J., & Hawkins, D. R. (1967). Sleep laboratory adaption in normal subjects and depressed patients ("first night effect"). *Electroencephalogr. Clin. Neurophysiol., 22,* 556–558.

Miles, L. E., & Dement, W. C. (1980). Sleep and aging. *Sleep Res., 2,* 119–220.

Monroe, L. (1967). Psychological and physiological differences between good and poor sleepers. *J. Abnorm. Psychol., 72,* 255–264.

Meyer, H. (1971). Sleep disorders in the elderly—A social medicine problem. *Praxis, 60,* 1041–1042.

Oliver-Martin, R., Cendron, H., & Vallery-Masson, J. (1975). Le sommeil chez les sujets ages: Description et analyse de quelques donnees recueillies das une population rurale. *Annales Medico-Psychologiques (Paris), 1,* 77–90.

Porter, R. J., Wolf, A. A., & Penry, J. K. (1971). Human electroencephalographic telemetry. *Am. J. EEG Technol., 11,* 145.

Prinz, P., Obrist, W., & Wang, H. (1975). Sleep patterns in healthy elderly subjects: Individual differences as related to other neurological variables. *Sleep Res., 4,* 132.

Prinz, P., Andrews-Kulis, M., Storrie, M., Bartol, M., Raskind, M., & Gerber, C. (1978). Sleep waking pattern in normal aging and in dementia. *Sleep Res., 7,* 138.

Rechtschaffen, A., Kales, A. (eds), Berger, R. J., Dement, W. C., Jacobson, A., Johnson, L. C., Jouvet, M., Monroe, L. J., Oswald, I., Roffwarg, H. P., Roth, B., & Walter, R. D. (1968). A manual of standardized terminology, techniques, and scoring system for sleep stages of human subjects. Washington, DC: US Government Printing Office Public Health Service.

Reinertshofer, Th, v. Oefele, K., Nedopil, N., & Ruether, E. (1984). Objective and subjective adaptation to the sleep laboratory. In *Abstracts of the 7th European Sleep Congress* (p. 262).

Roffwarg, H., Muzio, J., & Dement, W. (1966). Ontogenetic development of the human sleep-dream cycle. *Science, 152,* 604–619.

Schmidt, H. S., & Kaelbing, H. (1971). The differential laboratory adaptation of sleep parameters. *Biol. Psychiatry, 3,* 33–45.

Thompson, L., & Marsh, G. (1973). Psychophysiological studies of aging. In C. Eisdorfer, & M. Lawton *The psychology of adult development and aging* (p. 122–148). Washington, D.C.: American Psychological Association.

Webb, W., & Swinburne, H. (1971). An observational study of sleep in the aged. *Percept. Mot. Skills, 32,* 895–898.

Webb, W., & Campbell, S. (1979). The first night effect revisited with age as a variable. *Waking and Sleeping, 3,* 319–324.

Webb, W. B. (1982). Sleep in older persons: sleep structure of 50- to 60-year-old men and women. *J. Gerontol., 37,* 581–586.

Williams, R. L., Agnew, H. W. Jr., & Webb, W. B. (1964). Sleep patterns in young adults: an EEG study. *Electroencephalogr. Clin. Neurophysiol. 17,* 376–381.

Williams, R., Karacan, I., & Hursch, C. (1970). *Electroencephalography of human sleep: Clinical applications* (pp. 1–169). New York: Wiley.

Williams, R. L., Hursch, C. J., & Karacan, I. (1972). Between-subjects variability and night-to-night variability in insomniacs and normal controls. *Sleep Res., 1,* 154.

Williams, R. L., Karacan, I., & Hursch, C. J. (1974). *EEG of human sleep: clinical applications.* New York: Wiley.

PART III
Psychogeriatric Disorders

11
Epidemiology of Psychogeriatric Disorders

Michael Shepherd

Almost 25 years ago a WHO Expert Committee produced a 50-page report on "Mental health problems of aging and the aged in their demographic . . . social and medical setting as a preliminary to discussing the possible means of protecting and promoting mental health and mitigating or curing mental illness in the aged" (WHO, 1959). In acknowledging the various issues raised by the well-established associations between senescence and mental ill-health, the tenor of the report was broadly optimistic. With reference to the expectations in Sweden that "the expected increase in the proportion of invalids in old age may have been more than offset by social and medical progress," the report concluded that "although the aging of populations creates certain serious problems, there has been a tendency to magnify the dangers that are likely to arise. The approach to the problems created by the increasing proportion of old people in many populations should be informed by the fact that such aging is a part of social progress."

A generation later this verdict is difficult to reconcile with the widespread concern aroused by the lengthening life-span not least by WHO which has been involved in the World Assembly on the Elderly. The senium has already been subdivided into the "troisième" and the "quatrième" ages on either side of the 75th year. Gerontology has emerged as a flourishing discipline. There has even been a revival of interest in the biological possibilities of extending the life-span (*Nature*, 1982), despite the observations attributed to Lemuel Gulliver concerning the immortal Struldbrugs whom he encountered in the country of Luggnagg during his travels. "When they come to fourscore years," wrote Jonathan Swift, they had not only all the Follies and Infirmities of other Old Men, but many more which arose from the dreadful Prospects of never dying. They were not only opinionative, peevish, covertous, morose, vain, talkative, but uncapable of Friendship, and dead to all natural affection, which never descended below their Grandchildren. The least miserable among them appear to be those who turn to Dotage and entirely lose their Memories; these meet with more Pity and Assistance, because they want many bad Qualities which abound in others.

This description foreshadows several of the problems posed by the sharply rising number of mentally disordered elderly people, to which the word "epidemic" is now freely applied. Indeed, the term "pandemic" was preferred by Morton Kramer in his jeremiad some years ago (Kramer, 1980). Such terms may be taken to indicate the relevance of an epidemiological approach to a major issue in public health, and in retrospect it is significant that the WHO Expert Committee report employed the noun "epidemiology" only once, and then in relation to suicide. Times have changed. In this chapter I propose to demonstrate not only that the epidemiological perspective has become indispensable for the psychiatrist concerned with the assessment and management of the mental illnesses of the senium, but that this perspective has been and should be adopted by representatives of a variety of related disciplines.

DESCRIPTIVE EPIDEMIOLOGY

I begin with descriptive epidemiology, a field that owes much to demography and medical geography. The contours of the situation are summarized in Table 11.1. These data make it apparent that the subject is an issue of global importance, recognized especially on the European continent.

TABLE 11.1 Development of the Age Structure in Europe from 1970 to 2000, Excluding the USSR, by Age Groups (%)

Age group	1970	1980	1990	2000
0 – 14	24.9	23.0	22.3	21.7
15 – 59	58.4	60.4	60.1	60.0
60+	16.7	16.6	17.6	18.3
60 – 74	12.9	11.9	12.3	13.2
75+	3.8	4.7	5.3	5.1

Source: Secretariat of the Economic Commission for Europe (ECE), Geneva. (1975). *Post-war demographic trends in Europe and the outlook until the year 2000. Economic Survey of Europe in 1974, Part II.* New York: United Nations.

One basic point needs to be established at the outset, namely, that while epidemiology has to do with populations, a senescent population can be regarded in two quite different ways: either as an arbitrarily defined, age-limited aggregate compared and contrasted with a chronologically younger population, or as the residue of a total population which has survived the hazards of youth and middle age to enter the senium. The objectives of the investigator will be in one of two directions, depending on the way in which he views the population: the first will tend to be the study of disease, the second of decrement.

NEUROEPIDEMIOLOGY

The recently founded subdiscipline of neuroepidemiology, which focuses on the dementias (Capildeo et al., 1983), is the most clearly delineated example of the former approach. After a long period of neglect these conditions have recently reanimated the attention of the neurologists, whose outlook is embodied in the clarion-call sounded in 1978 by Professor Fred Plum. His particular target was the Alzheimer-senile form of dementia because it accounts for more than 50% of dementia over the age of 65. To Plum this is "an increasingly prevalent neurological disease . . . an epidemic that can be prevented only by successful attention of science and especially neurobiology to solving the problems that manifest themselves predominantly in the aging brain . . . Alzheimer disease, like parkinsonism, may turn out to be a specific neurochemical system degeneration, perhaps be susceptible to at least temporary improvement with pharmacotherapy . . . fundamental neuroscience now shares responsibility to our future public health comparable to that shouldered by microbiology a half century ago" (Plum, 1979). The spectacularly successful elucidation of the pathogenesis of kuru by Gajdusek and his colleagues has encouraged the advancement of etiological hypotheses in terms of neurochemistry, immunology, virology, and genetics but biologically-oriented neuroepidemiological research in this field is hampered by two clinical obstacles: first, dementia is a syndrome that results from several disease processes and, second, Alzheimer's disease remains a diagnosis by exclusion so that, as Gajdusek and his colleagues point out, "Until criteria are established for diagnosis, it seems almost pointless to attempt an epidemiological analysis. . . . At this stage there does not even appear to be any reliable information on the accuracy of clinical diagnoses in a large enough series of patients with Alzheimer's disease. Therefore, no estimate is available on the degree of case ascertainment that might be expected from population surveys" (Masters et al., 1981).

In the present state of knowledge the development of longitudinal studies with case controls designed to identify risk factors represents perhaps the most promising approach to causation via epidemiology, but its potential must be severely limited until more diagnostic precision can be obtained (Sluss, 1980).

CLINICAL EPIDEMIOLOGY

This observation may serve as a pointer to the need for an intensification of work in the important field of clinical epidemiology, especially in what Morris has called "completing the clinical picture" (Morris, 1957). Some of this has been directed to the delineation of particular syndromes, which include the varieties of psycho-organic reactions, morbid preoccupations with the themes of decline and death, the psychiatric links with physical illness, and the environmental strains of isolation. All these conditions, though not unknown among members of younger age groups, present themselves more prominently by virtue of their efflorescence in the senium.

One fundamental reason for expanding knowledge in this sphere is the significance for classification, a topic of particular concern to epidemiologists, and one that is poorly developed in psychogeriatrics, as may be demonstrated by the differences between the schemata of ICD9 and DSM III. In addition, the prospects of clinical epidemiology have been extended by the study of the large captive populations of chronic psychiatric patients whose declining mortality rate has enabled large-scale observations to be made on the later states of the natural history of their disorders. Manfred Bleuler, for example, has pointed to the surprising improvement in his unique series of schizophrenics, and suggested that schizophrenia may be associated with anoxic cerebral changes (Bleuler, 1978). Again, Ciompi has reported that patients with an earlier neurotic or depressive illness improve in their later years, a finding which appears to reflect primarily the influence of social or environmental factors (Ciompi, 1969).

Such factors also exercise a key role in the outcome of mental disorders arising in the senium. As Whitehead and Hunt have recently shown, the 5-year prognosis of those conditions necessitating admission to a hospital is poor (Whitehead & Hunt, 1982), but the extramural milieu clearly plays a major role in both the patients' symptomatology and their capacity for adaptation. It was for this reason that some years ago I recommended and outlined a research design for phase 4 of the WHO study of Mental Health Services in Pilot Study Areas. The earlier, monitoring exercises had already demonstrated the growing size of the burden, the pressure on beds and on community services, and the need for rationalizing the available facilities. My proposal was based on a prospective investigation of discharged psychogeriatric patients whose subsequent fates could be compared as they passed through the extramural services of the various areas. The demographic and epidemiological information collected in these areas indicates a wide diversity of facilities whose relative effectiveness and efficiency could thus be evaluated.

DRUG EPIDEMIOLOGY

The above applies mainly to the institutionalized elderly. Community surveys, however, reveal a large extramural reservoir of all but the most severe degrees of mental disorders in old age (Magnussen et al., 1982). The key medical agent concerned with their care is the primary care physician, who may acknowledge the significance of psychosocial factors in the genesis of these conditions but all too often relies exclusively on medication in their management, so much so that the prescription of psychotropic drugs to the elderly has become one of the major aspects of another new subdiscipline, that of "drug-epidemiology." Population-based figures show a seemingly universal picture. In a recent survey of the Canadian province of Saskatchewan, for example, the over-60s constitute some 16% of the population but receive 42% of all psychotropic drugs prescribed; more than half the people in this age group were taking these drugs, twice the proportion for people of all ages (Saskatchewan Alcoholism Commission, 1981). The same trend is evident in the United Kingdom concerning the prescription of sedatives, hypnotics, neuroleptics, and antidepressants, as well as the large array of "cerebral vasodilators and activators," all of them scientifically dubious yet widely employed.

The most striking effect of this therapeutic fashion has been an iatrogenically induced epidemic of adverse pharmacological effects, some more incapacitating than the disorder being treated. It may be mentioned that from a biological standpoint the increased susceptibility of the elderly to the unwanted effects appears to be related to a change in the pharmacokinetics and an impairment in the homeostatic mechanisms of old age. From an epidemiological standpoint it represents a major hazard to be weighed against the possible advantages of medication.

PSYCHOSOCIAL EPIDEMIOLOGY

In the ascertainment of mental illness in the population at large, epidemiologists rely on traditional techniques, laying particular emphasis on such issues as sampling and standardized methods of assessment. In disorders of the senium, however, a particular problem arises from the need to study "decline" or "decrement" as well as disease, for while the study of "decline" has to do with psychobiological variation, epidemiology, per se, deals only with the pathological part of that variation. The remainder is normal variation, partly a physiological adaptive response to environment, and partly a failure of homeostasis. In operational terms, therefore, as several workers have acknowledged, a dimensional rather than a categorical model of dysfunction becomes imperative in distinguishing between mental health and ill-health in the aged by means of the epidemiological method.

The methodological problems of this task have been analyzed by Cooper and Schwartz (1982) who point out that "mental health must . . . be defined in terms of psychological rather than of physiological functioning." They stop short, however, of extending their discussion to the sphere of yet another subdiscipline, that of psychosocial epidemiology. While drawing attention to the "shortage of accurate reliable measures" they make no mention of intelligence, although the borderlands between decrement and disease are sharply illuminated by recent developments in psychology. Here the atheoretical psychometric mode of enquiry, based on statistical theory, has been superseded by modern cognitive psychology which favors a more active concern with functional mechanisms. According to this approach, whereas the fluid, and to some extent the crystalized, cognitive abilities developed in the early years represent a genetically regulated process of maturation, aging is not so much an orderly, unidirectional process of decline as a disorderly, multidirectional process resembling, in military terms, a rout rather than a retreat. The end state of later years thus becomes dependent on the stability of the psychobiological systems underlying intellectual performance, which in turn is subject to a variety of environmental influences, including disease and dysfunction. In these circumstances, psychometrics are less useful than the concept of intelligence developed by Welford as an extension of Bartlett's work on the analysis of skills in real life situations, where performance is affected by not only bodily changes but also such forces as motivation, social prestige, and expectations, and the development of methods of coping with situations and problems.

This concept leads naturally from the psychological to the social component of psychosocial epidemiology, which focuses, over and above the formal increase in failing faculties, on what has been called "the real pathology of old age . . . pain, disablement, frustration, boredom, lack of purpose and loss of identity and self-respect, all of which lead to dissatisfaction with the quality of life" (Tulloch et al., 1979). Most of these features have been confirmed by recent surveys of old people, and many of the problems are summarized in the so-called "environmental docility" hypothesis, according to which, "As the competence of the individual decreases, the proportion of behaviour attributable to environmental, as compared with personal characteristics increases" (Amann, 1981). This is not, however, to demean the role of those personal attributes, among which the subject's sense of well-being emerges as the most important (Garritt et al., 1978). As a number of studies on elderly populations have shown, it is via the concept of self-rated health status that the interests of social gerontologists and epidemiologists overlap (Tissue, 1972). The evidence makes it clear that the subjects' state of health, as assessed by medical examination, is closely related to the level of the perception, but this in turn is an essentially subjective response related more closely to general health than to verifiable criteria of the physical and mental condition. Such findings constitute the twin basis of Mark Abrams' conclusion, based on a detailed survey of a group of 1,600 individuals over 65, that ". . . any substantial progress in raising the life satisfaction of elderly people depends largely upon providing better and more extensive health services for them and upon providing them with equivalents of the support already available to many through proximity to good neighbours and friends" (Abrams, 1978).

CONCLUSION

Here, then, is a practical note on which to terminate this brief survey. From it emerges the fact that a number of disciplines—demography, neuropsychiatry, psychology, sociology, pharmacology, gerontology—all employ the epidemiological method to study the etiology, clinical features, and management of mental disorder in old age. It is hoped that their joint efforts will contribute to knowledge and to effective action.

REFERENCES

Abrams, M. (1978). *Beyond three-score and ten* (p. 23). Age Concern Research Publication. Worcester, London: The Trinity Press.

Amann, A. (1981). *The status and prospects of the aging in Western Europe.* Occasional paper No. 8. European Centre for Social Welfare Training and Research. Vienna.

Bleuler, M. (1978). *The schizophrenic disorders.* New Haven, London: Yale University Press.

Capildeo, R., Haberman, S., Benjamin, B., & Rose, F. C. (1983). Why neuroepidemiology? *Psychological Medicine, 13,* 15–16.

Ciompi, L. (1969). Follow-up studies on evolution of former neurotic and depressive states in old age: Clinical and psychodynamic aspects. *Journal of Geriatric Psychiatry, 3,* 90–106.

Cooper, B., & Schwartz, R. (1982). Psychiatric case-identification in an elderly urban population. *Social Psychiatry, 17,* 43–52.

Garritt, T. F., Somes, G. W., & Marx, M. B. (1978). Factors influencing self-assessment of health. *Social Science and Medicine, 12,* 77–81.

Kramer, M. (1980). The rising pandemic of mental disorders and associated chronic diseases and disabilities. In E. Strömgren, A. Dupont, & J. A. Nielsen (Eds.), *Epidemiological research as basis for the organization of extramural psychiatry* (pp. 382–397). *Acta Psychiatrica Scandinavica,* Suppl. 28, Vol. 65.

Magnussen, G., Nielsen, J., & Buch, J. (1982). Epidemiology and prevention of mental illness in old age. *Nordisk Gerontologisk Tidskrift,* Suppl.

Masters, C. L., Gajdusek, D. C., & Gibbs, C. J. (1981). Problems of case ascertainment and diagnosis in the epidemiology of dementia occurring in geographic isolates and worldwide. In J. A. Mortimer & L. M. Schuman (Eds.), *The epidemiology of dementia* (pp. 155–170). New York: Oxford University Press.

Morris, J. N. (1957). *Uses of epidemiology.* Edinburgh, London: Churchill Livingston.

Nature (1982). News and views: The elixir of life. *Nature, 296,* 392–393.

Plum, F. (1979). Dementia: an approaching epidemic. *Nature, 279,* 372–373.

Saskatchewan Alcoholism Commission, Research Division (1981). *Central nervous system, prescription drugs, and elderly people: An overview of issues and a Saskatchewan profile.* Final Report.

Sluss, T. K. (1980). *A method of investigating risk factors for senile dementia—Alzheimer's type in the Baltimore Longitudinal Study.* Doctoral thesis. The John Hopkins University, Baltimore, Maryland.

Swift, C. G. (1981). Psychotropic drugs and the elderly. In G. Tognoni, C. Bellantuono, & M. Lader (Eds.), *Epidemiological impact of psychotropic drugs* (pp. 232–238). Amsterdam: Elsevier.

Tissue, T. (1972). Another look at self-rated health among the elderly. *Journal of Gerontology, 27,* 91–94.

Tulloch, A. J., & Moore, V. (1979). A randomized controlled trial of geriatric screening and surveillance in general practice. *Journal of the Royal College of General Practitioners, 29,* 733–742.

Whitehead, A., & Hunt, A. (1982). Elderly psychiatric patients: A 5-year prospective study. *Psychological Medicine, 12,* 149–157.

World Health Organization (WHO). (1959). *Mental Health Problems of Aging and the Aged.* (Technical Report Series No. 171). Geneva.

12
Depression, Alcoholism, and Other Functional Syndromes

Felix Post

In reviewing the present state of knowledge of depressions and other functional psychiatric disorders, the various conditions will be dealt with in the order in which they are associated with increasing disruption of emotional and other personality functions. To avoid overlap with other chapters, classification, epidemiology, and the various treatment modalities will be dealt with only cursorally. Equally, the areas of gerontopsychiatry in which there has been little increase of knowledge, and to the extent the author is aware, no research is in progress, will be treated only briefly.

PERSONALITY DEVIATIONS

The subject of personality disorders in old age and its relationship to lifelong personality deviations from statistical norms has recently been thoroughly dealt with by Gurland (1984). Adopting Gurland's distinction between personality disorders per se and conditions secondary to personality deviations, in neither area has there been much recent increase in knowledge. The effects of aging on abnormal personalities are of marginal clinical relevance. However, the late development of dependence on alcohol and senile seclusion are of considerable clinical importance.

The Aging Deviant

Like statistically normal individuality, deviant personality is only minimally altered by aging of the central nervous and neuroendocrine systems. Slowing in the interneuronal circuitry and the related decline of learning ability and of memory for new or recently acquired material, together with age-linked changes in patterns of social interaction, may well be factors in the often reported slight shifts with increasing age from extraversion to introversion. The deviant personality with its poor integration in social networks is especially vulnerable to introverting effects of aging.

The traditional senile personality change presents as a caricaturing of potentially maladjustive traits with increased narrowing and withdrawal toward and, in a literal sense, into the self: suspiciousness, surly irritability, avariciousness, moodiness, hypochondriasis, to name only a few. Whether marked character changes of this type occur without causative dementia of old age does not seem to have been investigated. Equally little is scientifically known about the later fate of lifelong deviants. There is an impression that inadequate personalities decline further, with marked deteriorations in standards of cleanliness, and with drifting from lodgings to institutions.

Less markedly inadequate persons may show increasing dependency on their relatives. Possibly, many aggressive personalities improve with aging; there certainly is the well documented decline of criminal tendencies. In a consecutive series of persons (mean age 80.6 years) referred to a psychiatric service from old age homes, only 15% were labelled as exhibiting personality disorders, but their resentment and lack of cooperation arising in an old age home would in most cases not have deserved the diagnosis of a personality disorder if seen by psychiatrists in other settings (Margo et al., 1980).

In a majority of paranoid illnesses of later life this condition develops slowly out of a personality which had been characterized by aloofness, suspiciousness, odd beliefs, and other eccentricities, as well as by a low marriage rate, and almost always by sexual maladjustment (first highlighted by Kay & Roth, 1961, and since then frequently confirmed). Earlier problems with sexual adjustment almost always form the background of complaints made by old people about their sexual functioning. In fact, old people rarely complain about sexual matters spontaneously, but the various ways in which declines in coital ability cause anxiety and phobic complications have recently been summarized by Kral (1984). Elderly male homosexuals, most of whom come to lead an isolated existence, have recently been recognized as a psychologically vulnerable group. To them, just the same as to heterosexual old people with social anxieties, much help can be given (Kimmell, 1977; Corby & Solnick, 1980).

Alcoholism

Many unstable persons enter old age with dependencies on sedatives and sleeping tablets, and in this age group disorders of attention, cognition, and mood are often due to the slower elimination of these substances than in younger subjects. However, the only addictive disorder that has been at all well studied is alcoholism.

It used to be thought that alcohol consumption decreased with rising age on account of greater financial stringency and increasing health consciousness (Mishara & Kastenbaum, 1980), and also that one-third of elderly alcoholics had started to become problem drinkers only after the age of 60 (Rosin & Glatt, 1971) mainly in relation to old age stresses and depressions. More recently, however, Wattis (1983) pointed out that alcoholism of the elderly is becoming a more serious problem as more heavily drinking cohorts move up into higher age ranges, and that smaller amounts of alcohol may result in higher blood concentrations. In a psychiatric screening ward, 23% of patients over 60 were alcoholics and many more were heavy drinkers. The incidence of alcoholism has been reported to peak between the ages of 45 and 50, but another peak occurs between 65 and 75, and by then the male–female ratio has fallen to 3:2 (Simon, 1980); in fact, a predominance of alcoholism in older women has been reported by Edwards et al. (1973).

Alcoholism is thus likely to become an increasingly important psychogeriatric disorder. It is often masked by other conditions, or hidden by collusion between members of the alcoholic's entourage, especially if they themselves are heavy drinkers (Wattis, 1981). Long-standing alcoholic abuse has also recently come into view as an important causal factor in late life dementias (see Wattis, 1983).

Dependency on alcohol is often induced in the elderly by solicitous relatives plying them with calming draughts for their attacks of distress, faintness, and weakness; alcohol can also induce depressive symptoms. Related to this, alcoholism of old people is often more easily managed than at younger ages. Older persons are more easily controlled by their relatives, provided they have been made to respond to discussions of the problem. Otherwise, and where aging drinkers live on their own, the only solution may be a transfer to a residential accommodation with good supervision. On the other hand, small amounts of alcohol may be beneficial (Mishara & Kastenbaum, 1980) and where the intake has gotten out of hand a therapeutic relationship may be all that is needed to put things right (Post, 1982).

Senile Seclusion

This is a condition which, on account of its nature and annual incidence of only 0.5 per 1,000 persons over 60, has been little studied (Macmillan & Shaw, 1966; Clark et al., 1975). A picture has emerged of old people with almost lifelong and increasing aloofness and hostility toward others, who have finally resorted to literally barricading themselves in their homes, rarely venturing outside. Some have their errands run by a relative who is often not allowed to cross the doorstep. Occasionally, the seclusion is shared by a sibling, usually a sister.

Members of the educated classes have been found to predominate, and when it could be tested, intelligence has usually been average or even above. Poverty has hardly ever been a problem—money has been found hidden in severely dilapidated homes which are often indescribably filthy and in an unhygienic state. Complaints about these conditions or terminal physical illness bring these people to hospitals, where many of them die soon after reception. In most, a formal psychiatric diagnosis is not applicable; a few were found to be paranoid in a setting of dementia, and there were also some who could be labelled as paranoid schizophrenics.

It has been claimed that senile recluses can be rehabilitated even without admission to hospital, and that their partners in seclusion quickly resume a normal outlook once they are set free from the patient's domination.

NEUROTIC DISORDERS AND SENILE DYSPHORIA

These two conditions will be dealt with in the same section because they seem to be identical or closely related, with a lowering of mood as the common denominator.

Patients with minor psychiatric disturbances, who account for the bulk of a general psychiatrist's or psychotherapist's work in younger adults, are only rarely seen by psychogeriatricians. Our recently acquired knowledge of these psychiatric disabilities, which hover on the borderlines of illness, has come from epidemiological studies and, to a lesser extent, from psychotherapists interested in the problems of older people.

Neuroses in Old Age

Earlier epidemiological investigations (as summarized by Bergmann, 1978) had noted that patients with neurotic illnesses were increasingly rarely referred to psychiatrists after they had reached the age of 45, but that there was evidence from general practice and community-based studies for a continuing high prevalence of minor psychiatric conditions. Quite recently, however, a German field study (Dilling et al., 1984) revealed that older people were afflicted by clinically significant neurotic and psychosomatic conditions considerably less often than the young, with prevalences of 26.0% in age group 15 to 44, of 23.3% in age group 45 to 64, but only of 16.9% in those over the age of 65. This last figure is very similar to the one given by Bergmann (1978) who reported and elaborated on his earlier findings in a sample of elderly community subjects, from which those diagnosed as organic and functional psychotics had been eliminated. Some neurotic problems were discerned, by means of semistructured interviews with the subjects and independent informants, in 45%, but in only 18% were they graded as disturbing or disabling, and in only 11% had such symptoms been noted for the first time after the age of 60.

Psychopathology

It has long been accepted that hysterics as they grow older no longer demonstrate their distress by conversion symptoms, and there is an impression that some of them tend to become chronic complainers. Nondelusional hypochondriasis, next to depression, is the most common minor psychiatric disorder in the elderly, and it may well present the mechanism by which anxiety is turned inward rather than outward in the form of sweating, tremor, palpitations, and hyperventilating, as seen in younger patients. In the elderly, histrionic as well as hypochondriacal conduct of recent origin quite often indicates an underlying "masked" depression or indeed a physical disease and not neurosis, but nothing has been published about the psychological history of patients employing this cry for help.

Obsessional symptoms rarely appear for the first time after the age of 60, but phobic developments are not infrequently seen, especially after losses of social support and physical breakdowns, like myocardial infarctions. Most patients with hypochondriacal, phobic, or more general anxiety complaints of late onset are concurrently also depressed. In contrast with longstanding neurotics, they are more often socially disadvantaged, and in comparison with early onset neurotics, they are afflicted more often and more severely with serious physical ill-health, and have higher mortality rates. These and other numerous factors associated with neurosis arising only late in life were analyzed from earlier data by Bergmann (1978), but there have been no more recent investigations.

Treatment

A recent overview of the role of psychotherapy in older patients was given by Kahana (1979), who pointed out that neurotic symptoms occurred in a disabling or distressing form in three kinds of cases. The psychological management of patients debilitated by dementing conditions, chronic physical ill-health, and social disintegration does not concern us here. Old people who develop neurotic reactions to recent situational problems usually also suffer from some form of depression, and their psychological management will be discussed later in this chapter. The third group of Kahana's neurotics consisted of essentially healthy aging persons, for whom therapy aimed at modifying attitudes and psychic structures may be rewarding.

There are numerous ways in which psychotherapeutic techniques have to be adapted to older patients. Procedures for increasing insight and life review should be applied only with caution, and greater stress should be laid on the patients' self-esteem and ability to deal with their anxieties (Ingebretsen, 1977). With a similar aim, dreams should be used not in a Freudian way, but should be altered in content by suggestion and autosuggestion toward the positive and hopeful (Brink, 1977). Busse (1976) indicated that the way in which the real problems underlying hypochondriacal complaints can be brought to the surface and dealt with is by allowing the patient's "organ recital" a full run during time-limited therapeutic sessions. In psychotherapy involving complaining old people negative countertransference in the younger therapist is very easily evoked and should be dealt with (Wilensky & Weiner, 1977). Many writers stress the need for psychotherapists working with elderly patients to use more directive methods and not to shy away from involving other family members and social agencies.

Group therapy has serious attendance problems, but one of the few controlled observations in this area found that attendants benefited equally from diffuse or more focalized therapy (Ingersoll & Silverman, 1978). Unlike sessions with younger patients, disturbances of an emotional kind during group sessions with elderly patients should be avoided; some patients may require individual sessions for a time (Krasner, 1977).

The treatment of phobic disorders may be facilitated by behavioral approaches (Brink, 1978). In fact, in the author's personal experience, behavioral methods are surprisingly effective even in very old people for the various types of agoraphobia, and it has been demonstrated (Garfinkel, 1979) that in vivo desensitization is more useful than the imaginal approach.

Senile Dysthymia or Dysphoria

It has long been accepted that, in keeping with the many vicissitudes of old age, depression is a common condition in the elderly. However, clinically based investigations (most recently summarized by Henderson & Kay, 1984) reported point prevalences of depression only of the order of 1 to 4%. Recent community studies using improved methodologies (e.g., Gurland et al., 1980) have confirmed that some 20% of the elderly report depressions, but that these were sufficiently severe to possibly require attention from community health workers in only some 13%. In line with earlier work, the point prevalence of major affective disorders was only 2.5%. Similar results were obtained by Blazer and Williams (1980) who discovered in nearly 15% of community elderly substantial depressive symptomatology. Applying the criteria for Major Depressive Episodes of the DSM III, only just under 4% were identified as suffering from clinical depressions, not always of a primary kind. The remaining 11% of Blazer and Williams' subjects exhibited only three or fewer DSM III criteria for the diagnosis of Major Depressive Episode. These workers hypothesized that these 11% represented old people hitherto described as suffering from senile demoralization, and they suggested the nonpejorative term of senile dysphoria with "dysphoria" being roughly equivalent to the DSM III "dysthymia." There is some overlap, but by and large major depressive episodes (unipolar and bipolar depressions) are equivalent to the endogenous depressions of earlier workers, while the dysthymias include their atypical and neurotic depressions.

Akiskal (1983) has attempted to analyze more finely the disorders which according to DSM III criteria should be classified as dysthymias in younger patients. His attempt to conceptualize depressive conditions which cannot be categorized as clearcut melancholic illnesses is, of course, only the latest of many theoretical speculations of mostly German and French psychiatrists. However, based on biological observations, Akiskal's conceptualizations seem relevant to elderly depressives. Later in this chapter we shall see that a considerable proportion of older patients make only incomplete recoveries after clinical depressions, and these may well be identical with Akiskal's chronic dysthymics; his characterologic dythymics may be equivalent to senile dysphorics. Also we noted earlier that 11% of Bergmann's (1978) elderly community subjects had neurotic symptoms arising for the first time during their sixties or later. This is the identical proportion of subjects labeled as dysphorics by Blazer and Williams (1980) using quite a different method of ascertainment, and most of Bergmann's late onset neurotics showed symptoms of depression. Might these late onset neurotics not be identical with Blazer and Williams' senile dysphorics, and some of them even with some of Akiskal's dysthymics?

Etiology

Regarding the causation of senile dysphoria-dysthymia, there is as yet very little published work concerned specifically with persons thought to be suffering from this disorder. However, research on the background of subjects suffering from "depression" will be briefly discussed in this section, as the great majority of persons assessed as "depressed" would have been exhibiting only minor depressive conditions. It has often been said that depression is a normal occurrence in people when they become aware of getting old, but that most of them lose their depressions as they adjust to the last stage of life. In a cohort study, Lehr (1982) found that over a period of 12 years mood levels remained steady or improved in 46.6% of her elderly subjects, and were lowered, to a trifling extent, in 53.4%. The number and severity of stresses registered by the researcher during the follow-through period did not correlate with lowering of mood levels, but these were affected much more by the subjects' conceptualizations of these stresses and by inadequate coping styles. Women had consistently lower mood levels than men. No doubt related to this, women have a higher monoamine oxydase activity than men throughout the life-span, and it has been shown that in both sexes this activity further increases with age (Robinson et al., 1977). Bereavement certainly is often followed by lasting depression, though only rarely coming to psychiatric attention. In one investigation (Bowling & Cartwright, 1982), one-half of widows still felt depressed five months after bereavement, and over a third of them were receiving from their family physicians psychopharmacological preparations. In general, personal arguments and subsequent loss of relationships were more frequently associated with minor depressions than ill health and financial stringencies, and these together with lack of relationships were more often found in "depressed" women, while men seemed more affected by lack of involvement in activities (Linn et al., 1980; Hale, 1982). In normals lowered mood is correlated with lowered levels of activity and self-confidence (Lehr, 1982), and it is obviously possible that some of the adverse experiences of depressed old people may be the result rather than the cause of their unhappy state.

Blazer and Williams (1980) found that their dysphorics shared with subjects suffering from major depressive episodes a frequently attested higher rate of social, economic, and physical health impairment, in comparison with mentally healthy old people. The stresses of old age alone seemed to have operated in well below half of their dysphoric subjects (4.5% of their community sample), while in 6.5% of their population dysphoria was associated with persistent or deteriorating medical conditions. Blazer and Williams interpreted dysphoria as due to a combination of diminished life satisfaction with periodic episodes of grief in response to social (e.g., bereavement), economic, and health losses.

A more factual etiological study was reported by Gillis and Zabow (1982). Their subjects were inmates of old-age homes, and they defined a first group of normals with high scores on a life satisfaction scale and with low scores on an equally well validated depression scale. A second group was ascertained as depressives on account of high scores on the depression scale, and, of course, also with low scores of life satisfaction. Finally, they regarded as dysphoric subjects who scored low on both the life satisfaction and the depression scales. They were unhappy, but not clinically depressed. Comparing these groups, it emerged that they did not differ by age, but while over 90% of normals and of dysphorics had become institutionalized for mainly social reasons, this was the case in only 42% of the depressives who were more often admitted for physical reasons. In comparison to both normal and dysphoric subjects, the depressives as a group had enjoyed significantly more education and larger incomes. Though dysphorics had

had slightly more education than normals, they had achieved even lower income levels during life than had the normal controls. Clearly circumscribed earlier depressive illnesses had, of course, been common in the depressives, but were registered for only 8% of the dysphorics, and for none of the controls. As might be expected, of those old people who had to enter a home, only 68% of normals had had much involvement with their families. Still fewer depressives (39%) had family ties, but only 16% of the dysphorics had maintained much family contact. Of these, 60% had had no family involvement whatever, a degree of isolation registered in only 35% of depressives and 13% of normal controls. This isolation, together with the lowered socioeconomic status of the dysphorics, was not the result of recent events, but seemed due to longstanding or even innate personality factors.

Treatment

If it is confirmed that senile dysphoria presents the end stage of an unsatisfying and unsatisfactory life, and corresponds to Akiskal's characterologic dysthymia, the chances for successful therapy are very limited. Possibly, a few dysphorics might belong in Akiskal's subgroup of subaffective dysthymia, and thus perhaps respond to antidepressants, but in the great majority only palliation through sociotherapeutic measures is likely to be applicable within the family or after entering an institution.

UNIPOLAR DEPRESSIONS

Symptomatology

It has long been thought that the depressions of later life not only last longer, but also recur with greater frequency than those of younger persons. However, the traditional view that they also became more severe with more agitation, suicidal risk, and delusional content has recently been challenged. Throughout life, people subject to attacks of severe depression have increased mortality, but survivors, against expectation, tend to experience amelioration of their symptoms (Ciompi, 1969). Certainly, in a consecutive series of hospitalized depressives over age 60 only a little over one-third exhibited severe melancholic symptoms, and in one-third there were no delusional or near delusional ideas of guilt, poverty, unworthiness, or physical illness. Furthermore, in terms of heredity, of precipitation by external events, and of response to either drug therapy or to electroconvulsive treatments, no clear distinction could be made between so-called endogenous and reactive or neurotic depressions. Where there were neurotic symptoms like anxiety, phobias, obsessions, or hysteria-like phenomena, these could usually be related to earlier minor flaws in personality structure

(Post, 1972). In a more recent series (Murphy, 1983), which also included a considerable number of outpatients and day-patients, 60% (rather more than in the earlier series) lacked the constellation of features usually associated with psychotic or endogenous depressions though satisfying Feighner's research criteria. Only 24% of patients were found to be suffering from depressive delusions or hallucinations.

Earlier Gurland (1976) had reported that the only significant difference in the symptomatology of young and old depressives lay in the greater prevalence of hypochondriasis with rising age. In an attempt to resurrect the concept of involutional depression, it was again largely the greater frequency of hypochondriacal symptoms that set late-onset depressives apart from early-onset cases (Pichot & Pull, 1981). However, a recent comparison of 31 patients (mean age 65 years), who had experienced their first depressions only after the age of 50, and of 60 patients (mean age 52 years) with earlier onsets, patients over the age of 50 (regardless of age at first attack) had more agitation, initial insomnia, and hypochondriasis; the late-onset patients showed not only more somatization and hypochondriasis (possibly related to their greater chronologic age), but with this less loss of libido, guilt, suicidal intent, and family history of depression. This last finding is in keeping with most genetic inquiries into late onset depression. The authors (Brown et al., 1984) conclude that further research into the genetic and biochemical basis of involutional depression is warranted.

Depression and Dementia

Until recently, two possible associations were conceptualized: (1) dementia with depressive admixtures, and (2) depressive illness complicated by symptoms suggestive of dementia. In other words, there were patients suffering from organic cerebral disorders and cognitive defects who exhibited a lowering mood level instead of apathy or euphoria, and there were other patients with depressions as well as with cognitive impairment, but with intact brains, the commonest form of "pseudodementia" seen in aged patients. More recently, there have been the two following developments. In the more severe depressions, cerebral changes in the form of derangements of neurotransmitter systems have become evident, and thus the borders between "functional" and "organic" have become blurred. Secondly, dementia is no longer used as a technical term for persistent or progressive cerebral deficits due to structural brain disease or deterioration, but the term is applied quite simply to any kind of cognitive impairment, which may or may not be reversible. One important example of recoverable cognitive impairment is that associated with depression. It has been proposed that to call this condition "pseudodementia" was illogical, terms like "dementia syndrome of depression" (Folstein & McHugh, 1978) being preferable.

The literature on pseudodementia and on its association with depressions of later life dates back to the beginning of the century. These past and numerous recent contributions will not again be reviewed here, as this has already been done in a thorough and scholarly fashion by McAllister (1983). Even more recently, Feinberg and Goodman (1984) have set out how the dementia syndrome of depression typically presents in one of four combinations: (1) a depressed patient superficially presents as a dement, but recovers completely; (2) depression with secondary dementia, where the patient is primarily depressed, but on investigation turns out to have an intellectual deficit (however, the syndrome is reversible by successful treatment of the depression—this, of course, is the condition which heretofore was called "pseudodementia"); (3) dementia presenting as depression, confirmed by investigation, but in spite of superficial appearances the investigator fails to define the presence of an affective disorder (the syndrome may be reversible or not reversible depending on the causes of the dementia); and (4) dementia with secondary depression, with the patient appearing demented (this is confirmed by investigation, which also confirms that concomitant depression is present; reversibility again depends on the etiology of the dementia). All this seems to be a fairly complete presentation of the clinical situations, with one addition: under (2), (i.e., the permutation that corresponds to the old term of depressive pseudodementia) the intellectual deficit is not only found on investigation, but is suspected on account of complaints of impaired memory or of confused behaviour.

Clinically, there is a strong impression that in patients with a dementia syndrome of depression the cognitive defects are limited to memory failures and possibly disorientation, but that fronto temporal lobe defects like dysphasia, dyspraxia, and finger dysgnosia are rarely if ever encountered. It is interesting, therefore, that as a result of preliminary studies it has been suggested that pseudodements may present cognitive defects as seen in subcortical dementia (Caine, 1981).

In conclusion, the status of depressive pseudodementia and its precise position on the organic-functional continuum still requires further research, as is indicated by several observations: No help in placing patients into either depression or senile dementia categories is likely to be forthcoming from tests for dexamethasone suppression. As reported by Coppen et al. (1983), out of 44 senile dements 20 registered as abnormal on the DST. It has been suggested, however, that DST nonsuppression in dementia reflects coexistent depression as measured by a specially designed rating scale (Katona & Aldridge, 1984). On the other hand, a number of psychometric studies have indicated that the mnestic difficulties of depressives (most marked in so-called pseudodements, but also psychometrically demonstrable in many severely ill depressives) are not only less severe than those of dements, but also that the dysfunctioning in dements is of a different and clearly pathological character. The learning and acquisition failures of depressives tend to correlate with the severity of their disorder, most evident when the depressed patient tries to remember random or unrelated events, but not when he begins to recall highly organized or related information that does not require the imposition of structure.

In contrast, memory failures in progressive dementia are characterized by the patient's inability to use relational properties to more effectively learn and remember information. Depressives have an easier access to previously acquired information, while dements have difficulty in "finding" what they have learned within their memories. It is this inaccessibility to previous knowledge that makes it difficult for them to appreciate continuing experience and events, which determines the encoding failures that result in failure of recent memory. Depressives fail at tasks that require sustained motivation and effort, and active processing operations. Dementing patients fail, despite sustained efforts, and equally on tasks which are in health accomplished automatically, requiring (in normals) little cognitive capacity of effort (Weingartner et al., 1982). That pseudodementia tends to resolve or improve after depression has been successfully treated was recently confirmed in an overdue validation study covering an observation period of two years (Rabins et al., 1984).

While all studies suggest that the dementia of depression is quite a different disorder than the dementia of Alzheimer, note has to be taken of an isolated report by Kral (1983) which concerns 22 patients between 62 and 78 years old, who were personally diagnosed and successfully treated by the author for depressive pseudodementia. Personal follow-up of 4 to 18 years (average 8 years) later revealed that 16 patients with or without further attacks of pseudodementia had developed Alzheimer-type dementias, and in three this diagnosis was confirmed postmortem.

Depression Associated with Brain Damage

At all ages, aside from causing cognitive and other impairment of personality functions, cerebral pathology may also be associated with affective disturbances, classically with affective blunting, apathy, or euphoria, but also with depression. Especially in older persons, fluctuating and temporary depression may occur when brain changes are of a biochemical rather than of a structural nature. Quite apart from the well-known depressant effects of certain deficiencies (e.g., in hypothyroidism or hypoxia) or of accumulating metabolites (e.g., in uremia), one wonders about indirect effects on the brain and on the effect of the many physical disorders which have been found so frequently to be in association with dysphoria and clinical depressions of the elderly. Among cerebrotoxic substances introduced from outside are, first of all, excessive alcohol and sedatives, but many medically prescribed preparations have also been shown to cause depression in the absence of any measurable cognitive defects (recently summarized by Salzman & Shader, 1979). Here we shall deal only with depression associated with common brain diseases and deteriorations of old age, omitting Huntington's chorea and other rare presenile dementias. It is difficult to establish the extent to which depressions associated with senile parkinsonism, cerebral infarctions, and Alzheimer's senile dementia represent understandable emotional reactions to damage and disability. There is, however, a good deal of evidence pointing toward depression as being causally related to damage of cerebral structures subserving affective functioning.

In Parkinson's disease dementia has been found to supervene in about one-third of patients, but depression is probably an even more frequent complication, and can also occur during treatment with L-dopa. There do not seem to have been any specific studies of all this in relation to old people, but the connection between depression in parkinsonism, the psychomotor symptoms of nonparkinsonian depressives, and the subcortical pathology of Parkinson's disease will no doubt be investigated more closely in the near future.

In the cases of multiinfarct dementia many earlier workers had strongly suspected that the incidence of clinical depression was higher than might be expected by chance. More recently (Robinson & Price, 1982), among 103 patients attending a stroke clinic (aged 63 to 11 years), who had been randomly selected, 30 were rated as having suffered from significant depression on a number of measures. None of them was still depressed at the end of one year after their strokes, but most had remained depressed on repeated serial ratings for from 7 to 8 months, without receiving any antidepressant treatments from the clinic.

Significantly, the highest risk for developing depression was between 6 months and 2 years poststroke. Demographic variables did not correlate with depression, nor did type of neurological deficit, global, or daily living impairment. However, patients with left hemisphere brain injury were significantly more depressed than those with right hemisphere or with brain stem infarctions. In relation to other work the investigators suggested that during the first 2 years left frontal lobe infarctions carried a high risk for depression. These workers did not look into the family histories of their organic depressives, but it is by now generally accepted that genetic and earlier personality factors in depressions (and in schizophrenia-like illnesses) related to brain disease are unimportant, suggesting that these complications are due to the cerebral pathology and its location.

In fact, Robinson et al. (1984) were able to demonstrate in a series of patients, each of whom had only a single stroke lesion, that depression was most severe and frequent with left anterior hemisphere infarcts. It was suggested that the relationship between presence and severity of depression and the cerebral location of stroke lesions might be linked with the neuroanatomy of biogenic amine containing pathways.

Turning to chronic brain syndromes not associated with focal cerebral damage, and thus in the older age groups most likely to be Alzheimer-type dementias, Miller (1980) found that, on clinical examination and in terms of scores on various measures, many chronic brain syndrome patients had important depressive components. For instance, on the Hamilton scale, depressives had a mean score of 28 points, while organics had a mean score of 18 points, with normals only scoring 5 points. Folstein et al. (1984) reported that 20% of patients with Alzheimer's dementia suffered from depressive episodes before or during the course of their decline, which was four times the rate reported in community surveys in the United States of America. They speculated that these depressive syndromes might be related to cholinergic defects resulting from a depletion of cells in the nucleus basalis of Meynert, or from the loss of cells in the locus ceruleus, both recently discovered in patients dying with Alzheimer's dementia. However, these speculations may be premature as Knesewich et al. (1983), during one year's follow-up, had failed to discover abnormal or increasing scores on the Hamilton and the Zung depression scales in early senile dements with no early histories of depression. It therefore still remains possible that the prodromal depressions of senile dementia, frequently described since Kraepelin's times, may occur only in patients with a depressive diathesis. Depressions in the setting of senile dementia have frequently been reported to be responsive to antidepressant therapies (e.g., Snow & Wells, 1981).

Causation

Etiological investigations have to address themselves to two different, but interrelated, questions: (1) What kind of people suffer from depressions in later life, and (2) What tends to precipitate in them a depressive illness?

Of the remote etiological factors the most important one is a proneness to depressive illnesses since earlier in life. Unfortunately, most studies have failed to look separately at elderly depressives with early and with late onsets of their conditions. Exceptions are genetic inquiries, most of which have indicated that early-onset cases yield considerably more frequent family histories of depression than late-onset patients, whose personalities have also been noted to have been more stable (summarized by Mendlewicz, 1976). Many authors have reported that, in comparison with healthy elderly people, depressives come from a background of greater social, economic, and physical health impairment (e.g., Blazer & Williams, 1980). Some of this was more closely examined by Murphy (1982) in a consecutive sample of all depressives over the age of 65 who had come for treatment as hospital, day, and outpatients from an urban area. Added to this series were the depressives found during the recruitment of normal control subjects from the same community. None of these belonged to the higher income groups, and, as expected, working class patients had more often experienced major social difficulties (25 as against 4%). Poor physical health was confirmed as being more common during the preceding year in Murphy's depressives, but previous reports to the effect that poor health was more often associated with a late as against an earlier onset of the first depression was not confirmed. Regardless of age at first attack, lower social class as well as severe economic and health impairments appeared to be interrelated and might reasonably be regarded as presenting increased vulnerability to depression in old age.

Inquiring into the more intimate social circumstances of her patients, Murphy discovered that in the presence of equally adverse external circumstances significantly more persons had succumbed to a depressive illness when they had also lacked all intimate and confiding relationships. Such a contact, which did not depend on its distance or frequency, seemed to protect old people from depression. This important finding was admittedly obtained by using a somewhat complex and intricate, but validated, technique, and it is of interest to note findings from Japan (Hasegawa, 1984). The author reported that in comparison with Western populations, the prevalence of major depression was much lower (between 0.9 and 1.9%), which he attributed to the continued preservation of extended family life in Japanese culture. Even in modern Tokyo, three-generation families living together had continued to be the pattern for 42% of the population, and 75% of the elderly of Japan shared their homes with children, with only 5% living alone. Moreover, Japanese men over 65 did not as a rule retire from the labor force, and if they did, they found plenty of meaningful occupations within the family household. Turning to the immediate precipitating factors of depression, earlier work (summarized elsewhere, Post, 1982) had indicated that these factors could be identified in from 65 to 80% of cases, even when great care had been taken to ignore events based only on self-report by the patients, or where these could possibly have been symptoms rather than causes of the depression. In a third of patients the following precipitating traumas were exit events: widowing, the moving away of children or close contacts, but also threats of loss, such as quarrels, or illness of a spouse, even though recovery took place. Next in importance was acute illness and the threat it implied. Retirement and recent financial or housing problems were less frequently encountered precipitating events.

Murphy (1982) employed a method derived from sophisticated recent studies of the role of disrupting life events in depression. These had been experienced during the year before interview by only 25 of 168 normal subjects, but during the year preceding the depression by 70 of 119 cases. Considering the total of stresses that had impinged upon her depressives,

Murphy concluded that there were only 15%, in whom the illness had come "out of the blue." However, even when disadvantaged background and recent losses seemed to have been at work in causing depressive breakdowns for the first time late in life, it must be obvious that social stresses, physical ill health, and losses of significant others or of status are the common lot of most old people, but only very few of them become clinically depressed.

Other vulnerability factors have, therefore, been looked for. Murphy (1982) had noted that two-thirds of her patients lacking intimate and confiding contacts had never in their lives been able to make any such contacts, and she concluded that longstanding personality problems must be seen as major vulnerability factors. We are not told, however, whether and to what extent this lack of intimate contacts was more often seen in late onset depressives. A good deal of work has been done recently in an attempt to discover variables that distinguish, in terms of etiology, late life depressions from those recurring at an earlier age. Apart from the relative paucity of genetic factors, we have already noted that with rising age there was a well authenticated increase of monoamine oxydase activity (Robinson et al., 1977), but other studies of intrinsic vulnerability factors for old age depression have rendered only suggestive, and so far unconfirmed, results. For this reason, these will only be summarized briefly.

We saw earlier in this chapter (pp. 233–234) that in depressives, even when not exhibiting "pseudodementia," cognitive impairment could often be psychometrically demonstrated. This was recently confirmed (Siegfried et al., 1984) in the showing that 50 depressives (average age 75, with Hamilton Depression Scores above 18) compared with 50 matched geriatric patients without depression performed significantly worse on a number of well-tried measures. After successful treatment with Nomifensine®, the depressives improved their scores significantly to the level of the nondepressed subjects. The greatest improvement of the depressives had been on the Critical Flicker Fusion Test, suggesting that a normalization of central nervous arousal had occurred. Earlier (summarized by Cawley et al., 1973) measurements of barbiturate sleep and sedation thresholds had suggested that cerebral arousal was lowered during severe depressions (after the age of 60, at any rate) to levels found in dementing cases, but that this lowering tended to be reversed after successful antidepressant treatment. This change correlated with improvement on certain cognitive measures.

It was postulated that the temporary decline of barbiturate tolerance and of cognitive functioning would be more marked in late-onset as compared with early-onset cases because it was indicative of an age-linked decrease of base line cerebral arousal in persons prone to clinical depression only in late life, as well as to the more frequent rate of recurrences in later life of all depressions. The prediction that in late-onset cases barbiturate thresholds and cognitive test scores would be lower on remission than those obtained in recovered early-onset depressives was only weakly supported. However, the depressives had lower scores than control subjects on a test of verbal intelligence, and also delayed auditory evoked cortical potentials similar to those obtained in aged dements (Hendrickson et al., 1979). Nine of 10 late-onset depressives, but only 1 case among early onset cases, had enlarged cerebral ventricles on computed tomography (Jacoby et al., 1981). The patients with enlarged ventricles also had decreased brain tissue densities similar to those of dements (Jacoby et al., 1983). Tomographies were not repeated after the patients had recovered, and it is not known whether these decreases of tissue densities portended permanent cerebral deterioration. Patients with late onset depressions had a much increased mortality rate, but their deaths were due to general rather than to cerebral causes (Jacoby et al., 1981).

Long duration of depression before treatment, higher age, and, probably related to this, the supervening of serious physical illnesses have often been confirmed as indicators of a poor prognosis in statistical terms, if not necessarily in individual cases. In patients over the age of 70, the presence of minimal organic signs such as partial disorientation and mild memory problems was found to be associated not with an increased mortality or with a later onset of dementia, but with less satisfactory outcome in terms of a lower discharge rate and impaired social adjustment. These patients were older, registered fewer precipitating events, and tended to have late rather than early onsets of their depressions (Cole & Hickie, 1976). However, when patients with minimal organic signs and with serious physical illnesses were excluded, it was reported (Cole, 1984) that patients who experienced their first attacks of depression only after the age of 60, at follow-up at 7 to 31 months (mean 18.1 months) had better outcomes than those with earlier onsets, possibly because they were less influenced by heredity and had previously more stable personalities. The outcome was no worse in patients with first attacks only after the age of 70. The death rate of late-onset cases was higher than in those with earlier illnesses, but that was solely due to their greater age, and patients with earlier onset more often pursued a chronic relapse course.

Especially in view of Caine's (1981) suggestion that dementia in depression may be related to subcortical pathology, and of Kral's (1983) finding of dementia supervening in many depressives after many years of follow-up, an investigation of cohorts of early- and late-onset depressives with repeated serial assessments up to the time of death, and where possible, to postmortem, is clearly needed. Such a study should settle the question of the extent to which some depressions in old age are precursors of dementia or are facilitated in certain persons under the impact of adverse life events or normal cerebral aging alone.

Treatment

It is realistic to discuss the management of the depressions of later life only against the background of their long-term course. Even before it had been recognized that clinical depressions in earlier life frequently left behind impaired mental health as well as a tendency to recur sooner or later, it had become clear that complete recovery from a depressive breakdown was, in spite of the introduction of modern treatments, uncommon in elderly patients. Adverse factors of the same kind as those precipitating depression, especially physical ill health and the associated higher age, were found to be correlated with a poorer long-term outcome (Post, 1972). The continued presence of close and intimate relationships did not, against expectation, improve long-term prognosis (Murphy, 1983). Earlier, and at a time when electroconvulsive therapy was the only specific form of treatment, only 31% of patients over the age of 60 were found to have made complete and lasting recoveries lasting longer than six years or up to the time of death (where this had occurred earlier); 29% suffered further attacks with good recoveries, but 17% remained continuously ill, and 23% became impaired by depressive invalidism of the same kind that characterized one of the subgroups of Akiskal's (1983) dysthymics. The results after the introduction of tricyclic antidepressants were only insignificantly better: only 26% of patients followed for three years after discharge from hospital remained completely recovered; 37% had further temporary breakdowns, 12% remained ill throughout, and 25% became dysthymic. In addition, the rate of attempted or of completed suicides was, in spite of the shorter observation period, nearly twice as high as in the earlier series. During this late period, elderly depressives were admitted to hospital far more often after treatment by their family doctors or in the outpatient clinic had failed. The failure to produce better results with drugs in addition to ECT might have been due to the greater intractability of patients requiring admission to a hospital (Post, 1972). However, in the more recent series studied by Murphy (1983) results during the year in which treatment was started were no better, even though these patients also included a large number not requiring hospital admission. While in Post's (1972) study symptomatology had not influenced outcome, Murphy (1983) found that patients who exhibited not only a distinct quality of depression, psychomotor changes, anorexia, weight loss, and guilt feelings, but also delusions of guilt, of bodily change or of illness, depersonalization, as well as occasional depressive hallucinations, presented a special case. These deluded psychotic depressives had a significantly poorer outcome than nondeluded psychotic and neurotic depressives. However, in this recent series ECT was used only sparingly and lithium not at all. Less than half of the psychotic depressives with delusions received ECT, which is regarded by some as the only treatment likely to benefit this type of patient.

The treatment of patients during the acute attack will be dealt with only briefly. In the section on neurotic disorders, we saw that psychotherapy was mainly directed to their depressive aspects. There have been only very few reports on psychotherapy applied to patients with major depressive episodes. In two large studies (Gerner et al., 1980; Jarvik et al., 1982) that compared various antidepressant drugs with placebo and with group therapies of either a psychodynamic or a behavioral type, it was confirmed that placebo treatment had no significant effect. Group therapy patients had a significant reduction of scores on the Hamilton Depression Scale (amounting to 33%); a reduction of 50% was achieved by antidepressant drugs during 26 weeks of observation. Pharmacotherapy patients either showed no response at all or a very marked one, while psychotherapy patients uniformly had a partial response. This suggested that psychotherapy alone was of limited benefit in the depressions of old age, but that it may well be useful in the many patients who fail to make good and lasting recoveries with somatic treatments. In the meantime, a pilot study has been reported (Sholomskas et al., 1983) that demonstrates the successful application of short-term interpersonal therapy (IPT) in the depressed elderly. This therapy was developed on the premise that depression, regardless of symptom patterns or of presumed biological vulnerability, occurred in a psychosocial and interpersonal context, and that understanding and renegotiating the problems associated with the onset of depression was important for the patient's recovery and probably also for the prevention of further episodes. This technique was employed by Sloane et al. (1984), and their preliminary impression was that IPT in contrast with nortriptyline treatment gave approximately equal improvement rates at the end of four months, that fewer IPT dropped out from treatment, and that only one patient recovered on placebo. The effect of more specifically directed cognitive behavior therapy, which may be as effective as drug treatment (Gelder, 1983), has not so far been reported in the case of older depressives.

Antidepressant drug treatment is discussed in Chapter 18 and little research has been done on electroconvulsive therapy with older patients. Studies by Fraser and Glass report that though in the long run electrode placements over the nondominant hemisphere produce as little objectifiable memory impairment as bilateral applications, there tends to be shorter postictal confusion (Fraser & Glass, 1978), and unilateral treatments were equally effective (Fraser & Glass, 1980). Three weeks after the last treatment, all but one of 29 patients studied had a good outcome. However, other researchers have reported much less satisfactory results, such as good initial responses in only 42% of cases, which had come down to 33% after six months (Karlinsky & Shulman, 1984). All researchers agree that only very few patients ultimately respond well to ECT rather than drugs as the first form of somatic therapy, but against expectation so-called neurotic depressives showed responses to ECT that were not significantly different from those achieved in psychotics (Post, 1972). Many psychiatrists no longer use ECT, but the majority view of psychogeriatricians is that this form of treatment remains invaluable especially for the very ill, and therefore gravely endangered patients, as well as for those for whom drug therapy has failed.

In keeping with the small proportion of aged depressives making complete and lasting recoveries, it has been recognized that maintenance treatment is required for most of them. In the course of three years, only 24% of patients required no further treatment; the remainder received episodically or continuously tricyclic and other antidepressant drugs, as well as lithium and sets of ECT (Post, 1972). Confirming strong clinical impressions, it has recently been demonstrated (Abou-Saleh & Coppen, 1983) that lithium prophylaxis is successful in the recurrent depressions of late life. In a few patients, the use of highly selective psychosurgery still remains indicated, though admittedly there have been no published reports. Social support alone, even in a day hospital, has been shown to be ineffective in the after care of older patients with only partial recoveries from major depressions (Smith & Cantley, 1983). Instead, the effects of brief psychotherapy and of cognitive therapy on the long-term course of old age depressions should be investigated. Finally, although a cautious, perhaps even pessimistic note has been sounded in this section, depressed old people nowadays have a better future than they did 40 years ago.

MANIC DISORDERS

Bipolar affective illnesses are not as uncommon in old age as used to be thought. In an English psychiatric teaching hospital with some 250 adult beds, a diagnosis of mania was confirmed from the records of 67 patients over the age of 60 for a ten-year period (Shulman & Post, 1980), and in a German psychiatric district hospital one-fifth of admissions for manic disorders were of patients over the age of 50 (Hoffmann et al., 1982). In the earlier series, the sex ratio was 2.7 females to 1 male. Well over half of the patients had had earlier attacks of depression, and in a considerable proportion three or more depressive episodes had occurred before the first manic attack. This observation casts doubt on the reliability with which bipolar affective illnesses are differentiated from unipolar depressions over relatively short time spans. In fact, more than 10 years had usually passed between the first depressive and the first manic attack, and the first manic episode had on an average occurred at the age of 59. All manics had recurrences, and among these there were usually also depressive episodes. Some case reports have been communicated recently (e.g., by Walter-Ryan, 1983) of patients experiencing their first affective illness in a manic form up to the ninth decade of life, with good responses to lithium, and sometimes with subsequent depression.

Symptomatology has been reported only in terms of unstandardized observations, but there is an impression that paranoid attitudes and irascible moods predominate over euphoria or elation, possibly because depression is never far away, and mixed manic-depressive states may be more frequent in the elderly with a mood of perplexity. Flights of ideas are often slow, suggesting incoherence. Thus, the differentiation of organic mental disorders or schizophrenic conditions may be difficult. The coexistence of physical, including neurological, symptoms is even more frequent than in depressions of late life, and the concept of secondary mania is often applicable.

In the most recent study (Glasser & Rabins, 1984), 42 manic admissions presented 4.9% of consecutive cases over the age of 60. Age at first attack with manic symptomatology was somewhat earlier than in Shulman and Post's report, but again in 7 of 42 cases mania might well have been secondary to a physical condition; in addition, 4 patients for the first time in life had become manic while being treated with tricyclic antidepressants. Earlier (Post, 1972) it was recorded that hypomanic features had apparently been precipitated by antidepressants in 5 of 92 patients over the age of 60.

Treatment also has not so far been systematically evaluated, but 24 of 27 manics over the age of 60 seemed to have responded well to lithium (Shulman & Post, 1980). Himmelhoch et al. (1980) reported a response rate of only 69%. The use of lithium in the elderly is discussed in Chapter 18, and also, without an evaluation, by Jefferson (1983).

PARANOID PSYCHOSES

Symptomatology

Without going into the earlier literature on paranoid illness of later life, it may be recalled that Roth (1955) had noted that a small minority, some 10% of older patients admitted to a mental hospital, were not suffering from either temporary or persistent cognitive impairment, or from an affective illness, but solely from delusions and hallucinations of a persecutory type. These patients were hardly ever discharged from hospital, and this differentiated them clearly from those with affective illnesses. Very much in contrast with temporarily confused and dementing patients, paranoids survived long periods of hospitalization. As these deluded and often also hallucinated patients did not exhibit any schizophrenic disintegration of personality, Roth suggested the diagnostic label of "late or senile paraphrenia," using this term in relation to symptomatology alone. Its course and etiology were more intensively investigated, and it was concluded that senile paraphrenia tended to occur in abnormal (mainly schizoid) persons, who were often further handicapped by deafness, and that the condition presented a late accession to the group of schizophrenias (Kay & Roth, 1961). This view has now been generally accepted.

Since then it has been shown (Post, 1966) and confirmed (Grahame, 1984) that there are three stable types of symptomatology in senile paraphrenia: (1) patients who exhibit only a few delusional ideas concerning their immediate surroundings or personal interactions, and sometimes also related hallucinations (cases of this type may only present after many years, or not at all, because the patients are usually managed by their families and neighbors); (2) the condition characterized by more widely spread delusions as well as by auditory, olfactory, and more rarely visual hallucinations, soon leads to disturbed behavior, which requires admission to hospital; and (3) the clinical picture very similar to that of younger paranoid schizophrenics, with delusions of bodily influence, of thought withdrawal, or thought insertion, and with an auditory hallucinosis, in which the patient reports voices talking about him in the third person or commenting on his actions (incongruity of affective expression, blunting, schizophrenic disorder of talk—formal thought disorder, or catatonic symptoms do not occur in these aged patients).

Any of these three clinical pictures may be seen in toxic psychoses, in the course of chronic organic psychoses, and also in illnesses which, in terms of their response to antidepressant drugs and of their course, belong to the unipolar or bipolar affective psychoses. Occasionally, "schizo-affective" remains an appropriate diagnostic label (Post, 1971), and even more rarely a paraphrenic picture becomes established in competently diagnosed affective patients (Logsdail, 1984). Paranoid illnesses is operationally defined as late or senile paraphrenia when the patient exhibits no organic-cerebral signs, and when any affective symptoms present do not respond to antidepressant remedies, but (along with the paranoid; schizophrenic-form, or schizophrenic symptoms) only to major tranquilizing drugs. (For details on these and many other points, see Post, 1984.)

Etiology

In comparison with the general population, there are slightly increased genetic risks for developing late paraphrenia (Kay, 1972), and the presence of sex linkage is suggested by the striking predominance of female over male cases (4:1), which has been universally reported. A far stronger predisposing factor is previous personality. As was mentioned earlier (p. 224), long-standing interpersonal and sexual adjustment is reported by the informants in the great majority of patients. Another clearly defined etiological factor is social deafness. This deafness is not related to aging, but due to long established middle ear pathology or otosclerosis, and may be a factor in prepsychotic personality development (Cooper, 1976; Cooper et al., 1976). Some psychodynamic mechanisms which may lead to paranoid thinking and experiencing have been suggested by Berger and Zarit (1978).

Treatment and Its Results

Relocation into more favorable surroundings of patients with only circumscribed paranoid symptoms is quite often successful, but the use of major tranquilizers (see Chapter 18) has turned late paraphrenia from an intractable into a manageable disorder, and paraphrenic symptoms also respond when they occur in a cerebral-organic setting. By judicious handling of patients with some social support, admission to hospital may be avoided in many, and discharge back to the community has become almost the rule. In an early series (Post, 1966), only 6 of 71 patients failed to respond to thioridazine by mouth; 22 continued to have some symptoms, but became fit for discharge, and symptoms were completely suppressed in 43 cases.

In the longer term, only 34% of patients surviving the first year remained completely symptom free; 38% had temporary relapses and 28% remained continuously psychotic (Post, 1980). Only 7 of 65 patients surviving more than one year failed to relapse when maintenance drug therapy was discontinued. It thus seems impracticable to institute drug holidays as has been advocated to avoid tardive dyskinesia. Fortunately, older patients seem to be little inconvenienced by their movement disorders (Mehta et al., 1977), which also occur in aged persons without exposure to major tranquilizing preparations (Blowers et al., 1981). Prognosis seems to depend primarily on the degree of success with which maintenance drug therapy can be carried through. This rests largely on the doctor and the team's skill in creating a relationship with these paraphrenics, and it is particularly difficult where the patient is deaf, or has never had any lasting good personal contacts.

A reappraisal of the etiology, mental mechanisms, and treatment of late paraphrenia, especially since the introduction of depot medication, seems overdue.

REFERENCES

Abou-Saleh, M. T., Coppen, A. (1983). The prognosis of depression in old age: The case for lithium therapy. *British Journal of Psychiatry, 143,* 527–528.
Akiskal, H. S. (1983). Dysthymic disorders: Psychopathology of proposed chronic depressive symptoms. *American Journal of Psychiatry, 140,* 11–20.
Berger, K. S., Zarit, S. H. (1978). Late life paranoid states: Assessment and treatment. *American Journal of Orthopsychiatry, 48,* 528–537.

Bergmann, K. (1978). Neurosis and personality disorder in old age. In A. D. Isaacs, F. Post (Eds.), *Studies in geriatric psychiatry* pp. 41–76. Chichester, New York, Brisbane Toronto: John Wiley.

Blazer, O., Williams, C. D. (1980). Epidemiology of dysphoria and depression in an elderly population. *American Journal of Psychiatry, 137,* 439–444.

Blowers, A. J., Bomson, R. L., Blowers, C. M., Bicknell, D. J. (1981). Abnormal involuntary movements in the elderly. *British Journal of Psychiatry, 139,* 363–364.

Bowling, A., Cartwright, A. (1982). Life after death: A study of the elderly widowed. London: Tavistock Publications

Brink, T. L. (1977). Dream therapy with the aged. *Psychotherapy 14,* 354–360.

Brink, T. L. (1978). Geriatric rigidity and its psychotherapeutic implications. *Journal of the American Geriatrics Society, 26,* 274–277.

Brown, R. P., Sweeney, J., Loutch, E., Kocsis, J., Frances, A. (1984). Involutional melancholia revisited. *American Journal of Psychiatry, 141,* 24–28.

Busse, E. W. (1976). Hypochondriasis in the elderly: A reaction to social stress. *Journal of the American Geriatrics Society, 24,* 145–149.

Caine, E. D. (1981). Pseudodementia. Current concepts and future directions. *Archives of General Psychiatry, 38,* 1359–1364.

Cawley, R. H., Post, F., Whitehead, A. (1973). Barbiturate tolerance and psychological functioning in elderly depressed patients. *Psychological Medicine, 1,* 39–52.

Ciompi, L. (1969). Follow-up studies in the evolution of former neurotic and depressive states. *Journal of Geriatric Psychiatry, 3,* 90–106.

Clark, A. N. G., Mankikar, G. D., Gray, I. (1975). Diogenes syndrome. A clinical study of gross neglect in old age. *Lancet, i,* 366–373.

Cole, M. G. (1984). Age, age of onset and course of primary depressive illness in the elderly. *Canadian Journal of Psychiatry, 28,* 102–104.

Cole, M., Hickie, R. N. (1976). Frequency and significance of minor organic signs in elderly depressives. *Canadian Psychiatric Association Journal, 21,* 7–12.

Cooper, A. F. (1976). Deafness and psyciatric illness. *British Journal of Psychiatry, 129,* 216–226.

Cooper, A. F., Garside, R. F., Kay, D. W. K. (1976). A comparison of deaf and non-deaf patients with paranoid and affective psychoses. *British Journal of Psychiatry, 129,* 532–538.

Coppen, A., Abou-Saleh, M., Milln, P., Metcalfe, M., Harwood, J., Bailey, J. (1983). Dexamethasone suppression test in depression and other psychiatric illness. *British Journal of Psychiatry, 142,* 498–504.

Corby, N., Solnick, R. S. (1980). Psychosocial and physiological influence on sexuality in the older adult. In J. E. Birren, R. B. Sloane (Eds.), *Handbook of mental health and aging* (pp. 893–921). Englewood Cliffs, N.J.: Prentice-Hall.

Dilling, H., Weyerer, S., Castell, R. (1984). *Psychische Erkrankungen in der Bevölkerung* (p. 58). Stuttgart: Enke.

Edwards, G., Hawker, A., Hensman, C., Peto, J., Williamson, V. (1973). Alcoholics known or unknown to agencies: Epidemiological studies in a London suburb. *British Journal of Psychiatry, 123,* 169–183.

Feinberg, T., Goodman, B. (1984). Affective illness, dementia and pseudodementia. *Journal of Clinical Psychiatry, 45,* 99–103.

Folstein, M. F., McHugh, P. R. (1978). Dementia syndrome of depression. In R. Katzman, R. D. Terry, K. L. Bick (Eds.), *Alzheimer's disease: Senile dementia and related disorders* (pp. 87–93) (Aging, Vol 7). New York: Raven Press.

Folstein, M. F., Robinson, R. G., McHugh, P. R. (1984). *Depression and neurological disorders: New treatment opportunities*. Paper read at the 14th CINP Congress, Florence.

Fraser, R. M., Glass, I. B. (1978). Recovery from ECT in elderly patients. *British Journal of Psychiatry, 133,* 524–528.

Fraser, R. M., Glass, I. B. (1980). Unilateral and bilateral ECT in elderly patients. *Acta Psychiatrica Scandinavica, 62,* 13–31.

Garfinkel, R. (1979). Brief Behaviour therapy with an elderly patient. *Journal of Geriatric Psychiatry, 12,* 101–109.

Gelder, M. G. (1983). Is cognitive therapy effective?: A discussion paper. *Journal of the Royal Society of Medicine, 76,* 938–942.

Gerner, R., Estabrook, W., Steuer, Jarvik, L. F. (1980). A placebo controlled double-blind study of imipramine and tradozone in geriatric depression. In J. O. Cole, J. E. Barrett (Eds.), Psychopathology in the aged (pp. 167–182). New York: Raven Press.

Gillis, L. S., Zabow, A. (1982). Dysphoria in the elderly. *South African Medical Journal, 62,* 410–413.

Glasser, M., Rabins, P. (1984). Mania in the elderly. *Age and Aging, 13,* 210–213.

Graham, P. S. (1986). Schizophrenia in old age (late paraphrenia). *British Journal of Psychiatry, 145,* 493–495.

Gurland, B. (1976). The comparative frequency of depression in various adult age groups. *Journal of Gerontology, 31,* 283–292.

Gurland, B. J. (1984). Personality disorders in old age. In D. W. K. Kay, & G. D. Burrows (Eds.), Handbook of studies in psychiatry and old age (pp. 308–318). Amsterdam, New York, Oxford: Elsevier.

Gurland, B., Dean, L., Cross, P., Golden, R. (1980). The epidemiology of depression and dementia in the elderly: The use of multiple indicators of these conditions. In J. O. Cole, J. E. Barrett (Eds.), *Psychopathology in the aged* (pp. 37–60). New York: Raven Press.

Hale, D. (1982). Correlates of depression in the elderly: sex differences and simularities. *Journal of Clinical Psychology, 38,* 253–257.

Hasegawa, K. (1984). The epidemiological study of depression in late life. Paper read at the 14th CINP Congress, Florence.

Henderson, A. S., Kay, D. W. K. (1984). The epidemiology of mental disorders in the aged. In D. W. K. Kay, G. D. Burrows (Eds.), *Handbook of studies on psychiatry and old age* (pp. 53–88). Amsterdam, New York, Oxford: Elsevier.

Hendrickson, E., Levy, R., Post, F. (1979). Averaged evoked responses in relation to cognitive and affective state of elderly psychiatric patients. *British Journal of Psychiatry, 134,* 494–501.

Himmelhoch, J. M., Neil, J. F., May, S. J., Fuchs, C. Z., Licata, S. M. (1980). Age, dementia, dyskinesias and lithium response. *American Journal of Psychiatry, 137,* 941–945.

Hoffmann, H., Rabich, D., Siegel, E. (1982). Manische Psychosen der zweiten Lebenshälfte. *Zeitschrift für Altersforschung, 37,* 417–421.

Ingebretsen, R. (1977). Psychotherapy with the elderly. *Psychotherapy, 14,* 319–332.

Ingersoll, B., Silverman, A. (1978). Comparative group psychotherapy for the aged. *Gerontologist, 18,* 201–206.

Jacoby, R. J., Dolan, R. J., Levy, R., Baldy, R. (1983). Quantitative computed tomography in elderly depressed patients. *British Journal of Psychiatry, 143,* 124–127.

Jacoby, R. J., Levy, R., Bird, J. M. (1981). Computed tomography and the outcome of affective disorders: A follow-up study of patients. *British Journal of Psychiatry, 139,* 288–292.
Jarvik, L. F., Mintz, J., Steuer, J., Gerner, R. H. (1982). Treating geriatric depression. A 26 week interim analysis. *Journal of the American Geriatric Society, 30,* 713–717.
Jefferson, J. W. (1983). Lithium and affective disorders in the elderly. *Comprehensive Psychiatry, 24,* 166–179.
Kahana, R. J. (1979). Strategies of dynamic psychotherapy with the wider range of older individuals. *Journal of Geriatric Psychiatry, 12,* 71–100.
Karlinsky, H., Shulman, K. (1984). The clinical use of ECT in old age. *Journal of the American Geriatric Society, 32,* 183–186.
Katona, C. L. E., Aldridge, C. R. (1984). Dexamethasone suppression test and dementia. *British Journal of Psychiatry, 144,* 333.
Kay, D. W. K. (1972). Schizophrenia and schizophrenia-like states in the elderly. *British Journal of Hospital Medicine, 8,* 369–376.
Kay, D. W. K., Roth, M. (1961). Environmental and hereditary factors in the schizophrenias of old age ("Late Paraphrenia") and their bearing on the general problem of causation in schizophrenia. *Journal of Mental Science, 107,* 649–686.
Kimmel, D. C. (1977). Psychotherapy and the older gay man. *Psychotherapy, 14,* 386–393.
Knesewich, J. W., Martin, R. L., Berg, L., Danziger, W. (1983). Preliminary report of affective symptoms in the early stages of senile dementia of the Alzheimer type. *American Journal of Psychiatry, 140,* 233–235.
Kral, V. A. (1983). The relationship between senile dementia (Alzheimer type) and depression. *Canadian Journal of Psychiatry, 28,* 304–306.
Kral, V. A. (1984). Sexual problems in old age. In D. W. K. Kay, G. D. Burrows (Eds.), *Handbook of studies in psychiatry and old age* (pp. 329–336) Amsterdam, New York, Oxford: Elsevier.
Krasner, J. D. (1977). Loss of dignity—Courtesy of modern science. *Psychotherapy, 14,* 309–318.
Lehr, U. M. (1982). Depression und "Lebensqualität" im Alter—Korrelate negativer und possitiver gestimmtheit. *Zeitschrift fü Gerontologie, 15,* 241–249.
Linn, M. W., Hunter, K., Harris, R. (1980). Symptoms of depression and recent life events in the community elderly. *Journal of Clinical Psychology, 36,* 675–682.
Logsdail, S. (1984). Affective illness changing to paranoid state. Report on three elderly patients. *British Journal of Psychiatry, 144,* 209–210.
McAllister, T. W. (1983). Overview: Pseudodementia. *American Journal of Psychiatry, 140,* 528–533.
Macmillan, D., Shaw, P. (1966). Senile breakdown in standards of personal and environmental cleanliness. *British Medical Journal, ii,* 1032–1037.
Margo, J. L., Robinson, J. R., Corea, S. (1980). Referrals to a psychiatric service from old people's homes. *British Journal of Psychiatry, 136,* 396–401.
Mehta, D., Mehta, S., Matthew, D. (1977). Tardive dyskinesia in psychogeriatric patients. A five year follow-up. *Journal of the American Geriatric Society, 21,* 226–228.
Mendlewicz, J. (1976). The age factor in depressive illness: some genetic considerations. *Journal of Gerontology, 31,* 300–303.
Miller, N. E. (1980). The measurement of mood in senile brain disease: examiner rating and self-reports. In J. O. Cole, J. E. Barrett (Eds.), *Psychopathology in the Aged* (pp. 97–122). New York: Raven Press.

Mishara, B. L., Kastenbaum, R. (1980). *Alcohol and old age.* New York: Grune and Stratton.
Murphy, E. (1982). Social origins of depression in old age. *British Journal of Psychiatry, 141,* 135–142.
Murphy, E. (1983). The prognosis of depression in old age. *British Journal of Psychiatry, 142,* 111–119.
Pichot, P., Pull, C. (1981). Is there an involutional melancholia? *Comprehensive Psychiatry, 22,* 2–10.
Post, F. (1966). *Persistent persecutory states in the elderly.* Oxford: Pergamon Press.
Post, F. (1971). Schizo-affective symptomatology in late life. *British Journal of Psychiatry, 118,* 437–445.
Post, F. (1972). The management and nature of depressive illnesses in late life: a follow-through study. *British Journal of Psychiatry, 121,* 393–404.
Post, F. (1980). Paranoid, schizophrenia-like and schizophrenic states in the aged. In J. E. Birren, R. B. Sloane (Eds.), *Handbook of mental health and aging* (pp. 591–615). Englewood Cliffs, N.J.: Prentice-Hall.
Post, F. (1982). Functional disorders II. Treatment and its relationship to causation. In R. Levy, F. Post (Eds.), *The psychiatry of late life* (pp. 197–221). Oxford, London, Edinburgh, Boston, Melbourne: Blackwell.
Post, F. (1984). Schizophrenic and paranoid psychoses. In D. W. K. Kay, G. D. Burrows (Eds.), *Handbook of studies on psychiatry and old age* (pp. 291–302). Amsterdam, New York, Oxford: Elsevier.
Rabins, P. V., Merchant, A., Nestadt, G. (1984). Criteria for diagnosing reversible dementia caused by depression. Validation by 2-year follow-up. *British Journal of Psychiatry, 144,* 488–492.
Robinson, D. S., Sourkes, T. L., Nies, A., Harris, L. S., Spector, S., Bartlett, D. L. (1977). Monoamine metabolism in human brain. *Archives of General Psychiatry, 34,* 89–92.
Robinson, R. G., Kubos, K. L., Starr, L. K., Rao, K., Price, T. R. (1984). Mood disorder in stroke patients. Importance of location of lesion. *Brain, 107,* 81–93.
Robinson, R. G., Price, T. R. (1982). Post-stroke depressive disorders: a follow-up study of 103 patients. *Stroke, 13,* 635–641.
Rosin, A., Glatt, W. M. (1971). Alcohol excess in the elderly. *Quarterly Journal of Studies on Alcoholism, 32,* 53–59.
Roth, M. (1955). The natural history of mental disorders in old age. *Journal of Mental Science, 101,* 281–301.
Salzman, C., Shader, R. I. (1979). Clinical evaluation of depression in the elderly. In R. Raskin, L. F. Jarvik (Eds.), *Psychiatric symptoms and cognitive loss in the elderly* (pp. 39–72). New York: John Wiley.
Sholomskas, A. J., Chevron, E. S., Pinsoff, B. A., Berry, C. (1983). Short-term interpersonal therapy (IPT) with the depressed elderly. Case reports and discussion. *American Journal of Psychotherapy, 37,* 55–66.
Shulman, K., Post, F. (1980). Bipolar affective disorders in old age. *British Journal of Psychiatry, 136,* 26–32.
Siegfried, K., Jansen, W., Pahnke, K. (1984). *Cognitive symptoms in late life depression and their treatment.* Paper read at the 14th CINP Congress, Florence.
Simon, A. (1980). The neuroses, personality disorders, drug use and misuses, and crime in the aged. In J. E. Birren, R. B. Sloane (Eds.), *Handbook of mental health and aging* (pp. 653–670). Englewood Cliffs, N.J.: Prentice-Hall.
Sloane, R. B., Staples, F., Bender, M., Razani, J., Schneider, L. (1984). *Psychotherapy vs. Nortriptyline for depression in the elderly.* Paper read at the 14th CINP Congress, Florence.

Smith, G., Cantley, C. (1983). Pluralistic evaluation: *A study in day care for the elderly mentally infirm*. Department of Social Administration, University of Hull.

Snow, S. S., Wells, C. S. (1981). Case studies in neuropsychiatry: Diagnosis and treatment of co-existent dementia and depression. *Journal of Clinical Psychiatry, 42,* 439–441.

Walter-Ryan, W. G. (1983). Mania with onset in the ninth decade. *Journal of Clinical Psychiatry, 44,* 430–431.

Wattis, J. P. (1981). Alcohol problems in the elderly. *Journal of the American Geriatric Society, 3,* 131–139.

Wattis, J. P. (1983). Alcohol and old people. *British Journal of Psychiatry, 143,* 306–307.

Weingartner, H., Cohen, R. H., Burney, W. E., Ebert, M. H., Kaye, W. (1982). Memory-learning impairments in progressive dementia and depression. *American Journal of Psychiatry, 139,* 135–136.

Wilensky, H., Weiner, M. B. (1977). Facing reality in psychotherapy with the aging. *Psychotherapy, 14,* 373–378.

13
Organic Brain Syndrome

Kazuo Hasegawa and Akira Homma

The demographic facts of an aging population are now well known. In 1983 in Japan, the number of elderly aged 65 years and over was 9.8% and it is estimated that it will be 18% in 2020. It is also becoming recognized that the rising number of those over 80 in particular will produce a very large increase in patients suffering from organic mental impairment. There is much less awareness, however, that the effects of this increase will impinge upon the practice of all branches of the medical profession caring for elderly patients and cannot be regarded solely as the responsibility of psychiatry. Furthermore several developments impel us to be concerned with organic mental disorders in all their aspects. Recent advances in the neurosciences have provided new methodological approaches and technical tools for the study of metabolic, vascular, electrophysiological, biochemical, and structural cellular changes in the brain associated with psychopathological states. Also, the current focus on chronic diseases and on critical care medicine has highlighted the problem of psychiatric manifestations of cerebral disorders resulting from cardiovascular, neoplastic, traumatic, and other diseases affecting the brain, either directly or indirectly as a result of systemic metabolic disturbances.

The prevalence of mental disorders in elderly medical and surgical inpatients is estimated to be between 40 and 50% (Schuckit et al., 1975; Chisholm et al., 1982). Delirium, dementia, and affective and anxiety disorders predominate. Delirium occurs in 30 to 50% of the elderly patients at some point during their hospitalization (Chisholm et al., 1982; Gillick et al., 1982). Particularly, delirium is one common reason why a patient would visit an emergency department. It is most important to diagnose delirium in the elderly because its occurrence usually points to the presence of an acute and potentially treatable somatic disorder. Also, a thorough evaluation of demented patients may be expected to result in diagnoses of potentially correctable disorders in approximately 15% (Wells, 1977).

The purpose of this chapter is to outline an organizing schema for the diagnosis and study of organic brain syndromes. This includes classification, definition of syndromes, and a general discussion of the etiologic factors and pathogenic mechanisms involved in the psychopathology of cerebral disorders.

DEFINITION

The standard nomenclature of the American Psychiatric Association defines organic brain syndrome as a constellation of psychological or behavioral signs and symptoms without reference to etiology. The essential feature of organic brain syndrome is a psychological or behavioral abnormality associated with transient or permanent dysfunction of the brain. The organic factor responsible for organic brain syndrome may be a primary disease of the brain or a systemic illness that secondarily affects the brain. Four of these organic brain syndromes are of primary importance in geriatric psychiatry. These are dementia, delirium, amnestic syndrome, and organic affective syndrome. These syndromes display great variability among individuals and in the same individual over time. Thus, organic brain syndromes are defined in terms of psychopathological symptoms and signs elicited by history, mental status examination, and observation of patient's behavior in nonlaboratory settings. Furthermore, organic brain syndromes include those aspects of mental functioning other than cognition, that is, motivation, affects, and impulse expression and control.

CLASSIFICATION

According to the latest revision of the American Psychiatric Association's Diagnostic Statistical Manual of Mental Disorders (APA, 1980), the organic brain syndromes can be grouped into ten purely descriptive psychopathological syndromes. They may be grouped as follows: those with global cognitive impairment—(1) delirium, (2) dementia; those with a relatively selective or circumscribed cognitive defect or abnormality—(3) amnestic syndrome, (4) hallucinosis; those involving personality, leaving cognition relatively intact—(5) organic personality syndrome; those resembling functional disorders—(6) organic delusional syndrome, (7) organic affective syndrome; those associated with ingestion or reduction in use of a substance—(8) intoxication, (9) withdrawal; and those constituting a residual category—(10) atypical or mixed organic brain syndrome.

This classification itself has several important respects from the one used currently as pointed out by Lipowski (1975, 1980). In DSM II, organic psychopathology such as that due to acute metabolic derangement, intoxication with drugs and poisons, and focal brain lesions in various sites finds no place. In addition, DSM II subdivides organic brain syndromes into "psychotic" and "nonpsychotic" and recommends an optional further subdivision into acute or reversible and chronic or irreversible syndromes. "Psychotic" and "nonpsychotic" are of little practical value in this area of psychiatry. Also, the division which designates that an acute brain syndrome is reversible and a chronic syndrome irreversible is misleading. A reversible syndrome may set in gradually in the course of a chronic illness, like pernicious anemia or hypothyroidism. An irreversible, "chronic," syndrome may come on acutely as a result of severe carbon monoxide poisoning or Wernicke's encephalopathy. Thus, this dichotomous classification has disadvantages as a basis for classification which faithfully reflects psychopathologic correlates of cerebral diseases.

Lastly, evidence of impairment of cognitive performance in a patient is usually regarded as presumptive evidence of cerebral dysfunction or disease. However, many clinicians have asserted that more or less global impairment of cognitive functioning is not the only possible manifestation of brain disorders. Disturbance of emotions, drives, impulse control and personality may sometimes result from lesions in circumscribed areas of the brain. Thus, the classification by DSM III breaks down the boundary between organic and functional mental disorders, taking into consideration that the concept of an organic brain syndrome has been for decades linked with that of cognitive impairment.

SUBCATEGORY OF ORGANIC BRAIN SYNDROMES

In this section, clinical features, etiologic factors, and pathogenic mechanisms involved in the psychopathology of the subcategory of the most common organic brain syndromes will be described.

Delirium

Delirium and dementia are by far the most common and important organic brain syndromes. DSM III presents a definition of delirium in the form of diagnostic criteria. The most important element in this set is the concept of clouding of consciousness, defined as "reduced clarity of awareness of the environment." Earlier, Lipowski (1967) defined "consciousness" as "that state of an organism which enables cognitive processes to occur," and "clouding of consciousness" as "a state characterized by a potentially reversible global impairment of cognitive processes of variable extent."

Lishman (1978) also suggests the definition that " 'clouding of consciousness' denotes the mildest stage of impairment of consciousness on the continuum from full alertness to coma." Thus, there remains some degree of disagreement about the precise meaning of this term, though the definition by DSM III is reasonably acceptable.

Clinical Features

The clinical features of delirium in the aged do not differ substantially from those in younger adults (Lipowski, 1980). These are described in some detail in the current nomenclature of DSM III and are summarized by Lipowski (1980) as follows: the patient manifests impairment in the area of directed thinking, registration, recent memory, and orientation, at least in the time sphere. There is evidence of disturbance in the mobilization, focusing, maintaining, and shifting of attention. Arousal is either reduced to less than normal wakefulness and alertness or heightened with increased but indiscriminate response to external stimuli. The patient's sleep and wakefulness cycle is altered with either insomnia and daytime drowsiness or diurnal rhythm reversal. Defects in cognition and attention tend to fluctuate unpredictably and without regularity during the day and become accentuated with insomnia at night. Behavioral manifestations include either decreased or increased psychomotor activity or wide swings from one to the other. Visual illusions and hallucinations are common, except in the aged, and abnormalities of other perceptual modalities may be present as well, accompanied by restlessness and fear. Persecutory delusions which are poorly systematized and fleeting may be present and intermixed with hallucinations. At any time, the patient may enter a lucid interval or a period of improvement in attention span, reality testing, and other symptoms and signs.

Two subtypes of delirium—one characterized by sluggish inertia or a stuporous state and the other by ceaseless and purposeless hyperactivity, hyperarousal, or agitation—have been described by Steinhart (1979) and Lipowski (1980). Lipowski (1980) also suggests the mixed subtype as a third clinical variant with features of both the hypoactive and hyperactive variants.

Several associated features may be seen in delirium. A whole range of emotions may be expressed by the patients. Fear, depression, apathy, rage, anxiety, and euphoria may all be exhibited. Psychotic symptoms such as threatening hallucinations and/or persecutory delusions are usually associated with hyperactive delirium and with increased autonomic symptoms and signs. It has been suggested that the individual differences in manifestation of associated features are dependent on premorbid personality, cultural background, and environmental setting (Kahn, 1971; Romano & Engel, 1944).

Clinical Course

There may be prodromal symptoms in which restlessness, hypersensitivity to stimuli, nocturnal visual hallucinations, difficulty in concentration and maintenance of a coherent train of thought, restlessness with poor sleep, and somnolence during the day predominate. However, the onset is usually rapid and often the first symptoms occur at night. Delirium lasts several days or a few weeks, rarely longer than a month. As a rule, there is a full recovery from delirium. If there is a coincidental illness, there may be death, although continuing pathology may also lead to dementia or other types of organic brain syndrome. Roth (1976) suggests that it might be expected that a number of persons with chronic recurrent delirious states arising from progressive systemic disease, such as cardiac or respiratory failure, would show a transition to demented states.

Etiology and Pathogenesis

Delirium may result from a wide range of factors, acting singly or in various combinations (Lipowski, 1980). In the absence of epidemiological data, one may only estimate that intoxication by medical drugs and substances of abuse, systemic metabolic disorders, and head trauma are the most common organic factors responsible for delirium. Purdie et al. (1981) conducted a retrospective review of 100 admissions to a general hospital with a diagnosis of delirium. A total of 44% of the patients were found to have a chronic organic brain syndrome with a superimposed acute insult which caused decompensation. The most common etiologic factors producing decompensation of a chronic organic brain syndrome were infection (in 23%) and environmental changes (in 17%). The most common etiologic factor causing delirium *de novo* was drug related. Table 13.1 presents a number of examples of the cause of delirium taken from the literature (Eisdorfer & Cohen, 1978; Ellis & Lee, 1978; Glickman & Friedman, 1976; Libow, 1973; Lipowski, 1980; Murphy, 1968; Roth & Myers, 1975; Simon & Cahan, 1963).

Yet, the susceptibility to the development of delirium varies considerably among individuals and across time. Specific predisposing factors include addiction to alcohol or drugs, advanced age, and cerebral damage sustained at any age and secondary to any cause (Doty, 1946; Hodkinson, 1973, 1976; Lipowski, 1967; Morse & Litin, 1969, 1971; Roth & Myers, 1975; Wells & Duncan, 1980). Psychological stress, sleep and sensory deprivation, prolonged immobilization, and severe fatigue are also likely to facilitate the onset, manifestations, and course of delirium in patients of all ages (Lipowski, 1980). Other researchers have noted that retirement problems and impairment of vision and/or hearing may be significant predisposing factors in the aged (Hodkinson, 1973; Morse & Litin, 1969). However, in

TABLE 13.1 Disorders Causing Delirium in the Aged

Disorder	Examples
Central nervous system disease	
Neoplasm	Primary intracranial neoplasm, metastatic neoplasm-bronchogenic carcinoma, breast carcinoma
Cerebrovascular disease	Arteriosclerosis, cerebral infarction, subarachnoid hemorrhage, transient ischemic attacks, hypertensive encephalopathy, vasculitis (lupus), cranial arteritis, disseminated intravascular coagulation
Infection	Neurosyphilis, brain abscess, tuberculosis, meningoencephalitis (bacterial, viral, fungal), septic emboli (subacute bacterial endocarditis)
Head trauma	Chronic subdural hematoma, extradural hematoma, cerebral contusion, concussion
Ictal and postictal states	Idiopathic seizures, space-occupying lesion, post-traumatic lesions, electroconvulsive therapy
Cardiovascular disease	
Hypoxemia	Respiratory insufficiency, anemia, carbon monoxide poisoning
Electrolyte disturbance	Kidney disease, adrenal disease, diabetes mellitus, diuretics, edematous states, inappropriate secretion of antidiuretic hormone, dehydration, starvation
Acidosis	Diabetic mellitus, kidney disease, pulmonary disease, chronic diarrhea
Alkalosis	Hyperadrenalcorticism, pulmonary disease, psychogenic hyperventilation
Hepatic disease	Acute hepatic failure, cirrhosis, chronic portahepatic encephalopathy
Uremia	Chronic glomerulonephritis, chronic pyelonephritis, acute renal failure, obstructive uropathy
Endocrinopathies	Hypothyroidism, thyrotoxicosis, "apathetic" hyperthyroidism, hypoglycemia, hyperglycemia, hypoparathyroidism, hyperparathyroidism, hypoadrenal corticism, hyperadrenalcorticism
Deficiency states	Hypovitaminosis-thiamine, nicotinic acid, vitamin B_{12}, folate deficiency, iron deficiency
Other disorders	
Trauma	Burns, surgery, multiple injury, fractures (fat embolism)
Sensory deprivation	Cataracts, glaucoma, otosclerosis, darkness ("sundown syndrome")
Exogenous toxins	Medications, alcohol, withdrawal syndromes, heavy metals, solvents, insecticides, pesticides, carbon monoxide
Temperature regulation	Exposure and accidental hypothermia, heat stroke, febrile illnesses

spite of the increased likelihood of the development of delirium in the presence of these predisposing conditions, there are no reliable prediction criteria and the ability to anticipate its development in any individual elderly person is limited (Lipowski, 1967).

As mentioned earlier, medications and drugs deserve special emphasis in the etiology of delirium in the aged. The use of various drugs by the elderly is pervasive, owing in part to the increased prevalence of illness in this age group. Extensive use of single and multiple drug regimens in the elderly has been documented in multicenter studies both in the United States and in Great Britain (Prien & Caffey, 1977; Williamson, 1978). Busse and Blazer have reported a high use of psychotropic medications and sedatives in the elderly (Busse & Blazer, 1980). Thus, drug use, especially of multiple drugs, appears to be commonplace among the elderly. Table 13.2 presents common examples of medications which have been reported as particularly likely to produce delirium in the elderly (Cohen, 1953; Davison, 1978; Eisdorfer & Cohen, 1978; Hasan & Mooney, 1979; Lipowski, 1980; Raskind & Storrie, 1980; Williamson, 1978).

Although delirium is occasionally due to an anatomical lesion which destroys brain tissue, attempts have been made to explain delirium in neurochemical terms. Yet, direct studies of cerebral metabolism in delirium remain to be carried out. Recent studies (Engel & Romano, 1959; Pro & Wells, 1977; Blass & Gibson, 1979; Nausieda et al., 1979; Lipowski, 1980) support the view that widespread derangement of cerebral metabolism, coupled with an imbalance of brain neurotransmitters, underlies delirium. Both cortical and subcortical structures are likely involved, as indicated by concurrent disorder of cognition and wakefulness.

Treatment

There is general agreement among clinicians that effective management of delirium ultimately rests on the identification and treatment of the underlying causative organic factors (Henry & Mann, 1965; Lipowski, 1967, 1980; Raskind & Storrie, 1980; Wolff & Curran, 1935). In addition to identifying and treating the underlying cause of the disorder, the management of delirium in the aged can be divided into five categories:

1. *Physiological support.* The severity of delirium is often related to a general physical condition and such illness in the elderly may be ameliorated by measures which improve the patient's physiological state (Harris, 1972). Principal among these measures are the maintenance of adequate hydration and nutrition and the correction of electrolyte imbalance.
2. *Environmental support.* Recommended manipulations of the patient's environment include having a relative stay with the patient, frequent

TABLE 13.2 Common Medications Causing Delirium in the Aged

Disorder	Medication	Common examples
Cardiovascular conditions	Antiarrhythmics	Procainamide, propranolol, quinidine
	Antihypertensives	Clonidine, methyldopa, reserpine,
	Cardiac glycosides	Digitalis
	Coronary vasodilatators	Nitrates
Gastrointestinal conditions	Antidiarrheals	Atropine, belladonna, homatropine, hyoscyamine, scopolamine
	Antinaeseants	Cyclidine, homatropine-barbiturate preparations, phenothiazines
	Antispasmodics	Methanthelene, propanthelene
Musculoskeletal conditions	Antiinflammatory agents	Corticosteroids, indomethacin, salicylate, phenylbutazone
	Muscle relaxants	Carisoprodol, diazepam
Neurologic-psychiatric conditions	Anticonvulsants	Barbiturates, carbamazepine, diazepam, phenytoin
	Antiparkinsonism agents	Amantadine, benztropine, levadopa, trihexyphenidyl
	Hypnotics and sedatives	Barbiturates, belladonna alkaloids, bromides, chloral hydrate, ethchlorvynol, glutethimide
	Psychotropics	Benzodiazepines, hydroxyzines, lithium salts, meprobamate, MAO inhibitors, neuroleptics, tricyclic antidepressants
Respiratory-allergic conditions	Antihistamines	Brompheniramine, chlorpheniramine, cyproheptadine, diphenhydramine, tripelennamine
	Antitussives	Opiates, synthetic narcotics
	Decongestants and expectorants	Phenylephrine, phenylpropanolamine, potassium preparations
Miscellaneous conditions	Analgesics	Dextropropoxyphene, opiates, phenacetin salicylates, synthetic narcotics
	Anesthetics	Lidocaine, methohexital, methoxyflurane
	Antidiabetic agents	Insulin, oral hypoglycemics
	Antineoplastics	Corticosteroids, mitomycin, procarbazine
	Antituberculosis agents	Isoniazid, rifampin

reorientation of the patient with calendars and clocks, leaving a light on at night to decrease nocturnal exacerbation, and providing adequate sensory stimulation by the use of a radio (Bayne, 1978; Lipowski, 1967).
3. *Nursing care.* Skilled nursing care is needed to modify or prevent disorganized behavior through orientation and by aiding in and maintaining communication. Nursing staffs also have important responsibilities to observe, record, and deal with fluctuations in the illness.
4. *Protection.* The restlessness, fear, and combativeness frequently seen in agitated elderly patients with delirium may lead to injury either to themselves or to others. Recommended precautionary measures include assignment of special duty nurses and placement of the patient in a room near the nurse's station.
5. *Medication.* Use of medication in the management of the aged with delirium is primary for sedation and sleep induction. The most commonly mentioned categories of medication are sedative hypnotics, neuroleptics, and benzodiazepines (Bayne, 1978; Lipowski, 1967, 1980; Moore, 1977; Wells & Duncan, 1980). Among the neuroleptics, haloperidol appears to be in vogue (Moore, 1977; Raskind & Storrie, 1980), but no established evidence indicates that any one major tranquilizer is more effective than any other or that one has fewer side effects than any other (Lipowski, 1980; Prien & Caffey, 1977).

Dementia

The definition of dementia in the description by DSM III is based on clinical symptoms alone, and carries no connotation as to prognosis. Dementia may be progressive, static, or remitting. The reversibility of a dementia is a function of the underlying pathology and of the availability and timely application of effective treatment. Thus, the patient with cerebral damage due to carbon monoxide poisoning is considered to be suffering from dementia, although the onset is acute and the course nonprogressive. Further, the patient with cerebral dysfunction due to hypothyroidism is appropriately diagnosed as having dementia, even though the dysfunction may be reversible and pathological alterations are lacking. Therefore, irreversibility and acuteness will not be considered for the diagnosis of dementia in this section.

Clinical Features

In the DSM III, the essential feature of dementia (Criterion A) is a loss of intellectual abilities of sufficient severity to interfere with social or occupational functioning. The remaining criteria are: (B) memory impairment; (C) one or more of the following: (i) impairment of abstract thinking, (ii) impaired judgment, (iii) other disturbances of higher cortical function (e.g. aphasia, apraxia, agnosia), (iv) personality change; (D) no clouding of consciousness; (E) evidence of a specific organic factor.

These features may frequently dominate the clinical picture, but focusing on them exclusively emphasizes the advanced stages of the dementing process; such an orientation is liable to neglect the clinical picture to be observed in early stages of the disease before severe defects are evident. In most accounts of dementia, memory impairment is considered to be the earliest and most persistent symptom, yet, early in the process of dementia, a variety of other symptoms may present and may capture the attention of the patient, his family, and his physician. Identification and evaluation of these initial symptoms of dementia are quite essential for the early diagnosis and treatment of dementia.

Storandt et al. (1984) have reported that a battery of four psychological tests successfully classified 98% of patients with mild dementia of the Alzheimer's type and healthy older persons by using discriminant function analyses. Berg et al. (1984) also have reported predictive features in mild senile dementia of the Alzheimer's type by using several indexes, such as clinical findings, psychometric tests, EEG, visual evoked potential, and CT measures. However, these procedures for discrimination would not be so advantageous in routine clinical trials. There is a need for more easily administered and less costly procedures such as rating scales, which can identify dementia in its early stages. Further research efforts should be directed toward clinical differentiation of persons with dementia from normal controls.

Clinical Course

According to Chapman and Wolff (1959), who have studied extensively changes in the highest integrative functions due to progressively larger focal lesions of the cerebral hemisphere in man, impairment common to diseases of the cerebral hemispheres falls into four categories: (1) the capacity to express appropriate feelings and drives; (2) the capacity to employ mental mechanisms (learning, memory, etc.) effectively for goal achievement; (3) the capacity to maintain appropriate thresholds and tolerance for frustration and failure, and to recover appropriately from them; and (4) the capacity to employ effective and modulated defense reactions. This delineation seems likely to reflect with fair accuracy progressive dysfunction in a patient suffering from a diffuse cerebral deteriorative disorder.

In most cases the symptoms gradually become apparent, but in some instances the dementia can be abruptly manifested during a period of stress due either to an upheaval in the patient's environment (e.g., the death of a spouse) or an intercurrent illness or injury. Also, a superimposed delirious state often unmasks a latent unsuspected dementia. Although usually slowly progressive, there have been several cases reported in which the clinical course was very malignant, with death occurring within 6 weeks of the time of onset of symptoms (Ehle & Johnson, 1977).

Symptoms and signs in the incipient phases of cerebral degeneration include a loss of interest in work, family, and vocation. Lability of affect or irritability is common, often with considerable increase in the overall anxiety level, particularly as the individual becomes aware of his falling powers. Decreased interest in goals and achievement is experienced, as well as diminished creativity, less motivation to stick to a task, trouble concentrating, and difficulty screening out disturbing environmental stimuli. The individual's characteristic defense mechanisms are utilized more frequently and more blatantly, often with less than normal effectiveness.

In this stage of the disease, many patients try to find a physical explanation for their feeling that "something is wrong." This hypochondriac tendency in a previously healthy elderly patient should raise the suspicion of cerebral degeneration. Thus, depression and anxiety may also constitute early features of the illness. Many of the early symptoms reflect the patient's emotional reactions to his declining mental acuity and differ little either qualitatively or quantitatively from those that occur in normal, healthy individuals who are exhausted, anxious, or face severe environmental pressure. Restlessness, fatigue, and lack of accustomed initiative are frequent subtle emotional changes experienced by the patient with Alzheimer's disease in the first stage of his illness (Stengle, 1943). These behavioral symptoms are usually better appreciated by the patient's family and co-workers than by the physician, so it is important to listen carefully and ask the appropriate questions of relatives if these early symptoms are to be recognized. The social behavior and personality of the patient during the initial phases of the disease most often show an accentuation of previous personality traits superimposed upon a background of apathy or euphoria (Roth & Myers, 1975).

Cognitive changes occur early and are frequently the presenting complaint of the patient or his family. Memory disturbances is by far the most common and is manifested by a significant difficulty in forming new memories (i.e., new learning ability or recent memory). Remote, well-established memories, on the other hand, are usually quite well retained. Though it is common, memory difficulty is not the only intellectual dysfunction. General problem solving ability wanes; this is particularly evident when the patient attempts to solve complex novel problems in which he cannot rely upon well established routinized skills. Comprehension and expression of complex ideas, thinking in an abstract fashion, and critical judgment are also dulled. Along with these higher level cognitive deficits, there is a definite loss of basic visual-motor integrative ability (constructional ability). Occasionally constructional apraxia is demonstrated in mental status testing, although testing in incipient phases such as memory difficulty is not definitely recognized. There is considerable variation in the presentation and course of the illness and in some cases the emotional changes are more dramatic than the intellectual, while in others the reverse is true.

As the disease progresses to a second stage, there is an accentuation of the emotional, social, and cognitive changes. The patient becomes increasingly self-absorbed and less concerned with the feelings and reactions of others. There is increased anxiety, and marked irritability with outbursts of anger may ensue. Depression often intensifies with the increasing awareness of diminished abilities. It is during this early phase of illness accompanied by depression that the patient often complains conspicuously of memory loss. Despite the complaint, definite memory loss may be difficult to demonstrate by available testing techniques. It is almost routine for the patient to complain specifically of loss of memory for recent events, often coupled with an avowal that memories for past events remain crystal clear. Kahn et al. (1975) suggest that the complaint that recent memory is lost is closely tied to feelings of depression and the cognitive set of depression in which everything current is denigrated. It is quite important to recognize these reactive emotional states because the dementia appears more severe than it is, and specific treatment of these states can produce a remarkable improvement in the patient's overall functioning.

During this phase of the disorder, the patient has trouble making plans, dealing with new situations, and initiating activity, and decisions and choices are avoided. Delayed recall and unreliability in calculations may be troublesome, as are slowed speech and understanding. Judgment also suffers, and frustration tolerance is usually even further reduced.

With a worsening of the condition, drives and feelings diminish. Appropriate dress and personal cleanliness may be ignored. Spontaneous speech decreases. There is a tendency to echo what is said to them (echolalia), comprehension is greatly reduced, and there is significant anomia. Difficulty in the execution of previously learned skilled movements also becomes prominent during this stage. Inattention and distractibility become very common at this stage. Personality changes are accentuated and insight becomes very tenuous. Personal warmth and concern for others often disappear. Now the defects of the function enumerated in the Diagnostic and Statistical Manual become readily apparent. Defective memory, particularly for recent events, is blatant. Time and space orientation are faulty. The patient is easily lost. Learning ability is markedly impaired. Some patients are restless and overactive, others lack energy.

It is usually in this phase of the disease that the motor and sensory neurological signs of brain dysfunction begin to appear. The appearance of specific neurological abnormalities does not depend upon duration of the disease process so much as upon the rapidity of the degenerative process and the extent and site of brain damage. Thus with rapidly progressive global disease such as Alzheimer's disease, signs of motor and sensory dysfunction may quickly assume prominence, whereas with more slowly progressive and more restricted diseases, the neurological examination may remain normal for long periods. Usually in this stage, primitive or infantile reflexes such as the shout, root, grasp, and palmomental begin to show themselves.

In the final stage of the disease, the patient becomes apathetic. There is blunting of all feelings. The patient is indifferent or unaware of people and situations. The patient now requires close care, and is grossly disoriented to time, place, and person. Recent and remote memory are defective. Calculations are impossible. The human substance of the personality is lost. If the patient remains in bed for any length of time, either because of apathy or intercurrent illnesses, flexion of the lower extremities begins to be experienced. Death usually results from nonspecific causes such as pneumonis, aspiration, or urinary infection and sepsis (Nielsen et al., 1977).

Mental Status Examination

An impression of a patient's mental status is generally discerned from the history, description of the patient's activities by family members, and results of general physical, neurological, and selected laboratory examinations. A formal mental assessment is also necessary to establish the presence of and to characterize the dementia. It is not essential to perform a detailed evaluation with all patients, but some such assessment of intellectual competence is necessary. For this purpose, a short screening mental status examination, performed rapidly is of practical value especially in routine clinical situations; this is useful for directing attention toward mental abnormalities.

The full clinical mental status examination is not described here. Most textbooks of neurology and psychiatry offer outlines for mental status evaluation.

At the time of testing, a careful evaluation of a patient's level of awareness is required. Abnormal awareness is associated with an inability to maintain coherent lines of thought, and can be separated into two basic types: depressed or fluctuating arousal associated with impairment in the level of wakefulness; and distractibility, a fully awake state with an inability to maintain attention. Mixtures of the types are common, but the differentiation between them is of considerable clinical significance.

Disturbed states of wakefulness such as lethargy or coma are common and relatively easy to identify. Considerably more difficult to demonstrate and understand is the inability to maintain a coherent line of thought in a state of full wakefulness. As mentioned before, this condition has been called delirious or acute confusional state. Unfortunately, this state is easily overlooked, leading to misinterpretation of other items of the mental status evaluation. While the patient can attend for short periods, this ability is rapidly lost and attention wanders.

Although observation is usually adequate to define the abnormality of wakefulness, formal testing is needed to quantify the awake-confused state. According to Cummings and Benson (1983), the digit span is most frequently used. At the rate of about one per second, the examiner recites a few numbers and immediately asks the patient to repeat them. If successful, a list with one more number is offered and so on until the patient makes an error. The "magic number seven plus or minus two" is considered normal. A patient failing at five or fewer digits has a significant attention problem.

For routine clinical practice, the clinician should use an examination that quickly probes wide areas of the patient's mentation. When an abnormality is identified, additional, more specific testing is necessary. If a rapid but more quantitative assessment of mental function is desired, the clinician may perform one of a variety of short standardized mental status examinations such as Hasegawa's Dementia Scale (Hasegawa et al., 1974; Hasegawa, 1983). The cognitive function test for the elderly with dementia should meet the following criteria: (1) it should require only a short time to complete; (2) tests requiring timing or speed are not suitable; (3) verbal tests are preferable to performance tests; (4) the test items should be answered by the normal elderly, but should be difficult for the demented aged. Based on these criteria, Hasegawa's Dementia Scale has been developed. The scale also has characteristics whereby each question has a differently weighted score and the weighted scores on the test have been standardized (Hasegawa et al., 1974). The scale comprises eleven questions as shown in Table 13.3. The scores of the scale vary from zero, representing complete failure, to 32.5 representing a full score.

The test's validity and reliability have been reported (Hasegawa, 1977; Fujita et al., 1979; Hasegawa et al., 1980; Karasawa et al., 1982; Hasegawa et al., 1984) and according to the results of a gerontopsychiatric epidemiological study conducted in the Tokyo metropolis (Hasegawa, 1977), the mean score on Hasegawa's Dementia Scale of the aged without dementia was 27.5, while that of the aged with dementia was 13.5. The mean score of those with mild dementia was 18.9, moderate dementia 12.2, and severe dementia 6.2. Also, the scores on Hasegawa's Dementia Scale correlated quite well with scores of other performance intelligence tests (Fujita et al., 1979). The correlation coefficients of the intercorrelations of all the tests ranged from 0.39 to 0.78. All of them were significant. These findings suggest the validity and reliability of Hasegawa's Dementia Scale as a screening test for the aged with dementia.

TABLE 13.3 Hasegawa's Dementia Scale for the Aged

1. What is the date today?	0, 3
2. Where are you? (Name of the place?)	0, 2.5
3. How old are you?	0, 2
4. How long have you been here?	0, 2.5
5. Where is your birthplace?	0, 2
6. When did World War II end?	0, 3.5
7. How many days are there in a year?	0, 2.5
8. Who is the Prime Minister?	0, 3
9. Subtract 7 from 100, then 7 from 93.	0, 2, 4
10. Name three and four digits in reverse order: 6-8-2, 3-5-2-9	0, 2, 4
11. Recall the five objects that were presented to you earlier	0, 0.5, 1.5 2.5, 3.5
	Total 32.5

Etiology of Dementia

Remedial Causes of Dementia According to the accumulated results in the studies by Wells (1977), a thorough evaluation of demented patients may be expected to result in diagnoses of potentially correctable disorders in approximately 15%. These disorders include instances of depression, drug toxicity, normal pressure hydrocephalus, benign intracranial masses, mania, hypo- and hyperthyroidism, pernicious anemia, epilepsy, and hepatic failure. As pointed out by Freemon (1981), the diagnostic effort in etiologic diagnoses should be directed toward the identification of treatable illnesses. A large number of medical and neurological diseases at least partially reversible by appropriate specific therapy can present as dementia.

Table 13.4 shows several treatable diseases which can present with progressive intellectual deterioration. The most common treatable causes of progressive intellectual deterioration are depression, chronic intoxication of certain depressant drugs, mass lesions, and normal pressure hydrocephalus. Mass lesions potentially amenable to therapy are subdural hematomas, particularly bilateral subdural hematomas in alcoholics, and benign neoplasmas, especially parasagitta meningiomas (Hunter et al., 1968). Normal pressure hydrocephalus and depression are so common that each will be discussed in separate sections.

With certain drugs chronic intoxication leads to progressive intellectual deterioration. For example, the anticonvulsant phenytoin taken for a prolonged period in excessive dosage can produce a clinical picture of dementia (Vallarta et al., 1978). Dementia may follow the chronic use of bromide (Tylden, 1971). Other single drug entities reported to cause reversible

TABLE 13.4 Remedial Causes of Dementia

Normal pressure hydrocephalus
Chronic drug intoxication
Mass lesions
  a. Frontal lobe tumors
  b. Subdural hematomas
Fungal meningitis
Hypothyroidism
Vitamin deficiency
  a. Vitamin B_{12} malabsorption
  b. Folic acid deficiency
  c. Pellagra
Tertiary syphilis
Liver or renal failure
Temporal lobe or psychomotor seizure status

---

dementia include methyldopa (Thornton, 1976), quinidine (Gilbert, 1977), and methotrexate (Pizzo et al., 1976). Phenacetin may produce dementia following long-term use, in addition to its well known renal toxicity (Murray et al., 1971).

Dementia following the prolonged use of several drugs taken simultaneously is more common than dementia produced by a single drug (Maruta, 1978). In a series of 60 consecutive demented patients, five had all mental symptoms resulting from a mixture of depressant drugs such as analgesics, hypnotics, and anticonvulsants. A few toxins can produce mental deterioration with chronic exposure. Most notable are the heavy metals such as lead (Asokan, 1974), mercury (Smith, 1978), and manganese (Banta & Markesbery, 1977). Anoxia associated with carbon monoxide poisoning can produce a chronic dementing illness which has the appearance of progression (Smith & Brandon, 1973).

Normal Pressure Hydrocephalus Progressive dementia that accompanies communicative hydrocephalus with a normal or nearly normal pressure of the cerebrospinal fluid has been recognized as a potentially treatable condition in recent years (Adams et al., 1965; Foltz & Ward, 1956; Hakim & Adams, 1965; Hill et al., 1967; Messert & Baker, 1966). In addition to the slowly progressive dementia, gait disturbance and incontinence have been observed in many of the reported cases. The condition may develop without recognizable preceding events or may follow subarachnoid hemorrhage, trauma, or chronic meningitis or may accompany neoplasmas.

The typical patient presents with dementia, abnormal gait, and frontal lobe signs. An occasional patient can appear uncooperative and aggressive (Crowell et al., 1973), but apathy and depression are more common. The earliest case is presented by mild headaches, forgetfulness, insomnia, and drop attacks (Rice & Gendelman, 1973; Botez et al., 1977).

For radiological evaluation, computed tomography (CT) scanning has largely replaced pneumoencephalography for evaluation of suspected normal pressure hydrocephalus. Sequential CT scanning to evaluate CSF flow can be performed following the injection of a radio-opaque substance such as metrizamide into lumbar subarachnoid space (Ostertag & Mundinger, 1978). Another diagnostic study using radioisotopes is termed cisternography. The isotope passes slowly over the cerebral convexities of patients with shunt responsive dementia (Alker et al., 1972).

It is difficult to determine which patients will improve following the neurosurgical shunt procedure. The series of reports shows several interesting facts (Messert & Wannamaker, 1974; Laws & Mokri, 1977; Stein & Langfitt, 1974; Magnaes, 1978). Patients with typical clinical characteristics have a greater chance of mental improvement following shunting than do those patients with atypical features. Also, those patients who have a demonstrable cause for their hydrocephalus have a greater likelihood of improvement. Detailed analyses of improvement after shunting have shown the presence of gait abnormality and apathetic inertia to be the best predictors (Jacobs et al., 1976; Gustafson & Hagberg, 1978).

Alzheimer's Disease and Senile Dementia Alzheimer's disease is a slowly dementing disorder associated with intraneuronal neurofibrillary tangles and argyrophilic plaques spread throughout the cerebral cortex. Neuronal death is followed by cortical atrophy with widened sulci and enlarged ventricles visible on CT scan. The clinical course is characteristic. Failing memory predominates the early phase of the disease, which is more slowly progressive than most other dementias. The end stage involves masked faces, increased muscle tone, flexed posture, sometimes myoclonus, and occasionally seizures. Autopsy studies have shown that the predominant histological basis for senile dementia is cortical atrophy with neurofibrillary tangles and argyrophilic plaques, indistinguishable from Alzheimer's disease (Todorov et al., 1975). Senile dementia with these histologic characteristics is called senile dementia of the Alzheimer type, abbreviated SDAT. The details of SDAT are described in Chapter 15.

Multiinfarct Dementia The view that brain parenchyma undergoes progressive attrition due to chronic hypoxia resulting from cerebral arteriosclerosis is not tenable. The diagnosis of "arteriosclerotic dementia" is frequently made in instances of gradual reduction of intellectual capacities, particularly if evidence of systemic, retinal, and cerebral arteriosclerosis is available. The degree of correlation between systemic, retinal, and cerebral arteriosclerosis has been reported to be of a low order (Alpers et al., 1948).

Equally, the correlation between the degree of cerebrovascular arteriosclerosis and dementia is limited. Also, no difference was found in the character, location, and degree of arteriosclerotic changes between demented and nondemented elderly persons (Raskin & Ehrenberg, 1956). Butler (1961) concluded that factors other than arteriosclerosis have to be advanced to explain the organic brain syndrome of many elderly persons.

Instead of the above-mentioned view, the evidence indicates that repeated infarction of the brain tissue may lead to dementia ("multiinfarct dementia") (Hachinski et al., 1974). In discussing lacunar infarcts, Fisher (1968) states, "there is no doubt that as the number of lacunes increases producing the lacunar state, mental deterioration occurs." These multiple infarcts are usually due to thromboembolic disease of the extracranial vessels or the heart, and are only infrequently due to atheromatous disease of intracranial vessels. When the small multiple infarctions are restricted to the deep frontal lobes, the term Binswanger's disease is sometimes used (Caplan & Schoene, 1978).

Other Identifiable Causes An unusual cause of dementia was described by Torvik and co-workers (1971) who in three elderly patients found widespread thromboses of small arteries and veins throughout the body but particularly in the brain. The main symptom had been progressive dementia, but cortical blindness and peripheral vascular disease were also observed. Heilman and Fisher (1974) reported a single case as "hyperlipidemic dementia." This patient, a diabetic with very high serum triglyceride, had originally been diagnosed as having arteriosclerotic dementia. Her mental status improved with only a low calorie and low cholesterol diet.

Other systemic disorders present with progressive intellectual deterioration. Dialysis dementia is a progressive, irreversible, and fatal psychotic organic brain syndrome. Its clinical manifestations are aggravated during hemodialysis and immediate postdialysis period. Some evidence suggests the symptoms are due to alminium accumulation in the brain tissue (Arief et al., 1979). Probably the only real treatment is renal transplantation, although diazepam produces transient improvement.

Head trauma is another significant identifiable cause of dementia. Severe dementia with neurological signs can result from a single episode of severe trauma; the mental defect is not progressive. Multiple minor blows can produce a cumulative effect—a very chronic, slowly progressive intellectual and personal impairment that has been extensively studied in boxers (Corsellis et al., 1973).

Chronic alcoholism is associated with many different dementing conditions. Korsakov's disease is relatively common, but it is classified as an amnestic syndrome. Subdural hematoma is common among alcoholics. After all these conditions are removed, however, another alcoholic dementia may remain. Though this clinical entity is unequivocal, clinical impression describes a mild but global dementia associated with moderate but reversible cortical atrophy (Fox et al., 1976; Carlen et al., 1978).

Creutzfeldt-Jacob disease is a rapidly progressive dementing illness with widespread neurological dysfunction, including ataxia, myoclonus, and cortical degeneration that is so severe that it can occasionally produce cortical blindness. The transmissibility of Creutzfeldt-Jacob disease has been determined by studies of kuru and scrapie (Gajdusek & Zigas, 1957; Hadlow, 1959; Gajdusek et al., 1966).

A large number of other degenerative brain conditions such as Huntington's chorea and Wilson's disease are characterized by progressive dementia. Pick's disease has symptomatology and course similar to Alzheimer's disease. In Pick's disease, atrophy is restricted to anterior frontal and inferior temporal cortices. The distribution of cortical atrophy visible on CT scan can suggest Pick's disease (McGeachie et al., 1979). Clinical differentiation can be attempted based upon the more severe memory loss, some elements of cerebral focal signs such as word searching and spatial disorientation, and a relatively mild degree of personality change in Alzheimer's.

In general, these disorders are named by eponym, and unequivocal diagnosis requires histological examination of brain tissue. Thus, although these disorders show clinical differences, it is likely necessary for the clinician not only to make extensive effort to specify the exact appropriate eponym but also to rule out treatable etiologies.

The Pseudodementias: Dementia Syndrome Associated with Psychiatric Disorders

Apparent intellectual impairment associated with psychiatric disorders, particularly depression, has been traditionally considered under the concept of pseudodementia (Madden, 1952; Kiloh, 1961); however, the literature on pseudodementia is somewhat confusing. The word "pseudodementia" is applied to two different groups of patients. The first group includes depressed individuals whose cognitive impairment improves when the depression is successfully treated. Pseudodementia has also been used as a more inclusive term encompassing all patients with apparent cognitive impairment secondary to psychiatric disturbances. Caine (1981) suggested four criteria to define and diagnose pseudodementia. First, there is intellectual impairment in a patient with a primary psychiatric disorder; second, the features of the syndrome resemble those induced by degenerative CNS disorders; third, the intellectual compromise is reversible; and fourth, the patient has no primary identifiable neurologic disease that can account for the cognitive changes. Although depression comprises a majority of pseudodementias, the syndrome can be produced by a number of psychiatric disturbances including mania, schizophrenia, hysterical conversion reactions, and Ganser syndrome.

The frequency of pseudodementia varies greatly depending on the methods of ascertainment. Most studies suggested a prevalence of approximately 10% among patients evaluated for a history of progressive intellectual deterioration (Marsden & Harrison, 1972; Seltzer & Scherwin, 1978; Smith & Kiloh, 1981; Smith et al., 1976). Follow-up studies, however, suggest that dementia is overdiagnosed and that as many as 20 to 50% of patients discharged from the hospital with a diagnosis of dementia may actually be suffering from a primary psychiatric disorder with pseudodementia (Nott & Fleminger, 1975; Ron et al., 1979). Thus, it is quite essential for the clinician to differentiate dementia syndromes associated with psychiatric disorders from primary psychiatric disturbances, particularly depression, in order to rule out treatable etiologies of dementia. Dementia syndrome associated with depression is discussed briefly below.

Depression is the final diagnosis of from 50 to 100% of pseudodementia among patients admitted for evaluation of progressive intellectual decline (Caine, 1981; Freemon, 1976; Good, 1981; Marsden & Harrison, 1972; Ron et al., 1979; Seltzer & Scherwin, 1978; Smith & Kiloh, 1981). Patients who become severely depressed or psychotic during recurrent depressive episodes in early and midlife may manifest a dementia syndrome when depression recurs at a more advanced age. Kay et al. (1955) found that 10% of patients over age 65 years who have affective disorders manifest prominent memory and intellectual deficits consistent with the diagnosis of dementia.

The features of intellectual deterioration include slowness of response, forgetfulness, disorientation, impaired attention, and disturbed ability to abstract and grasp the meaning of situations (Caine, 1981; Folstein & McHugh, 1978; McHugh & Folstein, 1979). Depressed mood and affect is usually apparent and the patient may express guilt, shame, and self-deprecatory feelings. Patients characteristically respond to direct questions with the answer "I don't know" or fail to make or complete a response. Signs of cortical impairment are not present. Thus, as pointed out by Cummings and Benson (1983), the dementia syndrome of depression closely resemble Parkinson disease with dementia, and has few similarities to a cortical degenerative process such as Alzheimer's disease.

Neuroendocrinological testing, such as the dexamethasone suppression test, has added a new dimension to the evaluation of depression. However, this evaluation cannot be relied on to distinguish depressive dementia from other dementias. Also, neuropsychological evaluation cannot be used to distinguish degenerative dementia from the dementia syndrome of depression. The poor performance on neuropsychological tests may mislead the clinician into making a diagnosis of organic brain syndrome, with the implication that the poor test results indicate structural brain damage. Such interpretation may lead to an abandonment of treatment efforts resulting in tragic consequences for depressed patients whose dementia would be reversible with the appropriate therapy (Cowdry & Goodwin, 1981). Depressive dementia is treated with the same interventions used in any severe depressive illness. The dementia syndrome of depression is one of the dementias that can be completely reversed, and the importance of looking for this syndrome among patients with progressive intellectual impairment cannot be overemphasized.

Recently Ravins and co-workers (1984) suggested the criteria for diagnosing reversible dementia caused by depression. Two-year follow-up by the prospective study confirmed the initial diagnosis and demonstrated that coexisting cognitive impairment and major depression are not usually precursory to progressive dementing illness. A past history of affective disorder, a subacute onset, a persistently depressed mood, a history of poor appetite and weight loss, and delusions of self-blame or physical ill health suggested that the patient is suffering a treatable cause of dementia. Also, the recently reported failure of the dexamethasone suppression test to distinguish between Alzheimer's disease and depression (Spar & Gerner, 1983) emphasizes that the clinical examination is the most specific diagnostic procedure now available.

Recent Epidemiological Studies of Dementia in the Aged in Japan

Though epidemiological aspects in psychogeriatrics are described in Chapter 11, some recent epidemiological studies of dementia in the aged in Japan are briefly presented here. According to the pioneering work by Kay and associates (1964) and also some recent Japanese epidemiological studies (Hasegawa, 1977; Karasawa et al., 1982), approximately 4 to 5% of elderly populations suffer from dementia. In Japan, approximately 10% of the population is 65 years and older. When roughly estimated, about 500,000 elderly people in Japan are inflicted with this malignant state of mental decline.

In order to confirm the findings regarding the prevalence rate of dementia in the aged living in the community as well as to establish adequate policies for caring for the demented elderly, the authors and associates carried out an epidemiological survey of age-related dementia in Kanagawa prefecture, located south to Tokyo metropolis. The subjects of the study were 1,800 people (age 65+) selected by random sampling from 224,492 elderly residents. There were no significant differences in the sex and age distributions of the subjects studied and those of the total population of Kanagawa prefecture. The survey was divided into two parts. The primary survey investigated general health status and screened 230 subjects as having suspected mental ill health. In the second survey, these 230 elderly people were visited at home and interviewed by a team composed of a psychiatrist and psychologist who performed the psychiatric examinations. The study mainly employed the diagnostic criteria of dementia according to DSM III. In addition, Hasegawa's Dementia Scale, already described in this chapter, was used for the intellectual assessment.

The results of the study revealed that 70 elderly people were suffering from age-related dementia, a prevalence rate of 4.8%. There were two characteristic findings in the study. First, the prevalence rate of dementia increased with the advancement of age, as shown in Figure 13.1. Above age 75 to 79 years, the prevalence rate showed a marked increase. Also, females exceeded males in the higher age group 75 years and older. Second, the study found a ratio of the prevalence rates of senile and vascular dementias of 24.3:41.3%—the senile dementia was much less prevalent than the vascular dementia. These findings are quite compatible with the results of the recent epidemiological studies in the Tokyo metropolis (Hasegawa, 1977; Karasawa et al., 1982) as shown in Table 13.5. In previous well-

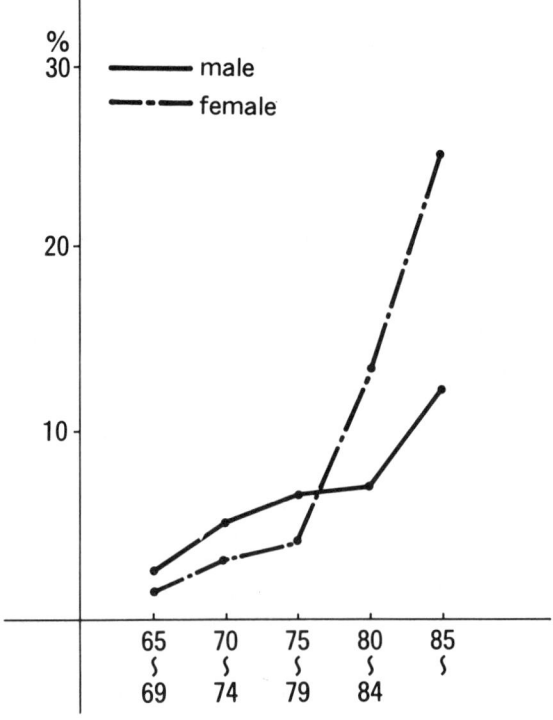

FIGURE 13.1 Distribution of prevalence rates of dementia in the aged according to age ($N=1507$).

TABLE 13.5 Three Recent Epidemiological Studies on Dementia in the Aged in Japan

Author	Hasegawa (1977)	Karasawa et al. (1982)	Hasegawa et al. (1984)
Year of study	1974	1980	1982
Subjects	4,716	4,502	1,507
Place	Tokyo	Tokyo	Kanagawa-pref.
Prevalence rate (%)	4.5	4.6	4.8
Age distribution (%)			
65–69	1.9	1.2	1.8
70–74	2.6	3.1	3.8
75–79	6.1	4.7	5.0
80–84	13.7	13.1	10.8
85+	26.8	23.4	20.8
Diagnosis (%)			
Senile dementia	1.2	0.6	1.2
Vascular dementia	2.7	1.7	2.0
Undifferentiated	0.6	2.3	1.6
Severity of dementia (%)			
Mild	1.5	1.9	2.4
Moderate	1.4	1.2	1.1
Severe	1.6	1.5	1.3

known reports (Kay et al., 1964; Bollerup, 1975; Broe et al., 1976) the prevalence rate of senile dementia appeared to be higher than that of vascular dementia, so the Japanese studies seem to point in the opposite direction. Although the results of the Japanese studies have to be interpreted cautiously, as pointed out by Gunner-Svensson and Jensen (1976), they are quite interesting and stimulating, suggesting the possibility of certain constitutional or genetic factors related to the etiology of senile dementia.

In the Kanagawa study, the deterioration of general physical functions was observed among many of the demented aged. Also, most of the aged with dementia (94.3%) had physical complications. Bedfastness was found in 28.6% of the aged with dementia, versus 1.1% in the total aged population. General physical functions deteriorated with the advancement of dementia, as shown in Figure 13.2. In the aged with dementia, various psychotic symptoms and problem behaviors were frequently observed. Sleep disturbance and waking the family at night were the most frequent psy-

2.9
Mild
(N : 35)
25.7%
8.6
17.1
11.4
34.3
Moderate
(N : 16)
12.5
37.5
25.0
25.0
Severe and very severe
(N : 19)
47.4
15.8
15.8
10.5
5.3
5.3
Total
(N : 70)
28.6
17.1
12.9
14.3
24.3
1.4
Bedfast
Sometimes in bed
Sometimes getting up
Getting up but slow
Active in the room
Active
Not specified

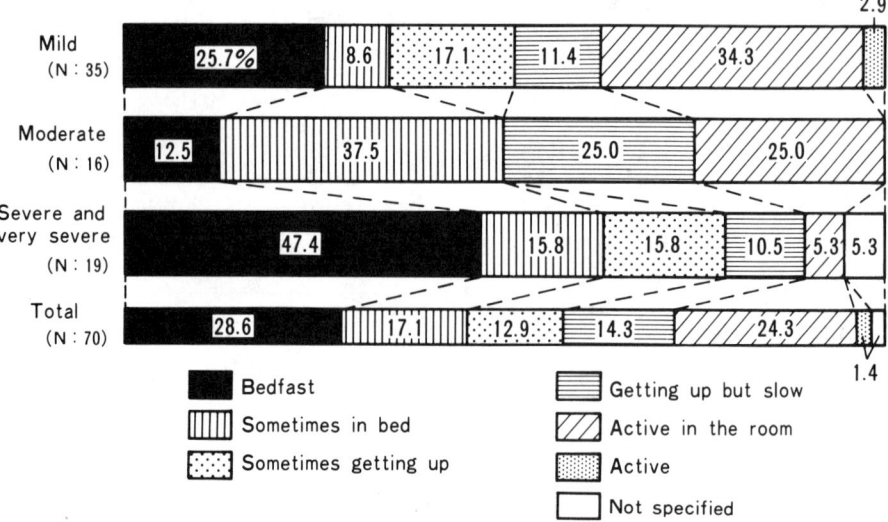

FIGURE 13.2 Degree of dementia and general activity of daily life (ADL).

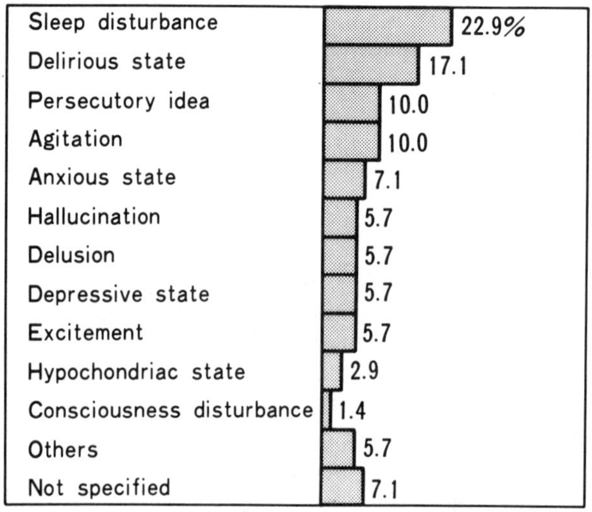

Sleep disturbance 22.9%
Delirious state 17.1
Persecutory idea 10.0
Agitation 10.0
Anxious state 7.1
Hallucination 5.7
Delusion 5.7
Depressive state 5.7
Excitement 5.7
Hypochondriac state 2.9
Consciousness disturbance 1.4
Others 5.7
Not specified 7.1

FIGURE 13.3 Associated psychotic symptoms (N=70).

chotic symptoms and problem behaviors, respectively, as shown in Figures 13.3 and 13.4.

Approximately 30% of the aged with dementia needed constant and total care. The families taking care of them were heavily burdened physically, psychologically, and economically. About 40% of the families admitted

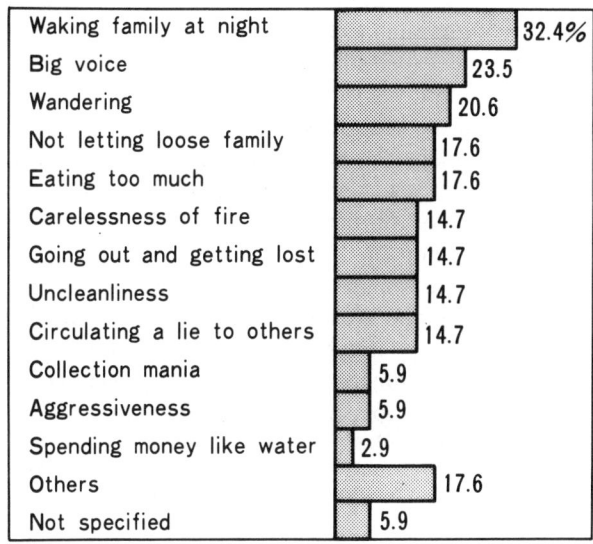

FIGURE 13.4 Problem behaviors (N=34).

problems within the family itself; i.e., difficulty in housekeeping, physical and mental exhaustion, insufficient sleep, economic burden, and intrafamilial discord.

The overall findings suggest that mental and physical care are required for the aged with dementia. Furthermore, in order to provide them with better nursing care, their individual needs must be clearly understood. It should be emphasized that an integrative network of social and medical services in the community be urgently established.

Treatment

The secondary behavioral features of dementia are the most treatable aspects of this disorder; the relief of these symptoms is essential for the adaptation of the aged with dementia within the community or family, as mentioned in the previous section. The care and treatment of the demented patient is principally based upon a thorough assessment of physical and psychological liabilities and assets coupled with a knowledge of premorbid personality characteristics. Treatment is aimed at restitution of those lost functions which are capable of restitution, reduction of the patient's need to employ those functions that have been lost, and maximal utilization of residual functions (Wells, 1977).

For the demented patient to fully utilize his remaining functions, psychopharmacological approaches may be employed to (1) relieve anxiety, (2) improve mood, (3) reduce paranoid and other psychotic symptoms, (4) control problem behaviors such as hyperactivity and assaultiveness, and (5) improve sleep. Symptomatic results with psychotropic agents are not as good as when they are employed in the functional psychiatric disorders. Yet, sometimes antipsychotic medications can be remarkably effective. The more acutely disturbed the patient, the more likely that the drugs will be helpful. They are not helpful and may even be deleterious for impaired memory or other intellectual deficits, or for impaired activities of daily living secondary to intellectual deterioration.

Interpersonal and environmental therapeutic approaches have become increasingly important in the treatment of the aged with dementia and families taking care of a demented patient and, in a sense, for the reduction of the patient's need for lost function described by Wells (1977). The details of drug therapy, psychotherapy, and day hospital care for the aged are presented later in this volume.

Amnestic Syndrome

Memory loss for specific items, an accentuation of the normal forgetfulness that afflicts us all, may be the initial symptom of a wide variety of medical, neurological, and psychiatric syndromes. True amnesia is a global forgetting of all events occuring over an identifiable time span. The essential feature of this disorder is a disturbance in short-term memory but not in immediate recall in a patient who is neither delirious nor demented. Impairment in short-term memory implies that the individual is either unable to consolidate memory into permanent storage or cannot retrieve memory from storage. New information cannot be retained for more than a brief interval and new memories cannot be laid down. DSM III chooses an arbitrary time of 25 minutes as the criterion for transfer of information from immediate memory into memory storage. Associated features include some impairment in remote memory and some degree of disorientation. Associated symptoms such as lack of initiative and emotional blandness may occur. Confabulation, namely filling memory gaps with inventive stories, is variably present.

Transient amnestic syndrome due to temporary dysfunction of certain portions of the limbic system is caused by head trauma, seizures, ischemia, and drugs. Destruction of these same areas causes permanent, ongoing memory deficits. Bilateral hippocampal infarction, herpes simplex encephalitis, and Korsakov's disease produce the vast majority of permanent memory disorder. The most common type of amnestic syndrome is Korsakov's disease, an amnestic syndrome secondary to thiamine deficiency, most common in alcoholics. This disorder almost always follows one or more episodes of Wernicke's encephalopathy, and pathologically involves the diencephalon and medial temporal lobes.

A careful study of patients with Korsakov's disease has demonstrated that, though often believed an irreversible and untreatable disorder, treatment results are often good. Approximately 25% of patients with Korsakov's disease recover fully, and another 25% recover to a significant degree (Victor et al., 1971). The time course of recovery is relatively variable, ranging from weeks to years.

Organic Affective Syndrome

The essential feature is a disturbance of mood resembling a depressive or a manic episode. This syndrome can be attributed to a clearly defined organic factor and does not meet criteria for delirium or dementia. The depressed type of organic affective syndrome is far more common than the manic type. The possible etiologic factors of the organic affective syndrome overlap those for delirium, and both syndromes may coexist in a specific patient. The organic affective syndrome is usually caused by toxic or metabolic factors. Certain substances, notably reserpin, methyldopa, and some of the hallucinogens, are apt to cause a depressive syndrome. Although reserpin induced depression was more common in the era of high dose reserpin therapy, even low dose reserpin can precipitate depression in a susceptible individual. Depression secondary to alpha methyldopa, clonidine, and more recently propranolol (Waal, 1967) has also been reported. Although diuretics such as thiazides and furosemide do not themselves affect mood, secondary hypokalemia can present as depression. The barbiturates, benzodiazepines, and the other sedative/hypnotic agents have also been implicated. The antipsychotic agents occasionally precipitate depressive signs and symptoms.

Endocrine disorders are also important etiologic factors and may produce either depressive or manic syndromes. Examples are hyper- and hypothyroidism, and hyper- and hypoadrenocorticalism. Carcinoma of the pancreas is sometimes associated with the depressive syndrome, possibly due to endocrine disturbance. Structural disease of the brain is a rare cause of the organic affective syndrome.

Treatment of the organic affective syndrome is directed toward correcting the underlying medical disorder or removing the causative toxic agent. Sometimes, of course, this is not possible. This problem is common in depression associated with Parkinson's disease or other neurologic disorders. In such cases, treatment with one of the tricyclic antidepressants is sometimes effective. Causes of the organic affective syndrome of the depressed type, are listed in Table 13.6.

TABLE 13.6 Causes of Organic Affective Syndrome, Depressed

Systemic illness	Neurologic disorder
Congestive heart failure	Parkinson's disease
Pulmonary, renal, and hepatic insufficiency	Intracranial mass lesion
	Huntington's chorea
Lupus erythematosus	
Acute intermittent porphyria	Toxic
Viral infection	Reserpin
Pancreas carcinoma	Alpha methydopa
Metabolic disorder	Clonidine
	Propranolol
Hypothyroidism	Bromide
Hyperadrenalcorticism	Ethanol
Hypokalemia	Barbiturates
Hypercalcemia	Diazepam
Pernicious anemia	Glucocorticoids
Acute intermittent porphyria	Digitalis

CONCLUSION

The organic brain syndromes are the most prevalent psychiatric disorders of later life. The majority of epidemiological studies find definite organic brain syndrome in approximately 5% of persons over age 65 (Hasegawa, 1977; Hasegawa et al., 1984). The behavioral and social consequences of these disorders will become even more important as the proportion of elderly persons in the population increases. Although the clinical management of organic brain syndrome, especially dementing illnesses, has often been associated with pessimism and even therapeutic nihilism, such a stance is no longer tenable. Many organic brain syndromes are treatable and even the patient with an irreversible dementia can benefit from a well-conceived therapeutic regimen. Wang (1977) suggests that dementia as a clinical syndrome can be viewed as a sociopsychosomatic disease and also emphasizes that many sociopsychological factors play an important contributory and complicating role in the development of the behavioral manifestations of intellectual deterioration. Early recognition and correction of these factors may help prevent the development of complications and slow the progression of deterioration.

REFERENCES

Adams, R. D., Fisher, C. M., Hakim, S., Ojemann, R. G., & Sweet, W. H. (1965). Symptomatic occult hydrocephalus with "normal" cerebrospinal fluid pressure. *New Eng. J. Med., 273,* 117–126.

Alkar, G. J., Glasauer, F. E., & Leslie, E. V. (1972). Long-term experience with isotope cisternography. *J. Amer. Med. Ass., 219,* 1005–1010.
Alpers, B. J., Forster, F. M., & Herbert, P. A. (1948). Retinal, cerebral and systemic arteriosclerosis. A histopathological study. *Arch. Neurol. Psychiatry, 60,* 440–456.
American Psychiatric Association. (1980). Diagnostic and statistical manual of mental disorders (3rd ed.) (pp. 101–162). Washington, D.C.: APA.
Arieff, A. I., Cooper, J. D., Armstrong, D., & Lazarowitz, V. C. (1979). Dementia, renal failure, and brain alminium. *Ann. Int. Med., 90,* 741–747.
Asokan, S. K., Vansant, J., Bassett, W. B., & Nardone, D. (1974). Delayed recognition of lead encephalopathy in two "moonshine" drinkers. *Southern Med. J., 67,* 1440–1442.
Banta, R. G., & Markesbery, W. R. (1977). Elevated manganese levels associated with dementia and extrapyramidal signs. *Neurology, 27,* 213–216.
Bayne, J. R. D. (1978). Management of confusion in elderly persons. *Can. Med. Assoc. J., 118,* 139–141.
Berg, L., Danziger, W. L., Storandt, M., Coben, L. A., Gado, M., Hughes, C. P., Knesevich, J. W., & Botwinick, J. (1984). Predictive features in mild senile dementia of the Alzheimer type. *Neurology, 34,* 563–569.
Blass, J. P., & Gibson, G. E. (1979). Carbohydrates and acetylcholine synthesis: Implications for cognitive disorders. In K. L. Davis, & P. A. Berger (Eds.) *Brain Acethylcholine and Neuropsychiatric Disease* (pp. 215–236). New York: Plenum.
Bollerup, T. R. (1975). Prevalence of mental illness among 70-year-olds domiciled in nine Copenhagen suburbs. *Acta Psychiatr. Scand., 51,* 327–339.
Botez, M. I., Ethier, R., Léveillé, J., & Botez-Marquard, T. (1977). A syndrome of early recognition of occult hydrocephalus and cerebral atrophy. *Quart. J. Med., 46,* 365–380.
Broe, G. A., Akhtar, A. J., Andrews, G. R., Caird, F. I., Gilmore, A. J. J., & McLennan, W. J. (1976). Neurological disorders at home. *J. Neurol. Neurosurg. Psychiatry, 39,* 362–366.
Busse, E. W., & Blazer, D. (1980). Disorders related to biological functioning. In E. W. Busse & D. Blazer (Eds.), *Handbook of geriatric psychology* (pp. 390–414). New York: Van Nostrand Reinhold.
Butler, R. N. (1961). Psychiatric aspects of cerebrovascular disease in the aged. *Proc. Assoc. Res. Nerv. Ment. Dis., 41,* 255–266.
Caine, E. D. (1981). Pseudodementia. Current concepts and future directions. *Arch. Gen. Psychiatry, 38,* 1359–1364.
Caplan, L. R., & Schoene, W. C. (1978). Clinical features of subcortical arteriosclerotic dementia (Binswanger disease). *Neurology, 28,* 1206–1215.
Carlen, P. L., Wortzman, G., Holgate, R. C., Wilkinson, D. A., & Rankin, J. G. (1978). Reversible cerebral atrophy in recently abstinent chronic alcoholics measured by computed tomography scans. *Science, 200,* 1076–1078.
Chapman, L. F., & Wolff, H. G. (1959). The cerebral hemispheres and the highest integrative functions of man. *Arch. Neurol., 1,* 357–424.
Chisholm, S. E., Denistron, O. L., Igrisan, R. M., & Barbus, A. J. (1982). Prevalence of confusion in elderly hospitalized patients. *J. Geront. Nursing, 8,* 87–96.
Cohen, S. (1953). The toxic psychoses and allied states. *Am. J. Med., 15,* 813–823.
Corsellis, J. A. N., Bruton, C. J., & Freeman-Browne, D. (1973). The aftermath of boxing. *Psychol. Med., 3,* 270–303.
Cowdry, R. W., & Goodwin, F. K. (1981). Dementia of bipolar illness: diagnosis and response to lithium. *Am. J. Psychiatry, 138,* 1118–1119.

Crowell, R. M., Tew, J. M., & Mark, V. H. (1973). Aggressive dementia associated with normal pressure hydrocephalus. *Neurology, 23,* 461–464.

Cummings, J. L., & Benson, D. F. (1983). *Dementia: A clinical approach* (pp. 15–34). Boston: Butterworth.

Davison, W. (1978). Neurological and mental disturbances due to drugs. *Age Ageing, 7(Suppl.),* 119–130.

Doty, E. J. (1946). The incidence and treatment of delirious reactions in later life. *Geriatrics, 1,* 21–26.

Eisdorfer, C., & Cohen, D. (1978). The cognitively impaired elderly: Differential diagnosis. In M. Strandt, I. C. Siegler, & M. F. Elias (Eds.) *The clinical psychology of aging* (pp. 7–42). New York: Plenum.

Ehle, A. L., & Johnson, P. C. (1977). Rapidly evolving EEG changes in a case of Alzheimer's disease. *Ann. Neurol., 1,* 593–596.

Ellis, J. M., & Lee, S. I. (1978). Acute prolonged confusion in later life as an ictal state. *Epilepsia, 19,* 119–128.

Engel, G. L., & Romano, J. (1959). Delirium: A syndrome of cerebral insufficiency. *J. Chronic Dis., 9,* 260–277.

Fisher, C. M. (1968). Dementia in cerebral vascular disease. In *Transactions of the sixth conference on cerebral vascular disease* (pp. 453–464). American Neurological Association. New York: Grune & Stratton.

Folstein, M. F., & McHugh, P. R. (1978). Dementia syndrome of depression. In R. Katzman, R. D. Terry, & K. L. Bick (Eds.) *Alzheimer's disease: Senile dementia and related disorders* (pp. 87–93). New York: Raven Press.

Foltz, E. L., & Ward, A. A. (1956). Communicating hydrocephalus from subarachnoid bleeding. *J. Neurosurg., 13,* 546–566.

Fox, J. H., Ramsey, R. G., Huckman, M. S., & Proske, A. E. (1976). Cerebral ventricular enlargement. Chronic alcoholics examined by computerized tomography. *J. Am. Med. Ass., 236,* 365–368.

Freemon, F. R. (1976). Evaluation of patients with progressive intellectual deterioration. *Arch. Neurol., 33,* 658–659.

Freemon, F. R. (1981). *Organic mental disease* (pp. 119–122). Lancaster, UK: MTP Press.

Fujita, M., Hasegawa, K., Takubo, E., Tobi, M., Watanabe, T., & Inoue, K. (1979). The comparative study on Hasegawa's brief intelligence scale and performance intelligence tests. *Jpn. J. Geront., 1,* 78–89.

Gajdusek, D. C., Gibbs, C. J., Jr., & Alpers, M. (1966). Experimental transmission of a kuru like syndrome to chimpanzees. *Nature (Lond.), 209,* 794–798.

Gajdusek, D. C., & Zigas, V. (1957). Degenerative disease of the central nervous system in New Guinea. The endemic occurrence of "kuru" in the native population. *N. Eng. J. Med., 257,* 974–978.

Gilbert, G. J. (1979). Quinidine dementia. *J. Am. Med. Ass., 237,* 2093–2096.

Gillick, M. R., Serrell, N. A., & Gillick, L. S. (1982). Adverse consequences of hospitalization in the elderly. *Soc. Sci. Med., 16,* 1033–1038.

Glickman, L., & Friedman, S. A. (1976). Changes in behavior, mood, or thinking in the elderly: Diagnosis and management. *Med. Clin. North Am., 60,* 1297–1313.

Good, M. I. (1981). Pseudodementia and physical findings masking significant psychopathology. *Am. J. Psychiatry, 138,* 811–814.

Gunner-Svensson, F., & Jensen, K. (1976). Frequency of mental disorders in old age. Examples of comparability of epidemiological investigations in relation to utility in planning. *Acta Psychiatr. Scand., 53,* 283–297.

Gustafson, L., & Hagberg, B. (1978). Recovery in hydrocephalus dementia after shunt operation. *J. Neurol. Neurosurg. Psychiatry, 41,* 940–947.

Hachinski, V. C., Lassen, N. A., & Marshall, J. (1974). Multi-infarct dementia: a cause of mental deterioration in the elderly. *Lancet, 2,* 207–210.

Hadlow, W. J. (1959). Scrapie and kuru. *Lancet, 2,* 289–290.

Hakim, S., & Adams, R. D. (1965). The special clinical problems of symptomatic hydrocephalus with normal cerebrospinal fluid pressure. *J. Neurol. Sci., 2,* 307–324.

Harris, R. (1972). The relationship between organic disease and physical status. In C. M. Gaitz (Ed.) *Aging and the brain* (pp. 163–177). New York: Plenum.

Hasan, M. K., & Mooney, R. P. (1979). Reversible toxic psychosis. *Am. Fam. Physician, 20,* 89–92.

Hasegawa, K., Inoue, K., & Moriya, K. (1974). The study on the brief intelligence scale for the demented elderly. *Seisinigaku (Psychiatry), 16,* 965–969.

Hasegawa, K. (1977). Mental health problems of the community-residing aged in Japan. Paper presented at the plenary session of the World Congress of Psychiatry, Honolulu, Hawaii.

Hasegawa, K. (1983). The clinical assessment of dementia in the aged: A dementia screening scale for psychogeriatric patients. In M. Bergener et al. (Eds.), *Aging in the eighties and beyond. Highlights of the twelfth international congress of gerontology* (pp. 207–218). New York: Springer Publishing Co.

Hasegawa, K., Homma, A., Sato, H., Aoba, A., Imai, Y., Yamaguchi, N., & Itami, A. (1984). An epidemiological study of age-related dementia in the community residing aged. *Gerontopsychiatry, 1,* 94–105.

Heilman, K. M., & Fisher, W. R. (1974). Hyperlipidemic dementia. *Arch. Neurol., 31,* 67–68.

Henry, W. D., & Mann, A. M. (1965). Diagnosis and treatment of delirium. *Can. Med. Assoc. J., 93,* 1156–1166.

Hill, M. E., Hougheed, W. M., & Barnett, H. J. M. (1967). A treatable form of dementia due to normal pressure communicating hydrocephalus. *Can. Med. Assoc. J., 97,* 1309–1320.

Hodkinson, H. M. (1973). Mental impairment in the elderly. *J. R. Coll. Physicians Lond., 7,* 305–317.

Hodkinson, H. M. (1976). *Common symptoms of disease in the elderly* (pp. 21–34). Oxford: Blackwell Scientific Publications.

Hunter, R., Blackwood, W., & Bull, J. (1968). Three cases of frontal meningiomas presenting psychiatrically. *Br. Med. J., 3,* 9–16.

Jacobs, L., Conti, D., Kinkel, W. R., & Manning, E. J. (1976). "Normal pressure" hydrocephalus. *J. Am. Med. Assoc., 235,* 510–512.

Kahn, R. L. (1971). *Psychological aspects of aging.* In I. Rossman (Ed.), *Clinical geriatrics* (pp. 107–113). Philadelphia: Lippincott.

Karasawa, A., Kawashima, A., & Kasahara, H. (1982). Epidemiological study of the senile in Tokyo metropolitan area. In H. Ohashi, K. Nakayama, M. Saito, & B. Saletu (Eds.) *The proceedings of World Psychiatric Association Regional Symposium Kyoto* (pp. 285–289). Tokyo: The Japanese Society of Psychiatry and Neurology.

Kay, D. W. K., Roth, M., & Hopkins, B. (1955). Affective disorders arising in the senium. *J. Ment. Sci., 101,* 302–318.

Kay, D. W. K., Beamish, P., & Roth, M. (1964). Old age mental disorders in Newcastle-upon-Tyne: Part I. A study of prevalence. *Brit. J. Psychiatry, 110,* 146–158.

Kiloh, L. G. (1961). Pseudo-dementia. *Acta Psychiatr. Scand., 37,* 336–351.
Laws, E. R., & Mokri, B. (1977). Occult hydrocephalus: Results of shunting correlated with diagnostic tests. *Clin. Neurosurg., 24,* 316–333.
Libow, L. S. (1973). Pseudo-senility: Acute and reversible organic brain syndromes. *J. Am. Geriatr. Soc., 21,* 112–120.
Lipowski, Z. J. (1967). Delirium, clouding of consciousness and confusion. *J. Nerv. Ment. Dis., 145,* 227–255.
Lipowski, Z. J. (1975). Organic brain syndromes: Overview and classification. In D. F. Benson, & D. Blumer (Eds.) *Psychiatric aspects of neurological disease* (pp. 11–35). New York: Grune & Stratton.
Lipowski, Z. J. (1980). *Delirium: Acute brain failure in man.* Springfield, Illinois: Charles C. Thomas.
Lishman, W. A. (1978). *Organic psychiatry.* Oxford: Blackwell Scientific Publications.
McGeachie, R. E., Fleming, J. O., Sharer, L. R., & Hyman, R. A. (1979). Diagnosis of Pick's disease by computed tomography. *J. Comp. Assist. Tomogr., 3,* 113–115.
McHugh, P. R., & Folstein, M. F. (1979). Psychopathology of dementia: implications for neuropathology. In R. Katzman (Ed.) *Congenital and acquired cognitive disorders* (pp. 17–30). New York: Raven Press.
Madden, J. J., Luhan, J. H., Kaplan, L. A., & Manfredi, H. M. (1952). Nondementing psychoses in older persons. *J. Am. Med. Ass., 150,* 1567–1570.
Magnaes, B. (1978). Communicating hydrocephalus in adults. *Neurology, 28,* 478–484.
Marsden, C. D., & Harrison, M. J. G. (1972). Outcome of investigation of patients with presenile dementia. *Brit. Med. J., 2,* 249–252.
Maruta, T. (1978). Prescription drug-induced organic brain syndrome. *Am. J. Psychiatry, 135,* 376–377.
Messert, B., & Wannamaker, B. B. (1974). Reappraisal of the adult occult hydrocephalus syndrome. *Neurology, 24,* 224–231.
Messert, B., & Baker, N. H. (1966). Syndrome of progressive spastic ataxia and apraxia associated with occult hydrocephalus. *Neurology, 16,* 440–452.
Moore, D. P. (1977). Rapid treatment of delirium in critically ill patients. *Amer. J. Psychiatry, 134,* 1431–1432.
Morse, R. M., & Litin, E. M. (1969). Post operative delirium: A study of etiologic factors. *Am. J. Psychiatry, 126,* 388–395.
Morse, R. M., & Litin, E. M. (1971). The anatomy of delirium. *Am. J. Psychiatry, 128,* 111–116.
Murphy, E. (1968). The confused elderly patient. *J. Irish Med. Assoc., 61,* 99–103.
Murray, R. M., Greene, J. G., & Adams, J. H. (1971). Analgesic abuse and dementia. *Lancet, 3,* 242–245.
Nausieda, P. A., Kaplan, L. R., Weber, S., Weiner, W. J., & Klawans, H. L. (1979). Sleep disruption and psychosis induced by chronic levodopa therapy. *Neurology, 29,* 553.
Nielsen, J., Homma, A., & B.-Henriksen, T. (1977). Follow-up 15 years after a geronto-psychiatric prevalence study. Conditions concerning death, cause of death and life expectancy in relation to psychiatric diagnosis. *J. Geront., 32,* 554–561.
Nott, P. N., & Fleminger, J. J. (1975). Presenile dementia: the difficulties of early diagnosis. *Acta Psychiatr. Scand., 51,* 210–217.
Ostertag, C. B., & Mundinger, F. (1978). Diagnosis of normal pressure hydrocephalus using CT with CSF enhancement. *Neuroradiol., 16,* 216–219.

Pizzo, P. A., Bleyer, W. A., Poplack, D. G., & Leventhal, B. G. (1976). Reversible dementia temporally associated with intraventricular therapy with methotrexate in a child with acute myelogenous leukemia. *J. Pediat.*, 88, 131–133.

Prien, R. F., & Caffey, E. M., Jr. (1977). Pharmacologic treatment of elderly patients with organic brain syndrome: A survey of twelve Veterans Administration Hospitals. *Compr. Psychiatry*, 18, 551–560.

Pro, J. D., & Wells, C. E. (1977). The use of electroencephalogram in the diagnosis of delirium. *Dis. Nerv. Syst.*, 38, 804–808.

Purdie, F. R., Honigman, B., & Rosen, P. (1981). Acute organic brain syndrome: A review of 100 cases. *Ann. Emerg. Med.*, 10, 455–460.

Ravins, P. V., Merchant, A., & Nestadt, G. (1984). Criteria for diagnosing reversible dementia caused by depression: Validation by two year follow-up. *Br. J. Psychiatry*, 144, 488–492.

Raskin, N., & Ehrenberg, R. (1956). Cerebral arteriosclerosis. *Am. Pract. Digest Treatment*, 7, 1095–1096.

Raskind, M. A., & Storrie, M. C. (1980). The organic brain syndromes. In E. W. Busse & D. G. Blazer (Eds.) *Handbook of geriatric psychiatry* (pp. 305–328). New York: Van Nostrand Reinhold.

Rice, E., & Gendelman, S. (1973). Psychiatric aspects of normal pressure hydrocephalus. *J. Am. Med. Ass.*, 223, 409–412.

Romano, J., & Engel, G. L. (1944). Physiologic and psychologic considerations of delirium. *Med. Clin. North Am.*, 28, 629–638.

Ron, M. A., Toone, B. K., Garralda, M. E., & Lishman, W. A. (1979). Diagnostic accuracy in presenile dementia. *Brit. J. Psychiatry*, 134, 161–168.

Roth, M. (1976). The psychiatric disorders in later life. *Psychiatr. Ann.*, 6, 57–98.

Roth, M., & Myers, D. H. (1975). The diagnosis of dementia. *Brit. J. Psychiatry* (Special Publication), 9, 87–99.

Schuckit, M. A., Miller, P. L., & Hahlbohm, D. (1975). Unrecognized psychiatric illness in elderly medical-surgical patients. *J. Geront.*, 30, 655–660.

Seltzer, B., & Sherwin, I. (1978). Organic brain syndromes: An empirical study and critical review. *Am. J. Psychiatry*, 135, 13–21.

Simon, A., & Cahan, R. B. (1963). The acute brain syndrome in geriatric patients. *Psychiatr. Res. Rep.*, 16, 8–21.

Smith, J. S., & Brandon, S. (1973). Morbidity from acute carbon monoxide poisoning at three year follow-up. *Brit. Med. J.*, 1, 318–321.

Smith, J. S., Kiloh, L. G., Ratnavale, G. S., & Grant, D. A. (1976). The investigation of dementia. *Med. J. Aust.*, 2, 403–405.

Smith, D. L., Jr. (1978). Mental effect of mercury poisoning. *Southern Med. J.*, 71, 904–905.

Smith, J. S., & Kiloh, L. G. (1981). The investigation of dementia: Results in 200 consecutive admissions. *Lancet*, 1, 824–827.

Spar, G. E., & Gerner, R. (1983). Does the dexamethasone suppression test distinguish dementia from depression. *Am. J. Psychiatry*, 139, 238–240.

Stein, S. C., & Langfitt, T. W. (1974). Normal pressure hydrocephalus. *J. Neurosurg.*, 41, 463–470.

Steinhart, M. J. (1979). Treatment of delirium—A reappraisal. *Int. J. Psychiatry Med.*, 9, 191–197.

Stengle, E. (1943). A study on the symptomatology and differential diagnosis of Alzheimer's disease and Pick's disease. *J. Ment. Sci.*, 89, 1–20.

Storandt, M., Botwinick, J., Danziger, W. L., Berg, L., & Hughes, C. P. (1984). Psychometric differentiation of mild senile dementia of the Alzheimer type. *Arch. Neurol.*, 41, 497–499.

Thornton, W. E. (1976). Dementia induced by methydopa with haloperidol. *New Eng. J. Med., 295,* 1222.
Todorov, A. B., Go, R. C. P., Constantinidis, J., & Elston, R. C. (1975). Specificity of the clinical diagnosis of dementia. *J. Neurol. Sci., 26,* 81–98.
Torvik, A., Endresen, G. K. M., Abrahamsen, A. F., & Godal, H. C. (1971). Pregressive dementia caused by an usual type of generalized small vessel thrombosis. *Acta Neurol. Scand., 47,* 137–150.
Tylden, E. (1971). Bromism. *Lancet, 4,* 924.
Vallarta, J. M., Bell, D. B., & Reichhert, A. (1974). Progressive encephalopathy due to chronic hydantoin intoxication. *Am. J. Dis. Child., 128,* 27–34.
Victor, M., Adams, R. D., & Collins, G. H. (1971). *The Wernicke-Korsakoff syndrome.* Philadelphia: F. A. Davis.
Waal, H. J. (1967). Propranolol induced depression. *Brit. Med. J., 2,* 50.
Wang, H. S. (1977). Dementia in old age. In C. E. Wells (Ed.) *Dementia* (pp. 15–26.) Philadelphia: F. A. Davis.
Wells, C. E. (1977). Diagnostic evaluation and treatment in dementia. In C. E. Wells (Ed.) *Dementia* (pp. 247–276).
Wells, C. E., & Duncan, G. W. (1980). *Neurology for psychiatrists* (pp. 45–64). Philadelphia: F. A. Davis.
Williamson, J. (1978). Prescribing problems in the elderly. *Practitioner, 220,* 749–755.
Wolff, H. G., & Curran, D. (1935). The nature of delirium and allied states: The dysergastic reaction. *Arch. Neurol. Psychiatry, 33,* 1175–1215.

14
Hypertension and Stroke

Yukito Shinohara

It is widely accepted that hypertension is a major contributory factor in the development of cerebrovascular disease (CVD), and is found in high frequency among CVD patients. It is also well known that the blood pressure is one of the prime determinants of cerebral blood flow (CBF) and the functions of blood-brain barrier (BBB). Therefore, the management of blood pressure is cardinal not only for the prevention of stroke but also for the treatment of acute and chronic CVD patients.

In this chapter, the relationships between hypertension and stroke will be described, primarily from the physiological and pathological viewpoints.

EFFECTS OF BLOOD PRESSURE ON CEREBRAL BLOOD FLOW AND BBB

Cerebral Circulation and Blood Pressure

The human brain is supplied with blood from several sources, including the two internal carotid arteries and the two vertebral arteries. It is generally accepted that in healthy adults the mean CBF is 50 to 60 ml/100 g brain tissue/min. Thus, assuming a brain weight of 1400 g, the total blood flow in the brain is about 700 to 850 ml/min. This represents about 15% of total cardiac output, even though the brain accounts for only just over 2 to 3% of total body weight. This suggests how important circulation to the brain is, compared with that to the other organs.

Although many factors are known to regulate the brain circulation, they may all be grouped together in terms of two important variables. These are the perfusion pressure at the level of the brain, which is almost equal to the systemic blood pressure, and the total resistance imposed upon the blood flow through the vessels of the brain (cerebral vascular resistance).

The perfusion pressure or the blood pressure head of the brain, which is the difference between the arterial and venous pressures at the level of the brain, is influenced mainly by the systemic blood pressure, and also partially by the local perfusion pressure of the extracranial vessels, which could be affected by stenosis or occlusion of these vessels. However, various investigations (Fog, 1937; Kety et al. 1950; Shenkin et al. 1950; Finnerty et al. 1954; Lassen, 1959) do not support the former belief (Monro, 1783) that blood flow in the brain passively follows changes in blood pressure.

Figure 14.1 shows a schematic view of the human cerebral circulation at normal blood pressure, when the diameter of the vessels is assumed to be normal. When the blood pressure drops, the blood flow in the brain is kept constant by dilation of the cerebral vessels, as illustrated in Figure 14.2. On the other hand, the cerebral vessels constrict to keep the blood flow constant when the blood pressure rises (Figure 14.3). This ability of the cerebral vessels to keep blood flow constant despite changes of blood pressure is called "autoregulation" of cerebral vessels.

CBF is, therefore, normally maintained at a fairly constant level within a mean arterial blood pressure (MABP) range of between about 50 and 150 mmHg (Figure 14.4). Recently it has been shown that when the blood pressure rises above a level of around 150 mmHg, a severe increase in blood flow in the brain may result (Ekström-Jodal et al., 1971/72; Lassen & Agnoli, 1973). The phenomenon of CBF increase at an extremely high blood pressure level was named "breakthrough," and an acute rise of blood pressure may develop "hypertensive encephalopathy" as described later.

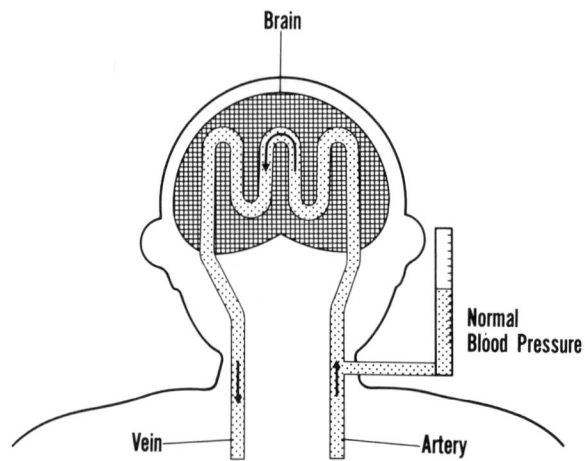

FIGURE 14.1 Schematic illustration of the blood flow in the brain. The diameter of the vessels is assumed to be normal at the normal blood pressure.

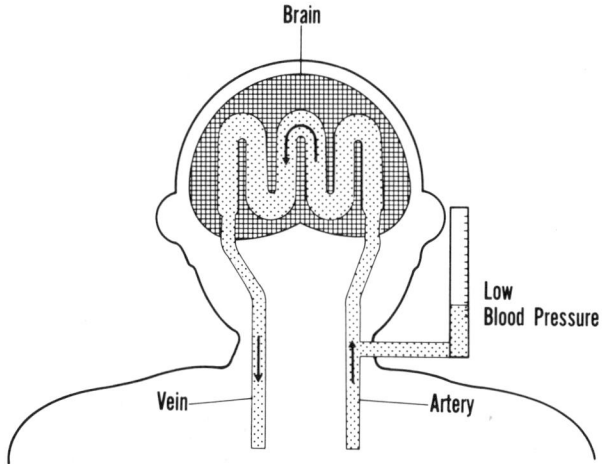

FIGURE 14.2 In comparison with Figure 14.1, this shows how the blood vessels in the brain dilate to ensure a constant flow of blood when the blood pressure falls.

In pathological conditions, such as cerebral infarction, hemorrhage, head trauma, diabetes, and probably in cases of severe arteriosclerotic changes of the blood vessels, and so on, autoregulation is easily destroyed. As shown in Figure 14.5 the blood flow then passively follows changes in blood pressure.

The real mechanisms of autoregulation whereby blood flow is maintained at constant levels despite large changes in perfusion pressure are not known,

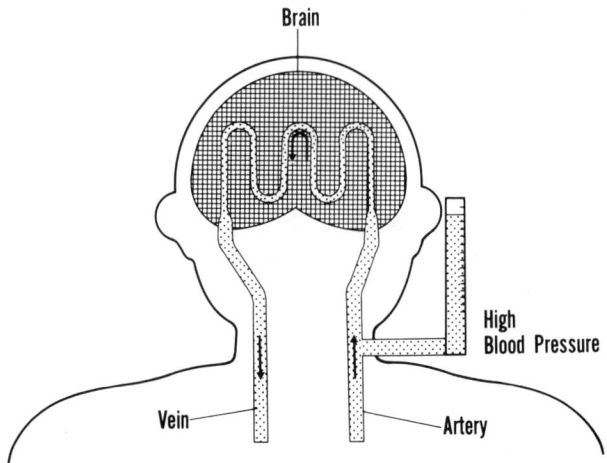

FIGURE 14.3 In comparison with Figure 14.1, the blood flow vessels constrict in order to maintain constant blood flow when the blood pressure rises.

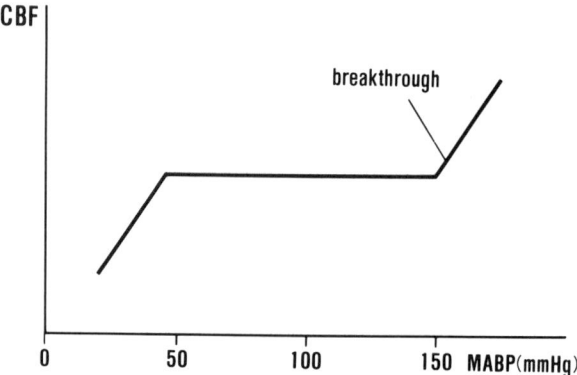

FIGURE 14.4 Normal autoregulation of cerebral blood flow (CBF). CBF is maintained constant over a wide range of mean arterial blood pressure (MABP).

although both neurogenic (James et al., 1969; Gotoh et al., 1971/72; Shinohara & Gotoh, 1975; Shinohara et al., 1978a) and myogenic (Lassen, 1964) mechanisms have been proposed.

Upper Limit of CBF Autoregulation in Hypertension

The question arises, is the upper limit of CBF autoregulation stable in various conditions such as chronic persistent hypertension without cerebrovascular disease? There is some evidence of a shift of the upper limit of CBF autoregulation to higher mean arterial pressures in hypertensive, as compared to normotensive, men (Strandgaard et al., 1973, 1976) and in hypertensive baboons (Strandgaard et al., 1975). Even after brief periods of chronic hypertension, both the upper and lower limits of autoregulation seem to shift to higher levels of mean arterial pressure (Figure 14.6). The lower limit of autoregulation does, however, appear to be displaced to a greater extent than the upper limit (Jones et al., 1976), although there is wide individual variation. Thus, there is a narrowing of the autoregulatory plateau in hypertensives as compared to normotensive controls.

The rate of elevation of blood pressure also seems to be very important for determining the relationship between CBF value and blood pressure level. It was reported that the CBF in baboons began to increase with a rise in blood pressure of up to 120 mmHg or more, if the rise occurred abruptly; in other words, autoregulation was maintained only until the blood pressure was 30 to 40% above the resting MABP value (Strandgaard et al., 1974) in this situation. In dogs and cats, similar findings have been reported; for example, an acute and moderate increase in arterial blood pressure within

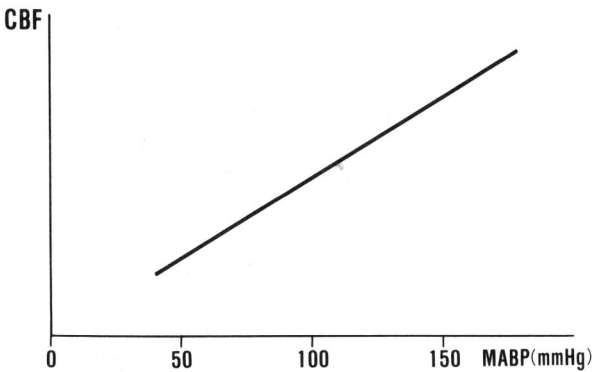

FIGURE 14.5 Disturbed autoregulation. When autoregulation is impaired, the CBF passively follows MABP.

the physiological range caused CBF to rise by 35 to 55% in dogs and by 40 to 60% in cats (Busija et al., 1980).

Accordingly, it is concluded that the upper limit of CBF autoregulation is determined not only by the MABP value but also by (1) rate of elevation of blood pressure, (2) resting CBF value, (3) presence of chronic hypertension, (4) species difference, and (5) probably the state of the autonomic nervous system of the cerebral vascular wall.

Effect of Severe Hypertension on Cerebral Vessels and BBB

It had been thought until recent years that an acute increase of blood pressure induces uncontrolled cerebral vasoconstriction and causes brain tissue ischemia. However, recent experimental studies have not supported this hypothesis, but have stressed the importance of forced dilatation of cerebral vessels and increased CBF (so-called breakthrough, as already described) at high blood pressure. Giese (1964) studied the intestinal (not cerebral) vessels of rats with angiotensin-induced hypertension and found alternating segments of dilatation and constriction (the sausage-string or bead-string phenomenon) in these vessels. Colloidal carbon was injected intravenously 1 hour before the angiotensin infusion was terminated and it was later found in the walls of arteries only at points of dilatation. This study suggested that the dilated segments represent areas where vascular contractility is overcome, causing endothelial necrosis, destruction of smooth muscle cells, and the formation of fibrin.

Direct observation of the pial arteriolar caliber and measurement of local CBF in cats (MacKenzie et al., 1976) indicated that pial arterioles con-

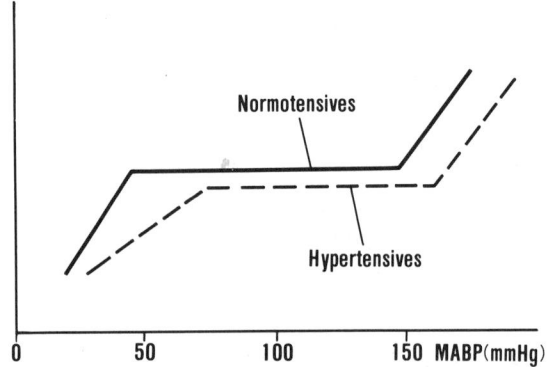

FIGURE 14.6 Autoregulation in normotensives and hypertensives. The upper and lower limits of autoregulation shift to the right.

stricted and CBF remained relatively constant as the blood pressure was increased by intravenous administration of angiotensin. They observed that arteriolar dilation appeared when MABP rose above 170 mmHg. In smaller arterioles (initial diameter less than 100 μm) a segmental dilatation (the sausage-string phenomenon) frequently preceded uniform dilatation of the vessels. This arteriolar dilatation was associated with a marked increase in local CBF, indicating that the upper level of autoregulation had been breached. It was also observed that hypertension produces dysfunction of the BBB since, in most of the animals examined, there was extravasation of protein-bound Evans blue into brain tissue in the area where CBF was increased (Johansson et al., 1974).

Hypertensive Encephalopathy

Hypertensive encephalopathy, one type of cerebrovascular disease, is the serious consequence of an inability of the cerebral vessels and BBB to cope with the strain of acute severe hypertension. It usually appears in relatively young adults who have developed an abrupt high blood pressure, as may occur with toxemia of pregnancy. There is often a tendency for misdiagnosis, but if acceptable criteria are employed, sudden blood pressure elevation produces characteristic clinical signs and symptoms, such as headache, nausea, vomiting, and seizures progressing to coma. Cerebral edema is the most ominous component of hypertensive encephalopathy, and its development may be related to a number of factors. BBB damage may occur even without a "breakthrough" of autoregulation in the brain (Johansson et al., 1974). A possible mechanism for the development of

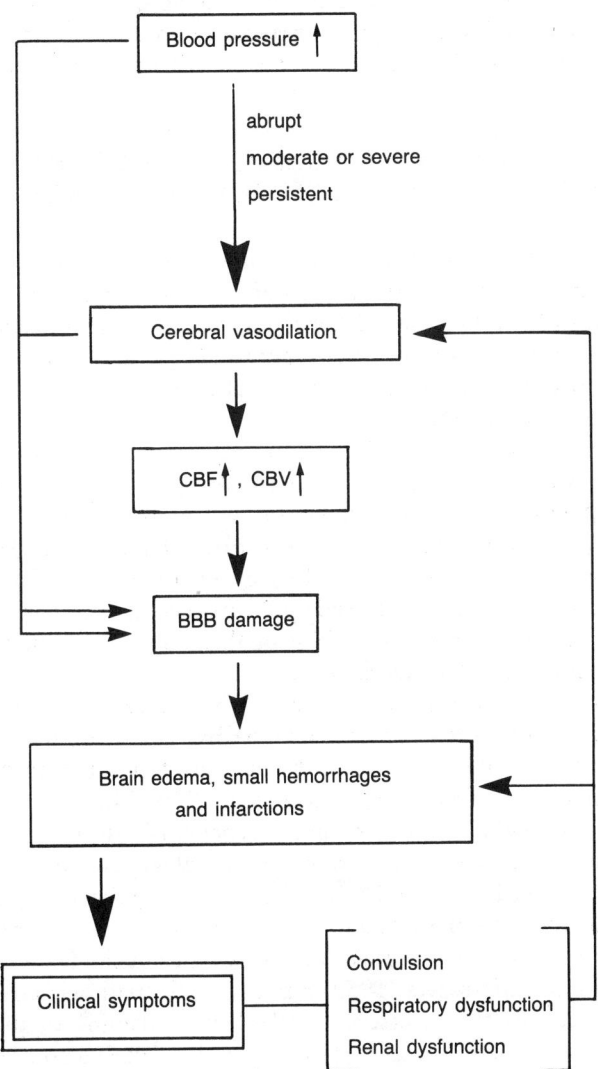

FIGURE 14.7 Possible mechanism of development of hypertensive encephalopathy (hypothesis).

hypertensive encephalopathy is shown in Figure 14.7. Probably sudden, moderate to severe, and persistent elevation of blood pressure induces cerebral vasodilatation with increased CBF and cerebral blood volume (CBV), which in turn produces BBB damage and brain edema. Clinical symptoms may be due mainly to brain edema and to small multiple hemorrhages and infarctions. Among the clinical symptoms, convulsion, respiratory and renal dysfunction, etc. aggravate brain edema and vasodilation, and a vicious circle of hypertensive encephalopathy is formed.

PATHOLOGICAL CHANGES OF CEREBRAL VESSELS AND STROKE IN PERSISTENT HYPERTENTION

It is generally believed that the most common and lethal cerebral complication of hypertension is cerebral hemorrhage. Hypertensive patients are, however, also subject to many other types of stroke. The concept "hypertensive encephalopathy" was described above, and this section will mainly be concerned with the pathological changes of cerebral vessels in patients with long-lasting hypertension.

It has been shown that a history of persistent hypertension is closely associated with stenotic lesions of the main cerebral arteries such as the carotid and vertebral arteries (Dickinson & Thomson, 1960; Evans, 1965). Actually, there is no doubt that arteriosclerotic changes of the vascular wall are greatly accelerated and intensified by hypertension. Such changes of cerebral vessels are generally considered to be related to cerebral infarctions, either through the reduction in CBF or through the production of small emboli from atherosclerotic plaques.

The abnormalities of the arterial wall, which have been variously named hyalinosis, angionecrosis, diffuse angiopathy, and hypertensive fibrinoid arteritis, are generally accepted as being almost peculiar to hypertensive patients (Scheinker, 1943; Feigin & Prose, 1959; Margolis, 1966). These changes in the cerebral vessels involve parenchymal arteries chiefly less than 2 to 8mm in diameter. Arteries within basal ganglia tend to be more frequently involved. It is also known that there are miliary aneurysms in the brain of patients with hypertensive cerebral hemorrhage. It is probable that these aneurysms are a late state of the process producing hyaline changes of cerebral arteries. Matsuoka (1952) interpreted the pathogenesis as follows: first angionecrosis of the arterial wall, then weakening of the wall, and subsequent true aneurysm formation. Margolis (1966) also noted that aneurysm formation was a prominent secondary feature in the focal arterial alteration. These changes seem to be related to the proximal cause of rupture and massive intracerebral hemorrhage, probably together with elevation of blood pressure.

It has long been known that small cysts in the white matter and deep gray matter of the hemispheres (basal ganglia, pons, thalamus, etc.) are observed in the autopsied brain of hypertensive patients (lacunar state). Most of these cysts have been considered to be the result of total occlusion of the small arteries supplying the affected area with resultant infarction (Fisher, 1965).

On the contrary, Cole and Yates (1968), after careful examination of a series of brains from normotensive and hypertensive subjects, made the following points: (1) large and small infarctions occur in the hypertensive group with only a slight preponderance over the normotensives; (2) large and small hemorrhages were mostly confined to the hypertensive population; and (3) in only three cases was a correlation of distinct ischemia and hemorrhagic lesions found. Therefore, this study suggested that the lacunar state of the brain in hypertensives was due to old minute hemorrhages only, casting doubt on the long-held hypothesis that the pathological processes underlying cerebral hemorrhage and infarction are related (Globus & Strauss, 1927). It also suggested the possibility that the progressive neurological deterioration in many hypertensive patients may be due to small hemorrhages (Ziegler, 1972).

Figure 14.8 shows a summary of pathological changes of cerebral vessels in persistent hypertension.

In patients with subarachnoid hemorrhage, it is known that rupture of the aneurysm is related to hypertension in about 60% of cases. Hypertension seems to influence not only the rupture but also the enlargement of these aneurysms.

Hypertension also produces several changes in cardiac function, including atrial fibrillation, which is one of the common sources of cerebral embolism.

Therefore, hypertension can be regarded as one of the main causes of almost all kinds of stroke.

HYPERTENSION AS A RISK FACTOR IN STROKE

Many investigations, including both prospective and retrospective epidemiological studies, have shown that hypertension is the most important contributor to stroke incidence compared with other factors such as atherosclerosis, heart disease, diabetes mellitus, cigarette smoking, taking oral contraceptives, etc. As different criteria were used for the determination of hypertension in the various studies, it is rather difficult to compare the various results. However, for example, the results of the People's Gas Light and Coke Company Study done on 1,329 men, 40 to 59 years old, who were healthy at the start of the study, showed over a 6-year observation period a five times higher death rate from cerebrovascular disease in the group with diastolic blood pressure values of 95 mmHg or more than in the group with values below 80 mmHg (Berkson & Stamler, 1965). A Build and Blood Pressure Study by the North American insurance companies (Society of Actuaries, 1959) also confirmed a marked increase in cerebrovascular accidents with rising blood pressure.

An epidemiological study in Georgia, USA, during an 87-month period

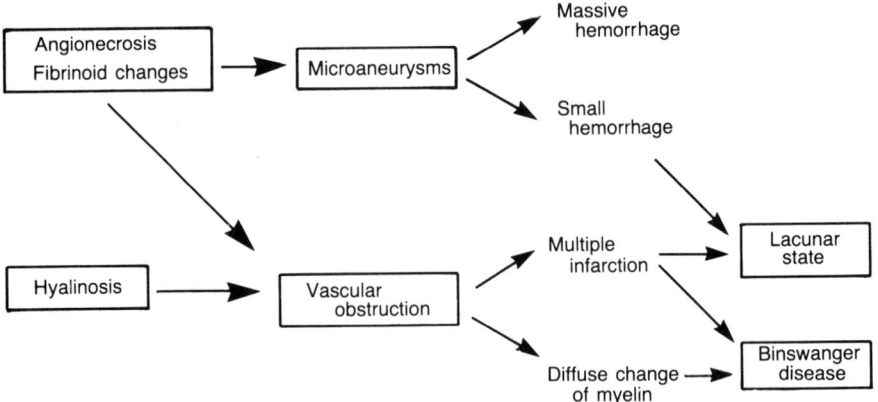

FIGURE 14.8 Pathologic changes of cerebral vessels in persistent hypertension.

revealed a clear relation between level of blood pressure and incidence of stroke (Heyman et al., 1971). A Canadian study in Manitoba (Rabkin et al., 1978a) showed that a stronger association with CVD was found for high systolic blood pressure than for diastolic blood pressure. This group (Rabkin et al., 1978b) also showed that after adjustment for age and systolic blood pressure, change in systolic blood pressure was significantly associated with subsequent cerebrovascular disease, primarily in men middle-aged or older. When considering systolic blood pressure after entry, changes from a measurement 5 years earlier were more important than systolic blood pressure changes over longer intervals. They concluded that in evaluating systolic blood pressure as a risk factor for stroke, the rate of change in systolic blood pressure is also an important factor.

In an extensive epidemiological study in Hisayama, Japan (Omae & Ueda, 1981), 1,621 people above 40 years of age were observed for 13 years, and 103 (23%) men died of stroke. The men who died of stroke included 0.9% of normotensives, 3.9% of borderline cases, and 11.3% of hypertensives (judged in the entry examination). According to this study, diastolic hypertension was more strongly related to the incidence of stroke. In the study in Hiroshima (Johnson et al., 1967), the age-adjusted morbidity ratios relative to the levels of systolic and diastolic blood pressure that preceded the development of stroke also demonstrate a marked increase in the risk of developing CVD in men and women who were hypertensive on entry into the study. Johnson et al. (1967) proposed that the level of diastolic blood pressure was a more useful indicator of increased risk for CVD than it proved to be for coronary heart disease in the same sample.

There are various results concerning hypertension as a risk factor of stroke, and it seems clear that hypertension (systolic, diastolic or both) must be considered an important risk factor in apopletic stroke.

The question next arises, what kind of stroke is associated with high blood pressure? As described before, it is generally believed that the most common and lethal of the cerebral complication of hypertension is cerebral hemorrhage, although the clinical differentiation of cerebral hemorrhage and occlusive CVD is often very difficult. In the Los Angeles study of male city employees, it was found that there was a 2% incidence of stroke among the normotensive population as compared to 9% among those with hypertension, the increased risk being more apparent in cerebral hemorrhage than in cerebral thrombosis (Chapman et al., 1966).

In the Framingham study, USA, it was reported that hypertension increased the probability of developing cerebral thrombosis about four- to fivefold over that of normotensive individuals (Kannel et al., 1965, 1970), and it was also shown that the relative risk of hemorrhagic stroke in hypertensive patients was no greater than that noted for the ischemic ones (Kannel et al., 1970). Therefore, hypertension appears to be the most common and potent precursor of cerebral hemorrhage and also cerebral infarction.

The occurrence of hypertension in stroke patients was also evaluated in retrospective epidemiological studies. During the years 1960 through 1967 in Israel (Lavy et al., 1973), 42% of 1,522 new stroke patients had hypertension. The frequency of hypertension among the stroke cases was higher in the 50-to-69 age group. The percentage of hypertensives was almost the same for the ischemic and hemorrhagic types of stroke. This study showed that hypertension plays an important role as a risk factor in the development of cerebral ischemia and hemorrhage alike. According to other investigators (Meyer et al., 1959; Gertler et al., 1968; Kurland, 1967; Prineas & Marshall, 1966; Baker & Katsuki, 1969; Louis & McDowell, 1970), 31 to 75% of stroke patients had hypertension. Therefore, hypertension seems to be one of the main characteristics of the stroke-prone individual.

It can be concluded from the above studies that there exists a very close and definite association between hypertension and hemorrhagic and ischemic CVD.

EFFECT OF HYPERTENSION ON CBF IN CVD PATIENTS

CBF in CVD Patients

It has been noted above that hypertension is related to the occurrence of CVD and also is frequently observed in patients with CVD. One might presume that the value of blood pressure is one of the important factors influencing CBF in CVD patients as well as in normal volunteers. However, our previous data (Shinohara et al., 1979, 1980) showed that the effects of age of the subjects, frequency of attacks, duration after onset, and the value of hematocrit on CBF are greater than that of blood pressure. Figure 14.9 shows the relationship between the mean hemispheric cortical blood flow value measured by means of the ^{133}Xe inhalation method and the blood pressure during CBF measurement in supratentorial occlusive CVD patients. In the acute stage (within 14 days after the onset of stroke), cortical blood flow values in both diseased and nondiseased hemispheres were rather low in patients with high blood pressure, as shown on the left side of Figure 14.9. However, in the subacute stage (from 15 to 28 days after onset) blood flow values were high in patients with hypertension. These relationships were statistically significant in both hemispheres (middle of Figure 14.9). In the chronic stage of stroke (more than 28 days after onset), the effects of hypertension on CBF became obscure. In the extreme acute stage of CVD, although a sudden change of blood pressure may influence CBF because of impaired autoregulation, under rather stable conditions of blood pressure (such as during the measurement of CBF) the size of cerebral damage, elevated intracranial pressure, increased cerebrovascular permeability, and other factors probably have a more important influence on CBF and the actual values of blood pressure may be less influential.

In the chronic stage, even if dysautoregulation of cerebral vessels still exists, resting blood pressure may have little effect on CBF value.

In contrast to the above result, as shown in Figure 14.10, a close relationship was observed between cortical blood flow value and blood pressure level in patients with brain stem infarction. These data indicate that the mechanism of autoregulation may be related to some part of the brain stem (Shinohara et al., 1978b), and also that the management of blood pressure is more important in patients with infratentorial cerebral infarction.

Autoregulation

As described above, brain damage can produce impairment of autoregulation in CBF. The extent of autoregulatory impairment in patients with cerebral infarction is illustrated in Figure 14.11, in which the vertical axis represents the "dysautoregulation index," i.e., changes in CBF divided by changes in perfusion pressure (effective MABP) during head-up tilting. As shown, the index is higher in patients with cerebral infarction than in controls, which means that autoregulation is more severely impaired in CVD patients. Figure 14.12 shows the relationship between dysautoregulation index and the duration after onset in patients with occlusive CVD. The number of cases is rather limited, but the figure indicates that improvement gradually occurs and the dysautoregulation index becomes normal 6 months after onset.

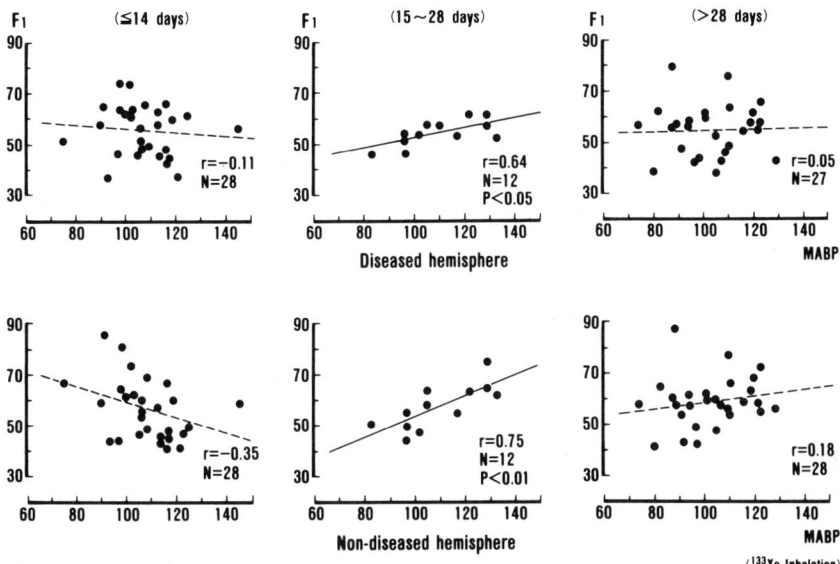

FIGURE 14.9 Relationships between mean cortical blood flow (F_1) measured by using the ^{133}Xe inhalation method and blood pressure in patients with supratentorial occlusive CVD. *Left:* Acute phase (within 14 days after onset). *Middle:* 15 to 28 days after onset. *Right:* More than 28 days after onset. *Upper:* Diseased hemisphere. *Lower:* Nondiseased hemisphere.

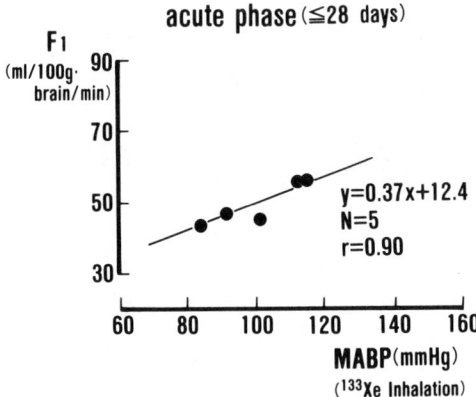

FIGURE 14.10 Relationship between mean cortical blood flow (F_1) and MABP in patients with brain stem infarction.

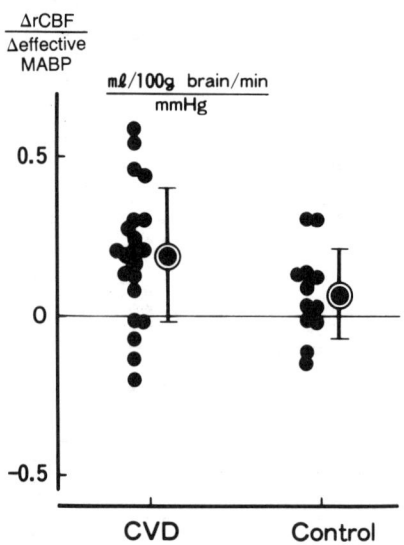

FIGURE 14.11 Dysautoregulation index in patients with cerebral infarction and controls.

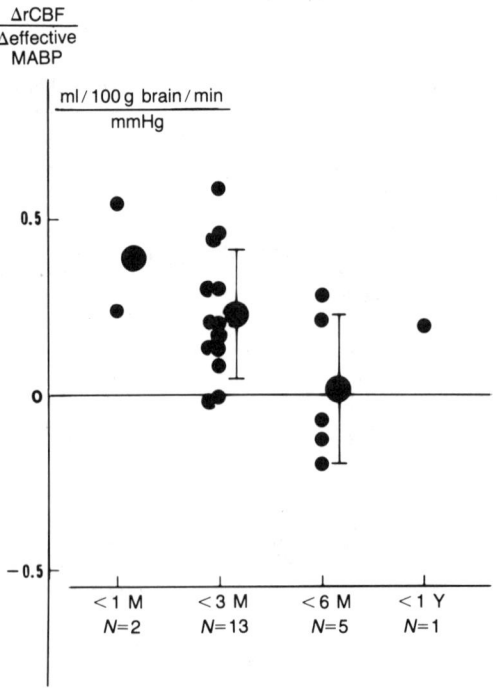

FIGURE 14.12 Dysautoregulation index (ΔCBF/Δeffective MABP) and duration after onset of cerebral infarction. M=month; Y=year.

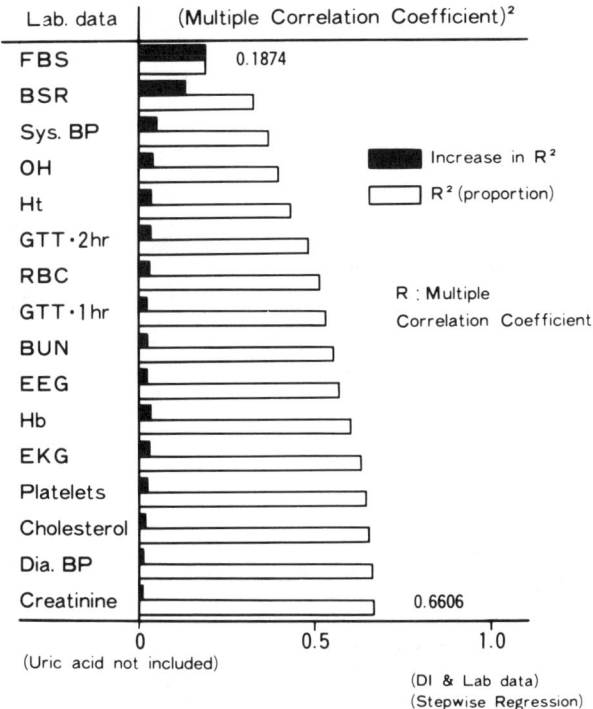

FIGURE 14.13 Multivariate analysis of factors influencing the cerebral dysautoregulation index in patients with cerebral infarction. R=multiple correlation coefficient.

The results of investigation of the factors influencing the degree of impairment of CBF autoregulation in patients with CVD, based on multivariate analysis, are summarized in Figure 14.13 (Shinohara et al., 1979). It can be seen that the effects of fasting blood sugar (FBS), blood sedimentation rate (BSR), systolic blood pressure, and orthostatic hypotension (OH) were greater than those of the other factors. The relationship was also examined between dysautoregulation and the single factor, hypertension; patients with hypertension showed more severe dysautoregulation than those without hypertension (Figure 14.14).

It is believed, therefore, that hypertension is at least one of the factors influencing cerebrovascular autoregulation in CVD patients. Even if MABP is maintained above 50 mmHg, patients with CVD may have a reduction in CBF and may complain of dizziness, fainting, and so on, with a decrease in blood pressure. These considerations are very important for an understanding of hypertension in patients with CVD and its treatment.

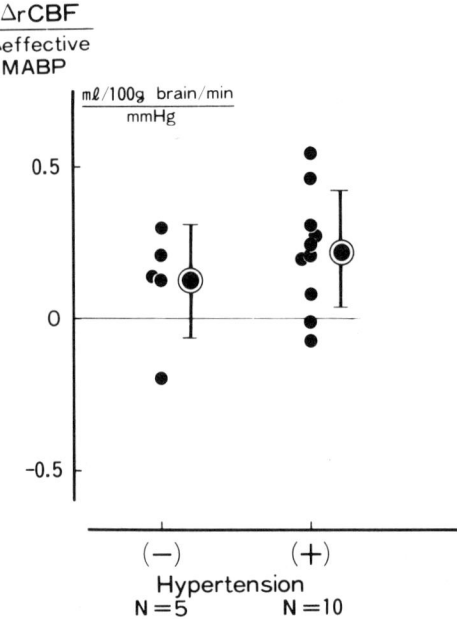

FIGURE 14.14 Effects of hypertension on autoregulation in patients with cerebral infarction. Hypertension: BP 150/95 or more.

TREATMENT OF HYPERTENSION

Treatment of Hypertension for Prevention of Stroke

Bearing the above considerations in mind, let us consider whether or not hypertension should be treated.

In animal studies using stroke-prone spontaneously hypertensive rats, it was proved that the control of hypertension by drug administration at an early age can reduce the occurrence of stroke (Yamori & Horie, 1975).

Colandrea et al. (1970) investigated the cardiovascular morbidity and mortality of systolic hypertension in the elderly over a period of about 48 months and concluded that isolated systolic hypertension was associated with an increased risk of cardiovascular complications. Many other reports (Waldek, 1977; Ikeda & Yokouchi, 1978; Veterans Administration Cooperative Study Group on Antihypertensive Agents, 1970) indicate that antihypertensive therapy may decrease the risk of cardiovascular complications and reduce subsequent mortality. In the investigation of the Veterans Administration Cooperative Study Group (1970), 380 male hypertensive patients were randomly assigned to either active antihypertensive agents or placebos for a 5-year period. Terminal morbid events occurred in 35 patients of the nontreated group as compared to 9 patients in the treated group. They concluded that treatment was more effective in preventing stroke and congestive heart failure than in preventing the complications of coronary artery disease.

Thus, no report has indicated that antihypertensive therapy had a deleterious effect on the prognosis or mortality in hypertensive patients. The only disadvantage is the transient side effects caused by medication. Therefore, hypertension should be detected early, treated adequately, and well controlled.

Treatment of Hypertension in CVD Patients

Full-scale discussion of the treatment of hypertension is beyond the scope of this chapter, but a brief note on the treatment of hypertension with cerebral dysfunction is in order.

Hypertensive Encephalopathy

The individual who becomes drowsy or semistuporous concomitant with an extreme rise in blood pressure (hypertensive encephalopathy) may represent an emergency. Hypotensive agents are recommended in such cases, the intention being to bring about a fairly abrupt fall in blood pressure, although care must be taken that this not be too extreme or too rapid, so that time is given for the arteriolar bed to dilate (Fazekas, 1966).

Acute Stage of Cerebral Hemorrhage or Infarction

It is usually considered that more than three-fourths of stroke patients have hypertension in the extreme acute stage. Usually this hypertension gradually improves with the course of illness. However, in cases with severe hypertension (e.g., more than 200 mmHg systolic pressure), it is probably necessary to control the blood pressure. Especially, in patients with cerebral hemorrhage or subarachnoid hemorrhage, hypotensive drugs are used to prevent enlargement of hematoma, rebleeding, and cerebral edema. The blood pressure level at which treatment is indicated is about 80% of the value of blood pressure in the extreme acute stage or around 180 mmHg systolic pressure.

In patients with occlusive CVD, hypertension is usually not treated in the acute stage unless the blood pressure is extremely high and labile or is tending to rise.

Chronic stage of stroke

A 4-year follow-up of occlusive CVD patients with hypertension revealed that a higher mortality rate (46%) and higher reoccurrence rate of stroke (44%) were observed in the untreated group than in the treated group (27%

and 20%, respectively) (Carter, 1970). It was also reported that the rate of reoccurrence of stroke within 2 years was much higher in patients with uncontrolled high diastolic blood pressure (e.g., more than 110 mmHg even after treatment) than in the well-controlled group (Beevers, 1973).

Therefore, the treatment of hypertension is necessary in patients in the chronic stage of CVD. As described already, cerebrovascular autoregulation may be impaired up to 6 months after a stroke, so a gradual and mild reduction in blood pressure is essential. The goal for the level of blood pressure is about 160 mmHg systolic pressure and less than 100 mmHg diastolic pressure. Clinical symptoms suggestive of blood flow disturbance, such as dizziness, fainting, angina pectoris, heart failure, and intermittent claudication should be checked frequently during the treatment. Particular attention must also be paid to orthostatic hypotension as a side effect of treatment. For these purposes, calcium antagonists, beta-adrenergic receptor blockers, and thiazide diuretics plus dihydroergotonine mesylate may be used for treatment.

REFERENCES

Baker, A. B., & Katsuki, S. (1969). Strokes: U.S. and Japan: A study of a Caucasian and oriental population. *Geriatrics, 24,* 83.

Beevers, D. G., Fairman, M. J., Hamilton, M. et al. (1973). Antihypertensive treatment and the course of established cerebral vascular disease. *Lancet, 1,* 1407.

Berkson, D. M. & Stamler, J. (1965). Epidemiological findings on cerebrovascular diseases and their implications. *J. Atheroscler. Res, 5,* 189.

Busija, D. W., Heistad, D. O., & Marcus, M. L. (1980). Effects of sympathetic nerves on cerebral vessels during acute moderate increases in arterial pressure in dogs and cats. *Circ. Res., 46,* 696.

Carter, A. B. (1970). Hypotensive therapy in stroke survivors. *Lancet, 1,* 485.

Chapman, J. M., Reeder, L. G., Borun, E. R., et al. (1966). Epidemiology of vascular lesions affecting the central nervous system: The occurrence of strokes in a sample population under observation for cardiovascular disease. *Am. J. Public Health, 56,* 191.

Colandrea, M. A., Friedman, G. D., Nichaman, M. Z., et al. (1970). Systolic hypertension in the elderly. An epidemiologic assessment. *Circulation, 41,* 239.

Cole, F. M., & Yates, P. O. (1968). Comparative incidence of cerebrovascular lesions in normotensive and hypertensive patients. *Neurology (Minneap.), 18,* 255.

Dickinson, C. J., & Thomson, A. D. (1960). A post mortem study of the main cerebral arteries with special reference to their possible role in blood pressure regulation. *Clin. Sci., 19,* 513.

Ekström-Jodal, Häggendal, E., Linder, L. E., et al. (1971/72). Cerebral blood flow autoregulation at high arterial pressure and different levels of carbon dioxide tension. *Eur. Neurol., 6,* 6.

Evans, P. H. (1965). Relation of longstanding blood-pressure levels to atherosclerosis. *Lancet, 1,* 516.

Fazekas, J. F. (1966). Cerebrovascular consequences of hypertension. Therapeutic implications. *Am. J. Cardiol., 17*, 608.

Feigin, I., & Prose, P. (1959). Hypertensive fibrinoid arteritis of the brain and gross cerebral hemorrhage. A form of "hyalinosis." *Arch. Neurol., 1*, 98.

Finnerty, F. A. Jr., Witkin, L., & Fazekas, F. F. (1954). Cerebral hemodynamic during cerebral ischemia induced by acute hypotension. *J. Clin. Invest., 33*, 1227.

Fisher, C. M. (1965). Lacunes: small, deep cerebral infarcts. *Neurology (Minneap.), 15*, 774.

Fog, M. (1937). Cerebral circulation. The reaction of the pial arteries to fall in blood pressure. *Arch. Neurol. Psychiatr., 37*, 351.

Gertler, M. M., Rusk, H. A., Whiter, H. H., et al. (1968). Ischemic cerebrovascular disease: The assessment of risk factors. *Geriatrics, 23*, 135.

Giese, J. (1964). Acute hypertensive vascular disease. II Studies on vascular reaction patterns and permeability changes by means of vital microscopy and colloidal tracer techniques. *Acta Pathol. Microbiol. Scand., 62*, 497.

Globus, J. H., & Strauss, I. (1927). Massive cerebral hemorrhage. Its relation to preexisting cerebral softening. *Arch. Neurol. Psychiatr., 18*, 215.

Gotoh, F., Ebihara, S., Tovoda, M., et al. (1971/72). Role of autonomic nervous system in autoregulation of human cerebral circulation. *Eur. Neurol., 6*, 203.

Heyman, A., Karp, H. R., Heyden, S., et al. (1971). Cerebrovascular disease in the biracial population of Evans County, Georgia. *Arch. Int. Med., 128*, 949.

Ikeda, M., & Yokouchi, M. (1978). Role of blood pressure in cerebrovascular disease in the aged. Abstract from the XIth International Congress of Gerontology, Tokyo (p. 37).

Johnson, K. G., Yamo, K., & Kato, H. (1967). Cerebral vascular disease in Hiroshima, Japan. *J. Chron. Dis., 20*, 545.

James, I. M., Millar, R. A., & Purves, M. J. (1969). Observations on the extrinsic neural control of cerebral blood flow in the baboon. *Circ. Res., 25*, 77.

Johansson, B., Strandgaard, S., & Lassen, N. A. (1974). On the pathogenesis of hypertensive encephalopathy. The hypertensive "breakthrough" of autoregulation of cerebral blood flow with forced vasodilation, flow increase, and blood-brain-barrier damage. *Circ. Res., 34*, 35 (Suppl 1), 167.

Jones, J. V., Fitch, W., MacKenzie, E. T., et al. (1976). Lower limit of cerebral blood flow autoregulation in experimental renovascular hypertension in the baboon. *Circ. Res., 39*, 555.

Kannel, W. B., Dawber, T. R., McNamara, P. M., et al. (1965). Vascular disease of the brain-epidemiologic aspects: The Framingham study. *Am. J. Public Health, 55*, 1355.

Kannel, W. B., Wolf, P. A., Verter, J., et al. (1970). Epidemiologic assessment of the role of blood pressure in stroke. The Framingham study. *JAMA, 214*, 301.

Kety, S. S., King, B. D., Horvath, S. M., et al. (1950). The effects of an acute reduction in blood pressure by means of differential spinal sympathetic block on the cerebral circulation of hypertensive patients. *J. Clin. Invest., 29*, 402.

Kurland, L. T., Choi, N. W., & Sayre, G. P. (1967). Current status of the epidemiology of cerebrovascular disease in stroke rehabilitation. In W. S. Fields & W. A. Spencer (Eds.), *Stroke rehabilitation: Basic concepts and research trends* (p. 3). St. Louis: WH Green.

Lassen, N. A. (1959). Cerebral blood flow and oxygen consumption in man. *Physiol. Rev., 39*, 183.

Lassen, N. A. (1964). Autoregulation of cerebral blood flow. *Circ. Res., 15* (Suppl 1), 201.

Lassen, N. A., & Agnoli, A. (1973). The upper limit of autoregulation of cerebral blood flow—on the pathogenesis of acute hypertensive encephalopathy. *Scand. J. Clin. Lab. Invest., 30,* 113.

Lavy, S., Melamed, E., Cahane, E., et al. (1973). Hypertension and diabetes as risk factors in stroke patients. *Stroke, 4,* 751.

Louis, S., & McDowell, F. (1970). Age: Its significance in nonembolic cerebral infarction. *Stroke, 1,* 449.

MacKenzie, E. T., Strandgaard, S., Graham, D. I., et al. (1976). Effects of acutely induced hypertension in cats on pial arteriolar caliber, local cerebral blood flow, and the blood-brain barrier. *Circ. Res., 39,* 33.

Margolis, G. (1966). The vascular changes and pathogenesis of hypertensive intracerebral hemorrhage. *Proc. Assoc. Res. Nerv. Ment. Dis., 41,* 73.

Matsuoka, S. (1952). Histopathological studies on the blood vessels in apoplexia cerebri. *Proc. 1st Int. Congr. Neuropath., 3,* 222.

McDowell, F., Potes, J., & Groch, S. (1961). The natural history of internal carotid and vertebral-basilar artery occlusion. *Neurology (Minneap), 11,* 153.

Meyer, J. S., Waltz, A. G., Hess, J. W., et al. (1959). Serum lipids and cholesterol levels in cerebrovascular disease. *Arch. Neurol., 1,* 303.

Monro, A. (1783). *Observations on the structure and functions of the nervous system.* Edinburgh: W. Creech.

Omae, T., & Ueda, K. (1981, September 20–25). Risk factors of cerebral stroke in Japan. 12th World Congress of Neurology. Kyoto, Japan.

Prineas, J., & Marshall, J. (1966). Hypertension and cerebral infarction. *Br. Med. J., 1,* 14.

Rabkin, S. W., Mathewson, F. A. L., & Tate, R. B. (1978a). Predicting risk of ischemic heart disease and cerebrovascular disease from systolic and diastolic blood pressures. *Ann. Int. Med., 88,* 342.

Rabkin, S. W., Mathewson, F. A. L., & Tate, R. B. (1978b). Long term changes in blood pressure and risk of cerebrovascular disease. *Stroke, 9,* 319.

Sheinker, I. M. (1943). Hypertensive disease of the brain. *Arch. Path., 36,* 289.

Shenkin, H. A., Hafkenshiel, J. H., & Kety, S. S. (1950). Effects of sympathectomy on the cerebral circulation of hypertensive patients. *Arch. Surg., 61,* 319.

Shinohara, Y. (1983). Cerebral vascular insufficiency. *Tokai. J. Exp. Clin. Med., 8,* 1.

Shinohara, Y., & Gotoh, F. (1975). Autoregulation of cerebral circulation in orthostatic hypotension. In T. W. Langfitt, L. C. McHenry, Jr., M. Revich, & H. Wollman (Eds.), *Cerebral circulation and metabolism,* New York: Springer-Verlag.

Shinohara, Y., Gotoh, F., & Takagi, S. (1978a). Cerebral hemodynamics in Shy-Drager syndrome. Variability of cerebral blood flow dysautoregulation and the compensatory role of chemical control in dysautoregulation. *Stroke, 9,* 504.

Shinohara, Y., Takagi, S., & Gotoh, F. (1978b). Factors influencing CBF and autoregulation in CVD patients. Effects of age, duration after onset and localization of lesion. *Jpn. J. Int. Med., 67,* 845.

Shinohara, Y., Takagi, S., & Kobatake, K. (1979). Multivariate analysis of factors influencing CBF and autoregulation in CVD. *Acta Neurol. Scand., 60* (Suppl. 72), 422.

Shinohara, Y., Takagi, S., & Kobatake, K. (1980). Factors influencing CBF in normal subjects and in patients with CVD. In J. S. Meyer et al. (Eds.), *Cerebral vascular disease,* Vol. 3 (International Congress Series, No. 532) (p. 152). Amsterdam: Excerpta Medica.

Society of Actuaries. (1959). *Build and blood pressure study,* Vol. 1. Chicago.

Strandgaard, S. (1976). Autoregulation of cerebral blood flow in hypertensive patients. The modifying influence of prolonged antihypertensive treatment on the tolerance to acute, drug-induced hypotension. *Circulation, 53,* 720.

Strandgaard, S., Jones, J. V., MacKenzie, E. T., et al. (1975). Upper limit of cerebral blood flow autoregulation in experimental renovascular hypertension in the baboon. *Circ. Res., 37,* 164.

Strandgaard, S., Jones, J. V., Sengupta, D., et al. (1974). Upper limit of autoregulation of cerebral blood flow in the baboon. *Circ. Res., 34,* 435.

Strandgaard, S., Olesen, J., Skinhoj, E., et al. (1973). Autoregulation of brain circulation in severe arterial hypertension. *Br. Med. J., 1,* 507.

Veterans Administration Cooperative Study Group on Antihypertensive Agents. (1970). Effects of treatment on morbidity in hypertension. II Results in patients with diastolic blood pressure averaging 90 through 114 mm Hg. *JAMA, 213,* 1143.

Waldek, S. (1977). Hypertension in the elderly. *Lancet, 1,* 1055.

Yamori, Y., & Horie, R. (1975). Experimental studies on the pathogenesis and prophylaxis of stroke-prone spontaneously hypertensive rats (SHR)—(2) Prohylactic effect of moderate control of blood pressure on stroke. *Jpn. Circ. J., 93,* 616.

Ziegler, D. K. (1972). Hypertensive vascular disease of the brain. In P. T. Vinken & C. W. Bruyn (Eds.), *Handbook of clinical neurology,* Vol. 11. Amsterdam: North-Holland.

15
Senile Dementia of the Alzheimer's Type

Barry Reisberg, Steven H. Ferris, Mony J. deLeon, Thomas Crook, and Nathaniel Haynes

Interest in senile dementia of the Alzheimer's type (SDAT) has been increasing exponentially among both laymen and clinicians over the course of the past several years. With respect to the former, a recent zenith was reached in the United States when Alzheimer's disease was front page news in the New York Times on two separate occasions within a 30-day period (Altman, 1984a, 1984b). With respect to the latter, a plethora of recent texts devoted specifically to Alzheimer's disease (Reisberg, 1981; Mace & Rabins, 1981; Corkin et al., 1982; Reisberg, London, et al., 1983) or to senile dementia and Alzheimer's disease (Katzman et al., 1978; Miller & Cohen, 1981; Shamoian, 1984; Wertheimer & Marois, 1984), are testimony to growing interest. Fortunately, clinical knowledge of this disease has increased proportionately to the remarkable increase in our society's awareness of the dimensions of the problem. In this chapter, we shall provide a brief historical background as to how this condition came to be neglected and recently, "rediscovered" among laymen and clinicians. This will be followed by a discussion of present knowledge with respect to diagnosis, prognosis, patient management, and caregiver management. Finally, we shall conclude with a discussion of the most promising directions with respect to future research.

PUBLIC AWARENESS OF SENILE DEMENTIA OF THE ALZHEIMER'S TYPE: HISTORICAL BACKGROUND

Alzheimer's disease is, of course, a mental disorder associated with old age. As such, it incorporates a dual stigma which may help to explain its apparently complete neglect among laymen until recently. It is a mental disorder, and disorders of the mind have always carried a special stigma in our society. It is also a geriatric disorder, and diseases associated with aging have traditionally been less well recognized in our society than diseases occurring in younger populations. It is only by invoking this dual stigma that a present-day reader can begin to understand why there exists, even today, no word among the hundreds of thousands of entries in the current unabridged dictionary of the English language which differentiates the progressive memory loss so commonly observed in aged persons from aging of other bodily organ systems. Webster's unabridged dictionary defines "senility" as: "1. the condition or quality of being senile; old age. 2. the characteristics of old age; weakness; infirmity of mind and body." (Webster's Dictionary, 1977a). It defines "senile" in much the same fashion, specifically as: "1. of old age. 2. showing signs of old age; elderly; weak in mind and body. 3. resulting from old age. 4. in physical geography, nearing the end of an erosion cycle" (Webster's Dictionary, 1977a).

Dementia is defined as "impairment or loss of mental powers," and only dementia praecox, "usually beginning in late adolescence," is listed as an example of a dementing disorder (Webster's Dictionary, 1977b). Alzheimer and Alzheimer's disease are nowhere mentioned in the current standard unabridged dictionary of American English. Perhaps the lay term most closely approaching what we would presently term Alzheimer's disease or senile dementia of the Alzheimer's type is "dotage", defined as, "1. feebleness or senility; childishness of old age; as, a venerable man, now in his dotage. 2. a doting, foolish or excessive fondness" (Webster's Dictionary, 1977c). Even "childishness of old age" does not, of course, distinguish in the lay mind dementia of the Alzheimer's type from the numerous other psychiatric and neurologic age-associated disorders, of which we need only mention involutional psychosis and emotional disorders associated with stroke as examples.

Hence, until very recently, there was no lay word that distinguished the dementia, with progressive loss of intellectual capacities, so commonly and tragically afflicting particularly elderly individuals from other age-related physical or mental disorders. The absence of a word for this condition naturally assisted society in ignoring the tragic dimensions of this illness. It was suffered in silence, and was not a subject for public discourse.

The very recent medical reawakening to the importance of this illness has resulted in a corresponding increase in lay understanding and awareness. The harbinger of this increased awareness appears to have been the formation of Alzheimer's disease support groups in various North American cities in the late 1970s. In 1978, perhaps the first national Alzheimer's disease society was formed in Canada. This was followed by the formation of the Alzheimer's Disease and Related Disorders Association in the United States, which held its first annual meeting in 1981. Growth in worldwide awareness of the illness since 1981 has been spectacular. Prior to 1981, there were no books that explained the true nature of this illness process to the lay public. Such books as existed (Freese, 1978; Galton, 1979) generally gainsayed the existence of the illness entirely. Dr. Freese's book is subtitled "A Factual Break-Through Guide to the Prevention and Cure of Senility—The Book that Makes Old Age Obsolete." Daily press recognition and treatment of the existence of the illness paralleled entirely that of the publishers. Hence, a major New York Times article on the subject in 1978 was entitled "Exposing the Myth of Senility" (Henig, 1978).

Given this history, it is understandable that the first books for the general public explaining the true nature of dementia of the Alzheimer's type, which appeared in 1981, had somewhat disguised titles (Reisberg, 1981; Mace & Rabins, 1981). The general public did not really begin to learn about the existence of the disease until 1982 (Meyer, 1982; Brozan, 1982a, 1982b). By 1983, recognition of the disease among the lay public had become general. In January of 1983, Marion Roach published a widely read and widely disseminated article in the *New York Times Magazine* describing her experience with her mother, an Alzheimer's victim (Roach, 1983). Political awareness of the importance of the illness began to increase to the extent that in March, 1983 the new Secretary of the United States Department of Health and Human Services, Margaret M. Heckler devoted her first press conference to the disorder. By the end of the year, President Reagan had announced the declaration of the first national Alzheimer's Disease Awareness Month. By 1984, national Alzheimer's societies existed in many European countries and the World Health Organization was paying increasing attention to the disorder (WHO Technical Report Series, 1986), now recognized universally as a major cause of death and suffering for mankind.

MEDICAL AWARENESS OF SENILE DEMENTIA OF THE ALZHEIMER'S TYPE: HISTORICAL BACKGROUND

Apparently the first physician to have recognized what has now come to be known as Alzheimer's disease was Aretaeus of Cappadocia in the second century A.D.. He distinguished an entity, "dotage," which began in old age, continued until death, and was characterized by "a torpor of the senses, and a stupefaction of the gnostic and intellectual faculties" (Adams, 1861). Galen, a contemporary of Aretaeus, distinguished the condition in much the same way (Galen, 1821–1833). Rush, in 1793, may have been the first to expand upon these brief definitions. He noted that, "I met with an instance of a woman between 80 and 90 who exhibited the marks of a second infancy, by such a total decay of her mental faculties as to lose all consciousness in discharging her alvine and urinary excretions. In this state of the body, a disposition to sleep succeeds the wakefulness of the first stages of old age" (Rush, 1793).

Prichard in 1837 described an entity which he termed "senile incoherence." He divided this entity into four successive stages: (1) impaired memory, (2) loss of reasoning power, (3) incomprehension, and (4) loss of instinctive action (Prichard, 1837). Although Folstein and coworkers (Folstein & Powell, 1984; Breitner & Folstein, 1984) have recently called attention to these descriptions, which they believe have merit, other subsequent investigators and observers have for the most part not maintained Prichard's nosology.

Esquirol's descriptions, published the year after Prichard's, have achieved greater permanence (Esquirol, 1838). Most present day observers would concur with his description of "demence senile" as an illness in which there occurs a weakening of the memory for recent experience and a loss of drive and will power. Clearly, Esquirol's observations that this condition appears gradually and may be accompanied by emotional disturbances were also accurate.

The neuropathologic triad of the disease entity which Kraeplin called "Alzheimer's disease" in honor of his pupil (Young, 1936) had been described by the early part of this century. Specifically, senile plaques were probably first described by Emile Redlich in 1892 (Redlich, 1898), neurofibrillary tangles by Alois Alzheimer in 1907 (Alzheimer, 1907), and granulovacuolar degeneration by Simchowitz in 1910 (Simchowicz, 1910). Binswanger had described an entity called "presenile dementia" in 1898 (Lipowski, 1980), and Alzheimer associated the clinicopathologic entity that we would today term "senile dementia of the Alzheimer's type" or, simply, "Alzheimer's disease" with this "presenile" state. Alzheimer believed that senile dementia was related to vascular arteriosclerotic factors. This view was challenged repeatedly over the next half-century, notably by the work of Simchowitz (1910), Grunthal (1927), Gellerstadt (1932), Margolis (1959), and Hirano and Zimmerman (1962). However, it was the work of Corsellis and Evans, replicated by Worm-Peterson and Pakkenberg, which overturned the arteriosclerotic theories of the origin of the most prevalent forms of senile dementia (Corsellis & Evans, 1965; Worm-Peterson & Pakkenberg, 1968), and the work of Corsellis (1962), and Tomlinson et al. (1968, 1970), Blessed et al. (1968), and Roth et al. (1966), which firmly established the current conceptualizations. These are that SDAT is a clinicopathologic entity, the pathologic component of which is notably associated with senile plaques, neurofibrillary tangles, and, as we now know from independent investigations, granulovacuolar degeneration (Woodard, 1962; Tomlinson & Kitchener, 1972; Ball & Lo, 1977).

Medical knowledge of the clinical concomitants of, SDAT has in many ways paralleled lay discovery of the illness. Beyond the brief description of

Esquirol, little was known before 1980. In 1980 and 1981 knowledge increased, apparently resulting in an explosion of knowledge between 1982 and 1984. The American Psychiatric Association's 1980 definition summarized knowledge until that time. It defined a new entity, primary degenerative dementia (which is synonymous with senile dementia of the Alzheimer's type) as follows:

> The essential feature is the presence of Dementia of insidious onset and gradual progressive course for which all other specific causes have been excluded by the history, physical examination, and laboratory tests. The Dementia involves a multifaceted loss of intellectual abilities, such as memory, judgement, abstract thought, and other higher cortical functions, and changes in personality and behavior.
>
> The onset is insidious, and the course is one of uniform, gradual progression. In the early stages memory impairment may be the only apparent cognitive deficit. There may also be subtle personality changes, such as the development of apathy, lack of spontaneity, and a quiet withdrawal from social interactions. Individuals usually remain neat and well-groomed and, aside from an occasional irritable outburst, are cooperative and behave in a socially appropriate way. With progression to the middle stage of the disease various cognitive disturbances become quite apparent, and behavior and personality are more obviously affected. By the late stage, the individual may be completely mute and inattentive. At this point he or she is totally incapable of caring for himself or herself. This stage leads inevitably to death. With senile onset, the average duration of symptoms, from onset to death, is about five years. (APA, 1980)

In 1981, the three stages or phases of the illness were described in greater detail and detailed case histories of the three phases were published (Reisberg, 1981). The following year more detailed descriptions of the evolution of the illness, incorporating seven stages from "healthy" or normal to severe dementia, were published (Reisberg et al., 1982). Implicit and explicit in these clinical staging instruments was a hierarchy of deficit in various cognitive and functional parameters. Publications in 1983 made these hierarchies more specific. Cole et al. published a hierarchic dementia scale with proposed hierarchies in cognitive, neurological, praxis, and other areas thought to apply to the dementia patient (Cole et al., 1983). Reisberg, London, et al., (1983; Reisberg, Schneck, et al., 1983) published concordant, seven-stage ordinal (hierarchic) deficits in concentration, recent memory, past memory, orientation, functioning and self-care, language, motoric functioning, and mood. Each of these seven-stage deficits was designed to correspond most closely to the previously published global description (Reisberg et al., 1982) of the progression of dementia of the Alzheimer's type.

Hence, by 1983, clinicians in disparate settings were independently concluding that Alzheimer's disease was probably a unique clinical as well as a unique neuropathological entity (Reisberg, 1983a). The word "unique," as opposed to "characteristic," is apposite. Dementia of Alzheimer's type had a characteristic onset and course, with a characteristic progression in terms of recent memory deficit, past memory deficit, orientation deficit, motoric deficit, mood changes, etc. Various investigators were concluding that the combination of those features in the absence of other features (Down's syndrome, choreiform movements, strokes, etc.) was probably unique. Analogously, neurofibillary tangles occurred in Alzheimer's disease as well as in some other illness entities (e.g. dementia pugilistica, Parkinsonian dementia), and senile plaques occurred in Alzheimer's disease as well as some other illness entities (e.g. kuru, Creutzfeldt-Jakob disease). However, the distribution, concentration, and broad nature of the pathology in Alzheimer's disease, in the absence of other pathologic features, was beginning to be seen as a unique process.

Consequently, by 1983, just at the time that lay recognition of the existence and importance of Alzheimer's disease was becoming general, clinicians were for the first time familiarizing themselves with the clinical features of this acknowledgedly common entity. The stage was set for continuing advances in 1984. The following section will focus on these most recent and perhaps most important advances.

SDAT: SELECT RECENT ADVANCES IN DIAGNOSIS AND STAGING

Function of Assessment Staging

The development of instruments such as the Global Deterioration Scale for Primary Degenerative Dementia (Reisberg et al., 1982) enabled clinicians in the course of a detailed clinical interview to (1) more accurately determine whether the patient's presentation was characteristic of one of the stages of normal aging or Alzheimer's disease, and, if so, (2) to stage the magnitude of severity of the illness. Subsequent work elucidated the prognostic concomitants of these stages, enabling clinicians to provide patients with accurate information as to whether their memory loss was consistent with normal aging, was a borderline condition, or, if consistent with the early stages of senile dementia of the Alzheimer's type, what the prognosis for persons at that stage was likely to be (Reisberg, Ferris, de Leon, et al., 1985; Reisberg, Ferris, Schulman, et al., 1986). Additional work elucidated the management needs of the patient at each stage, as well as the management needs of their caregivers (Reisberg, 1984).

The multiaxial concordant clinical assessments on the Brief Cognitive Rating Scale (BCRS) enabled clinicians to assess in a detailed and iterative manner the magnitude of change, if any, of patients on clinical parameters, in the course of pharmacologic treatment trials or other therapeutic interventions (Reisberg, 1983b). It was hoped that these multiaxial assessments would also help in the differential diagnosis of Alzheimer's disease. However, although it was indeed demonstrated that Alzheimer's patients tended to present with relatively concordant ordinal magnitude of deficit across each of the axes, the degree of concordance was not shown to be sufficient to readily enable clinicians to differentiate dementia of the Alzheimer's type from, for example, dementia associated with alcohol abuse. For other disorders such as the pseudodementia of geriatric depression, BCRS axis concordance may have been more useful; however it was clear that more expeditious and rapid clinical staging and diagnostic instruments were necessary.

Such an instrument has recently been developed. It is known as Functional Assessment Staging (FAST) for Alzheimer's disease (Reisberg, Ferris, Anand, de Leon, et al.). The FAST assessment instrument (Table 15.1) enables clinicians to accomplish the following heretofore difficult or impossible tasks in the assessment of the aged patient with cognitive impairment:

1. Rapidly determine whether or not the nature of the dementing process is consistent with uncomplicated senile dementia of the Alzheimer's type, both in terms of its present manifestation, as well as in terms of the evolution of the illness process.
2. Stage, in a relatively detailed fashion, even the most severe patients with dementia of the Alzheimer's type.
3. Differentiate various complications of Alzheimer's disease from the natural progression of the illness.
4. Accomplish all of the above with sufficient facility such that preliminary determinations as to diagnosis, differential diagnosis, and complicating factors can be made on the basis of information provided by family members, in many cases even over the telephone, prior to the actual examination of the patient.

These advances are possible for several reasons, notably:

1. Alzheimer's disease is a consistent and pervasive dementing process, the progression of which invariably has a definable consistency.
2. Dementing processes associated with other etiologies proceed differently.
3. Many functional activities in all twentieth century societies are universal, and hence it is possible to describe functional decrements in universal terms.

TABLE 15.1 FAST (Functional Assessment Stages) In Normal Aging and Alzheimer's Disease (AD)

Global deterioration scale stage	Clinical diagnosis	FAST characteristics
1. No cognitive decline	Normal	No functional decrement either subjectively or objectively manifest
2. Very mild cognitive decline	Normal for Age	Complains of forgetting location of objects; subjective word finding difficulties
3. Mild cognitive decline	Borderline impairment	Decreased functioning in demanding employment settings evident to co-workers; difficulty in travelling to new locations
4. Moderate cognitive decline	Mild AD	Decreased ability to perform complex tasks such as planning dinner for guests, handling finances, and marketing.
5. Moderately severe cognitive decline	Moderate AD	Requires assistance in choosing clothing; may require coaxing to bathe properly.
6. Severe cognitive decline	Moderately severe AD	(a) Difficulty in putting on clothing properly (b) Requires assistance bathing; may develop fear of bathing (c) Decreased ability to handle mechanics of toileting (d) Urinary incontinence (e) Fecal incontinence
7. Very severe cognitive decline	Severe AD	(a) Ability to speak limited to less than six words (b) Intelligible vocabulary limited at most to a single word (c) Ambulatory ability lost (d) Ability to sit up lost (e) Ability to smile lost (f) Ability to hold up head lost

The functional assessment stages of normal aging and dementia of the Alzheimer's type have been enumerated in such a way as to be optimally concordant with the corresponding Global Deterioration Scale (GDS) stages. These FAST stages are described below. The approximate prognostic concomitants of these stages are also described below.

FAST Stage 1: No subjective or objective functional decrement.

The aged subject's ostensible and subjective functional abilities in occupational, social, and other settings remain intact in comparison with their performance five to ten years previously.

Diagnosis: Normal cognitive functioning.

Prognosis: Excellent for continued adequate cognitive functioning.

FAST Stage 2: Subjective functional decrement. No objective evidence of decreased performance in complex occupational or social activities.

The most common age-related functional complaints are the forgetting of names and locations of objects, and decreased ability to recall appointments. These subjective decrements are generally not noted by intimates or co-workers. Complex occupational and social functioning is not compromised by the subjectively observed decrements.

Diagnosis: Cognitive functioning compatible with normal aging.

Prognosis: Excellent for continued adequate cognitive functioning.

Commentary: These subjective symptoms are very common in elderly individuals. They may also be troubling and may lead the individual to consult with a physician. The symptoms may be associated with primary affective disorder or primary anxiety, and symptoms of these conditions should be carefully looked for. In many cases no condition other than normal aging is found.

FAST Stage 3: Objective functional decrement of sufficient severity as to interfere with complex occupational and social tasks.

This is the stage at which an individual may begin to forget important appointments for the first time in their lives. Similarly, a professional who may have been able to write hundreds of articles or reports over the course of his or her adult years for the first time now finds him or herself unable to finish a single report. Functional decrement may also become manifest in complex psychomotor tasks, such as ability to travel to novel locations.

Individuals at this stage have no difficulty with routine tasks, such as marketing, handling their finances, or travelling to familiar locations. They may retire from demanding occupational and social settings, whereupon their deficits may no longer be manifest.

Diagnosis: Cognitive functioning compatible with borderline functioning secondary to a variety of possible conditions including incipient Alzheimer's disease.

Prognosis: The three- to four-year prognosis appears to be benign with respect to further cognitive deterioration in more than 80% of cases.

Commentary: Although clinically these symptoms may appear subtle, they can be of sufficient magnitude as to considerably alter a patient's lifestyle. They can be sufficiently alarming as to result in an emergency visit to a physician or clinic.

FAST Stage 4: Deficient performance in the complex tasks of daily life.

At this stage individuals have difficulty returning with the correct items and proper amounts of foodstuffs and similar material when marketing. Unless supervised, they have difficulty balancing their checkbooks and may make significant financial errors. Functioning in other complex areas is also compromised. One patient at this stage scheduled a dinner party and instructed half the guests to arrive on a particular day and other guests to arrive on the following day. Another patient at this stage ostensibly continued to function as an attorney, in partnership with her husband. Although she was able to independently travel to and from her office on a daily basis, she could not recall when queried the names or details of any of the "cases" she supposedly was continuing to work on. In actuality, her husband had taken on her work.

Patients at this stage can still function independently in the community, since they can dress, bathe, choose their own clothing, travel to familiar locations, etc. However, independent community functioning is compromised. One woman at this stage lived alone and continued to pay her own rent; however, when queried, she underestimated the amount of her rent by 50%. This same woman incorrectly stated she lived in a hotel, when in actuality she resided in an apartment house.

Diagnosis: Cognitive functioning consistent with mild Alzheimer's disease.

Prognosis: If only properly and carefully diagnosed cases are considered, and if one excludes questionable cases, then none of these patients ever show recovery of their former abilities. A significant minority—27% in our series—do not demonstrate notable decline, however, over the subsequent three- to four-year interval. Twenty-seven percent of patients at this stage were deceased at follow-up and an equal percentage were institutionalized. The remaining subjects (approximately 18% in our series) continue to reside in the community three to four years later, although their clinical status has notably deteriorated.

Commentary: Many of these patients continue to function independently in a community setting, although their symptoms may lead to financial and other difficulties. Family members may become alarmed by the symptomatology at this stage and may bring the patient to the physician for diagnosis for the first time. An unusually stressful situation may result in increased anxiety in these patients and, occasionally, an emergency visit.

FAST Stage 5: Deficient performance in such basic tasks of daily life as choosing the proper clothing to wear.

At this stage patients can no longer function independently. The caregiver must assist not only in managing financial affairs and in marketing, but must also assist the patient in choosing the proper clothing for the season and for the occasion. The patient will frequently wear obviously incongruous clothing combinations unless the caregiver intervenes. This deficit in choosing the proper clothing is virtually pathognomic of this stage. Less characteristically, some patients at this stage begin to forget to bathe regularly unless reminded. Sometimes coaxing as well as reminding to bathe is necessary. Another functional deficit which frequently becomes manifest over the course of this stage is difficulty driving an automobile. The patient may inappropriately speed up and slow down the vehicle, mistakenly go through a stop sign or stoplight, or even collide with another vehicle for the first time in many years. Frequently, the patient is sufficiently alarmed by these deficits to voluntarily discontinue driving, though occasionally, coercion by the spouse or other caregiver is necessary.

Patients at this stage are still capable of putting on their clothing properly, once it has been selected for them, and once bathing are capable of washing themselves and even of adjusting the bathwater properly.

Diagnosis: Cognitive functioning consistent with moderate Alzheimer's disease.

Prognosis: A minority of patients, even at this stage, do not show deterioration over the subsequent three- to four-year interval. Most, however, either are found to be deceased, institutionalized, or, if in the community, deteriorated.

Commentary: Crying episodes or other emotional disturbances, including hyperactivity and a variation in diurnal rhythm (sleep disturbance), frequently result in crises and physician intervention at this stage.

FAST Stage 6: Decreased ability to clothe, bathe and/or toilet oneself.

In uncomplicated Alzheimer's disease these functional deficits generally proceed in an ordinal manner with the evolution of the illness process. Five distinct ordinal functional substages can be identified and these stages are described below. It should be noted that distinctions between the substages may be less marked than those between the integer functional stages. Hence, stages 6(a) and 6(b) occasionally become manifest simultaneously. Also, in unusual circumstances in uncomplicated Alzheimer's disease, the strict ordinality of progressive functional deficit may be violated with respect to the functional substages and, for example, (uncommonly) stage 6(b) may precede 6(a).

Substage 6(a): Decreased ability to put on one's clothing properly.

Initially in this substage, many patients will begin to put their regular clothing on over their nightclothes. Other patients, for the first time in their adult lives, will experience difficulties in tying their shoelaces properly, in buttoning and/or zipping their clothing, in putting on neckties, or in putting shoes on the proper feet. As the illness advances caregivers provide increasing assistance with the mechanics of helping the patient to clothe themselves properly.

Substage 6(b): Decreased ability to handle the mechanics of bathing.

At this stage patient's ability to properly adjust the bath water declines. Difficulties in entering and exiting from the bath, in washing properly, and in completely drying oneself may also become manifest. As noted previously, fear or resistance to bathing sometimes precedes actual deficits in bathing.

Substage 6(c): Decreased ability to handle the mechanics of toileting.

Patients at this stage begin to forget to flush the toilet. They also may begin to forget to wipe themselves properly when toileting and may develop difficulty in properly pulling up their underclothing, pants, or dress. The caregiver begins to assiste the patient in handling the mechanics of toileting.

Substage 6(d): Urinary incontinence.

Occasionally, this occurs virtually simultaneously with stage 6(c), but more frequently, there is a discernable interval of a few to several months between these substages. The urinary incontinence occurs at this stage in the absence of infection or other genitourinary tract pathology. It appears to be entirely the result of decreased cognitive capacity to respond to urinary urgency with appropriate toileting behavior.

Substage 6(e): Fecal incontinence.

This substage may also become manifest simultaneously with the preceding substage (urinary incontinence), or even at the same time that difficulties with the mechanics of toileting becomes evident to the caregiver. More frequently this substage is temporarily discreet. The mechanism, like that of urinary incontinence, appears to be decreased cognitive capacity.

Diagnosis: Cognitive functioning consistent with moderately severe Alzheimer's disease.

Prognosis: Each of six patients whom we followed at this sixth stage were institutionalized or deceased at the time of the follow-up after approximately four years.

Commentary: Agitation and overt psychotic symptomatology frequently produce crises at this stage which may result in medical contact. Other symptoms such as the onset of incontinence may also produce crises. Violence and/or incontinence may lead the family to consider institutionalization for the patient.

FAST Stage 7: Loss of speech, locomotion, and consciousness.

This is the last stage of Alzheimer's disease. Although some patients succumb earlier in the course of the illness to social hazards (e.g. vehicular accidents, assaults, becoming hopelessly lost) or infections for which persons with decreased cognitive capacity have an increased susceptibility, the majority of Alzheimer's patients survive until some point in this seventh stage.

Substage 7(a): Vocabulary becomes limited to fewer than a half-dozen words.

There is a progressive loss of vocabulary and of speech abilities with the progression of Alzheimer's disease. Reticence and a paucity of speech are frequently noted in the fourth and fifth GDS stages. In the sixth GDS stage the ability to speak in complete sentences is gradually lost. Subsequent to the development of incontinence, speech becomes circumscribed to single word productions and spoken vocabulary becomes limited to only a few words.

Substage 7(b): Intelligible vocabulary becomes limited to a single word.

The final spoken word for the Alzheimer's patient is variable. For some patients, the spoken vocabulary becomes limited to the single word "yes." For other patients the final spoken word is "no." One woman's final word was "okay," which she repeated in response to all verbalization-provoking phenomena. Hence, if she wanted to toilet, express anxiety, express the affirmative or the negative, she said "okay." As the illness progresses, the ability to speak even this final single word is lost. However, months afterward, the patient may suddenly articulate the seemingly forgotten final word, only to return to a state of obliviousness with respect to intelligible speech. After intelligible speech is lost, vocalizations become limited to grunts or screams.

Substage 7(c): Loss of ambulatory ability.

Neuropathologic studies indicate that the motor cortex is spared except in the most severe(late) stages of Alzheimer's disease. Perhaps this late cortical deterioration accounts for the loss of ambulatory ability at this late point in the evolution of the disease. Lesser forms of ambulatory disturbance, however, are not uncommonly observed at earlier stages of the disease. These less severe loco-motor disturbances may be the result of decreased cognitive capacities, and resultant psychomotor changes, rather than destruction of the motor cortex per se (Reisberg, London et al., 1983; Brun & Englund, 1981). For example, inappropriate gait speed (the patient either walks too quickly or too slowly) is not infrequently noted in the earlier stages of the disease. In the sixth stage the patients may begin to ambulate more deliberately or to take smaller steps. Assistance in walking up and down staircases is generally required prior to the loss of all ambulatory ability.

The onset of ambulatory loss is somewhat varied. Some patients simply take progressively smaller and slower steps. Others begin to tilt forward, backward, or laterally when ambulating. Twisted gaits have also been noted.

After ambulatory abilities are lost, other voluntary motoric abilities become compromised. Several months to years afterwards, many surviving patients develop contractures, although it is not certain at this time whether these are in some instances preventable by aggressive physical therapy.

Substage 7(d): Loss of ability to sit up independently.

After Alzheimer's patients have lost the ability to ambulate without, and subsequently even with, assistance, they are still capable of sitting in a chair unassisted. Several months after ambulatory ability is lost, the ability to sit up unassisted is lost. At this point, they are still capable of smiling, chewing, grunting, and grasping.

Substage 7(e): Loss of ability to smile.

At this stage Alzheimer's survivors can generally still move their eyes and may appear to show deliberate ocular movements in response to stimuli. Grasp reflexive ability is also preserved as is the ability to swallow in many patients. Patients at this stage are still capable of holding their head up independently.

Substage 7(f): Loss of ability to hold up head.

One of the few Alzheimer's survivors at this stage continued to move her eyes, although ocular movements were not readily associated with exogenous stimuli. This patient was fed with a pipette. She continued to cry out, however there appeared to be little association between her grunts and cries and exogenous phenomena.

Many of the symptoms in the earlier stages and substages of Alzheimer's disease appear to be the functionally definable endproducts of accumulative pathology which is recognizable, albeit less distinct, earlier in the illness process. Similarly, the stuporous and the comatose states, which may ultimately be observed in the final substage of the disease may be related to progressive electrophysiologic slowing (Reisberg, Schneck, et al., 1983; McAdam & Robinson, 1956; Weiner & Schuster, 1956) and progressive decrements in cerebral metabolism (Freyham et al., 1951; Ferris et al. 1980; de Leon et al. 1983), which are known concomitants of the illness.

Diagnosis: Cognition and functioning consistent with severe Alzheimer's disease.

Commentary: Pathologic passivity frequently replaces earlier agitation in this stage. Nevertheless, some patients become agitated or psychotic for the first time. Not infrequently, family members will consult physicians for the first time with respect to a crisis, which may or may not result in institutionalization.

Alzheimer's disease is not generally noted on death certificates as a cause of death. Hence, a certain circularity occurs with respect to the demise of Alzheimer's victims. Since Alzheimer's disease cannot be the cause, another cause is ascribed. Nevertheless, a recent study by Sulkava et al. indicated that 14% (3 of 22) of the Alzheimer's patients whom he followed to autopsy ultimately died of no obvious immediate cause other than this disease, "suggesting a failure in the central regulation of vital functions, such as "respiration' " (Sulkava et al., 1983). He concluded that "since Alzheimer's disease is also a 'malignant' disease which drastically diminishes the patient's life expectancy it should always be mentioned in the death certificates of these patients."

Relationship of Functional Hierarchy in Alzheimer's Disease to Normal Human Development

The hierarchical nature of the clinical symptomatology in dementia of the Alzheimer's type has been noted by at least two groups of independent investigators (Reisberg et al., 1982; Cole et al. 1983; Reisberg, Schneck, et al., 1983). De Ajuriaguerra et al. (1964) have suggested that the functional decline in degenerative dementia approximates the childhood developmental stages in reverse. Our observations when viewed retrospectively appear to be in agreement with this hypothesis (Table 15.2).

Interestingly, the extent to which stages are separated in normal human development also provides an indication of their degree of disparateness in dementia of the Alzheimer's type. Hence, the stages at a certain point merge and overlap in normal aging. Similarly, the borderlines between the FAST

TABLE 15.2 Correspondence Between Functional Assessment Staging (FAST) Deficits in Aging and Alzheimer's Disease and Normal Human Development

FAST stage	Approximate age at which function is acquired
1	Normal adult
2	Normal aged adult
3	Young adult
4	7 years to adolescence
5	5 to 7 years
6(a)	Approximately 5 years[a]
(b)	Approximately 4 years[a]
(c)	Approximately 48 months[b]
(d)	Approximately 36–54 months[c]
(e)	Approximately 24–36 months[a,b,c]
7(a)	Approximately 15 months[a,b]
(b)	Approximately 12 months[a,b]
(c)	Approximately 12 months[a,b]
(d)	Approximately 6–9 months[a,b]
(e)	Approximately 8–16 weeks[a,b]
(f)	Approximately 4–12 weeks[a,b]

Sources: [a] Eisenberg (1975). [b] Vaughan (1969). [c] Pierce (1975).

stages in Alzheimer's disease are subtle rather than abrupt. However, just as in the normal aging process, the midpoints and extremes of some of the stages may be very separate from the stage immediately preceding it; similarly, the midpoints and extremes of some of the FAST stages in the disease may be temporally quite removed. Finally, the total duration of the normal developmental stages does not differ strikingly from the total duration of the degenerative stages in Alzheimer's disease. In this regard it is interesting to return to the APA's Diagnostic and Statistical Manual's definition, cited earlier, which states, "with senile onset, the average duration of symptoms, from onset to death, is about five years" (APA, 1980). Particularly, if we take into consideration the fact that approximately 50% of AD cases do not present until the fifth or sixth stage, this temporal course of degeneration is not markedly different from the converse developmental course. Also to be taken into consideration is the fact that the vast majority of Alzheimer's patients do not survive the full course of the illness process. Many succumb in the sixth stage, and many others, perhaps the majority, succumb in the early part of the seventh stage. Some Alzheimer's patients succumb relatively early in the course of the illness process in the fifth, or even the fourth, stage. Death in the fifth stage from such tragedies as vehicular accidents can sometimes be clearly traceable to Alzheimer's disease. Death in the fourth stage may be less readily related to the Alzheimer's disease process.

If the above two factors are taken into consideration, namely, the relatively, late presentation of many Alzheimer's cases, and the mortality rate of many patients over the course of the illness process, the APA's estimated survival time of five years is not very different from the estimated illness duration at each stage in Table 15.3. Indeed, if we assume that the average patient presents at the end of the fourth stage or beginning of the fifth stage, and dies at the end of stage 7(a) or the beginning of stage 7(b), which are likely to be accurate estimates, then the average duration of illness from Table 15.3 would be exactly 5 years.

The other major developmental phenomena which also apply to the FAST are the relative, rather than absolute, ordinal hierarchy of both normal human development, from a functional standpoint, and ordinal degenerative change in dementia of the Alzheimer's type. That normal human development proceeds in an ordinal fashion is, of course, indisputable. However, individuals will occasionally violate the normal developmental hierarchy. Hence whereas very few, if any, infants will speak many words before they can sit up, and no infants speak before they can smile, some infants will be capable of saying a few words before they can walk without assistance. Similarly, some Alzheimer's patients may still be able to utter intelligible words at the point when they have lost the ability to ambulate.

TABLE 15.3 Approximate FAST Stage Duration in Subjects with Normal Aging and Alzheimer's Disease

FAST stage	Estimated duration[a]
1	50 years
2	15 years
3	7 years
4	2 years
5	18 months
6(a)	5 months
(b)	5 months
(c)	5 months
(d)	4 months
(e)	10 months
7(a)	12 months
(b)	18 months
(c)	12 months
(d)	12 months
(e)	18 months
(f)	not applicable

[a] In subjects who survive and progress to the subsequent deterioration stage.

Even more subtle, is the distinction in Alzheimer's patients between loss of ability to put on clothing properly and loss of ability to bathe properly. Developmentally, of course, these distinctions may also be subtle. Hence, although the progression of functioning in Alzheimer's disease, like that in normal aging, is unquestionably ordinal, occasional minor variations occur with respect to the precise hierarchy, particularly for adjacent substages. Major hierarchical violations, however, are indicative of other or confounding pathology.

FAST: Utility in the Staging of Severe Dementia

At the stage at which Alzheimer's victims lose the ability to put on their clothing properly [stage 6(a)], they may, for reasons related to behavioral disturbance as well as cognitive deficit, achieve only baseline(zero) scores on most psychometric and even mental status evaluations. Hence, test measures may be less useful in differentiating patients from this point onwards. At the point when patients lose the ability to speak, in the early part of the seventh stage, test measures and mental status assessments are uniformly of no value in differentiating patients according to the magnitude of severity of the illness process. Hence, the FAST staging procedure enables us to distinguish at least 11 ordinal stages of Alzheimer's disease, in an expeditious fashion, beyond the point at which other assessment procedures may no longer be of value.

The importance of this development for Alzheimer's research is difficult to overestimate. One example of its utility for research being conducted at present, however, might be instructive. A recent detailed scholarly paper by an eminent group of investigators compared various neuropathological changes in the brains of victims of "Alzheimer's presenile dementia," "senile dementia of the Alzheimer's type," and "Down's syndrome of middle age" (Mann et al., 1984). They noted that:

> When compared with age matched controls the severity of neuropathological changes was greatest in the younger patients with Alzheimer's disease, but this fell with age such that by 90 years the level of change in Alzheimer's disease approached that in old age alone. There were only slight differences in the extent of these pathological changes in those patients with Down's syndrome when compared with others of similar age with Alzheimer's disease. It is concluded that the presenile dementia of Alzheimer's disease, the senile dementia of the Alzheimer type and Down's syndrome in middle age all form an age-related continuum of pathological change.

Of course an alternative explanation might be that the magnitude of severity of the illness process in their groups may not have been comparable. This was not assessed in their otherwise extensive investigations, nor is it assessed in similar studies at this time. The FAST staging of the magnitude of Alzheimer's disease severity provides a means of remedying these obvious deficiencies in contemporary studies.

FAST: Utility in the Differential Diagnosis of Dementia

In conjunction with information about the onset, course, and presentation of SDAT, the FAST staging procedure is useful in the diagnosis as well as staging of uncomplicated Alzheimer's disease. It is also of great value in identifying extraneous treatable complications of Alzheimer's disease and in the differential diagnosis of Alzheimer's disease from other dementing disorders of later life (Table 15.4).

With respect to illnesses complicating an otherwise consistent Alzheimer's picture, the following examples might be cited.

1. Inability to market or handle finances at the time when a person can still function adequately in a demanding employment setting should lead the clinician to consider the possibility of a focal cerebral process associated with, for example, acalculia, or a "pseudodementing" process such as depression.

TABLE 15.4 Differential Diagnostic Considerations of FAST Nonordinality

FAST stage	FAST characteristics	Differential diagnostic considerations: particularly if FAST stage occurs early (nonordinally) in the evolution of dementia
1.	No functional decrement, either subjectively or objectively, manifest	
2.	Complains of forgetting location of objects; subjective work difficulties	2. Anxiety neurosis; depression
3.	Decreased functioning in demanding employment settings evident to coworkers; difficulty in traveling to new locations.	3. Depression; subtle manifestations of medical pathology
4.	Decreased ability to perform complex tasks such as planning dinner for guests, handling finances, and marketing.	4. Depression; psychosis; focal cerebral process (e.g. Gersman syndrome)
5.	Requires assistance in choosing proper clothing; may require coaxing to bathe properly.	5. Depression
6.	(a) Difficulty putting on clothing properly	6. (a) Arthritis; sensory deficit; stroke; depression
	(b) Requires assistance bathing; may develop fear of bathing	(b) Arthritis; sensory deficit; stroke; depression
	(c) Inability to handle mechanics of toileting	(c) Arthritis; sensory deficit; stroke; depression
	(d) Urinary incontinence	(d) Urinary tract infection; other causes of urinary incontinence
	(e) Fecal incontinence	(e) Infection; malabsorption syndrome; other causes of fecal incontinence
7.	(a) Ability to speak limited to one to five words	7. (a) Stroke; other dementing disorder (e.g. diffuse space occupying lesions)
	(b) Intelligible vocabulary lost	(b) Stroke; other dementing disorder (e.g. diffuse space occupying lesions)
	(c) Ambulatory ability lost	(c) Parkinsonism; neuroleptic induced or other secondary extrapyramidal syndrome; Creutzfeldt-Jakob disease: normal pressure hydrocephalus: hyonatremic dementia; stroke; hip fracture; arthritis; over medication
	(d) Ability to sit up independently lost	(d) Arthritis; contractures
	(e) Ability to smile lost	(e) Stroke
	(f) Ability to hold up head lost	(f) Head trauma; metabolic abnormality; other medical abnormality; overmedication; encephalitis; other causes

2. Inability to put on clothing properly at the time when a patient can still choose the proper clothing to wear, can occur in depression. It can also, of course, occur as a result of cerebral focal pathology, such as stroke, CNS metastasis, etc. Arthritis, a fracture, or other physically debilitative processes can also result in this presentation.

3. Inability to handle mechanics of bathing when the SDAT patient is still capable of choosing the proper clothing for the season and the occasion commonly results from arthritis or other physical debilities.

4. The development of urinary incontinence prior to the anticipated ordinal stage might indicate that the patient has developed a urinary tract infection which might respond to appropriate intervention with antimicrobial agents.

5. The development of fecal incontinence prior to the anticipated ordinal stage might be indicative of a gastrointestinal infection. It might also be indicative of one of the numerous other possible causes of incontinence in the elderly which should be investigated in an appropriate fashion.

6. Premature loss of speech in what is otherwise an uncomplicated Alzheimer's type presentation should lead the clinician to strongly suspect the possibility of focal cerebral pathology, in particular cerebral infarction. This might be indicative of either a primary multiinfarct dementia, or of a mixed degenerative dementia with coexisting cerebrovascular pathology.

It should be noted that cerebral infarction may occur even in the absence of evidence for infarction on the computed tomography (CT) scan. A nuclear magnetic resonance (NMR) scan may occasionally reveal a large or small infarction which is entirely invisible on the CT scan (Sipponen et al., 1983). In any event, NMR may be particularly useful in differentiating senile dementia of the Alzheimer's type from multiinfarct dementia and mixed degenerative and infarction dementias (Besson et al., 1983). Even in the absence of any neuroradiologic evidence for infarction, either on CT or NMR, the clinician should carefully search for other evidence of focal pathology, such as asymmetric reflexes or other asymmetric sensory or motor abilities. Such asymmetry can help to confirm a clinician's suspicion of focal phenomena in, for example, an Alzheimer's patient who may be incapable of toileting without some assistance but who is still continent and who has recently lost all ability to utter intelligible speech.

7. Premature loss of ambulatory ability in otherwise uncomplicated Alzheimer's disease occurs as a result of cerebral infarction; CNS metastatic disease; other primary causes of dementia including notably Creutzfeldt-Jakob disease, normal pressure hydrocephalus, metabolic dementias; hip or leg fractures; arthritis; severe peripheral vascular disease; primary or secondary parkinsonism; overmedication; or other causes. Many of these etiologies have been discussed, are well known, or are self-evident. At least one requires further elaboration.

Creutzfeldt-Jakob disease may be a more frequently encountered dementing illness than is often recognized. A literature review yielded 121 confirmed cases of Creutzfeldt-Jakob disease who died in England and Wales in the decade from 1970–79, and 31 probable cases (Will & Mathews, 1984). Three presentations of Creutzfeldt-Jakob disease could be distinguished. Of these, by far the most common was the subacute form, rapidly leading to a helpless condition and early death. In the intermediate form, the terminal stages were identical but were preceded by a prolonged period of focal or diffuse neurological signs. In the amyotrophic form progressive dementia was accompanied or followed by extensive neurogenic muscle atrophy. Naturally, since focal signs and neurogenic muscular atrophy are not part of the constellation of Alzheimer's disease, clinicians should have little difficulty distinguishing these latter forms from dementia of the Alzheimer's type. Gait disturbance, specifically ataxia, was a presenting symptom in 19% of subacute cases in the series reviewed by Will and Mathews. Hence, gait disturbance can be a useful early differentiating sign between the common subacute form of Creutzfeldt-Jakob disease and dementia of the Alzheimer's type. Other frequent differentiating symptoms between these two conditions include dizziness, visual disturbance, and involuntary movement which occurred at presentation in 11%, 9%, and 5% of subacute CJD patients, respectively, but which do not occur as part of the presentation of SDAT.

Ataxia as a differentiating feature in the diagnosis of dementia, and more particularly in the differential diagnosis of subacute Creutzfeldt-Jakob disease and Alzheimer's disease, recently achieved some importance in a case which came to broad public attention (Altman, 1984c). George Balanchine, the noted choreographer, developed ataxia as an initial symptom in a subsequently progressive dementing process, which resulted in his demise. Creutzfeldt-Jakob disease was revealed at autopsy.

8. Premature development of a comatose state in an Alzheimer's patient may occur from many causes. Etiologies which should be prominently considered include overmedication, intercurrent illness, a cerebrovascular accident, and head trauma. Aspiration should always be suspected late in the illness. This can lead to unconsciousness and apparent "foaming at the mouth" which can be mistaken for a seizure.

SENILE DEMENTIA OF THE ALZHEIMER'S TYPE: SELECT RECENT ADVANCES IN MANAGEMENT

The development of stage specific decriptions of normal aging and progressive senile dementia of the Alzheimer's type has enabled clinicians to determine the corresponding management needs of the patient. The stage

TABLE 15.5 Care Needs of the Alzheimer's Patient and the Patient's Family

Global stage	Impact on the patient	Impact on the family	Nursing needs	Care recommendations
1	None	None	None	None
2	Subjective discomfort; no overt emotional symptoms	Family is less concerned about subjective deficits than the patient	None	Reassurance with respect to benign prognosis
3	Anxiety may be manifest	Retirement and patient's withdrawal from demanding tasks are considered by the family unit	None	"Tactical" withdrawal from situations which have become, by virtue of their complexity, anxiety-provoking
4	Denial and emotional withdrawal	Family takes over finances and associated responsibilities, begins to supervise the patient	Independent survival still attainable.	Assistance toward goal of maximum independence; financial supervision; structured and/or supervised travel; identification bracelets and labels may be useful
5	Denial and emotional withdrawal with occasional tearfulness and anger.	Family begins to take on the emotional burden of the patient's illness. Supervision and care of the patient begins to become a full-time responsibility	Patient can no longer survive in the community without assistance. Needs continuous supervision with respect to travel and social behavior	Part-time home health care assistance is frequently very useful in assisting the patient's caregiver. Driving becomes hazardous and should be discontinued. Family may require guidance in handling patient's emotional outbursts
6	Personality and emotional changes occur. These are quite variable and include: (a) delusional behavior, e.g. patients may accuse their spouse of being an imposter; may talk to im-	Caregiver is frequently forced to devote his/her entire life to the care of the patient who in return, cannot recall the kindness shown to them, and may occasionally even forget the spouse's	Patient requires assistance with basic ADL. Early in this stage, assistance with dressing and bathing is required. Subsequently assistance with continence be-	Full-time home health care assistance is frequently very useful in assisting the patient's caregiver. Strategies for assistance with bathing, toileting, and in the management of incontinence should be discussed with the family. Need for tranquilization and appropriate adjustment of major tranquilizers, if these

TABLE 15.5 (*Continued*)

Global stage	Impact on the patient	Impact on the family	Nursing needs	Care recommendations
	aginary figures in the environment, or in the mirror; (b) obsessive symptoms, e.g. person may continually repeat simple cleaning activities; (c) anxiety symptoms, agitation, and even loss of willpower because an individual cannot carry a thought long enough to determine a purposeful course of action. Denial occasionally entirely protects against the emotional impact of the illness on the patient.	identity. Emotional burden becomes unbearable. Institutionalization considered	comes necessary as well	are prescribed should be addressed. Emotional stress in the caregiver should be minimized with supportive techniques.
7	Screams and other verbal outbursts as well as panting become a means of communication and must be distinguished from true distress. Pathologic passivity also develops.	Acceptance and coping mechanisms begin to mitigate the emotional trauma and distress.	Early in this stage, assistance with feeding as well as dressing, bathing and toileting is required. Subsequently, assistance with ambulation and finally purposeful movement becomes necessary.	Full-time assistance in home or institutional setting is a necessity. Strategies for locomotion should be explored. Need for tranquilization frequently evaporates. Specific needs are quite variable but most frequent causes of death and disability to be avoided are aspiration pneumonia and traumatic or decubital ulceration. Soft food diet is generally tolerated, however, nasogastric feeding is frequently necessary during crises.

specific care requirements of the Alzheimer's patient have recently been published (Reisberg, 1984). These management needs and recommendations are outlined in Table 15.5.

The affective symptoms that develop in the Alzheimer's patient most commonly in the fifth global deterioration scale stage are somewhat characteristic of this illness, just as we have seen is the case with respect to the other symptomatology of the Alzheimer's patient. Table 15.6 outlines the affective symptoms which are, and which are not, commonly part of the presentation of the Alzheimer's patient.

The psychotic and psychosis-like symptomatology of the Alzheimer's patient is also characteristic. These symptoms occur most frequently in the sixth Global Deterioration Scale stage. A rating instrument designed to specifically assess these characteristic psychotic symptoms in the Alzheimer's patient has been published (Reisberg & Ferris, 1985).

The neuropharmacology of the Alzheimer's disease brain is unique. Disproportionate deficits in the cholinergic system are well known (Bartus et al. 1982). Other neurotransmitter systems, such as the noradrenergic system, may also be disproportionately affected (Bondareff, 1981). Interrelationships between the parkinsonian syndrome and Alzheimer's disease have been observed (Hakim & Mathieson, 1978; Boller et al., 1980). Hence, the response profile and side effect profile of the Alzheimer's patient to neuroleptics and antidepressants are likely also to be unique. These unique relationships are amenable to investigation at this time.

TABLE 15.6 Affective Symptoms of Alzheimer's Disease[a]

Symptoms that occur in the affective syndrome of Alzheimer's disease		
Occur frequently	Tend not to occur	May occur
Episodes of tearfulness	Guilt feelings	Somatization
Irritability	Suicidal ideation	Sleep disturbance
Anger	Appetite disturbance	
Suspiciousness	Pervasive dysphoria	
Pacing		
Agitation		

[a]Rule 1: Information with respect to symptomatology in the Alzheimer's patient must come from the caregiver. Denial protects against full realization of symptomatology in the patients themselves.

A past history or family history of affective disorder is no more common in the Alzheimer's patient than in the general population.

CONCLUSION

Impressive and major strides have been made over the past few years in our understanding of senile dementia of the Alzheimer's type. Notably, advances have been made in the clinician's ability to diagnose, differentially diagnose, and manage the illness. Unfortunately, we do not at this time have treatments for the primary cognitive symptoms of the illness. Neither do we have at present treatments which affect the fundamental etiologic process of Alzheimer's disease. Nor, indeed, do we know the cause of the process. It is hoped that future advances will bring us closer to the understanding and treatment of the basic mechanisms of this major illness.

REFERENCES

Adams, F. (Ed.). (1861). *The extant works of Aretaeus* (p. 103). London: *The Cappadocian,* Sydenham Society.

Altman, L. K., (1984a) New brain study technique reveals an Alzheimer defect. *New York Times,* August 24, p. 1.

Altman, L. K. (1984b). Alzheimer's disease linked to damaged areas of brain. *New York Times,* September 7, p. 1.

Altman, L. K. (1984c). The mystery of Balanchine's death is solved. *New York Times,* May 8, p. C1.

Alzheimer, A. (1907). Uber eine eigenartige Erkrankung der Hirnrinde. *Allgemeine Z. Psych. Psych. Ger. Med., 64,* 146–148.

American Psychiatric Association (1980). *Diagnostic and statistical manual of mental disorders* (3rd ed.), (pp. 124–126) Washington, DC: American Psychiatric Association.

Ball, M. J. & Lo, P. (1977). Granulovacuolar degeneration in the aging brain and in dememtia. *J. Neuropathol. Exp. Neurol., 36,* 474–487.

Bartus, R. T., Dean, R. L., Beer, B., & Lippa, A. S. (1982) The cholinergic hypothesis of geriatric memory dysfunction: A critical review. *Science, 217,* 408–417.

Besson, J. A. O., Corrigan, F. M., Foreman, E. I., Ashcroft, G. W., Eastwood, L. M. & Smith, F. W. (1983). Differentiating senile dementia of Alzheimer type and multiinfarct dementia by proton NMR imaging. *Lancet, ii,* 789.

Blessed, G., Tomlinson, B. E., & Roth, M. (1968). The association between quantitative measures of dementia and of senile changes in the cerebral gray matter of elderly subjects. *Br. J. Psychiatry, 114,* 797–811.

Boller, F., Mizutani, T., Ruessman, R., et al. (1980). Parkinson's disease, dementia, and Alzheimer's disease: Clinicopathologic correlations. *Ann. Neurol., 7,* 329–335.

Bondareff, W., Mountjoy, C. Q., & Roth, M. (1981). Selective loss of neurons of origin of andrenergic projection to cerebral cortex (nucleus locus ceroleus) in senile dementia. *Lancet, i,* 783–784.

Breitner, J. C. S., & Folstein, M. F. (1984). Familial Alzheimer dementia: A prevalent disorder with specific clinical features. *Psychol. Med., 14,* 63–80.

Brozan, N. (1982a). Coping with travail of Alzheimer's disease. *New York Times,* Nov. 29, p. B10.

Brozan, N. (1982b). Coping with an ailment of the aging. *International Herald Tribune,* Dec. 2.
Brun, A., & Englund, E. (1981). Regional pattern of degeneration in Alzheimer's disease: Neural loss and histopathologic grading. *Histopathology, 5,* 549–564.
Cole, M. G., Dastoor, D. P., & Koszycki, D. (1983). The hierarchic dementia scale. *J. Clin. Exp. Gerontol., 5,* 219–234.
Corkin, S., Davis, K. L., Growdon, J. H., Usdin, U., & Wurtman, R. J., (Eds.). (1982). *Alzheimer's disease: A report of progress in research, Aging, Vol. 19.* New York: Raven Press.
Corsellis, J. A. N. (1962). *Mental illness and the ageing brain* (Monograph No. 9). London: Maudsley.
Corsellis, J. A. N. & Evans, P. H. (1965). The relations of stenosis of the extracrainial cerebral arteries to mental disorders and cerebral degeneration in old age. *Proceedings of the Fifth International Congress on Neuropathology,* 546.
de Ajuriaguerra, J. Rey, M., Bellet-Muller, M. (1964). A propos de quelques problèmes posées par le deficit operatoire des viellards atteints de démence degenerative en début d'évolution. *Cortex 1,* 232–256.
de Leon, M. J., Ferris, S. H., George, A. E., et al. (1983). Positron emission tomography studies of aging and Alzheimer's disease. *Am. J. Neuroradiol., 4,* 568–571.
Eisenberg, L. (1975). Normal child development, In A. M. Freedman, H. R. Kaplan & B. J. Sadcock (Eds.), *Comprehensive textbook of psychiatry/II* Vol. 2 (pp. 2036–2054). Baltimore MD: Williams & Wilkins.
Esquirol, J. E. D. (1838). *Des Maladies Mentales.* Paris: Balliere.
Ferris, S. H., deLeon, M. J., Wolf, A. P., et al. (1980). Positron emission tomography in the study of aging and senile dementia. *Neurobiol. Aging, 1,* 127–131.
Folstein, M. F., & Powell, D. (1984). Is Alzheimer's disease inherited?: A methodologic review. *Integrative Psychiatry, 2,* 163–170.
Freese, A. S. (1978). *The end of senility.* New York: Arbor House.
Freyham, F. A., Woodford, R. B., Kety, S. S. (1951). Cerebral bloodflow and metabolism in psychosis of senility. *J. Nerv. Ment. Dis., 113,* 449–456.
Galen (1821–1833). De symptomatum differentis liber, In C. G. Kuhn, (Ed.). *Opera Omnia,* (p. 200–201) Leipzig: Knobloch.
Galton, L. (1979). *The truth about senility—And how to avoid it.* New York: Thomas Y. Crowell.
Gellerstedt, N. (1932–1933). Our knowledge of cerebral changes in normal involution of old age. *Ups.-Lak/Foren Forh, 38,* 193.
Grunthal, E. (1927). Clinical and anatomical investigations on senile dementia. *Z. Gesamte Neurol. Psychiat., 111,* 763.
Hakim, A. M., & Mathieson, G. (1978). Basis of dementia in Parkinson's disease. *Lancet, ii,* 729.
Henig, R. M. (1978). Exposing the myth of senility. *New York Times Magazine,* Dec. 3, p. 158, ff.
Hirano, A., & Zimmerman, H. M. (1962). Alzheimer's neurofibrillary changes: A topographic study. *Arch. Neurol., 7,* 227–242.
Katzman, R., Terry, R. D., Bick, K. L. (eds.). (1978). *Alzheimer's disease: Senile dementia and related disorders, Aging* Vol. 7. New York: Raven Press.
Lipowski, Z. J. (1980). Organic mental disorders: Introduction and review of syndromes. In H. I. Kaplan, A. M. Freedman, & B. J. Sadcock (Eds.), *Comprehensive textbook of psychiatry,* Vol. 2 (pp. 1359–1392). Baltimore, MD: Williams & Wilkins.

Mace, N. L., & Rabins, P. V. (1981). *The 36-hour day*. Baltimore: The Johns Hopkins University Press.
Mann, D. M. A., Yates, P. O., Marcyniuk, B. (1984). Alzheimer's presenile dementia, senile dementia of Alzheimer type and Down's syndrome in middle age form an age related continuum of pathological changes. *Neuropathol. Appl. Neurobiol. 10*, 185–207.
McAdam, W., & Robinson, R. A. (1956). Senile intellectual deterioration and the electroencephalogram: A quantitative correlation. *Br. J. Psychiatry, 102,* 819.
Margolis, G. (1959). Senile cerebral disease: A critical survey of traditional concepts based upon observations with newer techniques. *Lab. Invest., 8,* 335–370.
Meyer, L. (1982). Aging prematurely. *Washington Post,* Jan. 8, p. 1.
Miller, N. E. & Cohen, G. D., (Eds.). (1981). *Clinical aspects of Alzheimer's disease and senile dementia,* Aging, Vol. 15. New York: Raven Press.
Pierce, C. M. (1975). Enuresis and encopresis. In A. M. Freedman, H. R. Kaplan, & B. J. Sadcock (Eds.), *Comprehensive textbook of psychiatry/II* Vol. 2 (pp. 2116–2125). Baltimore, MD: Williams & Wilkins.
Prichard, J. C. (1837). *A treatise on insanity and other disorders affecting the mind* (pp. 69–80). Philadelphia: Haswell, Barnington, and Haswell.
Redlich, E. (1898). Ueber miliare sklerose der Hirnrinde bei seniler Atrophie. *Jahrb. F. Psychiatr., 17,* 208–216.
Reisberg, B. (1981). *Brain failure: An introduction to current concepts of senility.* New York: Free Press/Macmillan.
Reisberg, B., (Ed.). (1983a). *Alzheimer's disease.* New York: Free Press/Macmillan.
Reisberg, B. (1983b). The Brief Cognitive Rating Scale and Global Deterioration Scale. In T. Crook, S. H. Ferris, & R. Bartus (Eds.), *Assessment in Geriatric Psychopharmacology* (pp. 19–35). New Canaan, CT: Mark Powley Associates.
Reisberg, B. (1983c). Clinical presentation, diagnosis, and symptomatology of age-associated cognitive decline, and Alzheimer's disease. In B. Reisberg (Ed.), *Alzheimer's disease* (pp. 173–187). New York: Free Press/Macmillan.
Reisberg, B. (1984). Stages of cognitive decline. *Am. J. Nurs., 84,* 225–228.
Reisberg, B., & Ferris, S. H. (1985). A clinical rating scale for symptoms of psychosis in Alzheimer's disease. *Psychopharmacol. Bull., 21,* 101–104.
Reisberg, B., Ferris, S. H., Anand, R., Buttinger, C., Borenstein, J., Sinaiko, E., & de Leon, M. J. (1984). Clinical assessments of cognition in the elderly. In C. A. Shamoian (Ed.), *Biology and treatment of dementia in the elderly* (pp. 15–37). Washington, DC: American Psychiatric Press.
Reisberg, B., Ferris, S. H., Anand, R., de Leon, M. J., Schneck, M. K., Buttinger, C., & Borenstein, J. (1984). Functional staging of dementia of the the Alzheimer's type. *Ann. N.Y. Acad. Sci.,* 435:481–483.
Reisberg, B., Ferris, S. H., de Leon, M. J., & Crook, T. (1982). The Global Deterioration Scale for Assessment of Primary Degenerative Dementia. *Am. J. Psychiatry, 139,* 1136–1139.
Reisberg, B., Ferris, S. H., de Leon, M. J., & Crook, T. (1985). Age-associated cognitive decline and Alzheimer's disease: Implications for assessment and treatment. In M. Bergener, M. Ermini, & H. B. Stahelin (Eds.), *Thresholds in aging* (pp. 255–292). London: Academic Press.
Reisberg, B., Ferris, S. H., Schulman, E., Steinberg, G., Buttinger, C., Sinaiko, E., Borenstein, J., de Leon, M. J., & Cohen, J. (1986). Longitudinal course of normal aging and progressive dementia of the Alzheimer's type: A prospective study of 106 subjects over a 3.6 year mean interval. *Prog. Neuropsychopharmacol. Biol. Psychiatry, 10,* 571–578.

Reisberg, B., Ferris, S. H., Sinaido, E., Borenstein, J., Anand, R., Buttinger, C., & de Leon, M. J. (1984). Aging and dementia of the Alzheimer's type (DAT): Longitudinal course of community residing subgroups (p. 164). *Collegium Internationale Neuro-Psychiopharmacologium, June 19–23, Book of Abstracts.*

Reisberg, B., London, E., Ferris, S. H., Borenstein, J., Scheier, L., & de Leon, M. J. (1983). The Brief Cognitive Rating Scale: Language, motoric and mood concomitants in primary degenerative dementia. *Psychopharmacol. Bull., 19,* 702–708.

Reisberg, B., Schneck, M. K., Ferris, S. H., Schwartz, G. E., & de Leon, M. J. (1983). The Brief Cognitive Rating Scale (BCRS): Findings in primary degenerative dementia (PDD). *Psychopharmacol. Bull., 19:* 47–50.

Roach, M. (1983). Another name for madness, (pp. 22–31). *New York Times Magazine,* Jan. 16.

Roth, M., Tomlinson, B. E., & Blessed, G. (1966). Correlation between scores for dementia and counts of "senile plaques" in cerebral gray matter of elderly subjects. *Nature, 209,* 109.

Rush, B. (1793). An account of the state of mind and body in old age, In *Medical inquiries and observations,* Vol. 2, (p. 311). Philadelphia, PA: Dobson.

Shamoian, C. A. (Ed.). (1984). *Biology and treatment of dementia in the elderly.* Washington, DC: American Psychiatric Press.

Simchowicz, T. (1910). Histologische studien uber die senile demenz. *Hist. Histopath. Arb., 4,* 267.

Sipponen, J. T., Kaste, M., Sepponen, R. E., Kuurne, T., Suoranta, H., & Sivula, A. (1983). Nuclear magnetic resonance imaging in reversible cerebral ischemia. *Lancet, i:* 294–295

Sulkava, R., Haltia, M., Paetau, A., Wilkstrom, J., & Palo, J. (1983). Accuracy of clinical diagnosis in primary degenerative dementia: correlation with neuropathological findings. *J. Neurol. Neurosurg., Psychiatry, 46,* 9–13.

Tomlinson, B. E., Blessed, G., & Roth, M. (1968). Observations on the brains of nondemented old people. *J. Neurol. Sci., 7,* 331–356.

Tomlinson, B. E., Blessed, G., & Roth, M. (1970). Observations on the brains of demented old people. *J. Neurol. Sci., 11,* 205–242.

Tomlinson, B. E., & Kitchener, D. (1972). Granulovacuolar degeneration of hippocampal pyramidal cells. *J. Pathol., 106,* 165–185.

Vaughan, V. C. (1969). Growth and development. In W. E. Nelson, V. C. Vaughan, & R. J. McKay (Eds.), *Textbook of pediatrics* 9th ed. (pp. 15–57), Philadelphia, PA: Saunders.

Webster's New Twentieth Century Dictionary Unabridged Second Edition (1977a). Collins/World, p. 1649.

Webster's New Twentieth Century Dictionary Unabridged Second Edition (1977b). Collins/World, p. 482.

Webster's New Twentieth Century Dictionary Unabridged Second Edition (1977c). Collins/World, p. 547.

Weiner, H., & Schuster, D. B. (1956). The electroencephalogram in dementia: Some preliminary observations and correlations. *Electroencephalogr. Clin. Neurophysiol., 8,* 479–488.

Wertheimer, J., & Marois, M. (1984). *Senile dementia: Outlook for the future.* Modern Aging Research, Vol. 5. New York: Alan R. Liss.

WHO Technical Report Series #730 (1986). *Dementia in later life: Research and action.* Geneva: World Health Organization.

Will, R. G., & Matthews, W. B. (1984). A retrospective study of Creutzfeldt-Jakob disease in England and Wales 1970–79 I: Clinical features. *J. Neurol. Neurosurg., Psychiatry, 47,* 134–140

Woodard, J. S. (1962). Clinicopathological significance of granulovacuolar degeneration in Alzheimer's disease. *J. Neuropathol. Exp. Neurol, 21,* 85–91.

Worm-Petersen, J., & Pakkenberg, H. (1968). Atherosclerosis of cerebral arteries, pathological and clinical correlations. *J. Gerontol. 23,* 445.

Young, A. W. (1936). Franz Nissl (1860–1918), Alois Alzheimer (1864–1915). In *Neurological biographies and addresses.* Foundation volume published for the staff to commemorate the opening of the Montreal Neurological Institute of McGill University (pp. 107–113). London: Oxford University Press.

PART IV
Strategies of Treatment

16
The Interface Between Internal Medicine and Psychogeriatrics

Hannes B. Stähelin

> But O' when wisdom brings no profit,
> to be wise is to suffer.
>
> SOPHOCLES, *King Oedipus*

Textbook descriptions of psychogeriatric patients suggest that these patients present clearly defined clinical pathological syndromes, signs, and symptoms which allow, after due differential diagnosis, a rather precise identification of the underlying illness. In reality, unfortunately, the diagnosis is often far from clear and a number of possible mechanisms and contributing factors have to be considered in the workup of the psychogeriatric patients. The interface of internal medicine and psychogeriatrics, however, does not only cover the differential diagnosis of a large variety of diseases contributing to or even causing confusion associated with mental deterioration in the elderly. In terms of effectiveness, internal medicine is the most important discipline involved in the treatment of conditions contributing to mental impairment of the psychogeriatric patient. Internal medical therapy may greatly improve the quality of life and is the most important tool in prolonging the life of the sick elderly. It is precisely this efficacy which places internal medicine and the geriatrician in a difficult and intricate relationship with biomedical, social, and ethical issues.

In considering the demented elderly patient we are faced with the mind–body problem and often forced to make moral judgments for which we are ill prepared. It is necessary that priorities be clearly set in the treatment and definition of therapeutic goals for the multimorbid patient, so common in geriatric medicine, and it is obvious that our position in the selection of priorities and therapeutic aims must take into account many moral and ethical questions. The complexity of the medical and moral facts defy our efforts to always make relevant judgments. The danger of oversimplification is commonly encountered, and one is tempted either to follow an existing set of principles or to settle medical issues by the principles of utility. The presence of a psychogeriatric illness also influences the ways in which the family, the physician, and other care-givers perceive a bodily illness. The first section deals with the above mentioned aspects of the interface of internal medicine with psychogeriatrics.

MIND–BODY INTERACTION

In general, the physician is aware of the close connection between mind and body. In affections of the central nervous system the relationship becomes even more obvious, influencing the patient and at the same time the reaction of society to the psychogeriatric patient. The mind–body problem occupies a central position for treatment of the psychogeriatric patient in internal medicine, which in a broader sense includes neurology and other related disciplines. From a theoretical point of view we assume that there is a relationship between a given thought, emotion, intention, or desire and a specific neurophysiological process (Rempää, 1973). Organic dementias themselves demonstrate the close connection between intact form as a prerequisite of an intact, functioning mind. Modern neurophysiological, and neurochemical techniques make it possible to correlate some mental phenomena with neurophysiological events. But the complexity of the pathological process in the psychogeriatric patient usually forecloses an identification of the underlying pathological mechanisms. A special difficulty lies in the fact that the early detection of psychogeriatric illnesses cannot be achieved from objective physical symptoms, despite great efforts made in the search for reliable symptoms.

Internal medicine, which deals with bodily illnesses, relies heavily on physical indicators of disease. In psychogeriatric illnesses the observable physical signs and symptoms turn out to be unspecific and poorly correlated with the degree of the illness. Tests of memory, judgement, and reasoning are much more sensitive tools in detecting diffuse alteration in brain function and largely surpass other available methods such as CT-scans, EEG, evoked potentials, and other electrophysiological or histopathological tools.

Performance on psychometric tests, however, is not only affected by medical conditions, but also by previous experiences, learning, life history, education, socioeconomic factors, and psychiatric disorders which all affect mental functions. Therefore, new research and therapeutic approaches emphasize a view of the entire patient (Bergener, 1983) taking psychological, social, and medical conditions into account. Another aspect of the interface of internal medicine with psychogeriatrics is in the consideration of brain failure as a medical problem similar to heart failure or respiratory insufficiency where it is reasonable to use drug intervention. This approach is successful in certain neurological illnesses such as Parkinson's disease and in all conditions where a bodily illness causes mental deterioration. Thus great scrutiny is necessary to detect the often hidden symptoms of a bodily disease masquerading as mental deterioration.

Diagnosis and Treatment: Moral and Ethical Questions

The mind–body interaction explains not only signs and symptoms of the psychogeriatric patient, but also has a profound influence on the approach of the family, the physician, and society as a whole toward the patient. The psychogeriatric patient is perceived differently from a patient with a bodily illness. The dementing process which alters mind and personality leads to a different judgement of the afflicted person by relatives and by the treating physician (Johnson & Johnson, 1983). It is less the knowledge of the irreversibility of the progressive course of the illness which determines our actions, which stress the family, and alientate the physician, but, rather, the problem of the overriding emphasis on "sapiens" in the evaluation of the quality of life of the debilitated elderly "homo sapiens" which becomes a mental barrier in the sober evaluation of the psychogeriatric patient. The psychogeriatric patient is no longer seen as "sapiens" and therefore there has to be a separate set of rules and ethical codes to apply to "homo-non-sapiens." Because of their mental condition, debilitated patients usually receive less complete and almost never exhaustive medical attention (Brown & Thompson, 1979). Hilfiker (1983) describes the prevalent diagnostic and therapeutic nihilism in the care of the debilitated elderly patient who is not brain dead but only supported by routine nursing care, a situation frequently encountered in nursing homes and hospital wards. Here the internist and geriatrician face the issue regarding which treatment is to be given and where to draw lines. Where mentally ill geriatric patients are concerned, the ethical rules for dying patients and intensive care offer no applicable guidelines.

The purpose of such rules is stated by Callahan (1980): "Ethical analysis and prescription . . . ordinarily represent an attempt to organize inchoate and disparate practices and jerry-built and ad hoc principles . . . into a coherent and structured moral system." Decisions regarding treatment are normally made according to a policy somewhere in between, on the one hand, a radical situation ethics, represented by Fletcher (1954), where there is rejection of fixed moral rules and principles, and, on the other hand, the ideas outlined by Ramsey (1970), where there are rigid moral rules with adherence to traditional medical and religious moral principles. According to Callahan (1980), a consensus on rules for treatment is in the process of being formulated for a number of issues, albeit in the absence of any agreement on the underlying theoretical principles. The limitations of a consensus without a firm theoretical foundation are obvious and at the core of ongoing discussion about the ethical dilemmas concerning brain failure in the elderly (Murphy, 1984). The lack of a commonly shared view of the problems of the terminally ill and the severely demented patient often prevents a fruitful discussion, and the decisions concerning treatment are often left solely in the hands of the physician or nurses. The question of what is in the interest of the patient is almost impossible to answer. Even though family care providers experience the patient as different from themselves or from the patient's own former state, they still assume the patient has views and expectations similar to their own. This however, is not likely to be the case.

The Problem of Priority

In view of the complex situation of the psychogeriatric patient requiring medical treatment we have to rely on recognizable ethical criteria that enable us to deal constructively with the plurality of principles (Rawls, 1971). To withhold treatment amounts to a judgment as to life and death. The President's Commission for the Study of the Ethical Problems in Medicine (1983) stated in this context that the drive to "stay in life" can conflict with another fundamental objective of medicine—the "relief of suffering."

Developments in medical care, legislation, and, among the concerned population, the promotion of living wills, argue against interference with a natural process of dying. In contrast is the example of Fox and Lipton (1983) in which it is emphasized that the decision for or against cardiopulmonary resouscitation must undergo great scrutiny. In an emergency situation where the physician is without knowledge of the patient's previous condition and views, since age per se does not affect prognosis, the decision to resuscitate must be made in favor of life.

Finally, the medical decisions are inextricably interwoven into several much larger general issues which contain ideas about the right of individual and actions to be carried out for the "common good" or "public interest." Decisions therefore are also based on a qualification of a patient in a broader sense, which subsequently leads to an evaluation of whether treatment is worth the economic, social, and moral costs. Thus, medical treatment again is dependent on assessments from both moral and medical points of view (Bayer et al., 1983).

The Decision to Treat

In the multimorbid elderly presenting with many symptoms, a single overall principle (e.g., maintain life by all means) does not appear to be adequate. In the presence of a far advanced primary degenerative dementia (senile dementia of the Alzheimer's type) the decision to withhold antibiotic treatment of pneumonia appears justified (Wanzer et al., 1984). Again reasonable accuracy of diagnosis and underlying psychogeriatric condition is always assumed but contrasts with the reluctance to perform extensive diagnostic procedures in the mentally impaired. Finally the decision, for example, whether to let debilitated patients die of thirst or starvation again addresses itself to the questions raised in the previous section. It remains doubtful whether the reliance on a "value history" (the values of a patient professed during a period of well-being) as suggested by McCullough (1984) would provide a solution.

The family's part in the decision regarding treatment will not be free from economic considerations, which in many cases are in conflict with a concern for the patient's welfare. Furthermore, the family is forced to renegotiate its relationship with the institutionalized psychogeriatric patient previously cared for at home (Johnson & Johnson, 1983). The growing awareness of psychogeriatric disturbances as a medical problem and not merely a sequela of aging in itself contributes to institutionalization, and accelerates the separation of the patient from the family. It is rather common for intercurrent bodily illnesses, which may aggravate mental impairment, to catalyze the process of separation from the family and a reason for institutionalization. Certainly, the general practitioner may play an important role in decision making and should also be involved in the decision regarding persons when hospitalized. As pointed out by Besdine (1983), the care of patients entering a hospital or nursing home will be assumed in all likelihood by physicians who are unfamiliar with the incoming resident's personality and preferences. Nevertheless, decisions to treat or not to treat can never be final and have to be reviewed continuously. In all cases relief of discomfort will be one of the prime goals of internal medicine in psychogeriatric patients. Factors influencing the decision to treat or not to treat include: the intention of the patient, the likely outcome with regard to psychogeriatric illness, life expectancy, quality of life, and nursing needs.

In the course of psychogeriatric illnesses it is the additional diseases which confront the treating physician and nursing team time and time again. For example, might not an intercurrent illness terminate a life which is by our standards, miserable? On the one hand, a condition such as urinary tract infection brings much discomfort but no vital threat and should correctly be treated with antibiotics. Decisions of this kind are very important especially since our diagnostic and therapeutic tools are rapidly growing and methods like endoscopy, noninvasive imaging, 24-h ECG monitoring, and laboratory analysis add to our capabilities to detect and influence diseases at an early stage. However, will they also contribute to prolonging periods of dementia? On the other hand, we should not forget that many elderly survive severe bodily illnesses with merely routine nursing care.

A physician may try to rely on the opinion of the patient's relatives. Family members, particularly children, experience ambiguous feelings. The helplessness felt when faced with mental illness may induce a desire for active therapy of all minor ailments or induce reproaches of neglect against nursing personal. However, the wish to shorten this miserable period of life may induce overtly pronounced death wishes. The family may also grossly overrate the effectiveness of any medical therapy, as illustrated by the case of a wife of a demented patient who stated that the administration of digitalis some years ago prevented the patient's timely death.

Davison (1984) defined one of the primary objectives of geriatric medicine as to prolong active life and shorten the time of dependency and illness before death. Internal medicine makes a very solid contribution to the health and well being of the elderly. But the question remains whether the elderly who are irreversibly impaired both bodily and mentally, should not receive treatment of concomitant diseases? As discussed above, the issue of "quality of life" remains a soft one and again the need to develop recognizable ethical criteria that account for the balance appropriate to the plurality of principles influencing and governing our social system emerges as a primary task of social gerontology and geriatrics.

CLINICAL ASPECTS

Internal medicine plays an important role in distinguishing primary dementing illnesses of the brain from correctable causes of progressive mental deterioration. Already in 1959 Engel and Romano (1959) pointed out that organic brain dysfunction in medically ill patients is common in geriatric units. Significant mental disturbances are observed in more than 50% of the medically ill (Kidd, 1962). According to Wells (1979, 1981) it is also important to distinguish between delirium and dementia. Confusional states are often associated with acute bodily illnesses and can be alleviated by treatment of the underlying disease. Seymour et al. (1980) suggest that from

8 to 20% of the elderly have an acute confusional state on admission to a hospital. Thus, it is particularly in the hospital setting that internal medicine plays an important role in the assessment and therapy of correctable causes of mental deterioration.

Potentially Reversible Mental Disorders

A strategy for dealing with a confused elderly patient is presented in Table 16.1. Life threatening conditions have to be dealt with first: hypoxia as a result of heart failure, pulmonary embolism, pneumonia or intoxication, hypovolemia as a result of a bleeding ulcer or aneurism, acidosis as a result of uncontrolled diabetes or sepsis, shock, hypoglycemia in diabetics, and Wernickes encephalopathy in alcoholics all require immediate medical or surgical therapy.

The next step is to carefully look for systemic disturbances that might produce or aggravate mental deterioration. An extensive overview of causes of potentially reversible mental changes in the elderly are given by Habot and Libow (1980) and by Wieck et al. (1982). Almost all conditions may cause pseudosenility under given circumstances; for example even gallstones may mimick a mental debility in the elderly (Copten, 1984). A previously well-compensated demented elderly person, e.g. with cognitive disturbances but autonomous within his social support system may respond to a new environment, to acute illness, or to a new medication with confusion (Ropper, 1979). Only slight metabolic changes precipitating mental deterioration suggest an underlying hidden pathology. Table 16.1 lists common, amendable medical conditions leading to deterioration in elderly subjects, especially if they already suffer from mental impairment. Dehydration plays an important role (Seymour, 1980) in producing confusional states. It is not always easily recognized in the elderly. A laxness of the skin, a dry tongue, and postural hypotension may not be reliable sings; Therefore, inspection of

TABLE 16.1 Strategy for Dealing with a Confused Elderly Patient

Life threatening conditions:	Hypoxia, hypovolemia, acidosis, Wernicke's encephalopathy, hypoglycemia
Bodily disturbances that can cause/aggravate mental deterioration:	Dehydration, urinary tract obstruction, infections, constipation, drugs, electrolyte imbalance, endocrine disorders, cardiac diseases, pulmonary diseases
Differential diagnosis of neurologic diseases presenting as dementia/confusional states	

the jugular vein in the supine horizontal position is mandatory. Dehydration may include both water and sodium depletion. Volume depletion is also suggested by a high blood urea/creatinine ratio and an elevated osmolality. Especially in the course of diuretic therapy adequate water and electrolyte intake has to be monitored in an elderly patient with mental impairment.

Acute confusional states in psychogeriatric patients may additionally be caused by urinary retention, again possibly a result of medication or obstruction in an indwelling catheter. Infections may induce dehydration in the absence of marked fever. Elevated body temperature may itself cause mental deterioration. Constipation is so common that an emerging fecal impaction leading to ileus is easily overlooked in the early stage.

Polymorbidity causes the elderly to be the leading consumer of medications. The most frequently prescribed are cardiovascular drugs, particularly diuretics, digitalis, and nitrates. In a survey of the very elderly (over 85 years) Knapp et al. (1983) reported that 58% were receiving three or more drugs. Six cardiovascular drugs accounted for 30% of all drugs prescribed. By a variety of mechanisms these drugs may cause confusion and/or dementia, as may the widely used benzodiazepines. Antidepressants, antiparkinson drugs and anticholinergic medication are to be ruled out in persons presenting symptoms of dementia and delirium. "Drug holidays" or, when more appropriate, a dosage reduction will give the answer.

Electrolyte imbalance follows as a result of diuretic therapy. It may result also from inadequate fluid intake, excessive water loss due to diarrhea, vomiting or uncontrolled diabetes mellitus. Diabetes insipidus or inappropriate antidiuretic hormone secretion are less common. Hyponatremia producing lethargy, headache, and anorexia may be difficult to diagnose in a psychogeriatric patient. Again this syndrome can be caused by drugs which induce inappropriate secretion of antidiuretic hormone or by some physical disease.

Uremia is not a rare condition in the elderly. In the psychogeriatric patient, however, the creatinine plasma level may be a poor indicator of renal function due to a large reduction of muscular mass. Impaired renal function alone or in combination with the age related decline may result from multiple factors reducing circulatory blood volume and glomerular filtration rate. Among those renal disorders that contribute to confusional states, drug induced renal failure is very important. Especially, the use of nonsteroidal antiinflammatory drugs may, in the presence of heart failure, lead to rapid deterioration (Clive & Stoff, 1984). Similarly, the combination of aminoglycosides and furosemid has the potential to induce renal failure and has to be carefully monitored.

Among the endocrine disorders, poorly controlled diabetes has to be considered. Hyperparathyroidism may be a cause of hypercalcemia and has to be differentiated from metastatic bone disease. Hypothyroidism mimics many symptoms of the demented patient. Laboratory evaluation of thyroidal hormones are mandatory in the differential diagnosis of dementias. An interesting observation is the fact that in the very old frail subject a large proportion (30%) show no detectable rise in TSH after stimulation with TRH. This suggests that very old people have a diminished TSH-reserve and may explain why they are less capable of coping with stress (Stähelin, 1982). Another corollary is that a diagnosis of hyperthyroidism may wrongly be based on the absence of a rise in TSH after stimulation, as in the presence of a nodular goitre. The diagnosis of hyperthyroidism may thus present difficulties.

A wide variety of cardiac diseases may play an important role in mental deterioration, although some conditions are amazingly well tolerated. In cases of bradycardia in a poorly mobile subject, a pacemaker often does not improve mental function, especially if the bradycardia is well tolerated, suggesting a sufficient cardiac output.

Preventive Medicine

There is, however, one vascular disorder where internal medicine can make a great contribution to the prevention of dementia in old age, and that is through hypertension control. Multiinfarct dementia is closely related to hypertensive artery disease. Other risk factors such as hyperlipidemia may also contribute through arteriosclerosis of the extracranial vessels and subsequent embolization. In a careful retrospective autopsy study we observed in multiinfarct dementia significantly greater signs of antecedent hypertension than in SDAT. An important conclusion is, therefore, that vigorous hypertension control may make a definitive contribution to the prevention of one cause of dementia in the elderly (Stähelin, 1984).

Differential Diagnosis of Neurologic Disorders

The final step in investigating symptoms of dementia is the exclusion of neurological causes. Subdural hematoma usually associated with falls, anticoagulant therapy, intracranial tumors or metastasis, posttraumatic confusional states lasting for prolonged periods of time, and subarachnoid hemorrhage or normal pressure hydrocephalus may be differentiated with the help of the CAT-scan. Lumbar puncture may be indicated in order to differentiate infectious diseases. The EEG can be used to exclude causes due to seizures and may assist in the diagnosis of Creutzfeldt-Jakob disease. A thorough medical workup of every patient suffering from confusion and/or

TABLE 16.2 Diagnostic Tests for the Evaluation of the Elderly Patient with Mental Impairment

Emergencies:	Routine *(cont.)*:
Hemoglobin, hematocrit, white cell count	ECG
Blood gas analysis	Chest X-ray
Quick test or PTT	CAT-scan of the head
Plasma glucose	X-ray of the abdomen
	Urine: glucose, cells (culture if indicated)
Routine:	
Complete blood count	Elective:
Serum electrolytes, BUN, creatinine, liver function, glucose, serum calcium, thyroid hormones	Lumbar puncture
	EEG
	Vitamin B_{12}, folate in plasma
Blood sedimentation rate	Test for syphilis
Quick test or PTT	Drug screening

dementia is the core of a good medical practice. A rapid complete workup is not only more efficacious but also more economical. Table 16.2 gives an overview of the different diagnostic tests.

CONCLUSIONS

In daily practice with the present state of the art, one should probably be less concerned with the clinical differentiation of primary degenerative and multiinfarct dementia since it may not be possible to make the clinical distinction between these two diseases with great confidence (Liston & La Rue, 1983), and in any case specific therapy is not available at this time. There is no question that for scientific reasons this distinction is important. At present it has little impact on the management of the psychogeriatric patient. It is, however, important to diagnose cryptic illnesses presenting as confusion or deterioration in a recently mentally-functioning demented patient (Larson, 1984). A careful recorded history of the patient's illness and a meticulous clinical investigation will allow a diagnosis.

The interface between internal medicine and psychogeriatrics has many facets which will often not be covered exhaustively. Its quintessence may, however, be summed up in a few lines: Geriatric medicine teaches us that there is often not much one can do to improve the life of a psychogeriatric patient. But the psychogeriatric illness is no excuse for not doing the little that one can.

REFERENCES

Bayer, R., Callahan, D., Fletcher, J., et al. (1983). The care of the terminally ill: Morality and economics. *N. Engl. J. Med., 309,* 1490–1494.

Bergener, M., & Stähelin, H. B. (1983). Multidisciplinary aspects of drug therapy in the elderly. In M. Bergener, U. Lehr, E. Lang, R. Schmitz-Scherzer (Eds.). *Aging in the eighties and beyond* (pp 126–135). New York: Springer Publishing Co.

Besdine, R. W. (1983). Decisions to withold treatment from nursing home residents. *J. Am. Ger. Soc., 31,* 602–606.

Brown, N. K., & Thompson, D. J. (1979). Non treatment of fever in extended care facilities. *N. Engl. J. Med., 300,* 1246–1250.

Callahan, D. (1980). Contemporary biomedical ethics. *N. Engl. J. Med., 302,* 1228–1233.

Clive, M. D., & Stoff, J. S. (1984). Renal syndroms associated with nonsteroidal antiinflammatory drugs. *N. Engl. J. Med., 310,* 563–572.

Copten, J., & Lendrum, R., Venables, C. W., James, O. F. W. (1984). Gallstones presenting as mental and physical debility in the elderly. *Lancet, i,* 1062–1063.

Davison, W. (1984). Grundlagen der Therapie im Alter. In M. Bergener & B. Kark (Eds.), *Therapie im Alter* (pp. 1–6). Darmstadt: Steinkopff.

Engel, G. L., & Romano, J. (1959). Delirium—a syndrome of cerebral insufficiency. *J. Chron. Dis., 9,* 260–267.

Fletcher, J. F. (1954). *Morals and medicine. The moral problems of: The patient's right to know the truth, contraception, artificial insemination, sterilization, euthanasia.* Boston: Beacon Press

Fox, M., & Lipton, H. L. (1983). The decision to perform cardiopulmonary resuscitation. *N. Engl. J. Med., 309,* 607–608.

Habot, B., & Libow, L. S. (1980). The interrelationship of mental and physical status and its assessment in the older adult: Mind—body interaction. J. E. Birren, & R. B. Sloane (Eds.). *Handbook of mental health and aging.* Chap. 29. Englewood Cliffs, NJ: Prentice-Hall

Hilfiker, D. (1983). Allowing the debilitated to die: Facing our ethical choices. *N. Engl. J. Med., 308,* 716–719.

Johnson, C. L., & Johnson, F. A. (1983). A microanalysis of "senility": The response of the family and the health professionals. *Culture Med. Psychiatr., 7,* 77–96.

Kidd, C. B. (1962). Criteria for admission of the elderly to geriatric and psychiatric units. *J. Ment. Sci., 108,* 68–73.

Knapp, D. A., Knapp, D. A., Michocki, R. J., Wiser, T. H., & Nuessle, S. J. (1983). Drugs prescribed for circulatory problems in the very elderly. *J. Clin. Exp. Gerontol., 5,* 57–66.

Larson, E. B., Reifler, B. V., Fatherstone, H. J., & English, D. J. (1984). Dementia in elderly outpatients: A prospective study. *Ann. Int. Med., 100,* 417–423.

Liston, H. E., & La Rue, A. (1983). Clinical differentiation of primary degenerative and multi-infarct dementia: A critical review of the evidence: Part I: Clinical studies. *Biological Psychiatry, 18,* 1451–1484.

McCullough, L. B. (1984). Medical care for elderly patients with diminished competence. *J. Am. Ger. Soc., 32,* 150–3.

Murphy, E. (1984). Ethical dilemmas of brain failure in the elderly. *Brit. Med. J., 288,* 61–2.

President's Commission for the Study of the Ethical Problems in Medicine and Biomedical and Behavioral Research. (1983). *Deciding to forego life sustaining treatment* (pp. 236–239). Washington, DC: U.S. Government Printing Office.

Ramsey, P. (1970). *The Patient as Person: Explorations in Medical Ethics.* New Haven, CN: Yale University Press

Rawls, J. (1971). *A Theory of Justice.* Cambridge: Harvard University Press.

Reenpää, Y., (1973). Ueber das Körper-Seele Problem. In H. G. Gadamer & D. Vogler (Eds.), *Neue Anthropologie* Band 5. Stuttgart: Thieme

Ropper, A. H. (1979). A rational approach to dementia. *Can. Med. Assoc., 121,* 1175–1190.

Seymour, D. G., Henschke, P. J., Cape, R. D. T., & Campbell, A. J. (1980). Acute confusional states and dementia in the elderly: The role of dehydration, volume depletion, physical illness, and age. *Age Ageing, 9,* 137–146.

Stähelin, H. B., Hew-Winzeler, A. M., Behrends, D., Seiler, W. O., & Ulrich, J. (1984). Unsolved clinical problems in advanced senile dementia. *Modern Aging Res., 5,* 269–277.

Stähelin, H. B., Staub, J. J., Hew-Winzeler, A. M., Seiler, W. O., & Girard, J. (1982). Die TRH-TSH-Regulation beim Hochbetagten und bei Patienten mit seniler Demenz. *Schweiz med Wschr, 112,* 1784–1786.

Wanzer, S. H., Adelstein, S. J., Cranford, R. E., et al. (1984). The physicians responsibility toward hopelessly ill patients. *N. Engl. J. Med., 310,* 955–959.

Wells, C. E. (1979). Diagnosis of dementia. *Psychosomatics, 20,* 517–522.

Wells, C. E. (1981) The organic brain syndromes. *Psychiatr. Clin. N. Am., 4,* 319–331.

Wieck, H. H., Brückmann, J. U., Lang, C., & Blaha, L. (1982) Senile dementia. In D. Platt (Ed.), *Geriatrics 1, Cardiology and vascular system, central nervous system.* Berlin: Springer Verlag.

17
Nutrition and the Elderly

Bertil Steen

Because the prevalence of acute and chronic disease rapidly increases with advancing age, and since a proper diet during disease is a prerequisite if the specific therapy is to have an optimal effect (Isaksson, 1975), the nutritional state of the elderly is of special importance. Thus the relatively high prevalence of disease and the special psychosocial conditions present in the higher age groups call for special attendance.

Items to be discussed in this respect include, not only the possibility of different needs for energy and nutrients in old age, but also the specific nutritional risks at this age and possibilities for intervention.

DIET

It is a widespread opinion that elderly people have less adequate dietary habits than the population as a whole. This seems not to be the truth, at least not in the eighth decade of life (Steen et al., 1977, Lundgren et al., 1987). Furthermore, elderly people seem to change their dietary habits in the same direction and in approximately the same degree as the population as a whole (Lundgren et al., 1987). Variation is great, however, and risk indicators and risk factors relating to less adequate nutrition exist.

Requirements

Energy

Energy metabolism decreases with advancing age, because of the decreasing number of cells in the organs, loss of metabolizing tissue, and reduced physical activity (Shock, 1972). Age related intracellular changes seem to play a minor role in this respect. In one study of healthy male individuals (McGandy et al., 1966) the average total energy expenditure was 2811 kcal/11.8 MJ and 1924 kcal/8.2 MJ at age 30 and 80, respectively. The proportion of energy expenditure due to physical activity was much higher in the young than in the old males in that study. On the other hand, energy expenditure due to basal metabolism showed just moderate decrease with age. These proportions can of course vary greatly between different populations due to differences in physical exercise habits. When discussing the energy requirements of the elderly it must be borne in mind that the elderly age-group is very heterogeneous. This is true for example of physical activity, degree of health and disease, and body weight, which might obviously change the requirements of both energy and some nutrients.

Protein

For practical purposes there seems to be no need for different protein recommendations for healthy elderly individuals than for younger age groups; the average need of protein may not be different in the healthy elderly (Cheng et al., 1978; Zanni et al., 1979). However, the present knowledge of protein requirements is based mainly on studies in younger populations, and there are some studies indicating differences in protein metabolism in the elderly compared to younger individuals. Both early studies (e.g., Kountz et al., 1951; Albanese et al., 1957) and more recent balance studies (Munro & Young 1978; Uyau et al., 1978) indicate that at least some elderly individuals require more dietary protein to maintain nitrogen balance. Werner and Hambraeus (1972) claimed that the elderly have a reduced tolerance to high protein loads, based on studies in which a daily protein intake of 100 g or more often resulted in a higher fecal nitrogen loss in elderly than in younger individuals. Some authors report a higher need for some amino acids in the elderly (Ackerman & Kheim, 1964; Tuttle et al., 1965). However, reports suggesting no higher needs in the elderly (Wehr & Lewis, 1966; Young, 1976) show that further studies are needed in this field.

Some of the existing controversies may be due to variations in the degree of health of the different populations under study. The need for dietary protein is often greater in disease states (Isaksson, 1973), which emphasizes its importance in elderly people. The protein situation is also related to the energy status. Thus, in a situation with low protein intake, there can be an increased need for energy to maintain nitrogen balance (Garza et al., 1976), and energy intake seems to have a greater effect on nitrogen balance than protein intake at marginal intakes of protein and energy (Calloway, 1975). This is of special importance in elderly with small food intakes, whether outside or inside the hospital. The common recommendation of daily dietary intake of protein of 0.8 g per kg body weight must be looked upon as a minimum in the higher age groups.

Thiamin

There are early studies suggesting an impaired utilization of thiamin in the elderly (Horwitt et al., 1948; Oldham, 1962). Therefore, the commonly used dietary allowances, such as the U.S. Recommended Dietary Allowances (Food and Nutrition Board, 1980), recommend higher allowances per 1000 kcal at low energy intakes.

Vitamin D

In its ninth edition the RDA for the first time recommend a dietary intake of vitamin D in adults of 5 μg a day, because some elderly people may have an insufficient intake of vitamin D and at the same time no access to sunlight (Food and Nutrition Board, 1980). Osteomalacia due to these factors can be one cause of skeletal rarefaction in the elderly (Exton-Smith et al., 1966).

Ascorbic Acid

Many studies (e.g., Andrews & Brook, 1966; Loh & Wilson, 1971) have shown low ascorbic acid levels in blood, especially in males. Although supplementation has been shown to increase the leucocyte levels (e.g., Burr et al., 1975), the clinical importance of the low blood levels and of supplementation is unclear.

Calcium

Most recommendations suggest a daily intake of calcium of 600–800 mg. The fact that a calcium balance can be maintained with lower intakes in some adults has produced even lower recommendations. Thus, FAO/WHO (1962) suggested a "practical allowance" for adults of 400 to 500 mg per day.

However, the efficiency of calcium absorption seems to decrease with advancing age (Avioli et al., 1965; Bullamore et al., 1970). This has been explained partially by vitamin D deficiency, since vitamin D treatment has been shown to increase absorption (Nordin, 1971). Furthermore, physical inactivity, common in house-bound elderly, may alter calcium balance.

Some evidence is now available that calcium levels below 500 mg per day may give rise to a negative calcium balance (Johnson et al., 1970; Linkswiler et al., 1974). Although there are indications that there is an increased need for calcium in older age groups, most authors do not feel that a recommendation to increase the recommended dietary allowances for these age groups is called for at present.

Iron

The recommended daily allowance for the higher age groups is 10 mg. However, the need for iron may be greater than that in some elderly people because of the high prevalence of iron losses from the gastrointestinal tract. The most common sources of such bleeding is an atrophic gastric mucosa and a diverticular colon.

Potassium

Inadequate dietary intake of potassium is one of many causes of potassium deficiency in the elderly. Others include diuretic treatment, secondary hyperaldosteronism due to conditions such as chronic heart disease or liver failure, and misuse of laxative or licorice. Often potassium deficiency is due to a combination of etiological factors in elderly patients.

Dietary Fiber

Dietary fiber—defined as the sum of the indigestible carbohydrate and carbohydrate-like components of food—has a relation to several conditions common in old age, such as constipation, cancer of the colon, and diabetes (for review see Burkitt and Trowell, 1975, Roth and Mehlman, 1978). The most commonly used dietary recommendations do not include dietary fiber. However, most elderly in industrialized countries should be recommended to increase their consumption of fiber-rich food items.

Water

Dehydration is especially dangerous in elderly persons because there is a deficit in thirst and water intake in the elderly as shown recently by Phillips et al. (1984). Such risks are especially obvious in the presence of infection with fever, diarrhea, and renal diseases (for review see Massler, 1979); severe symptoms, such as mental confusion and circulatory insufficiency, may result.

Dietary habits

Although knowledge of the dietary habits of elderly populations is scarce for many parts of the world, there exist several dietary surveys from countries such as Sweden, Great Britain, and the United States. Of special importance are such broad population studies that include not only data on intake of energy and nutrients and meal habits, but also sociopsychological and medical data.

These dietary surveys have used many different methods of different validity, so special attention must be given to the methods used. This is also true regarding the degree of representativeness of the population samples under study. The principal methods used are weighing, and record and interview methods (for review see Roine and Pekkarinen, 1968). The most suitable methods in epidemiological work are interview methods (for review see Marr, 1971, and Steen, 1977a). The importance of validity tests in dietary surveys has been underlined by, for example, Isaksson (1980), who suggests that comparisons of nitrogen analyses of 24-hour urine samples and the calculated dietary intake of protein should be performed. On the basis of such tests Steen et al. (1977) showed that the dietary history method, originally described by Burke (1947), was more valid than the commonly used 24-hour recall method.

Results from dietary surveys of elderly people in Sweden and Great Britain are very much in agreement, and show that dietary habits were on average good in these age groups, but that variation was great, with standard deviations being in the order of 25% regarding intakes of energy and nutrients (Panel on Nutrition of the Elderly, 1972; McLeod et al., 1974a, 1974b, 1975; Rinder et al., 1975; Steen et al., 1977; Committee on Medical Aspects of Policy, 1979; Lundgren et al., 1985). As examples, data from the Swedish study will be given. Average energy intakes were 9.8 MJ and 8.1 MJ for males and females, respectively, corresponding well to the British studies. As mentioned earlier, variation was great regarding nutrient intakes in spite of sufficient average intakes. Thus, not less than 18% of the subjects showed protein intake values below 0.7 g per kg body weight, and riboflavin intake in the lowest decentile group of both sexes was below the minimum recommendation value of 0.4 mg per 1000 kcal per day. The ascorbic acid situation seemed to be much better in Sweden than in Great Britain, where about 5% of the subjects had less than 10 mg of ascorbic acid daily. However, the regional variation was considerable. Taking all studied nutrients together, it may be generally concluded that a substantial proportion of subjects showed intakes below recommended standards, although the average intake values were rather high.

Malnutrition

Obvious undernutrition seems to be uncommon in the elderly in Europe. In the British studies mentioned earlier 3% of the probands aged 65 and over were judged to be malnourished. Six years later the incidence in the same probands had increased to 7%. It was, however, very uncommon that the condition was not associated with nonnutritional disease.

During the last few years attention has been drawn to "hospital malnutrition," reported from many countries, such as Denmark (Hessov, 1977), Sweden (Steen, 1980), Great Britain (Hacket et al., 1979), and the United States (Steffee, 1980). For the elderly, chronically ill patients in hospitals and nursing homes especially the dietary problem seems to be largely a quantitative one, with an urgent need to consume enough energy, rather than a qualitative one. Such patients may have many reasons for an inadequate intake of food, including disease per se, inadequate drug therapy, physical or mental handicaps, low physical activity, bad meal environment, poor dental state or oral hygiene, and an unsuitable distribution of meals throughout the day.

Obesity

It is well known that very old people are usually thin. Sometimes the explanation is given that this depends on a selective mortality of fat people. However, at least to some degree, the explanation is a decreasing amount of body fat in the same individuals, apparently starting somewhat earlier (age 75) in females than in males. This fact has an obvious bearing when discussing indications for the therapy of obesity in the elderly (for review see Steen, 1985a). The risks of obesity are still under debate, especially when speaking of elderly individuals and populations. While it is generally agreed that obesity is associated with a number of major conditions common in higher age groups, such as coronary heart disease (Gordon & Kannel, 1973), hypertension (Kannel et al., 1967), cerebrovascular disease (Heyden et al., 1971), glucose intolerance (Gordon, 1969), and osteoarthritis of the weight-bearing joints (Leach et al., 1973), the relation to mortality is still somewhat obscure.

Recently, Andres (1980) reviewed a number of population studies regarding the relation between obesity in the aged and mortality, and found that the hypothesis that obesity is a graded variable in its impact on mortality, and that even minor degrees of obesity are detrimental, could not be supported by data from the studies reviewed. However, crude relation analyses between obesity and mortality have to be interpreted with great caution. Possible confounding factors such as tobacco smoking are important in this respect, and such factors can be different in different regions of the world.

The understanding of obesity requires knowledge of many different etiological and pathophysiological aspects of the condition. In geriatric medicine the nutritional and physical activity aspects are the most relevant. The nutrient density of the food is especially important in a low-energy consumer group of individuals such as the elderly. Ordinary food in most industrialized countries has a low nutrient density because of a high proportion of fat and refined sugar. Therefore, intake of the same type of food in old age as earlier in life might give either too much energy, too little essential nutrients, or both. It is thus important to realize that malnutrition means undernutrition, overnutrition, or both at the same time, because undernutrition of essential nutrients can be combined with overnutrition of fat, refined sugar, and energy.

Some studies have shown a relationship between social factors and obesity in old age. The socioeconomic status is inversely related to the prevalence of obesity, especially in females (Burnight & Marden, 1967; Bray, 1978). Loneliness also seems to have some relation to both decreased and increased appetite, as shown by Mellström and Steen (1981).

Treatment of obesity in old age should be instituted with great caution, demanding more rigorous indications before intervention. This is especially true in the oldest age groups, since physiological aging seems to be related to a progressive loss of body fat. Surgical methods should be avoided, and drug therapy is questionable. The methods of choice are to try changes of diet, physical activity, and sometimes behavior. An attractive principle is to use large amounts of dietary fiber as an adjunct in the treatment (Albanese, 1980).

BODY COMPOSITION

Knowledge of the human body composition is essential in both gerontology and geriatric medicine. The measurements of the amounts of body fat and body cell mass is of value when judging the net effect of energy intake and expenditure, and the body cell mass is a better reference than body weight or body surface area when judging an individual's energy exchange and work performance.

Some authors still use the concept of "lean body mass," that is, body weight minus adipose tissue. However, since the body is not a simple two-compartment system, and since "lean body mass" is a heterogenic body compartment, many authors nowadays prefer the concept of body cell mass as a better estimate of the metabolically active tissue than lean body mass (Moore et al., 1963).

As demonstrated by several studies (Allen et al., 1960; Burmeister & Bingert, 1967; Forbes & Reina, 1970; Novak, 1972; Shukla et al., 1973) body cell mass decreases with age. In one longitudinal study body cell mass decreased by on average 1 kg and 0.6 kg for males and females, respectively, between the ages of 70 and 75 (Steen et al., 1979), but decreased significantly during the period 70 to 79 years of age only in males (Steen et al., 1981).

Many studies show an increase of body fat with age, especially when expressed as a percentage of body weight. However, in the eighth decade of life, body fat changes seem to be rather small (Steen et al., 1985).

Changes in the amount of body water, especially in certain situations, may be of very high importance in the elderly. In the eighth decade of life, where body weight is decreasing rather markedly in both sexes, a longitudinal study covering ages 70 to 81 (Steen et al., 1985) showed that a major cause of this decrease of body weight was a decreasing amount of body water, especially extracellular water. This seems to be a feature of normal aging, although it may be counteracted by changes in cardiac and renal function that increase the amount of body water, also in individuals without obvious signs of heart of kidney disease.

SPECIFIC NUTRITIONAL ASPECTS

Data from the literature regarding the influence of *dental state* upon the dietary intake are contradictory and somewhat confusing (for review see Steen, 1985b). Many authors have found that elderly people with a poor dental state experienced difficulty in ingesting items such as meat and hard foods but few have found a similar relationship between dental state and the intake of energy and nutrients.

The *nutrition-immunity* interactions in old age have been discussed in detail, especially the last few years. It has been shown that dietary supplementation in elderly people with nutritional deficiency results in an improved immunocompetence in terms of cutaneous hypersensitivity, lymphocyte proliferation response to nitrogens and antigens, and alterations in T cell subsets (Chandra, 1985).

Also, the relationship of dietary factors to cerebral function is a matter of investigation and debate. However, administration of lecithin and choline have failed to benefit patients with Alzheimer's disease in short-term studies. The possibility that long-term treatment may retard the progression of the disease is still under investigation. Clinical trials of tryptophan in depression are inconclusive, but studies using tyrosine are more encouraging (Huff & Growdon, 1985).

PUBLIC HEALTH ASPECTS

The public health basis for nutrition intervention programs varies from country to country because of different demographic, social, psychological, and medical factors, apart from the nutritional status of the population. Also, attitudes toward the elderly themselves are major obstacles to the possibility of sticking to world-wide nutritional intervention programs. (Selby & Schechter, 1982; for review see Steen, 1977b).

Well-known groups of elderly people at special risk of developing malnutrition are those elderly with lower education and lower income levels (Steen et al., 1977b); those housebound; those bereaved; those having no regular cooked meals; those with physical disability, depression and other mental disorder; and those in the lowest social classes who receive a supplementary benefit (Panel on Nutrition of the Elderly, 1972; Committee on Medical Aspects of Food Policy, 1979; Exton-Smith, 1980).

Some social factors and characteristics of the elderly population are of special importance in this context, at least in most industrialized countries, namely, the predominance of females, social isolation, misuse of alcohol, and housing, including facilities for storage and cooking of food.

There is a general agreement that elderly people should be helped to lead independent lives in their own homes for as long as possible (United Nations, 1982). This requires support from society and the family and/or voluntary bodies. Home-help services are very important (International Federation on Aging, 1975; Mellström & Steen, 1981).

The Report of the World Assembly on Aging held in Vienna in 1982 (United Nations, 1982) offers some pointers for the future. According to that report special attention should be paid to the improvement of the availability of sufficient food stuffs; fair and equitable distribution of food; public education, including for the elderly, in correct nutrition and eating habits; provision of health and dental services for early detection of malnutrition and improvement of mastication; studies of the nutritional status of the elderly at the community level; and the extension of research on the role of nutritional factors in the aging process to communities in developing countries.

REFERENCES

Ackerman, P. G., & Kheim, T. (1964). Plasma amino acids in young and older adult human subjects. *Clin. Chem., 10,* 32.
Albanese, A. A. (1980). *Nutrition for the elderly.* New York; Alan R. Liss.
Albanese, A. A., Higgons, R. A., Orto, L. A., & Zavattaro, D. N. (1957). Protein and amino acid need of the aged in health and convalescence. *Geriatrics, 12,* 465.
Allen, T. H., Anderson, E. C., & Langham, W. H. (1960). Total body potassium and gross body composition in relation to age. *J. Gerontol., 15,* 348.
Andres, R. (1980). Influence of obesity on longevity in the aged. In C. Borek, C. M. Fenoglio, D. W. King (Eds.), *Aging, cancer and cell membranes* (p. 238). Stuttgart: Thiene.
Andrews, J., & Brook, M. (1966). Leucocyte-vitamin C content and clinical signs in the elderly. *Lancet, i,* 1350.

Avioli, L. V., McDonald, J. E., & Lee, S. W. (1965). The influence of age on the intestinal absorption of 47 Ca in women and its relation to 47 Ca absorption in postmenopausal osteoporosis. *J. Clin. Invest, 44,* 1960.

Bray, G. A. (1978). Definition, measurement, and classification of the syndromes of obesity. *Int. J. Obesity., 2,* 99.

Bullamore, J. R., Gallagher, J. C., Wilkinson, R., Nordin, B. E. C., & Marshall, D. M. (1970). The effect of age on calcium absorption. *Lancet, ii,* 535.

Burke, B. S. (1947) The dietary history as a tool in research. *J. Am. Diet. Assoc., 23,* 1041.

Burkitt, D. P., & Trowell, H. H. (1975). *Refined carbohydrate foods and disease.* New York: Academic Press

Burmeister, W., & Bingert, A. (1967). Die quantitativen Veranderungen der menschlichen Zellmasse zwischen dem 8. und 90. Lebensjahr. *Klin Wochenschr, 45,* 409.

Burnight, R. G., & Marden, P. G. (1967). Social correlates of weight in an aging population. *Milbank Mem, Fund. Q., 45,* 75.

Burr, M. L., Hurley, R. J., & Sweetnam, P. M. (1975). Vitamin C supplementation of old people with low blood levels. *Geront. Clin., 17,* 236.

Calloway, D. H. (1975). Nitrogen balance of men with marginal intakes of protein and energy. *J. Nutr., 105,* 914.

Chandra, R. K. (1985). Nutrition-immunity infection interactions in old age. In R. K. Chandra. (Ed.), *Nutrition, immunity and illness in the elderly* (pp. 87–96). New York: Pergamon Press.

Cheng, A. H. R., Gomez, A., Bergan, J. G., Lee, T. C., Moncheberg, F., & Chichester, C. O. (1978). Comparative nitrogen balance study between young and aged adults using three levels of protein intake from a combination wheat-soy-milk mixture. *Am. J. Clin. Nutr., 31,* 12.

Committee on Medical Aspects of Food Policy. (1979). *Nutrition and health in old age* (Dept. Health Social Security Report on Health and Social Subjects No. 16). London: HMSO

Exton-Smith, A. N. (1980). Nutritional status: diagnosis and prevention of malnutrition. In A.N. Exton Smith, F. I. Caird (Eds.), *Metabolic and nutritional disorders in the elderly* (p. 66).

Exton-Smith, A. N., Hodkinson, H. M., & Stanton, B. R. (1966). Nutrition and metabolic bone disease in old age. *Lancet, ii,* 999.

FAO/WHO (1962). Calcium requirements. *Report of an FAO/WHO expert committee on calcium requirements* (WHO Tech Rep Series 230). Rome: FAO.

Food and Nutrition Board. (1980). *Recommended dietary allowances* (9th ed.). Washington, D.C.: National Academy of Sciences

Forbes, R. M., & Reina, J. C. (1970). Adult lean body mass declines with age: Some longitudinal observations. *Metabolism, 19,* 653.

Garza, C., Scrimshaw, N. S., & Young, U. R. (1976). Human protein requirements: The effect of variations in energy intake within the maintenance range. *Am. J. Clin. Nutr., 29,* 280.

Gordon, E. S. (1969) Obesity: gluttony or genes? *Postgrad. Med., 45,* 95.

Gordon, T., & Kannel, W. B. (1973). The effects of obesity on cardiovascular disease. *Geriatrics, 28,* 80.

Hacket, A. F., Yeung, C. K., & Hill, G. L. (1979). Eating patterns in patients recovering from major surgery—a study of voluntary food intake and energy balance. *Br. J. Surg., 66,* 415.

Hessov, I. (1972). Energy and protein intake in elderly patients in an orthopedic surgical ward. *Acta, Chir, Scand., 143,* 145.

Heyden, S., (1971). Hames, C. G., Bartel, A., Cassel, J. C., Tyroler, H. A., & Cornoni, S. C. (1971) Weight and weight history in relation to cerebrovascular and ischaemic heart disease. *Arch. Intern. Med., 128,* 956.
Horwitt, M. K., Liebert, E., Kreisler, O., & Wittman, P. (1948). *Investigations of human requirements for B-complex vitamins* (NRC Bull. No. 116). Washington, D.C.: Nat. Acad. Sci.
Huff, F. J., & Growdon, J. H. (1985). Nutrition and neuropsychiatric illness. In R. K. Chandra (Ed.), *Nutrition, immunity and illness in the elderly* (pp. 203–212). Oxford, England: Pergamon Press.
International Federation on Aging: (1975) *Home-help services for the aging around the world.* Washington, D.C.: author.
Isaksson, B. (1973). Clinical nutrition. Requirements of energy and nutrients in diseases. *Bibl. Nutr. Diet., 19,* 1.
Isaksson, B. (1975). Future trends in clinical nutrition. *Bibl. Nutr. Diet, 21,* 163.
Isaksson, B. (1980). Urinary nitrogen output as a validity test in dietary surveys. *Am. J. Clin. Nutr., 33,* 4.
Johnson, N. E., Alcantara, E. N., & Linkswiler, H. M. (1970). Effect of protein intake on urinary and fecal calcium and calcium retention of young adult males. *J. Nutr., 100,* 1425.
Kannel, W. B., Brand, N., Skinner, J. J., Jr., Dawbeer, T. R., & McNamara, P. M. (1967). The relation of adiposity to blood pressure and development of hypertension. *Ann. Intern. Med., 67,* 48.
Kountz, W. B., Hofstatter, L., & Ackerman, P. (1951). Nitrogen balance studies in four elderly men. *J. Gerontol., 6,* 20.
Leach, R. E., Baumgard, S., & Bloom, J. (1973). Obesity: Its relationship to osteoarthritis of the knee. *Clin. Ortop., 93,* 271.
Linkswiler, H. M., Joyce, C. L., & Arnaud, C. R. (1974). Calcium retention of young adult males as affected by level of protein and of calcium intake. *Trans. N.Y. Acad. Sci., 36,* 333.
Loh, H. S., & Wilson, C. W. M. (1971). Relationship between leucocyte ascorbic acid and hemoglobin levels at different ages. *Int. J. Vitamin Nutr. Res., 41,* 259.
Lundgren, B. K., Steen, B., & Isaksson, B. (1987). Dietary habits in 70 and 75-year-old males and females. Longitudinal and cohort data from a population study. *Näringsforskning* (in press).
Marr, J. W. (1971). Individual dietary surveys. Purposes and methods. *World Rev. Nutr. Diet, 13,* 105 (Karger, Basel).
Massler, M. (1979). Geriatric nutrition II: Dehydration in the elderly. *J. Prosthet. Dent., 42,* 489.
McGandy, R. B., Barrows, C. H., Jr., Spanias, A., Meredith, A., Stone, J. L., & Norris, A. H. (1966). Nutrient intakes and energy expenditure in men of different ages. *J. Gerontol., 21,* 581.
McLeod, C. C., Judge, T. G., & Caird, F. I. (1974a). Nutrition of the elderly at home. I. Intakes of energy, protein, carbohydrates and fat. *Age Ageing, 3,* 158.
McLeod, C. C., Judge, T. G., & Caird, F. I. (1974b). Nutrition of the elderly at home. II. Intakes of vitamins. *Age Ageing, 3,* 209.
McLeod, C. C., Judge, T. G., & Caird, F. I. (1975). Nutrition of the elderly at home (III). Intakes of minerals. *Age Ageing, 4,* 49.
Mellström, D., & Steen, B. (1981). Some examples of relations between social factors and dietary habits in 70-year-old people. In E. Beverfelt, A. C. Julsrud, H. Kjoerstad, & A. M. Nygård (Eds.), *Nordisk gerontologi.* Oslo: Hammerstad Boktrykkeri.

Moore, F. D., Olesen, K. H., McMurrey, J. D., Parker, H. V., Ball, M. R., & Boyden, C. M. (1963). *The body cell mass and its supporting environment.* Philadelphia, London: Saunders.
Munro, H. N., & Young, U. R. (1978). Protein metabolism in the elderly. *Postgrad. Med., 63,* 143.
Nordin, B. E. C. (1971). Clinical significance and pathogenesis of osteoporosis. *Br. Med. J., 1,* 571.
Novak, L. P. (1972). Aging, total body potassium, fat-free mass and cell mass in males and females between ages 18 and 85 years. *J. Gerontol., 27,* 438.
Oldham, H. G. (1962). Thiamine requirements of women. *Ann. Ny. Acad. Sci., 98,* 542.
Panel on Nutrition of the Elderly (1972). *A nutrition survey of the elderly.* (Dept, Health Social Security Report on Health and Social Subjects No. 3). London: HMSO.
Phillips, P. A., Rolls, B. J., Ledingham, J. G. G., Forshing, M. L., Morton, J. J., Crowe, M. J., & Wollner, L. (1984). Reduced thirst after water deprivation in healthy elderly men. *N. Eng. J. Med., 311,* 753.
Rinder, L., Roupe, S., Steen, B., & Svanborg, A. (1975) 70-year-old people in Gothenburg. A population study in an industrialized Swedish city. General presentation of the study (I). *Acta Med. Scand., 198,* 397.
Roine, P., & Pekkarinen, M. (1968). Methodology of dietary studies. In G. Ritzel (Ed.), *Richtlinien gesunder Ernährung.* Inter Z. Vit. forsch, Vol. 31, Beiheft II.
Roth, H. P., & Mehlman, MA (Eds.) (1978). Symposium on role of dietary fiber in health. *Am. J. Clin. Nutr., 31,* 1.
Selby, P., & Schechter, M. (1982). *Aging 2000: A challenge for society.* Lancaster, Boston, The Hague: MTP Press Ltd.
Shock, N. W. (1972). Energy metabolism, caloric intake and physical activity of the aging. In L. A. Carlson (Ed.), *Nutrition in old age.* Symposia of the Swedish Nutrition Foundation (p. 12). Uppsala: Almqvist & Wiksell.
Shukla, K. K., Ellis, K. J., Dombrowski, C. S., & Cohn, S. H. (1973). Physiological variation of total-body potassium in man. *Am. J. Physiol., 224,* 271.
Steen, B. (1980). Intake of protein in geriatric long-term care patients. *Akt. Gerontol., 10,* 515.
Steen, B. (1985b). Nutrition. In M. S. J. Pathy *Principles and practice of geriatric medicine.* (pp. 241–261). Chicester, England; Wiley. Ltd.
Steen, B. (1977a). Nutrition in 70-year-olds. Dietary habits and body composition. A report from the population study of 70-year-old people in Gothenburg, Sweden. *Näringsforskning, 21,* 201.
Steen, B. (1985a). Obesity in the aged. In R. Watson (Ed.), *Handbook on nutrition in the aged.* Boca Raton, FL: CRC Press.
Steen, B. (1977b). *Public health aspects of nutrition of the elderly: Report on a study.* Copenhagen: WHO
Steen, B., Isaksson, B., & Svanborg, A. (1979). Body composition at 70 and 75 years of age. A longitudinal population study. *J. Clin. Exper. Gerontol, 1* 185.
Steen, B., Isaksson, B., & Svanborg, A. (1981). Body composition at 70, 75, and 79 years of age. A longitudinal population study. *Proceedings from Twelfth International Congress of Nutrition,* San Diego (p. 102).
Steen, B., Isaksson, B., & Svanborg, A. (1977). Intake of energy and nutrients and meal habits in 70-year-old males and females in Gothenburg, Sweden. A population study. *Acta Med. Scand., (Suppl) 611,* 39.

Steen, B., Lundgren, B. K., & Isaksson, B. (1985). Body composition at age 70, 75, 79, and 81. A longitudinal population study. In R. K. Chandra (Ed.), *Nutrition, immunity and illness in the elderly* (pp. 49–51). New York: Pergamon Press.

Steffee, W. P. (1980). Malnutrition in hospitalized patients. *JAMA, 244,* 2630.

Tuttle, S. G., Basset, S. H., Griffith, W. H., Mulcare, D. B., & Swendseid, M. E. (1965). Further observations on the amino acid requirements of older men. *Am. J. Clin. Nutr., 16,* 229.

United Nations (1982). *Report of the world assembly on aging,* Vienna, United Nations, New York, Uyau, R., Scrimshaw, N. S., & Young, V. R. (1978). Human protein requirements. N-balance response to graded intakes of egg protein in elderly men and women. *Am. J. Clin. Nutr., 31,* 779.

Wehr, R. F., & Lewis, G. T. (1966). Amino acids in blood plasma of young and aged adults. *Proc. Soc. Exp. Biol. Med., 121,* 349.

Werner, I., & Hambraeus, L. (1972). The digestive capacity of elderly people. In L. A. Carlson (Ed.), *Nutrition in old age.* X Symposia of the Swedish Nutrition Foundation (p. 55). Uppsala: Almqvist & Wiksell.

Young V. R. (1976). Protein metabolism and needs in elderly people. In M. Rockstein, M. L. Sussman (Eds.), *Nutrition, longevity, and aging* (p. 67). New York: Academic Press Inc.

Zanni, E., Calloway, D. H., & Zezulka, A. Y. (1979). Protein requirements of elderly men. *J. Nutr., 109,* 513.

18
Drug Therapy in the Elderly—Biochemical, Pharmacological, and Clinical Considerations

Christof Hesse and Kevin O'Malley

Elderly persons already account for a significant portion of all patients seen in medical practice. They represent a rather heterogeneous group of human beings (Dengler, 1982), consisting of persons of various chronological and biological age; those with or (rarely) without concomitant disease; smokers and nonsmokers; those found in various physical states as a result of differences in nutrition and with very dissimilar levels of physical and intellectual competence.

The definition of a "gerontopharmacology" seems, however, justified by several common and important factors that differentiate this patient group from that of younger adults:

- Elderly patients sometimes react to drug treatment in ways unexpected and different than younger adults.
- Pharmacokinetic parameters in the elderly differ from those in a younger adult population.
- Elderly patients, for the most part, suffer from more than one disease concurrently. This condition is usually referred to as "multimorbidity."

Following a short survey of our present knowledge of special biological and pharmacological conditions in treating the elderly, selected classes of drugs and their application in geriatrics will be discussed. Finally, consequences of this treatment for the elderly will be described.

BIOLOGICAL CHANGES IN THE ELDERLY

Tissue characteristics and physiological processes vary considerably over the lifetime of an individual. The greatest changes are seen in the very young and the very old. Ideally, terms such as "very young" and "very old" are best used with reference to the biological age of the individual. Because this is not practicable we use chronological age instead. This could be the reason for the great biological and pharmacological variability found in groups of elderly of similar calendar years.

Among the many important age-related changes, the following are of particular relevance to our considerations: Body weight normally decreases with increasing age, and concomitantly adipose tissue doubles at the expense of functional parenchyma (Gregerman et al, 1962; Forbes & Reina, 1970; Novak, 1972). Body water decreases (Edelman & Leibman, 1959). Cardiac output decreases by 30 to 40%, and splanchnic and renal function deteriorates nearly linearly with age (Brandfonbrener et al., 1955; Bender, 1965; Sherlock et al., 1950). There are also some functional changes in the gastrointestinal tract which theoretically could interfere with drug absorption. For example, a decrease in gastric acid output with a subsequent increase in the gastric pH, could affect ionization and thus the solubility of drugs. There is a sound probability that the number of absorbing cells will be reduced with age. Finally, an increased incidence of duodenal diverticles, due to bacterial colonization in the small intestine, appears to be the principal cause of malabsorption of some substances in the elderly.

The situation associated with different protein fractions and enzyme systems is not so straightforward. Plasma albumin decreases by 10%, while the globulin fraction increases (Woodford-Williams et al., 1964; Goldman, 1971; Leask et al., 1973). Alpha-1-acid glycoprotein, which binds basic drugs, tends to increase with aging, but there is some debate as to what is caused by aging per se and what is caused by the common pathological conditions found in this age group. There is essentially no change in the activity of the conjugation enzyme system (glucuronidation, sulfatation, acetylation), whereas the activity of the mixed functional oxidase system decreases and that of the monoaminooxidase system increases with advancing age. These changes have important implications for drug therapy as they are the basis for pharmacokinetic changes (absorption, distribution, transport, metabolization, and excretion).

There are many pharmacodynamic factors that change with aging. The more important of them include receptor function, homeostasis, postreceptor biochemistry, and structural changes (see O'Malley & Kelly, 1983). Beta-adrenoceptor response decreases with age but the response to the anticoagulant effect of warfarin increases. Diminished homeostatic responses are a hallmark of aging and cause the body to be less able to counteract perturbations caused by drugs. Thus the elderly are likely to have increased responses and a greater tendency to adverse drug reactions. Structural changes, for example, in the vascular system and the kidney have shown implications for the circulatory action of drugs.

GENERAL PHARMACOKINETIC OBSERVATIONS

Absorption

Although a lowered rate of absorption could be expected from the data cited above, studies employing such different drugs as Propicillin, indomethacin, Paracetamol, sulfamethizole, aspirin, Practolol and quinine showed no significant differences in the elderly compared with younger adult probands (see Stevenson, 1979, for a review). Data from a few very old patients (over 75 years of age) suggest such a possibility in the case of the tetracyclic antidepressant maprotiline (Bergener et al., 1984). According to these data, a diminished absorption should be found only in very old patients and then only to a small or moderate degree. Further studies in all classes of drugs are certainly necessary and justified.

Distribution

As a consequence of the changes noted above, the actual volume of distribution (V_d) of a given drug changes with age. The way it changes depends on the chemical nature of the drug: For lipid soluble drugs (i.e., diazepam, Chlormethiazole), V_d will increase, and consequently serum levels will decrease, while for the more polar drugs (distribution mainly in the body water, e.g., digoxin, Propicillin K), V_d will decrease and serum levels will increase. The changes in serum level, however, also depend largely on the unaltered or altered elimination half-life of the drug under consideration.

Plasma Protein Binding

The effect of altering the plasma protein binding of a drug depends on the degree to which the individual drug is normally bound to plasma proteins. If only a small portion of a drug is so bound, a change of about 30% in plasma protein will not materially affect the amount of free drug in circulation and consequently the distribution and elimination of the drug occurring from the free fraction in the serum. The reverse situation applies for a highly bound drug (90% to 95% or more): in this case a small change in the amount of bound drug (about 10%) will free considerably more of the drug for redistribution or elimination. Furthermore, if the protein-bound portion of a drug with a small V_d is reduced, the rate of drug clearance will be increased. The plasma clearance will remain unchanged, but the amount of free drug per unit of volume of plasma will be greater. If, however, a drug has a large V_d, more of it will partition into the tissue if the protein-bound amount decreases. As before, plasma clearance remains unchanged.

The impact of altered protein binding could become significant if more than one drug were competing for the binding sites. This is a situation encountered very often in the elderly, in the treatment of more than one disease with the administration of several drugs simultaneously.

Metabolism and Elimination

As with absorption and distribution, there are a number of physiological changes in the elderly that may have consequences for metabolism and excretion of drugs. A diminished renal clearance is likely to have consequences for drugs that are excreted mainly over the renal route in a largely unchanged state, as is the case with digoxin. Although renal clearance of digoxin is the major route of elimination in healthy young probands, the extrarenal (mostly biliary) route of excretion is more important in the elderly or in patients with renal impairment (Whiting et al., 1979). There are other drugs excreted mainly or exclusively over the renal route whose dosage should be reduced when given to elderly or renally impaired patients: aminoglycosides (e.g., streptomycin, gentamicin, kanamycin, tobramycin, amikacin, and sisomycin), tetracyclines (with the exception of doxycycline), colistin, lithium, procainamide, methotrexate, ethambutol, and phenobarbital.

Urine, usually thought of as a medium for the disposal of drugs from the body, must be given special consideration as part of a system in which a minimal concentration of a drug should be achieved. This is very important in the treatment of infections of the urinary tract. Ball, Viswan, Mitchard, and Wise (1977), could show, with Mecillinam and amoxicillin (unpublished results), that elderly persons with a serum creatinine that is normal for their age and who therefore have normal renal function had an apparent serum half-life that was 3 to 4 times longer than that of a young control group. Urinary concentrations of the drugs, in this case, were consequently low—in some cases, lower than the minimum inhibitory concentration—and this resulted in a failure to clear the infection.

As with absorption and distribution, there are metabolic changes in the elderly which could influence drug metabolism. Although, until now, there have been no studies on the human microsomal oxidative liver metabolism, extrapolations from animal data (Kato et al., 1962, 1964) suggest that mixed functional oxidation might be reduced with increasing age. The studies of O'Malley et al., 1971, on antipyrine lend further support to this hypothesis. The induction of oxidizing enzymes seems to be lowered in the elderly (Salem et al., 1978; Stevenson, 1977; Padgham & Richens, 1974), although the evidence is not yet convincing. All of these studies have been performed with the measurement of test-drug metabolism. Another method could be to follow up the fraction of an endogenous compound oxidized through the mixed functional oxidases in urine. Such measurements were taken by Hildebrand (1975) with 6-β-hydroxicortisole. A follow-up with such a system of measurement would facilitate the assessment of the enzyme induction possible in nearly every case of treatment and give a data base from routine treatment.

Drugs that are metabolized over nonoxidative routes in younger adults and in the elderly seem to have similar plasma half-lives. Such reactions involve acetylation, glucuronidation, sulfation, and reduction. Compounds metabolized through nonoxidation are often opposed to oxidized drugs ("Type I" compounds as compared to "Type II" compounds).

While establishing that single-dose pharmacokinetics is of use in determining the influence of the various pharmacokinetic mechanisms of the drug in an organism, studies of steady-state concentrations are of much greater clinical relevance. Apart from the benzodiazepines and the tri and tetracyclic antidepressants, which will be treated separately and in more detail later, positive correlations have been found in phenytoin (Houghton et al., 1975) and propranolol (Feely and Stevenson, 1978), while there was no correlation in the case of chlorpropamide (McLaren et al., 1978). In conclusion, it can certainly be said that the pharmacokinetic parameters change, in part, with advancing age, but that the changes are not dramatic. The resulting differences, if any, are normally an increase of up to double the steady-state serum level. Such changes can, however, gain clinical importance in the case of drugs with a narrow therapeutic range, such as digoxin and the tri and tetracyclic antidepressants or lithium. Further studies in clearly defined elderly populations, including consideration for the problem of enzyme induction in the elderly and designed as long-term investigations, are certainly necessary.

SPECIAL CLASSES OF DRUGS

A heterogeneous collection of drugs has been grouped under the collective term "geriatrics." They have, or are claimed to have, one or more of the following effects:

- They lead to a better brain perfusion through vasodilation.
- They counteract or prevent arteriosclerosis by lowering the serum lipid level.

- They help supply the brain with nutrients or with oxygen by economizing metabolism or cell function, which results in better mental performance.

According to data published by the German social insurance agencies, this group of drugs is prescribed to about 40% of all elderly patients in Germany (Kukuk, 1983). In the prescription rate to elderly patients, this figure compares with 43% for cardiac glycosides.

These figures show that "geriatrics" are frequently prescribed in medical practice and that the cost of these prescriptions is in no case a minor consideration for the community. On the other hand, almost everybody who cares about his or her reputation as a scientist doubts whether "geriatrics" really have the effect claimed by their manufacturers or, indeed, any effect at all beneficial to the patient. The reason for this is that not only do pharmaceutical firms sometimes claim illusory effects for a drug, but also that many studies without controls or with very little control have been performed with "geriatrics," and the results published. It is unfortunate that those studies could not stand up to sound scientific criticism nor could their results be reproduced by other groups.

Problems also arise in the effort to produce sound clinical studies involving the "geriatrics" because of the nonexistence, or at least near nonexistence, of validated and usable measuring instruments for aged patients. The psychometric tests used have usually been validated with university students between 18 and 30 years of age. Another question is whether the tests actually gauge the variables that they claim to measure. An alternative which is sometimes employed is the "Nürnberger Alters Inventar" (NAI) according to Oswald and Fleischmann (1985), which has been validated in use with elderly people.

Comparability of controlled studies suffers from the fact that, until now, there has been no generally accepted protocol for such investigations. Long-term studies (i.e., longer than 3 months) are very seldom performed. Certainly the value of this heterogeneous group of drugs can only be assessed by joint international long-term studies, beginning with monosubstances and extending, if necessary, to combinations. In this way, interactions which are advantageous (if any exist) can be found.

As a survey of the literature (Kukuk, 1983) has shown, there certainly are drugs among the "geriatrics" that are effective. Of these, procaine seems to act as a weak and reversible blocker of monoaminooxidase and, therefore, as a mild antidepressant, counteracting the physiologically elevated level of monoaminooxidase in the elderly.

Among the "nootropic" drugs papaverine, cyclandelate, nicotinic acid, Piracetam, and Hydergine®, the last three substances seem to offer the most attractive possibilities for treatment of the elderly. Of these, Hydergine® and, to a slightly lesser degree, Piracetam seem to show the better results. The exact mechanism in the action of these drugs is not yet known. Therefore, further biochemical and controlled clinical studies should be performed with this medication. We can, however, anticipate that therapy with the "geriatrics" will develop to a selective and, as far as possible, specific therapy within the framework described later in this chapter.

Hypnotics and Tranquilizers

Sleep patterns and vigilance change with advancing age (Spiegel, 1982) and complaints of insomnia become more common in elderly patients. This has also been reflected in practice where the number of prescriptions of hypnotics ranks relatively high among all prescriptions written for the aged (Freeman, 1979; Davison, 1984; Weber, 1984). The drugs usually prescribed are clomethiazole (seldom in Germany), the barbiturates and, above all, the benzodiazepines.

There are many side effects which can result from treatment with hypnotics and some of these are severe. The following have been described: daytime drowsiness, paradoxical excitement (Gibson, 1966), nocturnal restlessness (Exton-Smith, 1967), and loss of equilibrium following the administration of barbiturates (MacDonald & MacDonald, 1977). Side effects with the use of barbiturates in the elderly occur with such high frequency that their use should be restricted to the treatment of epilepsy. Drowsiness and sedation following the administration of clomethiazole or diazepam are more than twice as common in patients over 70 years old than in those under the age of 40 (Boston Collaborative Drug Surveillance Program, 1973). Immobility, inanition and incontinence after long-term administration of nitrazepam have been reported only in the elderly (Evans & Jarvis, 1972).

In a study of compliance behavior in the aged, Weber (1984) found that the hypnotic medication was never voluntarily given up by the patient, while 25% of the cardiac glycosides, 22% of the psychopharmaca, and 33% of the antihypertensive drugs were taken irregularly, to cite just a few examples. This shows that the patient feels a necessity for the hypnotic medication. There could be several reasons for this, ranging from unjustified expectations of the duration of sleep at night through changes in the sleep–waking cycle (daytime naps) to physical inactivity during the day. There are certainly sound reasons for the prescription of a hypnotic, for example, in the treatment of a depressive state, but a prescription based only on symptoms should be avoided. In the use of hypnotics there is always the danger of addiction. The duration of treatment with a hypnotic should be as short as possible. In rare cases where prolonged treatment is necessary, drug-free periods (drug-holidays) should be planned by the doctor. It is good practice to use the sedating side effects and the long metabolic half-life of the tricyclic and some of the tetracyclic antidepressants by giving the antidepressive medication as a single dose in the evening. This should make an additional hypnotic unnecessary.

Similar guidelines apply to daytime sedation in crisis management: The prescription period of the benzodiazepine tranquilizers which are normally used should be as short as possible, and the dosage should be held to the absolute minimum required.

Clomethiazole

In contrast to the practice in England and Australia, clomethiazole is seldom prescribed as a hypnotic in Germany (Triggs, 1979). Besides its tranquilizing and hypnotic effects, it has marked anticonvulsant properties. Clomethiazole is extensively metabolized in the liver during a rather short half-life (about 4 hours). One of the side effects is the danger of breathing depression, especially after intravenous infusion, and this drug has a relatively addictive potential. The pharmacokinetic effects of clomethiazole in the elderly (Triggs, 1979) differ from those encountered in younger adults in that with the former group there is a higher biovailability (i.e., reduced first-pass effect), a reduced degree of protein plasma binding, and a reduction of binding to the cellular elements of the blood. This results in a greater area under the curve (AUC) and thus an exposure to higher drug levels than those in younger adults. Although clomethiazole seems to be a good drug for the treatment of delirious states and sometimes for status epilepticus, its use with the aged has its limits.

Barbiturates

Most barbiturates have a long elimination half-life, show a tendency to physical addiction with deliriant or convulsive symptoms on withdrawal, a high potential for enzyme induction, and are extremely dangerous in overdose. They are therefore not recommended for the treatment of insomnia.

Benzodiazepines

The benzodiazepines are among the most widely prescribed drugs in the Western world, used across the whole adult age range. They are characterized by production of a remarkably low organ toxicity in younger adults and therefore possess a broad safety margin. Epidemiological data, however, indicate that, in spite of this low toxicity, their widespread use is not without problems (Boston Collaborative Drug Surveillance Program, 1973;

Greenblatt et al., 1977). Benzodiazepines constitute about 50% of prescription drugs associated with clinical problems of psychotropic origin found in the elderly (Freeman, 1979). Among many reviews, the latest has been published by Greenblatt et al. (1983). As clinical research with the benzodiazepines has shown, their differential clinical effects are fewer than claimed by the pharmaceutical manufacturers. This is no surprise, since the long-acting N-desmethyldiazepam is a common metabolite of many benzodiazepines with at least the clinical effect of diazepam and a very long elimination half-life. As in all other drugs with an oxidative (Type-I) metabolism and a long elimination half-life, the interindividual variability of disposition time of N-desmethyldiazepam is extremely great.

An interesting fact in this connection is that the oxidation of diazepam to the N-desmethyl compound does not decrease with advancing age. However, the initial drug distribution in the different compartments of the body seems to change as a function of age (Klotz et al., 1975). Metabolic pathways which do not employ the mixed functional oxidase system typically do not show any decrease with advancing age. Therefore, the prescription to elderly patients of benzodiazepines which are metabolized by means of glucuronidation or conjugation (e.g., oxazepam, lorazepam) should be encouraged from a pharmacokinetic viewpoint. The benzodiazepines seem to be one of the few groups of drugs where sensitivity to the medication increases with advancing age. As Castleden and George (1979) show, the aging brain seem to have a higher sensitivity to benzodiazepines than is the case with younger adults, judging by side effects common in the elderly but rather seldom seen in younger patients. The authors discuss the possibility that sensitivity of the benzodiazepine receptors increases with advancing age.

Antidepressives and Lithium

The incidence of depressive disorders increases with advancing age and in recurrent depressive disease the frequency of episodes also increases (Braithwaite et al., 1979). Taking the Schildkraut hypothesis as a possible explanation for this fact, the biological findings correlate well with the clinical results (e.g., Gottfries et al., 1979): With advancing age, the biosynthesis of the neuro-transmitting monoamines declines, while the activity of brain monoaminooxidase increases. The resulting imbalance between production and metabolism thus leads to an increased vulnerability of the elderly to depressive disorders.

The correlation between dosage, serum level in steady state and clinical effect in antidepressives has been discussed in many papers. Drugs with a terminal dimethylamino group (e.g., amitryptiline, imipramine, clomipramine) coexist in the body with their first metabolite (nortriptyline, desipramine, N-desmethylclomipramine) in comparable concentrations. The parent compound is considered to act more on the serotonergic receptors, while the first metabolite has a more noradrenergic character. In this case, no correlation of serum level in steady state and no clinical effect with the sum of these elements for the two substances can be expected to exist. Therefore, the first and nearly classic studies were performed with nortriptyline (e.g., Asberg et al., 1971). Our own experience has shown and many studies have reported a very loose interindividual correlation of dosage with serum level in steady state. In a fixed-dose regimen, there was a 15- to 20-fold span between the patient with the lowest and the one with the highest serum level. This finding makes no sense in terms of analytical accuracy or precision, which amounts to about 10% relative. Asberg et al. (1971) found a curvilinear, inversely U-shaped correlation of the serum level of nortriptyline with clinical outcome in endogenous-depressive patients. Although their findings are still controversial, the concept of a therapeutic window has already been adopted by many groups.

In a study with maprotiline (Bergener et al., 1984) we also found an inversely U-shaped correlation of serum level with clinical effect, accompanied by a high degree of statistical certainty ($p \leq 0.01$). According to our data, in younger adults and elderly patients, persons anywhere between 18 and 80 years of age, the best clinical effect, based on a Hamilton Rating, was achieved with a dosage between 200 ng/ml and 300 ng/ml of maprotiline. The dosage necessary for a given serum level in the elderly was about 2/3 of that in younger adults. There was no difference between the two groups in the correlation of serum level with the clinical findings. These findings provide strong support for the concept of a "geriatric dosage" in the application of antidepressives. Maprotiline is unique in that it acts nearly exclusively on noradrenergic receptors.

The classic antidepressives have cholinergic side effects and a quinidinelike action on the heart. They can thus show cardiotoxicity. Nortriptyline is generally considered the most toxic of these compounds, but until now data have been scarce. The second generation antidepressives (e.g., mianserine, maprotiline, nomifensine, dibenzepine, doxepin) are usually said to have fewer side effects but sometimes also to be less active as antidepressive drugs than amitriptyline or clomipramine. The quinidinelike action of the tricyclics can sometimes be exploited in the treatment of the elderly for the correction of arrhythmias. In any case, heart action must be monitored carefully in antidepressive treatment.

The tri and tetracyclic antidepressants are as effective in the elderly as in younger patients. The same applies to lithium for prophylaxis in recurrent depressive disorders. Treatment with lithium must be followed carefully through the determination of serum levels. In the body, lithium behaves chemically like sodium, and every change in sodium turnover will have its corresponding effect on serum lithium. Two side effects of lithium treatment are a depression of thyroid function and a special kind of tremor. Lithium is excreted unchanged by way of the kidneys and its elimination rate depends on renal function. Treatment with indomethacin has been reported to reduce renal clearance to about 50 to 60% of pretreatment values (Frölich et al., 1979). This is one of the few cases where interaction can achieve great clinical importance.

In my opinion, therapy with tri- and tetracyclic antidepressants could therefore profit considerably from therapeutic drug monitoring.

COMPLIANCE

Adherence to medical advice, either in the adaptation of personal life style or in drug treatment, is the prime prerequisite for successful drug therapy. However, as mentioned in the section on the benzodiazepines, compliance with drug prescription is not generally observed by elderly patients (Kunze, 1982; Stähelin, 1984; Weber, 1984). Of the reported noncompliance, the major part was by intention (72%) and characterized by a lower drug intake than was prescribed or by simply failing to take the medication (Weber, 1984). Most of the patients whose noncompliance was intentional considered their prescriptions unnecessary. Antibiotics, antirheumatics, antihypertensives and cardiac drugs ranked among the medication which patients most frequently failed to take.

Various environmental and personal factors could be expected to influence patient compliance. Among these are four areas where a change might bring improvement:

1. "Child-proof" packages have turned out to be also "Granny-proof" (Atkinson et al., 1978): 25 out of 37 patients were unable to open child-proof packages, although the proper way to do this had been demonstrated to them.
2. Patients often experience difficulties both in reading and understanding the manufacturers' printed instructions accompanying the drugs, as well as the doctors' oral instructions. Of the information provided by the physician, 37% to 60% is lost at once; the more information is given, the more it is lost (Weber, 1984). Drug containers with missing or incorrect labels were also a cause of noncompliance.
3. Treatment patterns with many drugs and a complicated schedule of drug intake seem to decrease compliance. The use of dispensers filled in the doctor's office by a nurse or by relatives can certainly improve compliance in this case.

4. Most patients expect a more partner-oriented relation to their doctor, while most doctors seem to prefer an authoritative approach (Kunze, 1982). Noncompliance can therefore also be a sign of (constructive) criticism of the doctor by the patient.

Finally, noncompliance could be one reason for the incidence of adverse drug effects, which, however, is lower for the elderly than extrapolated from the data relating to younger adults (Dengler, 1982).

CONCLUSION

As we have seen, the elderly patient certainly does not exist as a single and sharply defined type. It is generally accepted that a natural variability increases with advancing age. However, there are some common characteristics which justify speaking of aged patients as one (rather heterogeneous) group:

1. There is a gradual reduction in lean body mass as well as in body water.
2. Active parenchyma declines with advancing age and is replaced by connective tissue or body fat.
3. Cardiac output and renal filtration rate decrease with advancing age.
4. The ability of the organism to maintain homeostasis is impaired through the process of aging.
5. Elderly patients often suffer from more than one disease concurrently (multimorbidity).

As we have tried to demonstrate in the preceding sections, drug therapy in the elderly is safe if carried out carefully; patients should not be deprived of their necessary drug treatment out of fear of adverse drug reaction (Stähelin, 1982). Stähelin has developed a general conceptual framework for drug therapy in the aged which probably provides the most sound basis for successful drug treatment:

1. Establish the most accurate diagnosis achievable.
2. Define the therapeutic goal.
3. Establish the hierarchy of medication required in treatment.
4. Select appropriate means to communicate the aim of treatment and medication to the patient: Prescribe a minimal number of drugs and tablets; ask about medication prescribed by other physicians and plan drug holidays.

5. Accept noncompliance as feedback so that you can improve your therapeutic goal.

REFERENCES

Boston Collaborative Drug Surveillance Program (1973). Clinical Depression of the Central Nervous System Due to Diazepam and Chlordiazepoxide in Relation to Cigarette Smoking and Age. *New Engl. J. Med., 288,* 277–280.

Braithwaite, R., Montgomery, S., & Dawling, S. (1979). Age, depression and tricyclic antidepressant levels. In J. Crooks & I. H. Stevenson (Eds.), *Drugs and the elderly* (pp. 133–143) London and Basingstoke: Macmillan.

Brandfonbrener, A. D., Landowne, M., & Shock, N. W. (1955). Changes in cardiac output with age. *Circulation, 12,* 557–566.

Burrowa, G. D., Vohra, J., Hunt, D., Slowman, J. G., Scoggins, B. A., & Davies, B. (1976). Cardiac effects of different tricyclic antidepressant drugs. *Br. J. Psychiat., 129,* 335–341.

Castleden, C. M., & George, C. F. (1979). Increased sensitivity to benzodiazepines in the elderly. In J. Crooks & I. H. Stevenson (Eds.), *Drugs and the elderly* (pp. 169–178). London and Basingstoke: Macmillan.

Davison, W. (1984). Grundlagen der Therapie im Alter. In M. Bergener & B. Kark (Eds.), *Therapie im Alter* (pp. 1–6). Darmstadt: Steinkopff Verlag.

Dengler, H. J. (1982). Summary and outlook. In M. Bergener & H. P. von Hahn (Eds.) *Influence of old age on the effect of drugs* (pp. 131–134) *Gerontology, 28,* Suppl. 1.

Edelman, L. S., & Leibman, J. (1959). Anatomy of body water and electrolytes. *Am. J. Med., 27,* 256–277.

Evans, J. G., & Jarvis, E. H. (1972). Nitrazepam and the elderly. *Br. Med. J., 1,* 10–12.

Exton-Smith, A. N. (1967). The use and abuse of hypnotics. *Gerontologia Clin., 9,* 264–269.

Feely, J., & Stevenson, I. H. (1978). The effect of age and hyperthyroidism on plasma propranolol steady state concentration. *Br. J. Clin. Pharmac., 6,* 446 P.

Forbes, G. B., & Reina, J. C. (1970). Adult lean body mass declines with age: Some longitudinal observations. *Metabolism, 19,* 653–663.

Freeman, G. K. (1979). Drug prescribing patterns in the elderly—a general practice study. In J. Crooks & I. H. Stevenson (Eds.), *Drugs and the elderly* (pp. 223–229). London and Basingstoke: Macmillan.

Frölich, J. C., Leftwich, R., Ragheb, M., Vates, J. A., Reimann, I., & Buchanan, D. (1979). Indomethacin increases plasma lithium. *Br. Med. J. 1,* 1115–1116.

Gibson, I. I. J. M. (1966). Barbiturate delirium. *The Practitioner, 197,* 345–347.

Goldman, R. (1971). Decline in organ function with age. In I. Rossman (Ed.), *Clinical geriatrics.* Philadelphia, PA: Lippincott.

Gottfries, C. G., Adolfsson, R., Oreland, L., Roos, B. E., & Winblad, B. (1979). Monoamines and their metabolites and monoamine oxidase activity related to age and to some dementia disorders. In J. Crooks & I. H. Stevenson (Eds.), *Drugs and the elderly* (pp. 189–198). London and Basingstoke: Macmillan.

Greenblatt, D. J., Allen, M. D., & Shader, R. I. (1977). Toxicity of high dose flurazepam in the elderly. *Clin. Pharmac. Ther., 21,* 355–361.

Greenblatt, D. J., Shader, R. I., & Abernathy, D. R. (1983). Current status of benzodiazepines. *N. Engl. J. Med., 309,* 354–358, 410–416.
Gregerman, R. I., Gaffney, G. W., & Shock, N. W. (1962). Thyroxine turnover in euthyroid man with special reference to changes with age. *J. Clin. Invest., 41,* 2065–2074.
Hildebrand, A. G., Roots, E., Speck, M., Saalfrank, K., & Kewitz, H. (1975). Evaluation of in vivo parameters of drug metabolizing enzyme activity in man following clemastine, phenobarbital or placebo administration. *Europ. J. Clin. Pharmacol., 8,* 327–336.
Houghton, C. W., Richens, A., & Leighton, M. (1975). Effect of age, height, weight and sex on serum phenytoin concentration in epileptic patients. *Br. J. Clin. Pharmacol., 2,* 251–256.
Kato, R., Vassanelli, P., & Chiesara, E. (1964). Variation in the activity of liver microsomal drug metabolizing enzymes in rats in relation to age. *Biochem. Pharmacol., 13,* 1037–1051.
Kato, R., Chiesara, E., & Frontins, G. (1962). Influence of sex difference on the pharmacological action and metabolism of some drugs. *Biochem. Pharmac., 11,* 221–227.
Klotz, U., Avant, G., Hoyumpa, A., Schenker, S., & Wilkinson, G. R. (1975). Effects of age and liver disease on the disposition and elimination of diazepam in man. *J. Clin. Invest., 55,* 347–359.
Kukuk, W. F. (1983). Zur klinischen wirksamkeit der "Geriatrika": Kritische durchsicht der literatur zu procain, nikotinsäure, papaverin, cyclandelat und piracetam. *Doctoral Thesis,* Düsseldorf.
Kunze, M. (1982). Psychological background of noncompliance in the elderly. In M. Bergener & H. P. von Hahn (Eds.) *Influence of old age on the effect of drugs. Gerontology* 28 1, 116–122.
Leask, R. G. S., Andrew, G. R., & Caird, F. I. (1973). Normal values for sixteen blood constituents in the elderly. *Age and Aging, 2,* 14–23.
MacDonald, J. B., & MacDonald, E. T. (1977). Nocturnal femural fracture and continuing widespread use of barbiturate hypnotics. *Br. Med. J., 2,* 483–485.
McLaren, I. H., Salem, S. A. M., & Shepherd, A. M. M. (1979). Studies on drug absorption and metabolism in the elderly. Personal communication, cited in: J. Crooks & I. H. Stevenson (Eds.), *Drugs and the elderly* (p. 58). London and Basingstoke: Macmillan.
Novak, L. P. (1972). Aging, total body potassium, fat-free mass and cell mass in males and females between the ages 18 and 85 years. *J. Gerontol., 27,* 438–443.
O'Malley, K., Crooks, J., Duke, E., & Stevenson, I. H. (1971). Effect of age and sex on the human drug metabolism. *Br. Med. J., 3,* 607–609.
O'Malley, K., & Kelly, J. G. (1983). Drug responses in old age. In P. Turner & D. Shand (Eds.), *Recent Advances in Clinical Pharmacology* (pp. 45–56). New York: Churchill Livingstone.
Oswald, W. D., & Fleischmann, M. (1985). Psychometrics in gerontological research. In M. Bergener, H. B. Stähelin, & M. Ermini (Eds.), *Thresholds in aging*—the 1984 Sandoz lectures in gerontology (pp. 241–254). London: Academic Press.
Padgham, O., & Richens, A. (1974). Quinine metabolism: A useful index of hepatic drug metabolising capacity in man? *Br. J. Clin. Pharmac., 1,* 352.
Salem, S. A. M., Rajjayaban, P., Shepherd, A. M. M., & Stevenson, I. H. (1978). Reduced induction of drug metabolism in the elderly. *Age and Aging, 7,* 68–73.

Sherlock, S., Bearn, A. G., Billing, B. H., & Paterson, J. C. S. (1950). Splanchnic blood flow in man by the bromsulfalein method: The relation of peripheral bromsulfalein level to the calculated flow. *J. Lab. Clin. Med. 35,* 923–932.

Spiegel, R. (1982). Aspects of sleep, daytime vigilance, mental performance and psychotropic drug treatment in the elderly. In M. Bergener, & H. P. von Hahn (Eds.), *Influence of old age on the effect of drugs* (pp. 68–82). *Gerontology, 28,* Suppl. 1.

Stähelin, H. B. (1982). Implications for prescribing practice. In M. Bergener, & H. P. von Hahn (Eds.), *Influence of old age on the effect of drugs* (pp. 123–130). *Gerontology, 28,* Suppl. 1.

Stevenson, I. H., Salem, S. A. M., & Shepherd, A. M. M. (1979). Studies on drug absorption and metabolism in the elderly. In J. Crooks & I. H. Stevenson (Eds.), *Drugs and the elderly* (pp. 51–64). London and Basingstoke: Macmillan.

Stevenson, I. H. (1977). Factors influencing antipyrine elimination. *Br. J. Pharmac., 4,* 261–266.

Triggs, E. J. (1979). Pharmacokinetics of lignocaine and chlormethiazole in the elderly; with some preliminary observations on other drugs. In J. Crooks, & I. H. Stevenson (Eds.), *Drugs and the elderly* (pp. 117–132). London and Basingstoke: Macmillan.

Weber, E. (1984). Zur Problematik der Compliance im Alter. In M. Bergener & B. Kark (Eds.), *Therapie im Alter* (pp. 7–17). Darmstadt: Steinkopff Verlag.

Whiting, B., Lawrence, J. R., & Summer, D. J. (1979). Digoxin pharmacokinetics in the elderly. In J. Crooks & I. H. Stevenson (Eds.), *Drugs and the elderly* (pp. 89–101). London and Basingstoke: Macmillan.

Woodford-Williams, E., Alvares, A. S., Webster, D., Lardless, B., & Dixon, M. P. (1964). Serum protein pattern in "normal" and pathological aging. *Gerontologia, 10,* 88–99.

19
Psychotherapy in Advanced Age

Götz Kockott

There has always been a very skeptical attitude toward psychotherapy in advanced age. In Freud's opinion (1942), after the fifth decade a person's mental mobility was too low for relearning, and life history material far too extensive for psychotherapy to have a reasonable chance of success. Although there have been several publications during the last two or three decades on successful treatment (which will be discussed in this chapter) there still remains a distinctly felt psychotherapeutic reservation toward this age group. Not without reason does one suspect that an attitude is behind this, in Anglo-American literature called "ageism", that is, a rejective attitude toward the elderly person. In the meantime the significance and the need for psychotherapeutic action in advanced age have been recognized. This activity, however, is only slowly gaining attention.

This chapter will discuss psychotherapy as defined by Strotzka (1975): the conscious and planned interactional process for the change of behavior disorders and suffering. Results of treatment for mentally ill elderly persons with neurotic development, depression, pathological grief reaction, and symptoms of anxiety will be described. These mental illnesses are often the result of age-specific problems which have gone psychologically unmastered. Treatment methods for elderly patients with other illnesses will also be discussed insofar as they seem accessible to psychotherapeutic methods (e.g., organic brain syndrome, heart disease). The abundance of methods describing procedures for further personality development of the mentally stable old person will not be discussed, nor will the important aspect of psychological guidance for the dying (Kübler-Ross, 1972). These subjects need separate consideration.

PSYCHOTHERAPEUTIC METHODS

First, some viewpoints will be discussed that are relevant to all methods of psychotherapy when applied in psychogeriatrics:

1. *Indication for therapy.* In principle, the indication for psychotherapy in advanced age is not any different than for other periods of life; it should, however, be approached with more reservation (see discussion). For the prognosis, the "age" of the neurosis is more important than age itself (Abraham, 1971; Bergmann, 1978). In advanced age acute neurotic disturbances are also more successfully treated.

2. *Therapy aims.* These should be kept at a modest (Hedri, 1968) and limited level (Muslin & Epstein, 1980; Wertheimer & Lobrinus, 1981). Often it is less important to help the individual with his problems of adapting himself to his environment than to adapt the immediate environment to the peculiarities of the patient (Ginzberg, 1950). Götestam (1980) formulated the following specific aims:

- increase in insight of the underlying causes of problems, as well as increase in facing reality as it is;
- symptom relief;
- relief to relatives, ideally as a temporary measure (e.g. through temporary admission to and treatment in a day hospital);
- deceleration or delay of deteriorative processes;
- adaptation of the patient to the situation in which he finds himself;
- increase in self-care skills (personal hygiene) and so-called daily life functions such as bathing, dressing, continence, and feeding;
- increase in active engagement in a wide field of activities;
- encouragement of the patient to be as independent as possible.

3. *Form of therapy.* The general opinion is that according to the limited aim psychotherapy should also be limited in time (e.g., Wertheimer & Lobrinus, 1981). In doing so, the therapist should be oriented toward the "here and now" and only when absolutely necessary should the whole life history be reviewed. Due to their many experiences of loss mentally ill elderly persons tend to quickly develop a dependency on the therapist, so that their own lack of independence is intensified. This dependence has to be accepted up to a certain degree. On the other hand, for precisely this reason psychotherapy is necessary, but with clear time limits or therapy sessions that are set far apart.

4. *Therapist–patient relationship.* The special situation here is the difference in age. Whereas in psychotherapy with younger persons the psychotherapist as a rule is older or at least of the same age, the situation with elderly patients is usually the reverse. This can evoke unusual transference

phenomena particularly for the therapist with which he first has to learn to deal. We have already noted that psychotherapy sessions should as a rule be set far apart due to the quick development of the elderly person's dependency on the therapist. In one approved method to keep up the therapist-patient relationship between sessions the therapist "steps out of his position of absolute neutrality" (Wertheimer & Lobrinus, 1981). He is more active and directive than is otherwise the case, particularly in psychodynamic psychotherapy; for instance, between sessions he has the patient fulfill small tasks that have been worked out together.

On the whole there is general agreement that for the large majority of elderly patients the usual psychotherapeutic method has to be adapted to the particularities of elderly people. There is controversy over some points however, such as how to deal with the tendency of elderly patients toward dependency—by encouragement or rejection—and whether the therapist should always be empathic or may also be confronting.

Psychoanalytic Oriented Psychotherapy

Individual Psychotherapy

The first psychotherapeutic effort in a form adapted to treatment of the aged was undertaken on a large scale by L. J. Martin (1944). Her form of therapy, practiced mainly in the 1930s, was very active, limited in time, had clearly defined aims, and was thus very similar to behavior-therapeutic methods. During the following two decades more psychoanalytically oriented forms of therapy were used. Grotjahn (1955) and more recently Radebold (1979) give a good theoretical background for this. Dodgen and Ransom (1967), Hiatt (1971), and Kahana (1979) report on successful therapies. The provisions for psychoanalytical treatment, however, severely restrict a potential number of patients. Besides the usual stipulations there may be no indication of organic brain syndromes. According to Kahana (1979) psychotherapy for the aged with the aim of changing ego structures is only possible if there is no other psychopathology apart from neurotic and reactive symptoms. Several other authors deal with the importance of the single aspect of analytical therapy forms adapted for the aged. The experiences are passed on very generally or in anecdotes (Pfeiffer, 1976; Pitt, 1974; Blau & Berezin, 1975; Weinberg, 1975; Langley, 1975; Verwoerdt, 1976; Bircher, 1981).

Group Psychotherapy

Group therapy has been widely applied in the field of gerontopsychiatry for approximately 30 years. Psychogeriatric centers not offering group activities are unheard of today. In spite of this general custom, literature dealing specifically with group psychotherapy with the aged is rare. In 1950, Silver gave information on his group psychotherapy studies with senile-psychotic women. Subsequently others (e.g., Linden, 1956; Rechtschaffen et al., 1954; Ross, 1959; Villa, 1976; Liederman et al., 1967) have reported on group psychotherapy with the aged. Some authors (Wolfe, 1970; Klein et al., 1965) give detailed descriptions of their procedures. On the whole, it seems that strictly psychoanalytical oriented group psychotherapy is possible for a small, very select group of patients. But for the vast majority of mentally ill elderly persons group therapies are carried out and modified according to the conditions of the institution, the degree of mental disturbance and the theoretical views of the therapist (e.g., Wächtler, 1982). These modifications pertain mainly to group structures (e.g., diagnostic or age homogeneity) and group styles. There is unity as to group size (at most 16, ideally 8 to 10 or less); furthermore, it is generally recognized that it is therapeutically helpful to have a few members in the group who are already closer to the therapeutic aim. They can serve as a model.

Family Therapy

There is one report in the literature on family therapy with the aged. Manaster (1967) briefly described his attempts to include family members in therapy of patients who were placed in or on the waiting list for a home for the aged. When invited to do so about half of the families attended therapy sessions. The sessions focused on an awareness of their own feelings, especially feelings about "putting their parents away," as well as a clearer understanding of the entire field of aging. The author reports positive results but fails to provide data to substantiate this statement.

Milieu Therapy

Milieu therapy in its strict sense is a psychodynamically oriented approach applied to entire wards. First described in 1953 by Jones, it has not been widely used in geriatric wards. It has been assumed that aged patients lack the necessary communication skills for such therapy. Wolff (1962, 1963, 1971) and Mishara (1978) have used milieu therapy as a control condition, however, with unsatisfactory results. Goldstein (1972) discussed advantages and disadvantages of a milieu therapeutic approach in a day hospital for the aged and concluded that it is a very difficult task for the staff, unless the approach is very well fitted to the specific institution. However, judging from the literature, it seems this form of therapy has not been given a fair chance (Götestam, 1980). Very often the term "milieu therapy" is used in a much broader sense and it becomes difficult to see the psychodynamic orientation behind the approach. Programs that structure the environment in a way that it becomes supportive and activating will be discussed in the next section since these methods are mainly behaviorally oriented.

Behavior Therapy

Even behavior therapists have been very reluctant to use their method with the aged. During the 1960s the first publications on this subject appeared in the United States (Lindsley, 1964; Filer & O'Connel, 1964; Cautela, 1966, 1969), but the applicability of various behavior therapy techniques have only been reported on a wider scale during the last ten years. However, a number of publications exist that describe forms of therapy used predominantly with the aged, but without specifically mentioning age, for instance the Token Economy Programme for chronic schizophrenic patients (Ayllon & Azrin, 1968).

Operant Techniques

So far operant techniques have been described more often than others, and they have wide application. They can influence intellectual loss in advanced age, even if only in a limited way (Murell, 1970; Hoyer, Labouvie, & Baltes, 1973; Birkhill & Schaie, 1975; Belluci & Hoyer, 1975). Institutionalized elderly patients have a strong tendency toward loss of activity and development of dependency. Accordingly, Old Age and Nursing Home therapy programs use, in addition to staff instructions, operant methods that provoke further activities and independency. Also Token Economy Programmes have often been used to alter social behavior (Mueller & Atlas, 1972; Nigl & Jackson, 1981; Hoyer et al., 1974).

Systematic Desensitization, Flooding

Relatively isolated but marked phobic symptoms are also seen in the aged, although infrequently. Apparently they can be treated with systematic desensitization or flooding as effectively as in younger patients.

Assertiveness Training

The often-used assertiveness training programs (e.g. Ullrich de Muynck & Ullrich, 1976) or individual variations of it are not suitable treatment methods for the aged because nonassertive behavior in elderly people is high and therefore we usually do not see generalization in therapy (Edinberg et al., 1977). So it has become customary, and certainly more efficient, to regain assertiveness by a multidimensional approach in the framework of a structured therapy with integration of role-play, shaping, and social reinforcement. This procedure is very significant in the treatment of inpatients, but it is also used particularly in the treatment of day patients.

Cognitive Approach

Only during the last few years has cognitive therapy, which turns to thought-content and cognitions, gained in stature. The assumption of cognitive therapy is that the patients, on account of incorrect assumptions, gain a distorted view of their environment and accordingly exhibit wrong reactions. Restructuring toward adequate cognition thus leads to an adequate view and change of behavior. To date there are only few positive reports on experiences (Sulz & Lauter, 1983), and a controlled investigation still does not exist for this form of therapy for the aged.

Change in the Environment

According to the fundamental views of behavior therapy, factors that maintain a certain behavior can be sought within the patient himself or in his environment. Consequently the behavior therapist will include the immediate social and other environments of the patient into his consideration of therapeutic protocol. Because the nursing staff has a meaningful role in relating to the elderly, particularly institutionalized patients, and is often included in treatment methods, it must be asked whether and which changes of attitude and behavior of staff seem due to behavior therapy programs and what effect this has on the aged patients. McReynolds and Coleman (1972), who were the first to pursue this question systematically, noticed that the nursing staff had a more optimistic attitude which presumably was due to their role change (new found importance), with corresponding effects on the patients. Richards and Thorpe (1978) arrive at very similar conclusions. There are quite a number of studies in the literature involving experimental evaluation of one or more factors in the environment and their effects on patient's behavior. These studies are all relatively well-designed and executed. In a series of publications McClannahan and Risley (1973, 1974, 1975a,b) presented the results of environmental changes in a nursing home for mainly aged persons. Attendance in various activities increased significantly more when it was announced and rewarded with a small amount of money (such as a quarter) than when it was rewarded with money or announcement alone, the last reward being by far the least successful. Availability of equipment such as puzzles and games increased activity significantly. Rewarding activity with prizes or snacks increased it. A store placed in the activity area where patients could shop increased attendance and participation in activities tremendously. Similar studies have been performed by Salter and Salter (1975) using reality orientation, activities of daily living (ADL), and recreational activities, by Wisocki (1977) for recreational activities, and by Jenkins et al. (1977), Götestam and Melin (1979) and Peterson et al. (1977) for other specific activities. All these studies found consistent changes in some dependent variable which was logically linked to the independent variable. Lindsley (1964) and Lawton (1970) stressed the importance of environmental prothetic help for the aged such as signs and calendars for the disoriented, support bars for the physically disabled, or family items to enhance recollections in those patients who suffer from impaired memory. This environmental treatment approach has been the cause of much optimism in recent years. Such programs should become standard strategies for increasing patients' activities and self-confidence.

Social Therapy

This term does not describe a form of therapy with a specific theoretical background, but the content of the treatment. Stindl et al. (1981) use the term in relation to the old person in two ways. On the one hand, they mean "the application of psychotherapy in the social environment" and refer, as does Radebold (1983), to a term of illness that includes social relations of illness and therapy. On the other hand they connect "real support of mental ill aged persons in the social environment." Here the main tasks are to reestablish social contacts and social contact ability with the family, with centers for the elderly and clubs, with provisions of financial and other help, for example, "meals on wheels," and, if unavoidable, to help procure a place in a home. In Anglo-American countries this work is done by specially trained social workers. One London field study using a convincing scientific method reports on the effectiveness of their work (Goldberg et al., 1970). In the control study, the work of specially trained social workers was compared with the usual care of Welfare Department Officers with regard to comparable populations. Changes in the sense of improvement in the patient's whole life situation were shown in both groups, but were significantly higher in the group with the specially trained social workers. More importantly, the effectiveness of sensibly planned sociotherapy for the aged became evident in this investigation. Unfortunately this study is so far the only one of its kind.

Special Therapy Approaches

Several special therapy approaches are used in institutions or outpatient facilities. In institutions these include "reality orientation," "remotivation," and "revitalization."

Reality orientation. With a so-called "classroom" approach or in a 24-hour program patients with symptoms of an organic brain syndrome relearn fundamental data as to time and place etc. by receiving repeated information provided by a specially trained staff.

Remotivation. This is a structured program carried out by nursing staff for very inactive chronic hospitalized patients. In about 12 "conversation" lessons the patients are asked to discuss topics of general interest, such as actual or historic events in world history.

Revitalization. Lehr (1979), uses this term for methods that increase creative locomotor behavior, such as dancing, gymnastics, or making music. Shapiro (1969) describes such a program that stimulates physically, mentally, and emotionally; making music is combined with physical exercises, memory training, and exercises for mental concentration. Frohne (1979) gives an overview of "music therapy" in the aged. Active reproduction of music is being reported in the literature, but there are no controlled data about the effect it has on the patients. Lehr (1979) believes dancing (Brüggemann, 1977) should also have a positive effect but again there are no data available to prove this statement.

The above-mentioned treatment methods will be discussed further in the sections pertaining to patients with organic brain syndrome and chronic hospitalized patients.

In an outpatient setting, special therapy approaches include building up self-esteem, and giving the patient training in care of self.

Building up self-esteem. Oberleder (1970) and Power et al. (1975) describe this intervention technique and believe that is especially suitable for handling crisis situations in elderly depressed and physically disabled people. One of the aims is to help the patient accept reality. In a therapy group the patients are asked to describe their appearance using a hand-mirror, and their emotions. The group assists with positive and negative corrections to their statements. Power et al. (1975) additionally provide body contact, ask the patients to help the staff to perform little tasks, and give them affirmations ("let me see your pretty eyes"). Similar methods have been used successfully by Brody et al. (1971) and Salter and Salter (1975).

Training in care of oneself. This is directed mainly to patients who are physically disabled (Parkinson's disease, multiple sclerosis, rheumatic arthritis, etc.) and who have organized groups by themselves. They usually work closely with the medical profession, give practical advice and mental support to patients with the same disease, and organize mutual help and meetings in which treatment methods can be discussed with specialists. One example of these groups is the German Parkinson Association (Deutsche Parkinson Vereinigung).

SYMPTOM-RELATED FORMS OF THERAPY

Depressive Syndromes

Nonpsychotic depression can be treated with individual psychoanalysis, providing that there are no signs of organic brain syndrome (Hiatt, 1971). Recently there have also been reports on psychoanalytical group therapy with this diagnostic group (Radebold, 1976). Problem-centered psychoanalytic therapy that deals with closed groups has the benefit, according to Wächtler (1982), of building up rather quickly a confidential relationship between patient and therapist. This form of therapy has proved to be useful under the time-limited conditions of day-hospital treatment. The procedure of Butler and Lewis (1977) used with depressive patients is considered controversial. Elderly people often feel the need for a life-review. According to Butler and Lewis (1977) it is important to do this in the context of a psychotherapeutic setting, so that a full, realistic review is accomplished. The aged individual can then be contented within himself and look back on a meaningful and fulfilled life. Butler and Lewis actively support their patients' endeavors toward this aim, and make suggestions for completion of life retrospects. These include visiting places and areas that were important in former times, completing a family history, collecting family photos and diaries, writing down one's own memories, one's life achievements. This can yield a lot of material that would need to be worked through psychoanalytically. Such a life-review can be painful and evoke anxieties—this is also the main point of criticism. Is it really possible to totally work through fears and anxieties, if, for instance, the result of this clarification process shows that one's whole life has been wrongly built up? Butler and Lewis are very optimistic: Whether a life-review is ultimately successful depends on the ability to work through earlier neurotic conflicts and negative sentiments psychotherapeutically. Some authors are very skeptical about this procedure; they do not see any sense in brooding over earlier traumatic events, faults, and losses and therefore find this method counterindicated (Hamilton & Cowdry, 1976). On the whole, one gains the impression that this drawing of balance can be a very healthy form of coping with age-specific problems for mentally stable old people. Indication for this form of therapy should certainly be used carefully for treatment of the mentally ill.

In the framework of behavior therapy, depressions are treated according to the model of Lewinsohn (1974) or, more recently, by a cognitive approach. One of the most prominent representatives in this field is Beck, who, together with colleagues, developed a treatment program for depression (Beck et al., 1981). This program has been examined in several controlled surveys and has proved effective in conjunction with other forms of therapy. With reference to the aged mentally ill person, there is no other literature apart from the above-mentioned report (Sulz & Lauter, 1983). Further investigations would be desirable.

Gauthier and Marshall (1977) deal with the topic of pathological grief. In social reinforcement in the form of care and sympathy, and in the silent conspiracy with which mourners are kept from all unpleasant memories, the authors see two main factors that play a part in the continuation of grief. In their interesting but certainly controversial therapy, the authors achieved significant improvement in the patients as well as in the relatives in approximately six sessions through a combination of instructions to the environment and flooding. One could call that a forced treatment for grief reaction. This forcing is questionable.

Phobias

Isolated phobias are rarely diagnosed in advanced age. They belong to the indication area of psychoanalytical individual or group therapy (Hiatt, 1971; Radebold, 1979; Wolff, 1970). Phobic symptoms occurring in advanced age can also be successfully treated with behavior therapy techniques such as systematic desensitization (Wanderer, 1972) or flooding (Thyer, 1981).

Organic Brain Syndromes

With this very large diagnostic group in the field of psychogeriatrics, psychoanalytical treatment is basically impossible (Hiatt, 1971). In reports on psychodynamically oriented individual or group therapy, great therapeutic restrictions are made with regard to patients with signs of organic brain syndromes. Often this diagnosis is a criterion for exclusion.

Nonanalytical psychotherapies are far better suited, particularly for distinctly marked symptoms of organic brain syndrome. Goldfarb (1969) therapeutically utilizes the need for dependency in his method and allows a parent-like relationship to develop from therapist to patient. In this way the patient feels protected, secure, cared for, and loses feelings of fear and insecurity. At the same time Goldfarb leaves the patient with the possibility of attaining small moral victories over the parent-like therapist. This method is undemanding of the patient and hardly time-consuming. Criticism is aimed at the broad applicability of this method. Outside of institutions, the presumed power of the therapist is not maintainable, and the method not applicable. Goldfarb defends himself by referring to the usefulness of such institutions in which a mentally disturbed person can lead a more human existence than he could living on his own. One has to view Goldfarb's method historically. It is to his merit to have been one of the first to take a psychotherapeutic interest in these patients. Berger (1978) describes group sessions for patients with obvious organic brain syndromes in which he incorporates all possibilities for activation, such as music and movement therapy, as well as word games for memory training, which could have certainly important consequences.

Within the framework of behavior therapy methods, a particular therapeutic procedure was developed for these patients, i.e., reality orientation. In a series of investigations on inpatients, evidence of effectiveness was furnished pertaining to the procedure adopted for patients with memory and orientation deficiencies (Hanley, 1981; Greene et al., 1976; Holden & Sinebruchow, 1978). Fundamental information pertaining to time and place are relearned by the hour "as in school" (classroom approach), or in a 24-hour program with trained staff, and constantly repeated. In this way the patients gain a wider radius of action. A series of studies showed evidence that not only was improvement of intellectual abilities achieved, but the so conditioned changes in social behavior became even larger (Citrin & Dixon, 1977; Folsom, 1968; Harris & Ivory, 1976; Barnes, 1974; Brook et al., 1975).

The 24-hour program is more effective than the hourly classroom procedure (Hanley et al., 1981), but age, the degree of disorientation, and physical restriction of movement are limiting factors for the success of this method (Zepelin et al., 1981); no improvement was evident in distinct senile dementia (Barnes, 1974; Zarit et al., 1982). Motivation by the therapist is an important factor for success (Brook et al., 1975). It is uncertain how long increased intellectual performance is maintained after the end of therapy; presumably it is dependent on the length of training (Barnes, 1974; Letcher et al., 1974). Even if first reports on this new method were too positive and enthusiastic, it has nevertheless been proved that for inpatients with moderate and severe psychorganic syndromes this method produces an improvement of orientation and social behavior, at least for a length of time.

There is another aspect to reality orientation—resensitization (Richman, 1969; Barns et al., 1973; Huber, 1973). In structured individual or group sessions the senses of those patients who have difficulty interacting with their environment will be trained. For visual resensitization, mobiles, paintings, and posters which change from time to time can be used; for auditory resensitization, records and also self-produced sounds and noises (clapping, whispering, etc.) can be used. Similarly, olfactory and gustatory resentization can be done. This approach was the main content of a much broader treatment program developed by Loew and Silverstone (1971) which also can be called milieu therapy. They reorganized a geriatric ward for 14 male patients with a mean age of 87.5 years. In comparison to controls, the experimental group showed a moderate increase in cognitive and social functioning after six months and were in a better mood. The authors came to the conclusion that: "the functioning of the very old can be influenced in a limited way by changes in social, psychological, and physical environment."

Chronic Hospitalized Patients

Chronic hospitalized patients do not belong to any uniform diagnostic group. After having been hospitalized for months or years, these patients develop certain common symptoms, such as inactivity, that can be attributed to this long-term hospitalization. These changes seem not to be treatable by psychoanalytical methods, and there is hardly any literature on this subject. Wolff (1970) describes results of psychoanalytically oriented treatment with 54 elderly patients in which treatment was suitably adapted to the aged population. His patients were hospitalized for an average of nine years. They were diagnosed as schizophrenics or neurotics and all showed additional symptoms of mild to moderate organic brain syndrome. Of this group, 34 patients improved significantly after weekly sessions over a period of at least three months with more insight into their problems, more interest in activities within the ward, and less disturbed short-span memory; 22 patients could be discharged, 12 of them into a nursing home. After one year the discharged patients were still able to cope adequately with their life situation outside the hospital. Unfortunately the results are presented to the reader in the form of a very general judgment. Neutral evaluation of success through data or independent reviewers would have been desirable.

Revitalization, mainly in the form of music therapy, has been used by Shapiro (1969). He describes in detail his experiences in treating elderly mentally ill persons with his method. His program had a transfer effect: People who took part in the Shapiro program also showed interest and took part in other activities. There exists no further evaluation and no data on the usefulness of such a therapy.

Gunn (1967) made an interesting observation regarding the effect of psychotherapy with chronic hospitalized patients. After one year of group psychotherapy, which has not been further specified, the use of antidepressants increased and at the same time the nursing staff reported less disturbed behavior of the patients. Gunn's interpretation is that the psychotherapy created a change from disturbed behavior to verbalization of depressed content. There exists no other literature with comparable observations.

Behavior therapy, in particular, has recently been adapted for this group of patients. Therapy programs have been developed with which activity and independence of inhabitants can be encouraged. Kennedy and Kennedy (1982) introduced such a program for especially inactive inhabitants. Other authors have proved that taking part in fitness training enhances activity (Adams & de Vries, 1973; DeCarlo et al. 1977; Elsayed et al., 1980; Libb & Clements, 1969; Sandel, 1978) and social interaction (Powell, 1974; Sandel, 1978). Motivation to take part was increased by a reward. Rewards were also used successfully to influence social behavior. It became evident that a direct offer of games and similar activities significantly increases participation in community ventures as compared with indirect offers (McClannahan & Risley, 1975). With home residents living a very withdrawn life a new approach to social contacts can be established by using the framework of a Token Economy Programme to reinforce each spoken word (Hoyer et al.,

1974), or else social interaction including verbal and nonverbal communication (Nigl & Jackson, 1981). Using social reinforcement Goldstein and Baer (1976) trained patients to write letters that were very likely to be answered and thus could break through the isolation of some home residents. Operant therapy methods seem to be superior to milieu therapy methods, involve shorter inpatient treatment, and increase transfer to day hospitals in which the patients experience more independence (Frank et al., 1982). These methods are clearly superior to the previously limited therapeutic potential.

For very inactive hospitalized patients, a specific method was developed in the United States for the improvement of social interactions—the structured program remotivation therapy. In twelve 30- to 60-minute sessions, topics of general interest relating to the reality of environment—current or historic world events, natural history topics, and the like—are discussed in a conversational, manner. This program has been carried out on a large scale in mental hospitals in the United States since the beginning of the 1960s. The nursing staff are trained as therapists in a 30-hour course to use this technique. In spite of its broad application in the United States, there is a paucity of literature on this topic. The staff's feeling that a bit of psychotherapy in its broadest sense is given to the patient in addition to body care is possibly the decisive reason for the positive attitude of the attendants toward use of the method. Whether or not this therapy is really of help and of help for what group of patients is still not certain.

Somatic Illness

It is well known that we face a so-called multimorbidity especially in the treatment of elderly people. Research is difficult if the question of the influence of these many somatic variables on mental state is to be answered. Studies that investigate the influence on only one dimension (one somatic parameter) are not satisfactory.

From a number of investigations we can assume that approximately 20 to 30% of people aged 65 and older are physically heavily disabled: bed ridden, use a wheel chair, or in need of assistance in walking (Streib & Orbach, 1967; Shanas, 1971). But there is very often a division between the medical and the subjective judgment regarding the level of health (Sachuk, 1970; Shanas et al., 1968; Lehr and Thomae, 1965). The majority of patients rate their own level of health more positively than would the medical profession. Many authors (Theissen, 1970; Schmitz-Scherzer, 1969; Lehr, 1967; Schreiner, 1969; Puschner et al., 1968) found correlations between negative judgment of health and low self-esteem, loneliness, passivity, and little planning for the future. These findings can be understood in the framework of the "cognitive theory of aging" (Thomae, 1970): For the elderly person's mental state it is much more important how the changes of life situations (and health) due to aging are received than the amount to which these changes objectively occur. Life history seems to be important in deciding how these changes are received. The burden of a somatic chronic illness can, but need not be, tremendous. Low self-esteem, anxiety, depression, increased sensitivity to rejection, and reduced attempts to engage in the usual activities of daily living may result. Self-esteem seems to depend strongly on the patient's mobility: hearing difficulties, blindness, athroses, and paralyses have a greater impact on the mental state than other chronic inabilities (Shanas et al., 1968). There is some literature on psychotherapy of patients disabled in these areas.

Disablement of the Senses

Hearing Difficulties. About 30% of elderly persons have hearing difficulties (Lauter, 1983). High frequencies especially cannot be heard, and therefore consonants are difficult to understand; this results in fragmented information reception and the elderly person retiring from social contact. Usually relatives are less understanding of people with hearing difficulties than of blind persons; this may lead to the patient's depressed retirement, suspicion, or even delusional ideas. The important psychotherapeutic task will be to create mutual understanding between the patient and his relatives and to find better ways to communicate using, for example, more visual communications such as gestures and written language.

Blindness. Evans and Jauregny (1981) used an interesting approach in treatment of elderly blind persons who lived very isolated and far apart from each other. With conference calls they treated them as a group using a cognitive behavioral oriented therapy form. After eight weekly conference calls the patients showed, in comparison to control, significant improvement in the variables loneliness, outside social contacts, and household activities.

Mobility

Inpatient Treatment (mainly). As already mentioned, chronically disabled hospitalized patients develop inactivity in addition to certain somatic inabilities. Via behaviorally oriented methods such as shaping, fading, and other individually adapted operant methods significant changes in dependent feeding behavior of an elderly woman have been achieved (Baltes & Zerbe, 1976), wheelchair patients have relearned how to walk to some extent (MacDonald & Butler, 1974) and nursing home residents have been motivated to bathe themselves more often (Rinke et al., 1978). These reports show interesting new possibilities for the treatment of similar physical disablement. A number of publications exist for therapy of incontinence. The varying results suggest that the less distinct the problem, the more differentiated, multidimensional, and intensive the treatment program, and the more favorable the outcome.

There is some literature on psychotherapy of patients with myocardial infarction. In the acute phase of anxiety, depression and problems in interaction with the nursing staff have to be dealt with (Köhle & Gaus, 1979). A strong and good therapist–patient relationship is crucial. In the rehabilitation phase, group psychotherapy seems helpful which is not only psychoanalytically oriented but also deals with the somatic illness directly and is combined with relaxation training etc. (Hahn, 1971).

According to Petzold and Reindell (1980) the treatment of choice for the socially adapted myocardial patient is relaxation training (autogenious training, I. H. Schulz), plus supportive psychotherapy with the aim of care of self; for the anxious-repressed patients, psychoanalytically oriented psychotherapy; and for the impulsive-dynamic patient, physical exercise treatment in groups. But there are no data to prove these statements. Godbole and Verinis (1974) compared two forms of short psychotherapy in elderly patients with somatic diseases, mainly diseases of the heart: the nonconfronting type (Goldfarb, 1969) and a confronting form (Garner, 1965). Assessment of improvement was made by questionnaires which were given to patients, nursing staff, medical doctors, and psychotherapists. Compared to a control group after treatment, both experimental groups were less depressed, recovered faster, and could be discharged earlier. The patient group with the confronting type of short psychotherapy did slightly better than the other experimental group.

An increasing body of data documents the effectiveness of regular, graduated programs of physical activity in the convalescence of cardiac patients (Naughton, Hellerstein, & Mohler, 1973). Yet, until recently little experimental attention had been paid to the psychological effects of exercise. Several studies (e.g., McPherson et al., 1967; Naughton et al., 1968) indicate that participation in physical activity programs can lead to an increased sense of well-being and decreased anxiety and depression in postinfarction patients. Hackett and Cassem (1973) further consider physical exercise to be the most potent antidote for depression available to the cardiac patient, and they recommend an appropriate program of physical conditioning beginning while the patient is still in the coronary care unit. They propose that physical conditioning acts to counter depression by restoring self-esteem, sense of independence, and feelings of self-sufficiency and accomplishment—in short, it restores patients' feelings of control over relatively stable factors in their lives.

Stroke. Most therapeutic interventions for stroke have been conducted in one of three ways. The first approach increases intellectual and physical stimulation of the patient in a structured, predictable, and supportive environment (e.g., Cohen, 1979; Davidson, 1963; Jones, 1975). A second general approach employs specific cognitive remediation programs (Gordon & Diller, 1983). A third intervention strategy applies conventional psychotherapies to enhance the patient's ability to cope with the psychological aftermath of stroke. Although supportive counseling for stroke patients has been advocated by a number of authors (e.g., Carlson, 1980; Charaton & Fisk, 1978; Fisher, 1961; Stonnington, 1980), group therapy is the most common psychotherapeutic intervention, presently used to facilitate coping in the poststroke patient. Reports of subjectively rated improvement among stroke patients and their families after group participation are common (D'Affliti & Weitz, 1974; Oradei & Waite, 1974; Piskor & Paleos, 1968; Singler, 1975; Watzlawick & Coyne, 1980). However, no controlled outcome studies have been published documenting the superiority of group therapy over no therapy or other therapy controls. In addition, it appears that the group therapies reported in the stroke rehabilitation literature have employed diverse procedures that have made it difficult to compare the therapies with one another.

Outpatient Treatment (mainly). Often elderly people have a strong fear of falling in addition to physical impairment of walking. For treatment the combination of physio-therapy and systematic desensitization seems necessary and has been successful (Discipio & Feldman, 1971; Feldman & Discipio, 1972).

A novel and promising outpatient intervention for the treatment of poststroke psychosocial disorders was developed by Griffith (1975). A community-wide plan was created in which teams of lay volunteers made routine visits to 31 stroke patients. These visits were made to stimulate patients' desire to recover and to encourage patients to make optimal use of their intellectual strengths by engaging in numerous games and tasks. Patient outcome was assessed by the family, doctors, speech therapists, and volunteers. Physicians reported that the general attitude and morale of nearly all of the patients had improved. Similarly, 21 patients showed improvement in speech. The success and cost effectiveness of this program suggests that it may represent an ideal posthospital rehabilitation program; it employs community resources to provide patients with social and cognitive stimulation that would not be possible in other settings.

It has already been mentioned that several authors developed methods to build up patients' self-esteem (Oberleder, 1970; Power et al., 1975; Brody et al., 1971; Salter & Salter, 1975). The methods are especially suitable for handling crisis situations in elderly depressed and physically disabled people and can easily be used in group therapy in an outpatient setting. Patient groups organized by the patients themselves have already been described.

The main goal of these associations is to enable the members to take better care of themselves. In Germany there exist approximately 15 well-organized patient associations for different somatic chronic disabilities, for example, Parkinson's disease, multiple sclerosis, and stroke.

GROUPS FOR RELATIVES

Introduced by family therapists, inclusions of relatives into the treatment is a rather new development. The first information on groups including relatives of mentally ill aged appeared only recently (Fuller et al., 1979; Rathbone-McCuan, 1976; Boviar et al., 1979; Zarit et al., 1982; Levine et al., 1983). The aim of this work is the enlightenment of relatives to the type of illness of the patient and the discussion of more adequate forms of dealing with the patient to ease living together. Lazarus et al. (1981) report on a very small group of relatives (four relatives of patients with Alzheimer's disease) and found limited effectiveness measured by means of questionnaires and compared to a control group with three relatives. Rönnecke (1978) has reported the first experiences from Germany. Another experience report from Germany has come from Hamburg (Klusmann et al., 1981; Bruder, 1983). An open group with a total of 16 relatives, mainly daughters (9) and daughters-in-law (3) met at two-week intervals. The majority of patients were psychoorganically disturbed and lived together with their relatives. Due to the situation the majority of participants were heavily burdened and in general able to maintain the home situation only with utmost energy. Keeping this aspect in mind, the group was primarily concerned with strengthening of ego functions and decreasing the relatives' feeling of guilt.

Groups for relatives will become important factors in psychogeriatric treatment, enabling a realistic assessment of the relatives' burden and their ability to cope. By this assessment, the decision for or against a patient's placement into a nursing home for instance, is facilitated.

DISCUSSION

Not every elderly person who seems to be changed needs psychotherapy. Old age brings with it typical tasks and problems the aged person has to deal with. For this he develops psychological adaptation techniques and coping strategies. With some of these he might be successful and not be impaired; only to the young he might seem "abnormal," for example in his severe rigidity, conservatism, or regression to personality-specific behavior patterns, which impresses as an increase of character traits (Lauter, 1983).

Christian Müller (1967) speaks in the same context of "normal neurotization" in old age. These persons in fact may occasionally need psychological advice but not treatment. If, for instance, rigidity means safeguarding against enormous stress and frustration, it would be fatal to try to change this therapeutically. That is why indication for psychotherapy with the aged should be decided on with the utmost care.

Psychotherapy with the aged has its peculiarities. Certainly many things make it more difficult. Often the capacity for insight is reduced by diminished ability to assimilate new experiences, particularly due to pathophysiological changes in the brain. On the other hand, it is frequently reported that especially in old age there is a greater readiness for critical self-reflection (Grotjahn, 1955; Müller, 1982). Maybe the demand of reality can be better accepted because it no longer threatens the narcissistic balance to such an extent (Karasu & Bourgois, 1980) or perhaps it is the pressure of the remaining lifespan (Müller, 1982). Thus the old person deals very differently with his psychic problems and psychotherapy accordingly has to be adapted individually. The old person's spontaneous tendency towards life balancing can help in finding a psychotherapeutic opening. In administering treatment the therapist never should forget that the approach of death is a reality. For Müller (1976), therefore, coming to terms with the knowledge that life will end is the central concern of every psychotherapy in advanced age.

A further reality is the loneliness of many aged patients—the therapist often becomes the most important or even the only person with whom to talk. According to general experience he has to be willing in this case to substitute for the lack of others and to accept his substitute role. But turning toward an old person by listening to him or having a helpful talk with him is by no means, not even for the aged, a form of psychotherapy that brings about fundamental changes of attitudes (Schulz, 1976; Mulligen & Bennet, 1977, 1978). Knowledge of psychology of aging and psychotherapeutic methods have to be added to general and ethical understanding.

In surveying the literature on this subject, there is still very little engagement for psychotherapists themselves. On the other hand, especially recently, the old person is uncritically offered all sorts of life-aid with a therapeutic approach. The aims are blurred and a lot of what is called therapy is at best pedagogical theory. This overenthusiasm can very easily bypass the exigencies of the aged. Kalish (1979) calls it a new form of agism: "The message of the New Age-ism seems to be that 'we' understand how badly you are being treated, that 'we' have the tools to improve your treatment, and that if you adhere to our program, 'we' will make your life considerably better." Müller (1976) points out another similar problem. In every psychotherapy with the aged he sees the underlying danger of wanting to "inject" uncritical optimism, thus joining into the defense against the knowledge that life must end and deceiving both patient and therapist. The aged patient easily sees through those games with nonexisting plans for the future and then feels deceived. Bearing this danger in mind, psychotherapy in advanced age should have the aim of finding a new meaning in old age, in the sense of "positive resignation" (Müller, 1976).

Efforts to prove the effectiveness of applied psychotherapies are very rare, a dilemma quite common to the area of psychotherapy. In most publications populations, therapy methods, and therapy content are vaguely described. Descriptions of success are general and have been examined with uncertain measures or not at all. The few authors who have tried to prove their success are Wolff (1970) with his psychodynamically oriented individual therapy and Lago and Hoffmann (1977, 1978) and Miller (1977) with their treatment of groups. Lately publications are increasing in which aspects of therapy are compared with each other using a controlled method, however almost exclusively in behavior therapy oriented literature. This is the only area in which scientific methods in a sense of control of therapy results are visible as prevailing efforts. In other areas the reports sometimes do not even rise above the realm of anecdotes. Psychotherapy research with the aged is particularly difficult (Mintz et al., 1981). The influence on therapy of external factors over which the therapist has no control is very large. The current methods of measuring success have not been standardized with regard to the population of the aged. But psychotherapy with the aged especially needs a scientifically well founded basis to convince not only critics but also those who bear the expenditure.

In summary, there is no reason to be pessimistic about psychotherapy in the aged if it is adapted to the particularities of elderly people. In inpatient services, mainly behaviorally oriented and milieu-therapeutic approaches have been used successfully as well as special therapy approaches such as reality orientation, remotivation, and revitalization. In gerontopsychiatric day hospitals group psychotherapy of different kinds, milieu and sociotherapy, have been applied widely and in outpatient services individual and group psychotherapy, psychodynamically or behaviorally oriented have been used with success. A rather new development is the organization of groups by the patients which focus on helping patients to cope with their disabilities. In working with the psychogeriatric population the following points should be kept in mind: Tender, loving care should be regarded as an integral part of any institutional setting for the aged; the physical and social environment of the patients should be stimulating; psychotherapy should be problem oriented; and the most supporting environment for the patient is his own home. Therefore therapy of psychogeriatric patients should aim to keep the patient at home as long as possible.

REFERENCES

Abraham, K. (1971). Zur Prognose psychoanalytischer Behandlung in vorgeschrittenem Lebensalter. *Psychoanalytische Studien, II,* 262–266. S. Fischer.
Adams, G. M., de Vries, H. A. (1973). Physiological effects of an exercise training regimen upon women aged 52 to 79. *J. Gerontol., 28,* 50–55.
Ayllon, T., Azrin, N. (1968). *The token economy: A motivational system for therapy and rehabilitation.* New York: Prentice Hall.
Baltes, M. M., Zerbe, M. B. (1976). Reestablishing self-feeding in a nursing home resident. *Nurs. Res., 25,* S. 24.
Barnes, J. H. (1974). Effects of reality orientation classroom on memory loss, confusion and disorientation in geriatric patients. *Gerontologist, 14,* 138–142.
Barns, E. K., Sack, A., Shore, H. (1973). Guidelines to treatment approaches *Gerontologist, 13,* 513–527.
Beck, A. T., Rush, A. J., Shaw, B. F., Emery, G. (1981). *Kognitive Therapie der Depression.* München: Urban u. Schwarzenberg.
Belluci, G., Hoyer, W. J. (1975). Feedback effects on the performance and self-reinforcing behavior of elderly and young adult women. *J. Gerontol., 4,* 450.
Berger, L. F. (1978). Activating a psychogeriatric group. *Psychiatr. Q., 50,* 63–66.
Bergmann, K. (1978). Neurosis and personality disorder in old age. In A D Isaacs, F. Post (Eds.), *Studies in Geriatric Psychiatry.* New York: Wiley.
Bircher, M. (1981). Psychotherapie im hohen Lebensalter—Erfahrungen mit Einzeltherapie bei geriatrischen und geronto-psychiatrischen Patienten. *Z. Gerontol., 14,* 48–60.
Birkhill, W. R., Schaie, K. W. (1975). The effect of differential reinforcement of cautiousness in intellectual performance among the elderly. *J. Gerontol., 5,* 578.
Blau, D., Berezin, M. A. (1975). Neuroses and character disorders, In J. G. Howells (Ed.), *Modern Perspectives in the Psychiatry of old age.* New York: Brunner/Mazel.
Bovier, Ph., Beroud, D., Cantin, R. (1979). Therapeutic mobilisation of the family of the aged psychiatric patient. *Med. Hyg., 37,* 1353, 3818–3822.
Brody, E. M., Kleban, M., Lawton, P., Silverman, H. A. (1971). Excess disabilities of mentally impaired aged. Impact of individualized treatment. *Gerontologist, II,* 124–133.
Brook, P., Degin, G., Mathes, M. (1975). Reality orientation, a theory for psychogeriatric patients: a controlled study. *Br. J. Psychiatry, 127,* 42–45.
Bruder, J. (1983). Zur Gruppenarbeit mit Angehörigen von dementen und nicht dementen alten Menschen. In H. Radebold (Ed.), *Gruppenpsychotherapie im Alter.* Göttingen: Vandenhoeck und Ruprecht.
Brüggemann, E. (1977). Tanz für den alten Menschen—Seniorentanz medizinisch gesehen. *Geriatrie, 7,* 395–397.
Butler, R. N., Lewis, M. I. (1977). *Aging and mental health positive psychosocial approaches.* St. Louis: Mosby.
Carlson, C. E. (1980). Psychosocial aspects of neurologic disability. *Nurs. Clin. North Am., 15,* 309–320.
Cautela, J. R. (1966). Behavior therapy and geriatrics *J. Gen. Psychol., 108,* 9.
Cautela, J. R. (1969). A classical conditioning approach to the development and modification of behavior in the aged. *Gerontologist, 9,* 109.
Charaton, F. A., & A. Fisk (1978). Mental and emotional results of stroke. *NY State J. Med., 78,* 1403–1405.

Citrin, R. S., Dixon, D. N. (1977). Reality orientation. A milieutherapy used in an institution for the aged. *Gerontologist*, 17, 39–43.
Cohen, S. (1979). Rehabilitation of the stroke patient. *Md State Med. J.*, 28, 82–83.
D'Affliti, J. Gr., Weitz, Gr. (1974). Rehabilitating the stroke patient through patient—family groups. *Int. J. Grouppsychother.*, 24, 323–332.
Davidson, R. (1963). The psychologic aspects of stroke. *Geriatrics*, 18, 151.
DeCarlo, T. J., Castiglione, L. V., Cavusoglu, M. (1977). A program of balanced physical fitness in the preventive care of elderly ambulatory patients. *J. Am. Geriatr. Soc.*, 25, 331–334.
Discipio, W. J., Feldman, M. C. (1971). Combined behavior therapy and physical therapy in treatment of a fear of walking. *J. Behav. Ther. Exp. Psychiatry*, 2, 151.
Dodgen, J. C., Ransom, J. E. (1967). Psychotherapy of a sexagenarian. *Dis. Nerv. System*, 28, 680–683.
Edinberg, M. A., Gleser, G. C., Karoly, P. (1977). Assessing assertion in the elderly: An application of the behavioral-analytic model of competence. *J. Clin. Psychol.*, 33, 869.
Elsayad, M., Ismail, A. H., Young, R. J. (1980). Intellectual differences of adult men related to age and physical fitness before and after an exercise program. *J. Gerontol.*, 35, 383–387.
Evans, R. L., Jaureguy, B. M. (1981). Group therapy by phone: a cognitive behavioral program for visually impaired elderly. *Soc. Work Health Care*, 7, 79–90.
Feldman, M. C., Discipio, W. J. (1972). Integrating physical therapy with behavior therapy. *Phys. Ther.*, 52, 1283.
Filer, R. N., O'Connel, D. D. (1964). Modification of aging persons in an institutional setting. *J. Gerontol.*, 19, 15.
Fisher, S. H. (1961). Psychiatric considerations of cerebral vascular disease. *Am. J. Cardiol.*, 7, 379–385.
Folsom, J. C. (1968). Reality orientation for the elderly mental patient. *J. Geriatr. Psychiatry*, 1, 291–307.
Frank, P. J., Klein, S., Jacobs, J. (1982). Cost—benefit analysis of a behavioral program for geriatric in patients. *Hosp. Community Psychiatry*, 33, 374–377.
Freud, S. (1942). Über Psychotherapie. Gesammelte Werke V S. Fischer.
Frohne, J. (1979). Musiktherapie mit alten Menschen. In H. Petzold & E. Bubolz (Ed.), *Psychotherapie mit alten Menschen*. Paderborn: Juntermann.
Fuller, J., Ward, E., Evans, A., Massam, K., Gardner, A. (1979). Dementia: supportive groups for relatives. *Brit. Med. J.*, 1, 1684–1685.
Garner, H. H. (1965). Brief psychotherapy. *Int. J. Neuropsychiatry*, 1, 616–622.
Gauthier, J., Marshall, W. L. (1977). Grief: a cognitive behavioral analysis. *Cognitive Therapy and Research*, 1, 39.
Ginzberg, R. (1950). Psychology in everyday geriatrics. *Geriatrics*, 5, 36–43.
Godbole, A., Verinis, J. S. (1974). Brief psychotherapy in the treatment of emotional disorders in physically ill geriatric patients. *Gerontologist*, 14, 143–148.
Goldberg, E. M., Morthery, A., Williams, B. T. (1970). *Helping the aged: A field experiment in social work*. London: Allen & Unwin.
Goldfarb, A. I. (1969). Institutional care of the aged. In E. W. Busse, & E. Pfeiffer (Eds.) *Behavior and adaptation in late life*. Boston: Little, Brown.
Goldstein, R. S., Baer, D. M. (1976). A procedure to increase the personal mail and number of correspondents for nursing home residents. *Behav. Ther.*, 7, 348.

Goldstein, S. (1972). A critical appraisal of milieu therapy in a geriatric day hospital. *J. Am. Geriatr. Soc., 19,* 693–699.
Gordon, W. A., Diller, L. (1983). Stroke: coping with a cognitive deficit. In T. G. Burish & L. A. Bradley (Eds.), *Coping with chronic disease.* New York: Academic Press.
Götestam, K. G. (1980). Behavioral and dynamic psychotherapy with the elderly. In J. E. Birren & R. B. Sloane (Eds.), *Handbook of mental health and aging.* New York: Prentice-Hall.
Götestam, K. G., Melin, L. (1979). Improving well-being for patients with senile dementia by minor changes in the ward environment. In L. Levi (Ed.), *Society Stress and Disease: aging and old age.* London: Oxford University Press.
Greene, J. G., Nicol, R., Janieson, H. (1976). Reality orientation with psychogeriatric patients. *Behav. Res. Ther., 17,*
Griffith, V. E. (1975). Volunteer scheme for dysphasia and allied problems in stroke patients. *Br. Med. J., 3,* 633–635.
Grotjahn, M. (1955). Analytic psychotherapy with the elderly. *Psychoanal. Rev., 42,* 419–427.
Gunn, J. C. (1967). Group psychotherapy on a geriatric ward. *Psychother. Psychosom., 15,* 26.
Hackett, T. P., Cassem N. H. (1973). Psychological adaptation to convalescence in myocardial in farction patients. In J. P. Naughton, H. K. Hellerstein, & I. C. Mohler (Eds.), *Exercise Testing and exercise training in coronary heart disease.* New York: Academic Press.
Hahn, P. (1971). *Der Herzinfarkt in psychosomatischer Sicht.* Göttingen: Vandenhoeck u. Ruprecht.
Hamilton, J. E., Cowdry, E. V. (1976). Psychiatric aspects, In F. U. Steinberg (Ed.), *Cowdry's the Care of the geriatric patient.* St. Louis: Mosby.
Hanley, I. G. (1981). The use of sign posts and active training to modify ward disorientation in elderly patients. *J. Behav. Ther. Exp. Psychiatry, 12,* 241–247.
Hanley, I. G., McGuire, R. J., Boyd, W. D. (1981). Reality orientation and dementia: a controlled trial of two approaches. *Br. J. Psychiatry, 138,* 10–14.
Harris, C. S., Ivory, P. B. (1976). An outcome evaluation of reality orientation therapy with geriatric patients in a state mental hospital. *Gerontologist, 16,* 496–503.
Hedri, A. (1968). Psychotherapie im höheren Alter. *Zeitschrift für Psychotherapie und medizinische Psychologie, 18,* 105–108.
Hiatt, H. (1971). Dynamic psychotherapy with the aging patient. *Am. J. Psychother., 25,* 591–600.
Holden, U. P., Sinebruchow, A. (1978). Reality orientation therapy: A study investigating the value of this therapy in the rehabilitation of elderly people. *Age ageing, 7,* 83–90.
Hoyer, W. J., Kanfer, R. A., Simpson, S. C., Hoyer, F. W. (1974). Reinstatement of verbal behavior in elderly mental patients using operant procedures. *Gerontologist, 14,* 149.
Hoyer, W. J., Labouvie, G. V., Baltes, P. B. (1973). Modification of response speed and intellectual performance in the elderly *Hum. Dev., 16,* 232.
Huber, R. (1973). Sensory training for a fuller life. *Nurs. Homes, 22,* 14–15.
Jenkins, J., Felce, D., Lund, B., Powell, C. (1977). Increasing engagement in activity of residents in old peoples homes by providing recreational materials. *Behav. Res. Ther., 15,* 429–434.
Jones, M. (1953). *The therapeutic community.* New York: Basic Books.

Jones, R. F. (1975). Stroke rehabilitation. Part I: general considerations. *Med. J. Austral.*, 2, 773–775.
Kahana, R. J. (1979). Strategies of dynamic psychotherapy with the wide range of older individuals. *J. Geriatr. Psychiatry*, 12, 71–100.
Kalish, R. A. (1979). The new ageism and the future models: A polemic. *Gerontologist*, 19, 398–402.
Karasu, I. B., Bourgeois, M. L. (1980). La psychothérapy chez le vieilard. *Ann. Med. Psychol.*, 138, 574–580.
Kennedy, R. W., Kennedy, A. B. (1982). Absence of purposeful behavior. Issues in training profoundly impaired elderly. In A. MacNeill Horton (Ed.), *Mental health interventions for the aging*. New York: Praeger.
Klein, W. H., LeShan, E. J., Furman, S. S. (1965). *Promoting mental health of older people through group methods*. New York: Mental Health Materials Center.
Klusmann, D., Gruder, J., Lauter, H., Lüders, I. (1981). *Beziehungen zwischen Patienten und ihren Familien-angehörigen bei chronischen Erkrankungen des höheren Lebensalters*. Hamburg.
Köhle, K., Gaus, E. (1979). Psychotherapie von Herzinfarkt—Patienten während der stationären und poststationären Behandlungsphase. In T. von Uexküll (Ed.), *Lehrbuch der psychosomatischen Medizin*. München, Wien, Baltimore: Urban und Schwarzenberg.
Kübler-Ross, E. (1972). *On death and dying*. New York: Macmillan.
Lago, D., Hoffman, S. (1977/78). Structured group interaction: An intervention strategy for the continued development of elderly populations. *Int. J. Aging Hum. Dev.*, 8, 311–324.
Langley, G. E. (1975). Functional psychoses. In J. G. Howell (Ed.), *Modern Perspectives in Psychiatry of old age*. New York: Brunner/Mazel.
Lauter, H. (1983). Psychologische Probleme im Alter. In E. Bönisch, J. E. Meyer (Hrsg.), *Psychosomatik in der klinischen Medizin*. Berlin: Springer
Lawton, M. P. (1970). Assessment, integration and environments for older people. *Gerontologist*, 10, 38–46.
Lazarus, L. W., Stafford, B., Cooper, K., Cohler, B., Dysken, M. (1981). A pilot study of Alzheimer patient's relatives discussion group. *Gerontologist*, 21, 353–358.
Lehr, U. (1967). Attitudes toward the future. *Human Development*, 10, 230–238.
Lehr, U. (ed.), (1979). *Interventionsgerontologie*. Darmstadt: Dr. D. Steinkopff Verlag.
Lehr, U., Thomae, H. (1965). *Konflikt, seelische Belastung und Lebensalter*. Köln, Opladen: Westdt. Verlag.
Letcher, P., Peterson, L. P., Scarbrough, D. (1974). Reality orientation: a historical study of patient progress. *J. Hospital and Community Psychiat.*, 25, 801–803.
Levine, N. B., Dastoor, D. P., Gendron, C. E. (1983). Coping with dementia: a pilot study. *J. Amer. Geriatr. Society*, 31, 12–18.
Lewinson, P. M. (1974). A behavioral approach to depression. In R. J. Friedman & M. M. Katz (Eds.), *The psychology of depression*. New York: Wiley.
Libb, J. W., Clements, C. B. (1969). Token reinforcement in an exercise program for hospitalized geriatric patients. *Perceptual and Motor Skills*, 28, 957–958.
Liederman, P. C., Green, R., Liederman, V. R. (1967). Outpatient group therapy with geriatric patients. *Geriatrics*, 22, 148–153.
Linden, M. E. (1956). Geriatrics. In S. R. Slavson (Ed.), *The fields of group psychotherapy*. New York: International Universities Press.

Lindsley, O. R. (1964). Geriatric behavioral prothetics. In R. Kastenbaum (Ed.), *New thoughts old age*. New York: Springer.
Loew, C. A., Silverstone, B. M. (1971). A program of intensified stimulation and response facilitation for the senile aged. *Gerontologist, 11*, 341–347.
MacDonald, M. L., Butler, A. K. (1974). Reversal of helplessness: Producing walking behavior in nursing home wheelchair residents using behavior modification procedures. *J. Gerontol., 29*, 97–101.
Manaster, A. (1967). The family group therapy program at Park View Home for the Aged. *J. Amer. Geriatric Soc., 15*, 302–306.
Martin, L. J. (1944). *A handbook for old age counselors*. San Francisco: Geertz Printing Co.
McClannahan, L. E., Risley, T. R. (1973). A store for nursing home residents. *Nursing Homes, 22*, 10–11.
McClannahan, L. E., Risley, T. R. (1974). Design of living environments for nursing home residents: recruiting attendance at activities. *Gerontologist, 14*, 236–240.
McClannahan, L. E., Risley, T. R. (1975a). Activities and materials for severely disabled geriatric patients. *Nursing Homes, 23*, 1–4.
McClannahan, L. E., Risley, T. R. (1975b). Design of living environments for nursing-home residents; Increasing participation in recreation activities. *J. Appl. Behav. Anal., 8*, 261–268.
McPherson, B. D., Paivio, A., Yuhasz, M. S., Rechnitzer, P. A., Pickard, H. A., Lefcoe, N. M. (1967). Psychological effects of an exercise program for postinfarct and normal adultmen. *J. Sports Med. and Physical Fitness, 7*, 95–102.
McReynolds, W. T., Coleman, J. (1972). Token economy: Patient and staff changes. *Behav. Res. Ther., 10*, 29.
Miller, E. (1977). The management of dementia: a review of some possibilities. *Br. J. Soc. Chin. Psychol., 16*, 77–83.
Mintz, J., Steuer, J., Jarvik, L. (1981). Psychotherapy with depressed elderly patients: research considerations. *J. Consult. Clin. Psychol., 49*, 542–548.
Mishara, B. L. (1978). Geriatric patients who improve in token economy and general milieu treatment programs: a multivariate analysis. *J. Consult. Clin. Psychol., 46*, 1340.
Mueller, D. J., Atlas, L. (1972). Resocialization of regressed elderly residents: a behavioral management approach. *J. Gerontol., 27*, 390–392.
Müller, Ch. (1976). Gedanken zur Psychotherapie und Soziotherapie im Alter. *Schweiz. med. Wschr., 106*, 1421–1425.
Müller, Ch. (1982). Psychotherapie in der Alterspsychiatrie. In H. Helmchen, M. Linden, U. Rüger (Ed.), *Psychotherapie in der Psychiatrie*. Berlin: Springer.
Müller, Ch. (1967). *Alterspsychiatrie*. Stuttgart: Thieme.
Mulligan, M. A., Bennett, R. (1977/78). Assessment of mental health and social problems during multiple friendly visits. *Int. J. Aging and Human Development, 8*, 43–65.
Murell, F. H. (1970). The effect of extensive practise on age differences reaction time. *J. Gerontol., 25*, 268.
Muslin, H., Epstein, L. J. (1980). Preliminary remarks on the rationale for psychotherapy of the aged. *Comprehensive Psychiatry, 21*, 1–12.
Naughton, J. P., Bruhn, J. G., Lategola, M. T. (1968). Effects of physical training on physiologic and behavioral characteristics of cardiac patients. *Arch. Physical Med. Rehab., 49*, 131–137.
Naughton, J. P., Hellerstein, H. K., Mohler, I. C. (1973). *Exercise testing and exercise training in coronary heart disease*. New York: Academic Press.

Nigl, A. J., Jackson, B. (1981). A behavior management program to increase social responses in psychogeriatric patients. *J. Am. Geriatric Soc., 29*, 92–95.
Oberleder, M. (1970). Crisis therapy in mental breakdown of the aging. *Gerontologist, 10*, 111–114.
Oradei, D. M., Waite, N. S. (1974). Group psychotherapy with stroke patients during the immediate recovery phase. *Amer. J. Orthopsychiatry, 44*, 386–395.
Peterson, R. F., Knapp, T. J., Rosen, J. C., Pither, B. F. (1977). The effects of furmituve arrangement on the behavior of geriatric patients. *Behavior Therapy, 8*, 464–467.
Petzold, F., & Reindell, A. (1980). *Klinische Psychosomatik*. Heidelberg: Quelle und Meyer.
Pfeiffer, E. (1976). Psychotherapy with elderly patients. In L. Bellak & T. B. Karasu (Eds.), *Geriatric Psychiatry* (191–206). New York: Grune and Stratton.
Piskor, B. K., Paleos, S. (1968). The group way to banish afterstroke blues. *Amer. J. Nursing, 68*, 1500–1503.
Pitt, B. (1974). *Psychogeriatrics*. London: Churchill Livingstone.
Powell, R. R. (1974). Psychological effects of exercise therapy upon institutionalaized geriatric mental patients. *J. Gerontol., 29*, 157–161.
Power, C. A., McCarron, L. T. (1975). Treatment of depression in persons residing in homes for the aged. *Gerontologist, 15*, 132–135.
Puschner, J., Schreiner, M., Tismer, K. G. (1968). Expansion und Restriktion in der Lebensthematik älterer Menschen. Ber. I. Kongr. Dt. Ges. Gerontol. Darmstadt: Steinkopff.
Radebold, H. (1976). Psychoanalytische Gruppenpsychotherapie mit älteren und alten Patienten. *Z. Gerontologie, 9*, 128–142.
Radebold, H. (1979). Der psychoanalytische Zugang zu dem älteren und alten Menschen. In H. Petzold, E. Bubolz (Eds.), *Psychotherapie mit alten Menschen*. Paderborn.
Radebold, H. (1983). Psychische Erkrankungen im höheren und hohen Lebensalter und ihre Behandlungsmöglichkeiten. In H. Reimann, H. Reimann (Hrsg.), *Das Alter; Einführung in die Gerontologie*. Stuttgart: Enke.
Rathbone-McCuan, E. (1976). Geriatric day care: A family perspective. *Gerontologist, 16*, 6.
Rechtschaffen, A., Atkinson, St., Freeman, J. G. (1954). An intensive treatment program for State Hospital Geriatric patients. *Geriatrics, 9*, 28–34.
Richards, W. S., Thorpe, W. L. (1978). Behavioral approaches to the problems of later life. In M. Storandt, I. C. Siegler, & M. F. Elias (Eds.) *The clinical Psychology of aging*. New York, London: Plenum Press.
Richman, L. (1969). Sensory training for geriatric patients. *Am. J. Occup. Ther., 23*, 254–257.
Rinke, C. L., Williams, J. J., Lloyd, K. E., Smith-Scott, W. (1978). The effects of prompting and reinforcement on self-bathing by elderly residents of a nursing home. *Behav. Ther., 9*, 873–881.
Rönnecke, B. (1978). Arbeit mit Angehörigen von Patienten einer gerontopsychiatrischen Poliklinik. In C. Müller (Hrsg.), *Gerontopsychiatrie, Vol. 7*. Düsseldorf: Janssen.
Ross, M. (1959). Recent contributions to gerontologic group psychotherapy. *Int. J. Group Psychother., 9*, 442–450.
Sachuk, N. N. (1970). Population longevity study: sources and indices. *J. Gerontol., 25*, 262–264.

Salter, C. D. L., Salter, C. A. (1975). Effects of an individualized activity program on elderly patients. *Gerontologist, 15,* 404–406.
Sandel, S. L. (1978). Movement therapy with geriatric patients in a convalescent home. *Hospital Community Psychiatry, 29,* 730–741.
Schmitz-Scherzer, R. (1969). *Freizeit und Alter.* Bonn: Phil. Diss. Universität.
Schreiner, M. (1969). *Zur zukunftsbezogenen Zeitperspektive bei alten Menschen.* Bonn: Phil. Diss. Universität.
Schulz, R. (1976). The effects of control and predictability on the physical and psychological well-being of the institutionalized aged. *J. Personality and Soc. Psychol., 33,* 563–573.
Shanas, E. (1971). Measuring the home health needs of the aged in five countries. *J. Gerontol., 26,* 37–40.
Shanas, E., Townsend, P., Wedderburn, D., Friis, H., Milhoj, P., & Stehouwer, J. (Eds.). (1968) *Old people in three industrial societies.* New York. Atherton Press. London: Routledge & Kegan Paul. Reprinted 1980. New York: Arno Press.
Shapiro, A. (1969). A pilot program in music therapy with residents of a home for the aged. *Gerontologist, 9,* 128–133.
Silver, A. (1950). Group psychotherapy with senile psychotic patients. *Geriatrics, 5,* 147–150.
Singler, J. R. (1975). Group work with hospitalized stroke patients. *Social Casework, 56,* 348–354.
Stindl, E., Kühl, K. P., Pilger, D., Kanowski, S. (1981). Nicht-medikamentöse Behandlung in der Gerontopsychiatrie. *Münch. med. Wschr., 123,* 79–83.
Stonnington, H. H. (1980). Rehabilitation in cerebrovascular diseases. *Primary Care, 7,* 87–106.
Streib, G. F., Orbach, H. L. (1967). Aging. In P. Lazarsfeld et al. (Eds.), The uses of sociology. New York: Basic Books.
Strotzka, H. (Ed.). (1975). *Psychotherapie: Grundlagen, Verfahren, Indikationen.* München: Urban und Schwarzenberg.
Sulz, K. D., Lauter, H. (1983). Stationäre Verhaltenstherapie der Depression—ein multimodaler Ansatz in der klinischen Praxis. *Psychiat. Prax., 10,* 33–40.
Theissen, Ch. (1970). Das Selbstbild des Alters als Spiegelbild des Altersbildes der Gesellschaft. *Ber. Kongr. Dt. Ges. Psychol.* Steinkopff, Darmstadt.
Thomae, H. (1970). Theory of aging and cognitive theory of personality. *Hum. Dev., 13,* 1–16.
Thyer, B. A. (1981). Prolonged in vivo exposure therapy with a 70-year-old woman. *J. Behav. Ther. Exp. Psychiatry, 12,* 69–71.
Ullrich-De Muynck, R., Ullrich, R. (1976). *Das Assertiveness-Trainings-Programm ATP; Einüben von Selbstvertrauen und sozialer Kompetenz.* München: Pfeiffer.
Verwoerdt, A. (1976). *Clinical Geropsychiatry,* Baltimore: Williams and Wilkins.
Villa, J. L. (1976). zit. nach Radebold, H.: Psychoanalytische Gruppenpsychotherapie mit älteren und alten Patienten. *Z. Gerontologie, 9,* 128–142.
Wächtler, C. (1982). Gruppentherapie in einer gerontopsychiatrischen Tagesklinik—erste Erfahrungen. *Psychother. med. Psychol., 32,* 122–126.
Wanderer, Z. W. (1972). Existential depression treated by desensitization of phobias: Strategy and transcript. *J. Behav. Ther. Exp. Psychiatry., 3,* 111.
Watzlawick, P., Coyne, J. C. (1980). Depression following stroke: Brief, problem-focused family treatment. *Family Process, 19,* 13–18.
Weinberg, J. (1975). Geriatric Psychiatry. In A. M. Freedman, H. J. Kaplan, & B. J. Sadock (Eds.) *Comprehensive Textbook of Psychiatry II.* Baltimore: Williams & Wilkins

Wertheimer, J., Lobrinus, A. (1981). Psychotherapie neurotischer Störungen beim alten Menschen: Eine Öffnung ins Leben. *Z. Gerontologie, 14,* 22–33.

Wisocki, P. A. (1977). *Sampling procedures: tools for stimulating the activity and interest of institutionalized elderly.* Paper presented at the American Psychological Association, San Francisco.

Wolff, K. (1962). Group psychotherapy with geriatric patients in a psychiatric hospital: Six-year study. *J. Am. Geriatr. Soc., 10,* 1077–1080.

Wolff, K. (1963). Individual psychotherapy with geriatric patients. *Dis. Nerv. System, 24,* 688–691.

Wolff, K. (1970). *The emotional rehabilitation of the geriatric patient.* Springfield, Illinois: Thomas.

Wolff, K. (1971). Individual psychotherapy with geriatric patients. *Psychosomatics, 12,* 89–93.

Zarit, S. H., Zarit, J. M., Reever, K. E. (1982). Memory training for severe memory loss: effects on senile dementia patients and their families. *Gerontologist, 22,* 373–377.

Zepelin, H., Wolfe, C. S., Kleinplatz, F. (1981). Evaluation of a yearlong reality orientation program. *J. Gerontol., 36,* 70–77.

PART V
Care and Services

20
Rehabilitation and Long-Term Care in the Elderly

Jean Wertheimer

DEFINITION OF REHABILITATION

The close relationship in the psychogeriatric and geriatric domains between somatic, psychological, psychiatric, and social elements calls for an analysis of the various components of each individual's predicament, followed by a synthesis from which the best therapeutic program may be deduced. The action thus planned and then put into effect aims at a "restitutio ad integrum" or, if this is beyond our reach, "ad optimum" (Rustemeyer, 1982). When we refer here to rehabilitation, that is what we mean.

Speaking very generally, the West German working group on rehabilitation (1970) gave the following definition: "Rehabilitation aims to help persons who are handicapped physically, psychically and spiritually, and who cannot overcome these handicaps by themselves, and also those who are threatened with being handicapped, to develop their aptitudes and energies to find an appropriate place in society, which primarily implies participation in working life" (Gadomski, 1980). While the greater part of this conception corresponds to the objectives of the rehabilitation of elderly persons, it is obvious that the latter part, referring to work, is not usually relevant to this category of the population. In geriatric medicine, the object is to arrive at the optimal quality of life. From this point of view, we might define rehabilitation as "the whole of medical, psychiatric, psychological, and social means that agree with an elaborate programme directed towards the restitution or maintenance of one's autonomy" (Wertheimer, 1981).

Four fundamental points are implied by this definition. The first is that of a *total approach* to the elderly person, whose situation must be evaluated with respect to every element of his predicament. The second indicates the need for *teamwork* to identify the aims pursued and the means necessary to work toward rehabilitation in a coordinated manner. The third is the need to be *realistic* in assessing the individual's residual capacities, which often presupposes a reasonable limit to therapeutic aspirations. The fourth and last point refers to *rehabilitation action,* which is simultaneously therapeutic and prophylactic, so that when optimal autonomy has been attained, efforts can be made to maintain it in the long term.

SOMATIC AND PSYCHIATRIC GERIATRICS

Somatic and psychiatric polymorbidity present us, at the outset, with the problem of making a distinction between physical and psychic geriatric rehabilitation. In adult medicine, the fields of somatic and psychological action may be quite distinct, even though some pathological conditions in this age group may display the same combined somatic–psychic pattern so common in old people. Among the latter, however, there are some typical characteristics such as a general slowing-up, heightened sensitivity to stress, modification of sensory functions, social isolation, etc., which affect relations with elderly people and call for special attitudes toward them.

The heterogeneity of the aged population is another factor influencing the matter of the somatic and/or psychiatric specificity of geriatric rehabilitation. Within the traditional age limits of geriatric medicine, there are quite different patterns of problems if, for example, we take the age groups from 65 to 70 years and 90 and over. In the former group, the needs are much more comparable to those found in the adult age group and are often so clearly defined that it is not particularly necessary to consider the individual as a whole. Physiotherapy alone may be sufficient for the rehabilitation of a 65-year-old patient after a hip operation. In the second group, the probable polymorbidity and also the risks entailed in immobilization will require a more comprehensive course of treatment, as in the case of a 90-year-old person with a fracture of the neck of the femur.

Another element to be considered is that of the nature of the institution in which the patient is to be treated. A geriatric hospital is likely to focus its rehabilitation efforts on physiotherapy, while a psychogeriatric hospital is predisposed by the special means it has available to give particular emphasis to questions of communication and relations (ergotherapy, organized activity, psychotherapy, etc.) Experience has demonstrated however that we cannot disregard the existence of a psychological problem in an old person undergoing a course of physical rehabilitation, and likewise we cannot neglect somatic conditions developing in a psychogeriatric case.

Although we must recognize that in the very structure of an organization for the care of old people there are specific functions, we must also realize that geriatric institutions as a whole are confronted by common problems. It is therefore necessary to meet both the specific needs of a patient and the larger needs relating to his psychological status and his social environment. The way to deal with such an ambiguous situation is not to make an all out effort to change the material infrastructure or to shuffle the rehabilitation personnel to correspond to the relative frequency of needs. Instead, the natural solution should be found in the "savoir-faire" and the "savoir-être" (Junod, 1984) which should be shared by all members of the team. They will all be able to listen to the patient, to be aware of his perception of himself, his reaction to what is being done for him, his motivations, and his emotional history. Through this experience, partly empirical, the team will be able to improve its action, composed both of technical acts and relational qualities.

The specificities of psychogeriatric rehabilitation emerge from two orders of reality. The first is the nature of the psychiatric pathology of conditions primarily affecting the emotional life of the patient (depression, manic states, delirious states) or mental operations (psychoorganic syndromes), which have repercussions on other structures of the personality. There is also a psychiatric polymorbidity which may be manifested in the same patient by depressive, delirious, and psychoorganic elements. The nature of the rehabilitation accomplished is also determined in part by the structures of the care given. There is a constant interaction between rehabilitation and the reality of the material circumstances in which it takes place, with the former seeking to adapt the organization to its needs while the latter, through its cumulative experience, working sometimes to modify and sometimes to develop the very concept of the rehabilitation sought. For example, the addition to a hospital of a home care unit and of a day hospital produces substantial effects on the carrying out of intrahospital rehabilitation programs, tending, among other things, to shorten the duration of hospitalization in exchange for an extension of extrahospital therapeutic measures.

GENERAL CHARACTERISTICS OF REHABILITATION

Several general concepts of geriatric rehabilitation are to be found in the literature. One is that of Steinmann (1979) who identifies three types of rehabilitation: preventive, global, and specific. The first of these aims is to maintain or improve the capacities of the healthy old person. The second is instituted when the patient is still in bed. Its objective is to restore as quickly as possible the skills and activities of the elderly patient. The third utilizes specific means which are determined by needs resulting from the particular pathology involved (hemiplegia, myocardial infarction, etc.) (Gamp, 1982).

Another conception is that of Hunt (1980) who characterized it by the use of the mnemonic word SPREAD, as follows: "*S* stands for specific control of underlying disease or impairment by medical, surgical, physical or psychological measures . . . *P* stands for prevention of secondary disability resulting largely from immobility and isolation . . . *RE* refers to restorative measures including physical and occupational therapy, remedial exercises, gait training, and bowel and bladder training. *AD* refers to the adaptation of the person to disability with or without changes in the underlying clinical process."

Among the determining factors for rehabilitation in geriatric medicine, four should be noted.

1. *The immobilization syndrome,* resulting from confinement to bed, is always a threat to a hospitalized elderly patient. Lachnit (1981) described the following symptoms:

- disturbances of neuromuscular coordination
- thrombosis and embolisms
- decubitus ulcers and maceration
- anorexia, difficulties in swallowing or breathing
- pneumonia resulting from hypostasis, diminution of vital capacity and the cough reflex
- incontinence, retention of urine, urinary infection
- constipation
- muscular atrophy, contractures, capsular shrinking
- arthrosis and ankylosis
- osteoporosis, fractures
- metabolic modifications typified by disturbances of nitrogen balance and calcium deficiency
- apathy, depression or agitation
- general debilitation

This impressive assortment of symptoms may be the consequence not only of confinement to bed but also of the absence of movement, stimulation, and social contacts which this entails, if not attended to by the early start of rehabilitation activities.

2. *Psychological regression,* the most serious form of which accompanies or triggers the immobilization syndrome, may result from the convergence

of psychic disturbances leading to dependency and institutionalization. Finding himself in a protective hospital environment, the patient is in danger of reverting to older forms of behavior, experiencing memories of a childhood which forever seeks to reassert itself, wanting to be washed, fed, clothed and to have no responsibility for control of the sphincters.

3. *The chronicity* of the greater part of geriatric disorders necessarily exerts a profound influence on rehabilitation, especially its duration.

4. *Polymorbidity* presents numerous problems to the medical and paramedical personnel. This often confounds the pursuit of correct diagnosis, since the interaction between several concomitant diseases produces atypical clinical pictures. This calls for an economical therapeutic strategy which entails the treatment of certain vital symptoms to the detriment of less important pathological manifestations. It indicates the precautions that must be taken in instituting the rehabilitation program.

Some general principles emerge from these premises:

1. Psychogeriatric and geriatric rehabilitation should be started early. If this is done, it can act as a prophylaxis against the immobilization syndrome and limit the risk of regression.
2. It serves to preserve optimal autonomy. Essential in acute situations, it is equally so in chronic cases. When the patient's condition requires long or even very long care, it is clear that he should be constantly encouraged to utilize his residual functions as fully as possible.
3. The duration of rehabilitation cannot be determined in advance and may continue for the lifetime of the patient. This principle, arising from chronic conditions, gives emphasis to the role of rehabilitation in tertiary prophylaxis and aims to limit the functional ravages of diseases in old age.
4. Rehabilitation is a multidisciplinary activity, carried out by a team including psychogeriatricians, somatic geriatricians, male and female nurses specializing in psychiatric and general care, auxiliary personnel, physiotherapists, psychologists, speech therapists, and social workers.

Behind these four fundamental principles is a deeper reality. Rehabilitation, which is necessarily complex since it is concerned with the totality of the individual and calls upon such a variety of professional skills, cannot be carried out successfully unless it is inspired by a common attitude—a philosophy of rehabilitation. This is marked by optimism in the efforts made to improve or maintain the patient's functions, by realism in not expecting the impossible, and by the determination of the whole team to work for the same objective, the benefit of each patient as a total individual.

GENERAL PSYCHOLOGICAL PROBLEMS

The occurrence of sickness in an old person presents psychological problems which relate to the risks of dependence, fear of the loss of autonomy, and fear of death. This period of confusion and uncertainty brings into question such values as self-esteem and belief in the importance of one's own existence. These phenomena provide both objectives and obstacles in the process of rehabilitation.

Attitudes Toward Health

According to Brody et al. (1983), attitudes toward health are influenced by the following factors: the degree of motivation, the perception of vulnerability to disease, the severity of symptoms, the belief in the efficacy of planned rehabilitation activities, the convictions concerning the physical, psychological, and economic costs involved, along with various personal characteristics, age, sex, socioeconomic status, etc. These authors emphasize that a great many old people suffer in silence without resorting to available medicosocial services, which runs counter to the assumption of hypochondria among the aged. This kind of resignation is explainable as a simple acceptance of discomfort as inherent in aging, pessimism about curative possibilities, the feeling that "nobody cares," a desire to avoid disturbing the health personnel and upsetting the family circle, poor understanding of the significance of symptoms, and a possible cognitive deficiency, impeding the expression of suffering.

Personality and Motivation

Involvement of the patient in the rehabilitation process depends upon factors in three different categories: recently occurring psychological events, those of longer standing, and the intervention of external events (Loebel & Eisdorfer, 1984). The psychological elements may be designated as "losses," resulting from such occurrences as somatic diseases, psychoorganic syndromes, and injuries to the patient's affective and relational life.

One important idea has been called "learned helplessness" (Hautzinger, 1978). The old person, suffering from a loss of faculties or capacities, recognizes that he can no longer act upon the outside world as he once did and can no longer deal effectively with situations of subjective importance which confront him. In the light of these considerations, the patient's commitment to rehabilitation procedures may be limited by the feeling that "the game is already lost."

The very nature of "psychiatric pathology" may greatly compromise hopes for rehabilitation. In chronic depression, loss of vitality and the turning inward upon one's self contribute to great difficulty in imagining a future. Prospects for rehabilitation do not have the same positive value to patients as they do to members of the therapeutic team. In cases of injury to the mnestic functions, the measures instituted encounter obstacles to learning due to short-term forgetfulness. These are only two of many examples.

Two psychological entities are constants which deserve more detailed analysis. One of these is *personality,* which, in the opinion of Havighurst (1968), is the key element in rehabilitation. We may recall the distinctions made by Reichard et al. (1982) who outlined profiles of some fairly well adapted aged persons (the Mature, the Rocking Chair, and the Armored) and some maladapted ones (the Angry and the Self-Hating types).

The other fundamental factor is *motivation.* As defined by Hesse and Campion (1983), motivation "refers to the need, drive or desire to act in a certain way to achieve a certain end." To these authors, this implies that the individual is either *pushed* by a need to minimize discomfort or *pulled* by a desire to achieve certain complex objectives. Motivation serves to diminish tension as a driving force, which postulates a regulator to determine at what point the tension becomes a problem. The sensitivity and responsiveness of this regulator may be modified by age or circumstances. Finally, the intensity of the motivation depends on the strength of the desire to achieve a particular result. Hesse and Campion noted that an elderly person may have a diminished capacity for development of his motivation because of psychiatric pathology, such as a confusional state, depression, or anxiety. In addition, the intensity of his motivation may be reduced, for example, when obtaining an improvement entails the acceptance of a permanent deficiency.

The Role of External Factors

External events should also be taken into account. Even at home, the aged person, because of his deficiencies, may find it harder and harder to cope with the environment. Lawton and Simon (1968) offer the hypothesis of "environmental docility." They consider that when the capacities of an individual diminish, the proportion of behavioral disorders due to existential conditions correspondingly increase. A change of scene entails dangers which may be vitally important. Difficulties in adaptation to an institution entail risks of psychological regression, depression, and loss of the will to live. It has been proven that mortality rates increase among aged persons transferred to nursing homes or geriatric or psychogeriatric hospitals and that those most at risk are patients suffering from psychoorganic syndromes and those in a poor general state of health (Blenker, 1967; Killian, 1970).

Hospitalization in a general hospital is also attended by considerable risks to the general condition of aged persons. Despite the success of a medical or surgical treatment, we find an overall increase in functional invalidity and a higher frequency of confusional states (Warshaw et al., 1982).

Psychology of the Attending Personnel

In cases of prolonged hospitalization, as the need for assistance increases, there is a diminution of cognitive capacities and of the faculty for exchanging information with the personnel. There is also both a qualitative and quantitative impoverishment of relational life (Hayslip & Panek, 1983). The conclusions of this study are that the duration of institutionalization is not responsible for these phenomena, the cause being attributed rather to the interaction between the therapeutic team and the patient. The psychological problems of the attending personnel are numerous. It is not easy to commit ourselves to a rehabilitation philosophy when we know that the objective is closer to a "restitutio ad optimum" than it is to a "restitutio ad integrum." We are compelled to recognize the limits of our own capacities while we must at the same time maintain the optimism and dynamism that we hope to transmit to the patient. The frontiers of individual functional capacity are often vaguely defined, which results in uncertainty as to the moment when rehabilitation, which has thus far been dynamic, must satisfy itself with an effort to conserve what has already been accomplished. Feelings of guilt may arise when one wonders if it was really right to modify objectives.

Also, and on a deeper level, the therapist sees behind the patient two images of intense personal concern to him, the image of his parents and the image of himself when he becomes old. His problem is to act in such a way that these intimate personal models help him in his perception of "the other" through their positive aspects, without disturbing the therapist–patient relationship by the conflictual aspects they may convey. A major part of the dilemma of the therapist gravitates around the intensity of the therapeutic commitment. Are we doing enough, too much, or not enough? This question is all the more difficult since one of the principles of rehabilitation is to stimulate the patient to regain his autonomy.

A study by Barton et al. (1980) clearly illustrates this difficulty. Observation of the regular personnel and the residents in a nursing home at the time of morning rounds shows that encouragement of independent forms of behavior predominated slightly among the residents, through the example presented by their own conduct, whereas the permanent personnel more commonly supported attitudes of dependence. Furthermore, the relatively independent attitudes of the residents stimulated the supportive reactions of the personnel, vis-à-vis the patients. The author concluded that in this institution independent conduct by patients was conserved by intrinsic factors unrelated to the behavior of the personnel while dependent conduct was directly maintained by the reinforcement given by the personnel. The complication of this problem is inherent in the fact that assistance which is useful in certain evolutive phases becomes harmful in others.

THE GENERAL STRATEGY OF REHABILITATION

The patient himself is at the heart of all these considerations. The first step in rehabilitation is the medical evaluation which analyzes each case in its broadest aspects, bringing together the somatic, psychological, psychiatric, and social components. Based on the abundance of information thus obtained, the doctor makes a synthesis which should include the following elements:

1. An inventory of deficits with an assessment of their importance and their functional and psychological consequences.
2. Data concerning the social context of the patient's life, including his housing conditions, the nature and frequency of his social contacts, and his economic situation.
3. An assessment of his relationships with his family, friends, and acquaintances and their affective and material effects on the organization of his day to day life.
4. An evaluation of the residual functions upon which the plan of rehabilitation can be based.

It is useful to make a distinction between the three following terms: *impairment*, referring to the type and seriousness of the condition, *disability*, relating to the seriousness of its functional consequences, and *handicap*, referring to the extent of permanent limitation in daily life (Rustemeyer, 1982). The key to the assessment, from the viewpoint of psychogeriatric and geriatric rehabilitation, is not the mere existence of a pathological condition but also the alteration of function which results from it (Kent, 1977).

In a second phase, the doctor determines the objectives and mobilizes the relevant members of the rehabilitation team. The questions he must consider at the outset are the following (Rustemeyer, 1983):

1. Can rehabilitation relieve the ill-effects on the patient's social environment or at least reduce them to an acceptable level?
2. Bearing in mind the expected residual handicap, would it be possible to adapt the remaining potential for living to the existing (modified if necessary) living accommodations available to the patient?
3. Is the necessary expenditure reasonably commensurate with the expected benefit?

The plan instituted must be personalized. The flexibility of the structures for rehabilitation must be such that this plan can be adapted to the complex predicament of each individual. The program must also be adaptable to long-term options. It will therefore not be followed rigidly as the case evolves, but will be modified to correspond to a changing reality.

In conducting the therapeutic action it is vital to stimulate the patient's motivation. To serve this purpose, it is essential to explain to the patient at the outset the purposes and methods of rehabilitation. As it proceeds, the work should avoid creating stress, following a rhythm that is not too rapid, with a program that is not overcharged. In terms of behavior, three means to reinforce motivation should be employed: Attention should be maintained at an optimal level, which can only be done if excessive demands are not made upon it; rest should always follow exertion and there should be a feedback of all progress made. The therapeutic personnel must therefore give close attention to the rhythm and intensity of all activity and the need for pauses and periods of rest, and should make sure to comment favorably on progress achieved (Davies, 1983).

THE INSTRUMENTS OF REHABILITATION

The various techniques utilized in rehabilitation of aged persons may be classified according to their general objectives, categorized by Steinmann as "global," "specific," and "preventive" (see page 409). Recourse to the structures of preventive rehabilitation are of concern not only for healthy old persons but also for those who have previously had the benefit of global and specific rehabilitation measures. Passage from one form of rehabilitation to the other is therefore a flexible matter. We shall nevertheless limit ourselves at present to describing the instruments of global and specific rehabilitation.

Nursing Care

The basis of rehabilitation in the hospital is nursing and the crucial activities of the nurse may be considered under the headings of technical care, relational activities, and readaptation to the ordinary acts of daily life. In terms of technical care, emphasis should be given to the importance of the position of the patient in his bed and to frequent mobilization, as an element in preventing the immobilization syndrome (see page 410). A serious aspect of this syndrome is the risk of decubitus ulcers, whose pathogenesis consists of permanent pressure on the same part of the skin surface, the five common localizations being the sacrum, the heels, the area of the trochanters, the malleoli, and the ischiatic tuberosities. These complications may be avoided by changing the patient's position frequently, making sure to prevent maceration resulting from perspiration and urinary incontinence, avoiding excessive pressure by using extra-soft pillows (Seiler & Stähelin, 1980), and protecting the heels with sheepskin pads.

Another technical job for the nurse is the fight against incontinence. She should encourage the patient to urinate at specific times, chosen on the basis of the physiological variation of diuresis and readily identifiable reference points during the day—after meals, before bedtime, etc. After an initial phase during which the patient is systematically taken to the toilet, personal autonomy is progressively developed by suggesting that he go to the toilet, pointing to where it is, and on occasion asking him if he needs to urinate (Gyselynck-Maubourg et al., 1978).

Development of the plan for patient care should be integrated into the rehabilitation program as a whole, and should always reckon with the patient in his entirety. One example among many of this point is in the theory of Myra Levine (1973). Based on the four principles of conservation, this fits easily into the philosophy of rehabilitation outlined above. It is concerned with the conservation of energy, by acting on nutritional and metabolic disturbances, conservation of structural integrity, by adapting the immediate environment to the patient's deficiencies, for example, by better lighting for a patient with poor eyesight, and conservation of the person and conservation of sociability.

The nurse also plays an important role in the application of the plan. The nurse is better placed than anyone else, as the process unfolds, to express judgment on adapting the intensity and rhythm of treatments to the individual. The nurse's observations will also help determine the capacities of the patient for carrying out the usual activities of everyday life, rising, washing, dressing, eating, etc. In the event of an apraxia in dressing, the nurse will cooperate with the ergotherapist in an effort at readaptation. The following two-phase technique was described by Gyselynck-Maubourg (1978). The first phase is carried out under controlled conditions. There is only one person in the room to help the patient, the bed has been made, the shutters are closed, and the nightclothes are out of sight. The first concern at this point is analytical, that is, to observe the patient's ability to put on each separate item of clothing. Next is the sequential aspect of dressing, to have the patient proceed spontaneously from one item of clothing to the next. In the second phase, variables that might distract the patient are progressively reintroduced into the environment, such as the presence of another nurse, or ordinary background noises, until the customary conditions for dressing have been reconstituted.

All the activities of the patient-care personnel, whether they are mediated through technical acts or consist only of communication, verbal or nonverbal, tend to stimulate the relational life of the patient. The organization of activities in the patient-care unit is of the utmost importance in this connection. It is vital for the personnel to maintain contact with the family so that they can be perceived as a harmonious component in the family–patient relationship. The general attitude should be one of "activating care," which implies: "Never do anything for the patient that he can do for himself; when you do help, do it in such a way that the help you give is also training the patient in self-help" (Rustemeyer, 1983).

Physical Therapy

The physical approach to the patient has two main aspects, one consisting purely of physiotherapeutic technique, while the other is a psychological approach through the intermediary of the body. This distinction is apparent if we compare the two extremes of electrotherapy and relaxation. It is less obvious if we speak of massage or of baths. The fact is that most physiotherapeutic acts have a considerable psychological component. One of the aims of physical therapy is to help restore the patient's confidence in himself through apprenticeship in movement and improved body awareness. The importance of the psychological and didactic roles of physiotherapy is shown in the work of Grannis (1981). This author asked a group of elderly patients and a group of physiotherapists to rank in their order of importance four assumed qualities of a physiotherapist: as a worker, as a teacher, as a person, and as a therapist. The patients put the idea of teaching first, ahead of personal qualities, thus emphasizing the importance they attached to regaining their autonomy. The physiotherapists listed personal qualities first, ahead of their role as teachers, stressing in this way their psychological role.

Active Physiotherapy

According to Weber (1983), the therapeutic objectives are increased strength, improved capacities for movement and coordination, training in muscular resistance, and the fight against spasticity. The more general aims are for optimal autonomy, general mobilization, and the resumption of walking, with or without auxiliary means.

Reeducation for walking follows a progressively graded course (Guicheux, 1981). It begins with readaptation in bed, with measures to prevent bedsores, systematic mobilization of the joints and a "functional positioning" aimed to prevent the risk of ankylosis. Kinesitherapy at this stage is mainly analytical, passively or actively, aiming to maintain the amplitude of articular movements and conserve muscular strength. Standing exercises are then begun, starting from a seated position on the edge of the bed, arriving at the vertical position progressively, using a sloping support, followed by balancing exercises, with lateral, anterior, and posterior pressures. Readaptation to walking then continues with the actual taking of steps, aided by a helper who places one hand in the corresponding hand of the patient, to serve as a cane, and provides support with the other hand beneath the patient's armpit or on the hip. This is followed by exercises with a four-leg walker, crutches, and finally between parallel bars. The readaptation then proceeds with a walk in a properly arranged garden. Depending on the nature of the disability, our ambitions may be limited to teaching the patient to walk with crutches or to use a wheelchair.

The prerequisites for active physiotherapy are good cooperation and the absence of any somatic contraindication. In psychogeriatrics, cooperation is basic. A study by Francet and Schwed (1981) analyzes the results of physiotherapy in 149 psychogeriatric patients. They observed that the majority of indications related to difficulties in walking, muscular weakness, disturbances of equilibrium, and rigidity. The principal treatments carried out consisted of active mobilization, readaptation to walking, passive mobilization, and neuromotor facilitation. Half of their results were good or excellent, one-quarter were poor, and one-quarter ineffective. The causes of failure, in diminishing order, were poor cooperation, the seriousness of multiple pathology, and lack of motivation.

The fight against spasticity in hemiplegic patients may benefit from the use of Bobath's technique (Weber, 1983) which utilizes the postural reflexes.

Passive Physiotherapy

Passive physiotherapy includes massage, hydrotherapy, and electrotherapy. Its objectives are analgesia, muscular relaxation, and improvement of the circulation in chronic articular conditions and arterial disorders. We shall not enter here into the details of these treatments. We should however recall certain precautions that should be taken. In massage, for example, kneading and percussion movements may cause ecchymoses in aged persons whose capillary systems are especially fragile. Too extensive hot mud packs or hot water baths may decompensate cardiac insufficiency. Carbon dioxide baths which have the merit of stimulating cutaneous heat receptors make it possible to use water at lower temperatures (Weber, 1983). In general, the duration of these treatments should be carefully determined, neither too long nor too short, and too many procedures should not be carried out simultaneously.

Some of these passive physiotherapy techniques are very useful in psychogeriatrics. Massage, taking the precautions noted, engenders a sense of relaxation which can be beneficial in states of anxiety or depression. The same is true of carbon dioxide baths, which have comparable psychiatric indications.

Physical Therapies with Psychotherapeutic Elements

Adapted group gymnastics harmonize several beneficial elements: mobilization of the joints, muscular exercise, body consciousness, the pleasure of physical action, and of group emulation. This technique therefore serves a double function, both social and physiological. The exercises respect the following rules: A session may consist only of exercises in chairs, if the physical condition of the participants so requires; at any time, each participant must feel free to interrupt or not to take part in an exercise; jumping, racing, suspensions, and violent or abrupt exercises are excluded; when the torso is bent, the head must not be brought lower than the hips; exercises that call for standing on tiptoes or on one leg are done only with support from the back of a chair or the hand of a partner (Durussel, 1978).

Ludotherapy is another form of physical treatment, consisting of a game played with balls, with the participants usually seated. Its main purpose is to combat apathy and the lack of cooperation which are characteristic of psychoorganic syndromes. The resulting animation stimulates the patients to emerge from their physical and psychic immobility and also favors the integration of a group. It mobilizes the joints, activates the reflexes, and creates a beneficial emulation arising from the spirit of competition (Müller et al., 1970).

Goldberg and Fitzpatrick (1980) describe a technique designated as "movement therapy" which utilizes dancing and works simultaneously on several levels: "Time (accelerating/decelerating), weight (increasing pressure/decreasing pressure), space (indirect/direct), and force (freeing/binding). Its use in a group of elderly institutionalized persons was rewarded by psychological improvement, and graded by scores for 'morale' and 'self-esteem.'"

Other approaches using a variety of physical therapy techniques are described in the literature. Among them is "motor animation" for groups of long-stay patients who no longer need highly active kinesitherapy (Thourault, 1981). The person conducting the sessions uses simple methods to enhance proprioceptive sensitivity by arousing awareness of the different positions of the body in space by ball games, games of skill, and dancing. He or she also leads exercises in equilibrium, seated and standing, and respiratory gymnastics. The objectives are the recovery of the body scheme and the encouragement of sociability.

Finally, we should refer to the application to old people of relaxation techniques such as yoga and sophrology. Schultz's autogenic training has proved its merits, especially in a modified and adapted form, in relation to functional disorders (Bircher-Beck & Scherler, 1972). This is also the case with the technique of J. de Ajuriaguerra and M. Cohen, which "uses the transferential relation which develops in the course of relaxation and, due to the evolution of the resistances characteristic of each patient, permits a modification of the structure of symptoms, a reinforcement of the bodily and psychic self and a better integration of relational life" (Richard et al., 1975).

Ergotherapy

The novelty of ergotherapy is in its method, making use of its action upon the outside world. It is differentiated in this respect from such kindred approaches as psychotherapy based on declarations based on one's perceptions, or physiotherapy based on the motor aspect of the activity. Two major categories of ergotherapy may be identified: functional and psychiatric. The former concentrates on the execution of movement, particularly of the upper extremities, through the use of specific techniques which often bring creativity into play, for example, weaving, or working with leather or wood. It is also concerned with the adaptation of handicapped persons to routine life, with exercise, and readaptation to day to day activities. Its function is also to act upon the environment by eliminating obstacles resulting from invalidity such as modifications of kitchen or bathroom facilities.

Psychiatric ergotherapy is focused on relational life and creativity. Through activities in the workshop, the patient is engaged in relationships both with the ergotherapist and other patients. In addition, the work accomplished may enable the patient to resume contact with the outside world, and learn again how to deal with it in the process of self-rediscovery, along with various capabilities.

In psychogeriatrics, functional and psychiatric ergotherapy are associated, in view of the demands of somatic and psychiatric polymorbidity. The workshop is a special vantage point from which, through manual activity, the patient, depending upon the extent of his regression, can proceed through four phases of rehabilitation (Wertheimer, 1984). Ergotherapy will first seek to capture the patient's attention. The aged patient who is not subjected to any stimulation at all moves about in a blurred and featureless world in which everything observed, thought, or felt has the same indifferent quality. To gain his attention is the basic starting point which can initiate the process of recuperation. It offers a choice, and initiates an embryonic movement in the direction of freedom. It indicates a certain opening up to what is going on in the outside world. In a second phase, the attention of the patient is supplemented by an intention. The object presented acquires new potentials, created by the imagination, spurred by the initial attention aroused. It becomes a subject for curiosity, observation, and even for anticipation. Ergotherapy in this phase opens the way for the perception of time. As he confronts the object, the patient begins to rediscover himself as a being with potentialities for action, capable of taking the world, or at least part of it, into the hands and the imagination, and transforming it. This initiates the third phase of reflection, in which the object reveals itself as a mirror, reflecting a dynamic image of the self. Finally, ergotherapy leads to action, which gives concrete form to the renewed capacity to cope successfully with the world, from which the aged patient had been wholly or completely excluded. The action may be performed for the self or for others, through the intermediary of individual activity or that of relational or cooperative activity.

Ergotherapy in demential states presents the problem of adapting the work to the residual capacities of the patient. The following methodology has been described by Pierrehumbert et al. (1976, 1978 a,b). The first stage consists of observation of spontaneous behavior. Five groups of activities have thus been identified: (1) activities carried out only for their own sake (stereotypes); (2) those seeking to obtain information from the outside world (manipulation of objects, for example); (3) those aiming to modify relations between the self and the world of objects (appropriation or rejection of objects); (4) those seeking to modify relations between the self and other persons (initiatives to make contact); and (5) those aimed at making transformations in the outside world (modifying the position, form, or nature of an object).

The second stage consists in suggesting to the patient an activity which analysis has indicated is within his reach, and thereafter attempting to move on to related but progressively more difficult tasks. The authors list a total of 106 activities, arranged in sequence according to increasing complexity. The objective of the method is to employ potential functions and if necessary substitute other functions for them. For example, a patient may not succeed in weaving, a task based on repetitions of complex sequences, when the teacher says, "now pass over this thread and then go under the next one." When the same activity is described in a simple rhythmic form, however, with the patient picking up the teacher's chant, "Over! Under! Over! Under!" she may learn to weave correctly.

Animation

To animate means to bring to life. This very general term covers everything involved in a rehabilitation effort designed to improve the patient's autonomy. It refers more specifically, however, to the rhythm with which this complex therapy is carried out. Animation is greatly concerned with timing. It introduces alternations between periods of activity and periods of rest, and also between different forms of activity. To the routine and natural rhythms of hospital life, determined by the physiological need to eat, sleep, etc., it adds others, which the patient is capable of controlling.

The general purposes of animation are definable both in terms of the individual and in terms of the institution. For the individual, the aim is to improve behavioral pathology and maintain or restore positive behavior and attitudes toward life, involving such fundamental elements as a sense of initiative, along with such specific interests as housework or cooking. Animation also has an impact on the institution. In providing conditions encouraging the development of the individual, it also offers a harmonious supplement to other therapeutic facilities in the establishment. It gives rise to a spirit of dynamism which enriches relationships between members of the personnel, between the patient-care personnel and the patients, and between the patients themselves. Animation should permeate the whole institution, manifesting itself by attitudes and acts of positive goodwill. The sitting room furniture should be arranged so that even the chairs will encourage natural and easy contacts. The lighting should be warm, engendering a sense of intimacy. The doors should be marked to show where they lead. The walls should have clearly visible calendars. Every section should have its own assortment of newspapers and magazines, as well as its own small library, radio corner, and television corner. In other words, the whole material organization of the institution should encourage an openness to others, facilitate better orientation in time and space and stimulate participation in the outside world.

The basic attitude of the personnel should demonstrate to the patient that he or she is recognized as an individual. This recognition, as time passes, will be enriched by conversations with the patient and family members and observation of the patient's behavior and habits. The patient should be able to discover among attendants a degree of complicity, an echo in resonance with his or her own feelings. The contact should also serve as a support for the patient's efforts to orientate himself with respect to the ward, to the institution, to the outer world, and to time, past, present, and future. There should be a consistent desire among the personnel to strengthen the patient's ties with reality. The patient should be helped to remember the day and date and the place where he is, and should be asked to give his address, to describe the neighborhood, and familiar itineraries, and should be encouraged to talk about past activities and projects.

Animation also includes bodily care, including haircuts and beauty treatments, which are important to maintain the patient's self-image.

Some patients may be integrated into animation groups (Wertheimer, 1984) by exercising their activities in special rooms, preferably not in the sleeping wards. The aim is to let the patient spend time with others and fill his or her day with a variety of activities. A day spent in this way is something like a sample of life outside the institution. It has its own rhythms, illustrating the importance of having a variety of occupations, such as reading newspapers, preparing meals, taking walks, and visiting exhibitions. Formation of a group of 8 to 10 persons makes possible renewed exchanges among them, and reinforcement of their self-images.

Psychotherapy

Psychotherapy is only mentioned in passing here because it is the subject of a separate chapter in this book. Its place in rehabilitation is clearly very important. Whereas most of the techniques discussed are designed to stimulate activity and exercise the means of communication, psychotherapy permits a direct approach to the affective and emotional life of the patient. According to Loebel and Eisdorfer (1984), it helps to develop a positive attitude and awaken hope. It makes it possible to express one's fears, to reduce feelings of guilt, to overcome the sense of loss, and it helps one to accept the process of aging.

Psychotherapy also plays an essential role vis-à-vis the family of an aged person with a chronic condition, giving the family the possibility of developing an authentic contact with the patient, a contact which would otherwise be distorted by unconscious feelings of fear and guilt. The impact of the psychotherapeutic action on the family will also have beneficial repercussions on the patient.

Language Therapies

The treatment of an aphasic patient should combine the general approaches to rehabilitation—physiotherapy, ergotherapy, management of social problems, etc.—with specific linguistic action. Sarno (1984) stressed this point as a vital element in a total approach to the patient's evolution. This evolution begins with a phase of "denial" or severe depression, followed by a stage of revolt by the patient against himself and then against others, and finally by a period of readaptation. After the acute phases and a spontaneous recuperation, "speech therapy" is best carried out in groups.

The same author found that there are specific techniques for the rehabilitation of patients with different types of dysarthria, the choice being determined by the nature of the deficit: "In practice, speech pathologists generally work primarily on the articulation of speech, rather than pitch, volume, rhythm, voice quality or rate. For this purpose, exercises that focus on particular classes of sounds requiring certain basic movement patterns are selected" (Sarno, 1984, p. 172).

In the Parkinsonian patient there is a specific difficulty in voice modulation. For example, the patient may not be able to speak in an interrogative manner or to express anger in his voice. This phenomenon occurs early in the disease. At the same time that the difficulty develops with the patient's own expressiveness, the patient begins to have trouble understanding that of others. Scott and Caird (1984) describe a therapy using visual, auditive, and tactile feedback mechanisms, leading to improved modulation of speech.

There appears to be no specific therapy, up to this time, for language disorders in senile dementia of the Alzheimer type.

Readaptation of the Memory

Various efforts to readapt the memory have been described in the literature (Treat et al., 1978). Lorayne and Lucas (1974), for example, used imaginary associations between things to be remembered and bizarre images. For example, if the patient has to remember that he left his eyeglasses on the bed, he might think of an enormous pair of glasses lying in bed asleep. Bower (1970) suggested making imaginary associations between a series of subjects to be kept in mind and the series of rooms in which one lives and customarily moves about.

Music and Art Therapies

Music therapy is fully integrated into rehabilitation programs. Its objectives are to reactivate emotional life through the connections, communicated by music, with positive events in the patient's past, the encouragement through music of contact with others and of social activities, and the release from psychomotor inhibitions through music (Schwabe, 1981). Music therapy may be divided into four types of activity: singing groups of 10 to 15 patients in a circle, for 45-minute periods twice a week; rhythmic instrumental improvisation groups of 8 to 10 patients, 30 to 40 minutes a week; dance groups of 15 to 20 patients, once or twice a week for 45-minute periods; receptive groups simply listening to music.

Fischer and Fischer (1977) described a therapy of artistic activity and noted, as have others, that cerebral lesions may favor the release of hitherto latent creative faculties. Their observation of a group of dements showed that drawing and painting had a revitalizing effect on the subjects who showed increased interest in ordinary daily activities. They found that the most seriously affected patients had a tendency to draw or paint from their own imaginations, although it was done in a stereotypical manner, while those patients less seriously affected preferred to copy.

Prosthetic Means

Old people are especially exposed to the risks of multiple sensory deficiencies. This indicates, on the one hand, that their immediate environment should be appropriately adapted and, on the other hand, that the necessary technical means should be available to them to minimize their handicaps.

To favor autonomous life at home, for example, the lighting should be good, the buttons and switches on domestic equipment should be clearly visible, as well as the controls on radio and TV sets. Containers of food and pharmaceutical products should be easy to handle, etc. There is no need to make a long list of the hazards that old people may encounter in day-to-day life, for they are quite obvious if we pay attention to them. Preventive readaptation of this kind becomes a matter of social values.

In the institutional milieu, we should make sure that the symbols used to designate various quarters, such as the toilets, are not too abstract and that they are adapted to the cultural reference points of the elderly patients.

Technology is constantly offering improved means to counteract difficulties in eyesight and hearing. Selwyn et al. (1982) have described some of these:

> Bilateral, directional hearing aids not only improve the user's hearing and understanding but also localize the sound, which may be necessary for a poor sighted or blind person who must use both ears to locate the source of sound... Bifocals often cause problems for the elderly because the reading-aid part of the lens may obscure the user's view of the floor or steps. To overcome this problem, single vision eyeglasses are available in flip-front designs, which allow the user to flip the front lenses up and out of the way of reading. (p. 260)

EVALUATING THE EFFICACY OF REHABILITATION

The very broad range of objectives in psychogeriatric and geriatric rehabilitation, with all its somatic, psychological, psychiatric, relational, and social dimensions, makes it very difficult to assess its effects. Should we undertake to evaluate changes in every one of these domains, or does the strong correlation between some of them make it unnecessary to do so? Some answers may be offered to this question.

In general terms, Pfeffer et al. (1982) consider that the ideal scales should be independent of socioeconomic status, level of formal education, and intelligence. According to Linn and Linn (1981), the fields to investigate should include life satisfaction, self-esteem, the locus of control, social participation, social adjustment, Activities of Daily Living (ADL), and Instrumental Activities of Daily Living (IADL). It is obvious that such an evaluation, in practice, would take a great deal of time and would encounter problems of cooperation in reconciling subjective assessments. In contrast, Wolinsky et al. (1984), in evaluating the needs of a sample of aged persons in the vicinity of St. Louis, used two distinct factors, one of them *global*—subjectively perceived health and sensory status, nutritional risk and scale of psychic health, and the other *functional*—ADL and IADL. Their observations demonstrated that these two factors were poorly correlated and should be evaluated separately. Furthermore, both should be examined in studies covering the state of health of the whole aged population in the community.

In the institutional framework, opinions converge on the usefulness and value of scales showing the degree of functional dependence, the principal ones being the ADL index (Katz et al., 1970), and the IADL index (Lawton & Brody, 1969). The former includes data on the following items: bathing, dressing, going to the toilet, transfer, continence, and feeding. The latter is concerned with more complex activities, such as ability to use the telephone, shopping, food preparation, housekeeping, laundry, mode of transportation, responsibility for one's own medication, and ability to handle finances. It also evaluates physical self-maintenance: use of the toilet, feeding, dressing, grooming, physical ambulation, and bathing. The ADL index seems better adapted for evaluation of long-stay services and the IADL to intensive rehabilitation and outpatient care.

THE REHABILITATION TEAM

The complete team consists of a psychogeriatric doctor, a geriatric doctor, male and female nurses specializing in psychiatric or general care, auxiliary personnel, ergotherapists, physiotherapists, psychologists, speech therapists, and social workers. Whenever several types of intervention are required, it is important that they be coordinated, so that they are all focused on a common objective in relation to the particular situation, while each has its specific objectives derived from the technical specialty involved. Their relationship to the patient simultaneously brings together and differentiates the members of the team. In addition to his or her specific activities, each member develops a special and individual relationship with the patient. Their respective personalities enter into play, multiplying the patient's points of reference and enabling him to have a richer and more varied social experience within the therapeutic context. The essential point in the common effort of the team as a whole is to avoid contradictions which would disturb the security of the patient and his family.

The concept of the team is a flexible one. In practice, we may distinguish between members working from within the hospital structure and those from outside.

The former part of the team is highly structured and characterized by its great frequency of interpersonal contacts. There is thus an uninterrupted observation of the patient, offering team members occasions to exchange their views and arrive at a more discriminating understanding of the case, with a constant review of the therapeutic aims and means.

In outpatient practice, the need to deliver a variety of services to the patient's home complicates the effort to coordinate the different aspects of rehabilitation. Depending upon the nature of local structures, services for treatment and care at home are more or less homogeneous.

Whatever the structure, it is essential for us to come as close as we can to a common action by exchanges of information and evaluation at clinical sessions for the presentation of cases and weekly evaluation meetings. Every effort must be made to avoid anarchy in the activities carried out for elderly people and in the attitudes of those responsible for these activities.

The doctor is the key to the activities of all members of the therapeutic team, establishing the objectives and activating the team as needs require. The doctor is in a central but not in a dominating position. In the terms used by Clark and Bray (1984), "First and foremost, leadership for the rehabilitation team is not an issue of absolutes but of practical necessities." The organization should be structured on a horizontal model in which the specific capacities of each member complement those of the others.

It must also be recalled that rehabilitation is a long-term activity. As it proceeds, the original situation necessarily changes so that the activity itself must evolve and if necessary be completely transformed. This is only possible if the observations of each member of the team are passed on to the others in frequent meetings.

PSYCHOGERIATRIC REHABILITATION AND MEDICOSOCIAL ORGANIZATION

The general aim of preserving optimal autonomy has profound effects on the organization of all the structures responsible for dealing with old people. The specificity of psychogeriatric rehabilitation justifies the existence either of specialized units or hospitals for the purpose. The latter must be capable of dealing with acute situations and medium-term rehabilitation (3 months). Since long-stay establishments specializing in psychogeriatrics are currently quite rare, the psychogeriatric hospitals have to take in chronic cases. General hospitals also have their share of psychogeriatric cases but are not well equipped to undertake rehabilitation programs. The suggestion of Warshaw et al. (1982) for the creation of small specialized acute units is quite relevant in this situation.

The establishment of a long-stay institution exposes the institution to the risk of being inundated by very serious psychogeriatric cases. It seems essential therefore to have an organization at the regional level which will be empowered to make rules for the allocations of serious, medium, and light cases and will also supervise and coordinate the admissions policies of nursing homes. Means should be found to avoid lapsing into an authoritarian approach which would fail to respect the freedom of these establishments and of candidates for admission. Limitation of the proportion of very serious cases is imperative to preserve the dynamism of rehabilitation and provide an appropriate atmosphere for animation.

In an ideal system, the specialized and general hospitals and the long-stay institutions would work in close cooperation with a specialized outpatient service. When this is done, the latter service can function both before and after hospitalization. It can thus facilitate either the maintenance of the patient at home or his return after treatment. This is most easily done if the service is connected with day hospitals (Wertheimer & Le-Dinh, 1983).

Caring for a patient at home also calls for the help of support services, such as housekeepers, "meals on wheels," and various voluntary agencies. Psychogeriatric rehabilitation, viewed in this broad context, implies the existence of a general medicosocial organization as part of our social structures, for it presupposes close coordination at every level.

In conclusion, long-term care in the domain of psychogeriatric rehabilitation is not limited to institutionalized care. When a team is entrusted with the care of an aged patient with psychic problems, it is quite likely that they will be responsible for him for the rest of his life. As the months and years go by, it is reasonable to expect that there will be many ups and downs, calling for a wide variety of therapeutic and medicosocial adjustments. The potentialities of all the various therapeutic and institutional means at our disposal are enhanced when unity exists in our concepts of health and rehabilitation policy. The resulting combination of elasticity in the use of our means of action and discipline in managing the various rehabilitation services helps make long-term care a dynamic enterprise.

REFERENCES

Barton, E. M., Baltes, M. M., & Orzech, M. J. (1980). Etiology of dependence in older nursing home residents during morning care: The role of staff behavior. *J. Pers. Soc. Psychol., 38*(3), 423–431.

Bircher-Beck, L. M., & Scherler, A. (1972). Utilisation du training autogène modifié en géronto-psychiatrie. *Schweiz. Arch. Neurol. Neurochir. Psychiatr., 110,* 275–278.

Blenker, M. (1967). Environmental change and the aging individual. *Gerontologist, 7,* 101–105.

Bower, G. H. (1970). Analysis of mnemonic device. *Am. Scientist, 58,* 496–510.

Brody, E. M. Kleban, M. H., et al. (1983). What older people do about their day-to-day mental and physical health symptoms. *J. Am. Geriatr. Soc., 31,* 489–498.

Clark, G. S., & Bray, G. P. (1984). Development of a rehabilitation plan. In T. F. Williams (Ed.), *Rehabilitation in the aging* (pp. 125–143). New York: Raven Press.

Davies, A. (1983). Back on their feet—behavioural techniques for elderly patients–1. *Nurs. Times, 79*(42), 49–51.
Durussel, J. (1978). Gymnastique et sport au 3ème âge. *Les Cahiers Médico-sociaux, 22*(4), 189–193.
Fischer, T., & Fischer, R. (1977). Nonverbal dialogue with the brain-damaged elderly. *Confinia Psychiatr., 20*, 61–78.
Francet, C., & Schwed, P. (1981). Evaluation des résultats de la physiothérapie en psychogériatrie. *Méd. Hyg., 39*, 4001–4005.
Gadomski, M. (1980). *Rehabilitation (Stuttg.) 19*, 20–23.
Gamp, R. (1982). Möglichkeiten und Grenzen der physikalischen Therapie in der Geriatrie. *Praxis, 71*(47), 1866–1870.
Goldberg, W. G., & Fitzpatrick, J. J. (1980). Movement therapy with the aged. *Nurs. Res., 29*(6), 339–346.
Grannis, C. J. (1981). The ideal physical therapist as perceived by the elderly patient. *Phys. Ther., 61*(4), 479–486.
Guicheux, S. (1981). Réadaptation à la marche d'un sujet âgé sans étiquette médicale précise. *Soins, 26* (23/24), 57–60.
Gyselynck-Mambourg, A. M., Ylieffe, M. & Delwaide, P. J. (1978). Revalidation en psychogériatrie. *Rev. gériatrie, 3*, 100–104.
Hautzinger, M. (1978). Altersdepression—Versuch einer psychologischen Begründung. *Z. Gerontol., 11*, 348–357.
Havighurst, R. J. (1968). A social–psychological perspective on aging. *Gerontologist, 8*, 67–71.
Hayslip, B., Jr., & Panek, P. E. (1983). Physical self-maintenance, mental status and personality in institutionalized elderly adults. *J. Clin. Psychol., 39*(4), 479–485.
Hesse, K. A., & Campion, E. W. (1983). Motivating the geriatric patient for rehabilitation. *J. Am. Geriatr. Soc., 31*(10), 586–589.
Hunt, T. E. (1980). Practical considerations in the rehabilitation of the aged. *J. Am. Geriatr. Soc., 28*(2), 59–64.
Junod, J. P. (1984). La formation du médecin en gériatrie. *Gaz. Méd.*, 75–79.
Katz, S., Downs, T. D., Cash, H. R., & Grotz, R. C. (1970). *Gerontologist, I*, 20–30.
Kent, S. (1977). Assessing function: A key to care of the aging. *Geriatrics, 32*, 83–88.
Killian, J. (1970). Effects of geriatric transfers on mortality rates. *Soc. Work, 15*, 19–26.
Lachnit, K. S. (1981). Möglichkeiten der Rehabilitation im geriatrischen Krankenhaus. *Akt. Gerontol., II*, 174–176.
Lawton, M. P., & Brody, E. M. (1969). *Gerontologist, 9*, 179–186.
Lawton M. P., & Simon B. B. (1968). The ecology of social relationships in housing for the elderly. *Gerontologist, 8*, 108–115.
Levine, M. E. (1973). *Introduction to clinical nursing.* Philadelphia: F. A. Davis.
Linn, M. W., & Linn, B. S. (1981). Problems in assessing response to treatment in the elderly by physical and social function. *Psychopharmacol. Bull., 17*(4), 74–81.
Loebel, J. P., & Eisdorfer, C. (1984). Psychological and psychiatric factors in the rehabilitation of the elderly. In T. F. Williams (Ed.), *Rehabilitation in the aging* (pp. 41–57). New York: Raven Press.
Lorayne, H., & Lucas, J. (1974). *The memory book.* New York: Ballantine.
Müller, C., Villa, J. L., & Wertheimer, J. (1970). La physiothérapie en psychiatrie et en gériatrie. *Méd. Hyg., 28*, 1736–1738.

Pfeffer, R. L., Kurosaki, T. T., Harrah, C. H., Jr., Chance, J. M., & Filos, S. (1982). Measurement of functional activities in older adults in the community. *J. Gerontol.*, 37(3), 323–329.
Pierrehumbert, B., et al. (1976). L'approche du réel chez le dément sénile. Fondements méthodologiques de l'ergothérapie en psychogériatrie. *Ann. Méd. Psychol.*, 134(2), 599–634.
Pierrehumbert, B., et al. (1978a). Ergothérapie intra-hospitalière et démence sénile. *Psychiat. Soc.*, 13, 85–92.
Pierrehumbert, B., et al. (1978b). Activité et réhabilitation dans les démences de la vieillesse. Propositions méthodologiques pour une ergothérapie en psychogériatrie. *Schweiz. Archives Neurol. Neurochir. Psychiatr.* 122(2), 315–371.
Reichard, S., Livson, F., & Petersen, P. G. (1982). *Aging and personality*. New York: Wiley.
Richard, J., et al. (1975). De l'application de la relaxation en gériatrie hospitalière. *Schweiz. Arch. Neurol. Neurochir. Psychiatr.*, 117(1), 157–169.
Rustemeyer, J. (1982). Rehabilitation und Alter. *Med. Welt*, 33(15), 561–565.
Rustemeyer, J. (1983). Rehabilitation—Physical and clinical aspects. In D. Platt (Ed.), *Geriatrics, Vol. 2*, (pp. 316–349). Berlin: Springer Verlag.
Sarno, M. T. (1984). Communication disorders in the elderly. In T. F. Williams (Ed.), *Rehabilitation in the aging* (pp. 161–176). New York: Raven Press.
Schwabe, C. (1981). Musiktherapie in der geriatrischen rehabilitation. *Z. Gesamte. Hyg.*, 27,(12), 937–940.
Scott, S., & Caird, S. I. (1984). The response of the apparent receptive speech disorder of Parkinson's disease to speech therapy. *J. Neurol. Neurosurg. Psychiatry*, 47, 302–304.
Seiler, W. O., & Stähelin, H. B. (1980). Aspects de la pathogénie, de la prophylaxie et du traitement des ulcères en décubitus. *Méd. Hyg.*, 38, 3966–3975.
Selwyn, D., Tandler, R., & Zampella, A. (1982). *Med. Instrum.*, 16(5), 259–260.
Steinmann, B. (1979). *La réadaptation du sujet âgé*. Forum Medici, Gérontologie pluridisciplinaire, Zyma Nyon.
Thourault, Y. (1981). L'animation motrice en service long séjour. *Soins*, 26(23/24), 67–68.
Treat, N. J., et al. (1978). Toward applying cognitive skill training to memory problems. *Experimental Aging Research*, 4(4), 305–319.
Warshaw, G. A., et al. (1982). Functional disability in the hospitalized elderly. *JAMA*, 248(7), 847–850.
Weber, S. (1983). Physikalische Therapie in der Geriatrie-Möglichkeiten und Grenzen. *Z. Gerontol.*, 16, 290–292.
Wertheimer, J. (1981). Readaptation in psychogeriatrics. In *The handicapped person in society: Proceedings of the Third European Regional Conference of Rehabilitation International* (pp. 172–174). Vienna.
Wertheimer, J., & Le-Dinh, T. (1983). Organisation sectorielle psychogériatrique: Service universitaire de Psychogériatrie de Lausanne. *Psychol. Méd.*, (15)8, 1297–1302.
Wertheimer, J. (1984). Animation dans les services de psychogériatrie. In preparation.
Wolinsky, F. D., et al. (1984). Measurement of the global and functional dimensions of health status in the elderly. *J. Gerontol.*, 39(1), 88–92.

21
The Psychogeriatric Day Hospital: Definition, Historical Development, Working Methods, and Initial Efforts in Research

Manfred Bergener, Erhard U. Kranzhoff, Joachim Husser, and Valentin Markser

DEFINITION

The psychogeriatric day hospital, providing inpatient care, is largely a clinical facility for the treatment of elderly people suffering from mental illness. The patients spend only the day there and for the evening and night return to their accustomed surroundings. A day hospital is designed to provide treatment during the day and is not to be confused with the day care home, especially common in England (whose responsibility it is to provide help to elderly people who need care), and the day center (places where elderly people can meet without requiring therapy or care).

BASIC CONCEPT OF THE DAY HOSPITAL AND THE HISTORY OF ITS FOUNDING

The first known article concerning a day hospital facility for the treatment of the mentally ill appeared in a Soviet journal. This article reported the founding of a day hospital "Don Kloster," in 1932 (Dzhagarov, 1937). At almost the same time, the first day hospitals in the Western world were opened. D. E. Cameron established such a facility at the Allan Memorial Institute in Montreal in 1946 (Cameron, 1947) and J. Bierer opened the first psychiatric day hospital in London, the Marlborough Day Hospital (Bierer, 1951). Although in the Soviet Union economic reasons were probably the chief motivating factor for the opening of the day hospital, the movement of the 1950s in the Western world was sparked by some doctors asking themselves: Why do patients who are mentally ill, but not bedridden, need a hospital bed? Why should they spend nights and weekends in a clinic, in which therapy at that time is limited to the most urgent physical care, the stand-by emergency service? (Finzen, 1981). Bierer, responding to the enthusiasm of the founding years, hoped that he could treat all patients in his day hospital, that it would be possible to advance the day hospital to a central position in psychiatric care within a reasonable period of time.

The day hospital in European countries, however, had quite a different development. While in England, in the 1970s, around 35,000 mentally ill patients were treated as day hospital patients, and there were about 100 psychiatric day hospitals (Finzen, 1974; Brocklehurst, 1982), the psychiatric day hospital in other countries developed only gradually. In spite of the demands of the Report of the Commission of Experts Concerning the Position of Psychiatry in the Federal Republic of Germany, 1975, and the positive experiences in other countries, Bosch and Steinhardt (1983), in their survey which is surely not exhaustive, counted 58 known day hospitals in the Federal Republic and West Berlin alone in 1982, six of which were exclusively psychiatric facilities.

WHAT IS THE FUTURE FOR THE PSYCHIATRIC DAY HOSPITAL?

The exuberant optimism of the founding period in the early 1950s, when many tended to believe that all mental illnesses could be treated in the day hospital, was followed by a period of experimentation. Generally speaking, psychogeriatric treatment in the day hospital consists of the following functions, rated differently as to their relative importance by the great majority of facilities which have accepted and practice them:

1. Stabilization of the goals achieved in therapy and initiation of rehabilitative measures following full inpatient treatment (henceforth referred to as inpatient treatment). Help is offered with the reintegration of patients into their accustomed social surroundings, with changes involving their social situation, and with the establishment of new social contacts.

2. Instituting a change in the tendency toward hospitalization (in the mainstay of inpatient treatment) and attempting to substitute day hospital treatment. Treatment in the day hospital has many advantages for the patient since, among other things, it keeps disturbing changes to a minimum and maintains the possibility of continuing existing social contacts.

3. Crisis intervention and the unburdening of the patient's relatives. An attempt is made to help those who have to deal with mentally ill family members.

Depending on whether the psychogeriatric day hospital is affiliated with a general hospital or functions independently, the areas indicated are evaluated differently. As regards contraindications and general medical requirements for treatment in the psychogeriatric day hospital, the following guidelines have proven themselves in most facilities:

1. The patient must be able to spend nights and weekends—possibly under the close supervision of relatives—without the risk of endangering himself or others.
2. The patient should not be severely limited in his mobility since he has to come to the day hospital every day.
3. The patient must not be impaired to the degree that he is unable to orient himself, especially in his immediate surroundings, and, because of the open character of the day hospital, to the degree that he requires constant supervision.
4. A specific diagnostic and/or therapeutic indication must be made to avoid patients and especially relatives considering the day hospital as a day center or something similar.
5. Persons under 60 years of age, as a rule, should not be admitted to the day hospital.

ORGANIZATION AND THERAPY PROGRAM AT THE MODEL PSYCHOGERIATRIC DAY HOSPITAL IN COLOGNE

The psychogeriatric Day Hospital of the Rheinische Landesklinik Köln opened in 1979. Through its affiliation with the General Psychiatric Hospital, the Day Hospital can take advantage of a great number of diagnostic and therapeutic facilities inherent in a clinic facility. At present, up to 27 patients can be treated in our day hospital. The unfavorable location of the day hospital with regard to transportation and the physical condition of the elderly people to be treated, however, make it necessary for a private bus firm to pick the patients up at home before 9 A.M. and drive them home again at about 4 o'clock in the afternoon. The day hospital operates from Monday to Friday. Each morning it offers a communal breakfast. Therapeutic activities are available from 9:30 A.M. to noon, and again from 1:30 P.M. to 4 P.M. During the lunch hour, the patients are able to keep to long established habits and rest up from the strain of the morning's activities in two quiet rooms.

The therapeutic team is composed of a doctor and two nurses who are on duty the whole day, and a psychologist, a social worker, a creative therapist, an occupational therapist, and a physical therapist who spend various amounts of time organizing the therapy program. In addition to the medical treatment of mental and somatic illnesses, individual and group therapy interventions, creative work with various materials, occupational and creative therapy, physical therapy with athletic activities, assistance and counseling with social problems are part of the daily program of therapy. On several afternoons in the month, when no therapy is scheduled, patients go for walks or make excursions, play social games, sing songs, listen to stories that are read to them and have an opportunity to make friends among themselves. Working in groups is at the heart of treatment in the day hospital. In the discussion group, which centers on the handling of problems, an attempt is made to instill a willingness to clear up conflicts, and patients are encouraged to seek contacts even outside the group. It is the goal of the weekly creative therapy to promote nonverbal modes of expression and thus give patients who are less than eloquent a possibility to open up. In another group, which meets twice a week, patients, through concentration and memory exercises, attempt to alleviate their cerebral-organic impairment or to become better acquainted with it, so that they can solve everyday problems in spite of their handicap.

In order to maintain the continuity of treatment, the day hospital operates a post-outpatient care service for a limited number of patients who are chronically ill. The continuing contact with personnel of the day hospital—even when this is infrequent—helps as a rule, to reduce the frequency of assignments to inpatient treatment.

Finally, an important part of the therapeutic task in the day hospital is the cooperation with and involvement of the relatives of the patient in treatment. The meetings with the patients' relatives, which take place at two-week intervals, under the guidance of the psychologist (in addition to almost daily telephone contacts), serve as an exchange of information on how to deal with the family member who is ill, how to promote understanding for the developing course of the illness, and how to achieve mutual responsibility for treatment. Furthermore, the relative's own role in the interaction with the patient can be worked out and support offered through the group.

DESCRIPTION OF PSYCHOGERIATRIC DAY HOSPITAL PATIENTS

Mindful of the indications and requirements mentioned above, 352 patients have been treated at the Psychogeriatric Day Hospital in Cologne during the 5 years since it opened at the end of 1979 (see Table 21.1). Most of these patients, that is, 55.4%, manifested symptoms of depression. The most frequent diagnosis was that of involution depression (32.4%), followed by senile organic psychosis (17.3%) and neurotic depression (15.9%). The smallest group consisted of patients with a dependency on alcohol and/or medication (3.4%) for whom day hospital treatment had to be weighed very critically in order not to provoke a possibly uncontrolled consumption of drugs.

Almost two-thirds of the patients (63.9%) came into the day hospital following inpatient treatment. On the basis of the organizational integration of the psychogeriatric day hospital into a clinical facility, the stabilization of the goals that had been achieved in therapy and the beginning of a gradual increase in strain following inpatient treatment were regarded by most patients as an indication of the need for treatment in the day hospital. The attempt to substitute day hospital treatment for inpatient treatment was made by 36.1% of the patients who were admitted through the clinic's common outpatient service to the psychogeriatric day hospital. As reports from the psychogeriatric day hospital to the psychiatric clinic of the Univer-

TABLE 21.1 Diagnosis Distribution, Mode of Treatment, and Time of Stay in the Psychogeriatric Day Hospital Over a Period of 4 Years

	On ward			Outpatient service			Total	
Diagnosis	No.	%	Time of stay (days)	No.	%	Time of stay (days)	No.	%
Schizophrenia	24	10.7	57.7	11	8.7	35.3	35	9.9
Organic psychosis	32	14.2	50.8	29	22.8	29.7	61	17.3
Involution depression	70	31.1	67.5	44	34.6	61.5	114	32.4
Reactive depression	15	6.7	39.2	10	7.9	45.4	25	7.1
Cyclothymia	17	7.6	41.5	8	6.3	50.3	25	7.1
Alcohol/medication dependency	9	4.0	28.8	3	2.4	39.0	12	3.4
Paranoid psychosis	17	7.6	34.6	7	5.5	45.3	24	6.8
Neurotic depression	41	18.2	48.4	15	11.8	63.1	56	15.9
	225	63.9	47.4	127	36.1	45.0	352	100.0

sity of Munich show (Ernst & Wächter, 1983), a change of institutional setting under these circumstances leads to a much greater emphasis on substitution than on the decrease of strain.

In determining the average time spent in the day hospital, no difference could be established between patients who were admitted through the outpatient service and patients who had previously had inpatient treatment. In particular, the previous inpatient treatment did not lead to a reduction in the time spent in the day hospital: At 47.3 days, the average time spent by these patients was even slightly longer than that of patients admitted directly through the outpatient service.

Tables 21.2 and 21.3 show the correlation of diagnosis with sex and living conditions. While, in the general population, of those 65 years old and older, 65% are women and 35% men, the proportion for patients during the time of observation in day hospital treatment was 72% and 28%, respectively. The predominance of women in the psychiatric institutions relative to their preponderance in the general population is also found (to the same degree) in other epidemiological investigations, although the causes of this phenomenon are still not sufficiently clear. Especially significant for the group of patients investigated was the relative preponderance of those living alone in comparison with the percentage of those over 65 years of age in the general population; as shown in Table 21.2, this can be explained simply through the high percentage of women living alone.

With regard to the eight diagnostic groups, schizophrenia was found especially often among women not living alone, cerebral-organic impairment among men not living alone and "involution depression," "paranoid psychosis" and "neurotic depression" among women living alone. The

TABLE 21.2 Sex and Living Situation: Day Hospital vs. Federal Republic of Germany

	Male (%)		Female (%)		Total (%)	
	Day hospital	FRG	Day hospital	FRG	Day hospital	FRG
Living alone	6.6	5.7	46.9	33.4	53.4	(39.1)
Not living alone	21.0	29.5	25.6	31.4	46.6	(60.9)
	27.6	35.2	72.4	64.8	100.0	(100.0)
	Male		Female		Total	
Living alone	+0.9		+13.5		+14.3	
Not living alone	−8.5		−5.8		−14.3	
	−7.6		+7.6		0.0	

TABLE 21.3 Diagnosis, Sex, and Living Situation

Diagnosis	Male				Female				Total	
	Alone		Not alone		Alone		Not alone			
	No.	%[a]	No.	%	No.	%	No.	%		
Schizo-phrenia	1	0.3 / 0.6	7	2.0 / 2.1	11	3.1 / 4.7	16	4.5 / 2.5	35	9.9
Organic psychosis	3	0.9 / 1.1	18	5.1 / 3.6	27	7.7 / 8.1	13	3.7 / 4.4	61	17.3
Involution depression	10	2.8 / 2.1	12	3.4 / 6.8	64	18.2 / 15.2	28	8.0 / 8.3	114	32.4
Reaction depression	2	0.6 / 0.5	10	2.8 / 3.3	5	1.4 / 3.3	8	2.3 / 1.8	25	7.1
Cyclothymia	—	0.0 / 0.5	8	2.3 / 1.5	8	2.3 / 3.3	9	2.6 / 1.8	25	7.1
Alcohol/medication dependency	3	0.9 / 0.2	5	1.4 / 0.7	3	0.9 / 1.6	1	0.3 / 0.9	12	3.4
Paranoid psychosis	—	0.4	1	0.3 / 1.4	16	4.5 / 3.2	7	2.0 / 1.7	24	6.8
Neurotic depression	4	1.1 / 1.0	13	3.7 / 3.3	31	8.8 / 7.5	8	2.3 / 4.1	56	15.9
	23	6.5	74	21.0	165	46.9	90	25.6	352	100.0

Chi² = 45.19; df = 21; $p < .002$; C = 0.337; C_{cor} = 0.374.

[a] "First" percentage no.: observed frequency; "second" percentage no.: expected frequency.

number of men not living alone who suffer from "involution depression," women not living alone where the diagnosis is "neurotic depression," and as women living alone who have "reactive depression" was unexpectedly low.

INITIAL EVALUATION AND EFFICIENCY OF DAY HOSPITAL PSYCHOGERIATRIC TREATMENT

> When we began to work on the project and applied ourselves to an improvement of the psychiatric care of those who are mentally ill, we didn't set out to make the care of these patients cheaper, but rather better.
>
> —Finzen (1983)

Efficiency and cost-effectiveness analyses often show these factors to be interdependent and decisive for the future of the psychogeriatric day hospital. Brocklehurst (1982) assumes that day hospital treatment in England (transportation included in the calculation) amounts to approximately 80% of the cost of inpatient treatment.

Based on the fact that the day hospital functions for only 40 hours a week, whereas a ward is operated 168 hours within the same period, there are economies in operating and personnel costs of the day hospital. Advocates of the psychogeriatric day hospital in the Federal Republic are therefore largely in agreement that dispensing with the hospital bed lowers investment and the cost of treating these patients. The question about the efficiency of the psychogeriatric day hospital is often considered, however, exclusively in terms of cost reduction in public health. Aside from the methodical difficulties in measuring efficiency, any reduction of efficiency due to the cost of treatment does not do justice to the significance and the inherent possibilities of the psychogeriatric day hospital.

In order to evaluate the status of psychogeriatric treatment in the day hospital as an essential element in the recommendations for reform of the report dealing with psychiatry in a large German city, we conducted several investigations at our day hospital with the more restrictive goal of extending our empirical knowledge of this subject. What we wanted to know was whether specific features could be identified, differentiating the patients treated in the day hospital from those receiving full inpatient treatment, chiefly with respect to social factors and those characterizing the history of illness. The idea here was to define more precisely the significance of the psychogeriatric day hospital as a link between outpatient and inpatient treatment. Table 21.4 shows important "characteristics," of three investigations that have been carried out dealing with this topic.

Investigation I

The first investigation compared a sample of patients (A) treated in the day hospital, who had been assigned directly from the outpatient service, with another group of day hospital patients (B) who had been transferred to the

TABLE 21.4 Sampling Overview

Investigation	Sampling	No.	Criteria	Methods
I	Day hospital (A) vs. day hospital (B)	23	Overall	Group comparison nonparametric correlation analysis
II	Day hospital (gen.) vs. ward (gen.)	76	Overall	Group comparison rank variance analysis
III	Day hospital (outpatient) vs. ward (outpatient)	84	Differentiated	Hierarchical cluster analysis

day hospital following inpatient treatment. It dealt, in this instance, with 23 patients who were investigated by means of overall criteria, 13 of whom had previously received inpatient treatment and 10 of whom had been assigned directly to the day hospital from the outpatient service. Of the 23 patients, 18 were women and 15 men, with an average age of 68 years. With regard to their family status, no significant clusters were found in any of the categories in Group A; in Group B, on the other hand, the great majority were widowed. The average time of stay of the 23 patients in the day hospital amounted to 42 days (i.e., there were no significant differences between Group A and Group B).

The patients were classified by diagnosis as follows: 70% suffered from affective psychosis, 17% from schizophrenia, and 13% from neurosis or personality disorders. The following instruments of investigation were used: AGP-System, Symptom Check List (SCL 90 R), Life Satisfaction Index (LSI), and Anticipation of Irreversibility Scale (AIS, Thomae & Kranzhoff, 1979).

What interested us in this investigation was chiefly the question: Were there differences between the two groups of patients at the time their treatment in the day hospital was begun—in other words, did those who had been primarily outpatients differ from the former full inpatients with respect to their symptoms when they were admitted to the day hospital?

For the analysis of the comparison between the groups, the nonparametric U-Test according to Mann and Whitney was employed (Diehl & Kohr, 1977). We found that at the time of admission to the day hospital (and also at the time of release), there were no statistically significant differences between the two groups of patients regarding the degree of severity of their mental symptoms, based on the AGP-System or the Self-Evaluation as well as the psychological variables (Life Satisfaction and Anticipated Irreversibility Scale).

From this evidence we concluded that possibly there was a group of psychogeriatric patients for whom treatment in the day hospital was indicated since they could no longer be treated in the outpatient service but needed not yet to be treated as inpatients, or no longer needed to be treated as such.

Investigation II

In a second investigation we compared an unselected group, i.e., without consideration for the mode of admission (Investigation I) of day hospital patients ($N = 35$) with a group receiving inpatient treatment ($N = 41$) over a period of 5 months to see which criteria were decisive for admission to the psychogeriatric day hospital or to an open psychogeriatric ward. For this purpose we employed the following instruments of investigation:

1. to record the social situation, the AGP-System; to record the socioeconomic status, social contacts, and mobility the Havighurst Role Repertoire was used;
2. to record the psychiatric situation, we employed the Overall Medical Opinion of the psychiatrist assigned to treatment for evaluation;
3. to record the psychological situation, as self evaluation, the Symptom Check List, the Life Satisfaction Scale and the Anticipated Irreversibility Scale were employed.

All three areas were quantified overall and divided into three degrees of severity which we characterized as light, moderately severe, and extremely severe strain. For statistical analysis we used the Model of Hierarchical Rank-Variance Analysis suggested by Schulze (1978).

We found, contrary to our expectation, no definitive criteria of admittance as defined by a higher degree of institutionalization (full inpatient vs. day hospital inpatient care) in the case of more severe psychiatric, social, or psychological strain. With regard to the objective social situation, patients under a high degree of strain were found principally among those who were in full inpatient treatment; this was true also for the evaluation of the degree of severity of illness attested to by the psychiatrist. It was interesting to discover contrary findings in the self-evaluation of the patients. More patients in the day hospital characterized themselves as severely impaired than did those on wards. When we considered the group of patients with low social status and lighter degree of illness, we found the same correlation: more members of this group were found in inpatient treatment. A possible explanation could be the lack of homogeneity of the full inpatient group with respect to the pretreatment they received.

Another possible explanation for this phenomenon might lie in the age structure. Patients under 65 years of age were distributed equally over the day hospital and the ward. In contrast, only 25% of those who were over 65 were found in the day hospital; on the ward the figure was 47%. In the group experiencing low social and psychiatric strain, this relationship was even more evident: 41%, or 55% of this group, was in inpatient treatment; in the day hospital group, however, the figure was only 16%. The question to what degree other criteria were of importance had remain open here.

Investigation III

As a result we carried out a third investigation, in which we intended to examine the theory that, instead of relying on the significance of overall criteria, another method of approach, namely, the use of a cluster-analysis technique, might help in defining conditional interrelationships as criteria affecting the decision for assignment to the various forms of treatment. In order to exclude possible pretreatment effects, we investigated only patients who had been assigned directly from the outpatient service to the day hospital or to inpatient treatment in two open psychogeriatric wards, operated for patients of both sexes. The investigation encompassed a period of 10 months, in which 84 patients were assigned directly from the outpatient service to both modes of treatment: 20 to day hospital treatment and 64 to inpatient treatment.

Our data consisted of information concerning the psychopathological, physical, and socioeconomic status as well as the variables of psychological strain, sex, and age. The data were subjected to a hierarchical cluster analysis, whereby the Clustan Program according to Wishart (1975) was employed.

A description of the sample, distributed over the day hospital and the ward, is presented in Table 21.5.

From the table it can be seen that a larger number of the younger age group (65 to 69 years old) was treated in the day hospital. The other age groups showed no difference between treatment in the day hospital and the ward. Widowed patients were slightly overrepresented on the wards. No difference was noted with respect to current living situations (i.e., living alone or with someone else).

With regard to psychiatric strain, we established a trend to slight or moderate strain, especially concerning psycho-organic, depressive, and apathetic syndromes, in day hospital patients, whereas the severe forms of these syndromes predominated with those treated as inpatients. Patients with good physical health were also predominant among those treated in the day hospital; patients with moderate or severe physical impairment were predominant on the wards. The findings of the cluster analysis point to an optimum solution of 7 clusters. In three of these clusters, the day hospital patients were overrepresented, i.e., twice as many day-hospital patients were found in these clusters compared with the number of patients in the total sampling. Two clusters show neither an over- nor underrepresentation of day-hospital or inpatients. Finally, two clusters show an underrepresentation of day hospital patients.

In the three clusters in which day hospital patients were overrepresented, we found the following common variables which, we assume, can be considered indicators for a day hospital treatment (see Table 21.6): "good somatic condition," "moderate psycho-organic syndrome," "light depressive syndrome," and "no necessity for aid in regulating financial affairs." With regard to age groups we found no evidence that younger patients should preferably be assigned to day hospital treatment. The multivariate analysis, consequently, is in contrast to the univariate analyses reported above.

Table 21.7 shows the characteristic items of both clusters in which day hospital patients were underrepresented: "moderate or severe physical im-

TABLE 21.5. Description of Sampling: Day Hospital vs. Full Inpatient Care

Variables	Day hospital (N = 20) No. (%)	Open wards (N = 64) No. (%)
Age:		
65–69	7(35)	11(17)
70–74	5(25)	24(38)
75–79	5(25)	17(27)
80 +	3(15)	12(19)
Gender:		
Male	5(25)	12(19)
Female	15(75)	52(81)
Marital status		
Unmarried	2(10)	5(8)
Married	9(45)	24(38)
Widowed	7(35)	32(50)
Divorced	2(10)	3(5)
Home situation:		
Living alone	9(45)	28(44)
Living with someone	11(55)	36(56)
Mortality:		
Deaths	8(40)	17(27)
Living situation:		
Help needed		
None	8(40)	23(36)
Some	4(20)	13(20)
Much	3(15)	6(9)
Can do nothing without help	5(25)	21(33)
Financial situation:		
Help needed		
None	9(45)	25(39)
Some	4(20)	2(3)
Much	2(10)	9(14)
Can do nothing without help	5(25)	19(30)
Paranoid syndrome:		
Light	2(10)	5(8)
Moderate	2(10)	11(17)
Psychoorganic syndrome:		
Moderate	15(75)	39(61)
Severe	0(0)	9(14)
Apathy:		
Moderate	12(60)	19(30)
Severe	2(10)	16(25)
Mental health:		
Good	14(70)	13(20)
Moderately good	5(25)	36(64)
Poor	1(5)	15(23)

TABLE 21.6 Day Hospital Patients Overrepresented

Cluster IV	Cluster (%)	Total (%)	Cluster I	Cluster (%)	Total (%)	Cluster II	Cluster (%)	Total (%)
Good mental health	100	32	Good mental health	100	32	65–69 years old	100	22
70–74 years old	100	35	75–79 years old	90	26	Moderate psychoorganic syndrome	88	25
Needed no help in handling financial affairs	75	48	Needed no help in handling financial affairs	70	48	Needed some help in handling financial affairs	19	8
Light depressive syndrome	63	18						
Light paranoid syndrome	25	8						
No. = 8			No. = 10			No. = 16		
Day hosp.: 210			Day hosp.: 208			Day hosp.: 184		
Open wards: 66			Open wards: 69			Open wards: 74		

Good physical health
Needed no help or only some help in the handling of financial affairs
Light symptoms of mental illness

TABLE 21.7 Day Hospital Patients Underrepresented

Cluster VII	Cluster (%)	Total (%)	Cluster III	Cluster (%)	Total (%)
Poor physical health	100	19	70–74 years old	100	35
Moderate paranoid syndrome	46	18	Moderately good physical health	93	49
Severe depressive syndrome	36	11	Light paranoid syndrome	22	8
Needed a lot of help in the handling of finanical affairs	27	14			
No. = 11 Day hosp.: 0 Open wards: 119			No. = 15 Day hosp.: 28 Open wards: 123		

> Poor physical health
> Moderate or severe symptoms of mental illness
> Need much help in handling financial affairs

pairment," "severe depressive or moderate paranoid syndrome," and "necessity for extensive aid in regulating financial affairs." These findings seem trivial. It must be emphasized, however, that age, sex and general living conditions did not seem to influence the various modes of treatment. Of the variables investigated, the medical and psychiatric indicators seemed to be the most significant. From the entire area of social and demographic variables, only the regulation of financial affairs had a significant influence. None of the other aids for the management of daily life appeared to be significant for the assignment to one of the two possible modes of treatment.

With regard to efficiency during the 4-year activity of the psychogeriatric day hospital, the length of stay of patients was investigated in detail with respect to the diagnostic relevance and mode of admittance (i.e., outpatients vs. ward). In reference to the first, it was shown that patients with the diagnosis "involution depression" and "neurotic depression" had a clearly longer stay, whereas patients with the diagnosis of "alcohol or medication dependence" had a clearly shorter stay than is expressed in the overall average time spent in treatment.

In reference to the other point, the analysis of diagnostic groups from Table 21.1 showed that particularly patients from three diagnostic groups—schizophrenic psychosis, senile organic psychosis, and involution depression—benefited from immediate day hospital treatment. Their average time of stay was 3 weeks (schizophrenic psychosis and organic psychosis), or 1 week less than the average stay for those of the same diagnostic groups receiving in-patient pretreatment. Patients in these diagnostic groups constituted a total of 60% of the patients treated in the day hospital during the time of observation. Patients with the diagnosis "neurotic depression," on the other hand, benefited little in terms of a shorter time of stay when they were treated directly as day hospital patients; the average stay for this subgroup amounted to 63 days in comparison to an average stay of 48 days for patients receiving inpatient pretreatment. On average, the time of stay was 1 or 1½ weeks shorter for patients with diagnoses of "reactive depression," "cyclothymia," "alcohol or medication dependency," and "paranoid psychosis" following inpatient treatment than for patients who had been assigned to the day hospital directly through the outpatient service.

During a 4-year observation, in the form of a reflection of the first years on the two following, all releases from the day hospital were ultimately compared with the releases from an open ward operated for both sexes (Table 21.8). Of the 75 patients who, in the course of 2 years, had been treated only in the psychogeriatric day hospital (i.e., without inpatient pretreatment) one patient died; of the remaining 74, 95.9%, or 71 patients, could be released to their former homes. In contrast, of those who were treated as inpatients, 5 died; there were only 77.1% who did not have to be transferred to another hospital or a home. Compared with the patients treated in the day hospital, of whom only 1.3% had to be accommodated in a home at the time of their release, 16% of those treated as inpatients could no longer maintain their own home. In examining the frequency of readmission or time between relapses, no significant difference could be established between the day hospital patients and those receiving inpatient treatment. Of 96 patients (42% of the 226 patients who could be released to go home) for whom a readmission was necessary within 2 years of their release, 82 were readmitted to the clinic within the first year, 14 within the second year. As Table 21.9 shows, a slight, although not significant, trend is found here

TABLE 21.8 Readmission to Outpatient vs. Full Inpatient Care

	Day hospital	On ward
	No.(%)	No.(%)
No readmission	40(53.3)	90(43.7)
Readmission within the first year	28(37.4)	54(26.2)
Readmission within the second year	3(4.0)	11(5.3)
Transfer to another hospital	2(2.7)	13(6.3)
Transfer to a home	1(1.3)	33(16.0)
Died	1(1.3)	5(2.4)
	75(100.0)	206(100.0)

TABLE 21.9 Readmission to Hospital Within the First and Second Year Following Release

	Day hospital No.(%)	On ward No.(%)	Total No.(%)
Readmission within the first year	28(90.3)	54(83.1)	82(85.4)
Readmission within the second year	3(9.7)	11(16.9)	14(14.6)
	31(100.0)	65(100.0)	96(100.0)

$\text{Chi}^2 = 0.88$; df = 1NS; $C_{cor} = 0.134$.

in that more day-hospital patients required readmission in the first year following their release than did those who had had full inpatient treatment.

To sum up the advantages or the place of the day hospital in the chain of treatment, we can say that the day hospital, as a link between outpatient and full inpatient care, treats patients with mental illnesses who can no longer, or not yet, be treated as outpatients, but also need no longer, or not yet, be treated as full inpatients, and as such functions more economically than the only alternative possibility of full inpatient treatment. In substance, the rehabilitation in day hospital treatment seems to be more efficient for patients belonging to specific diagnostic groups, i.e., endogenous depression, schizophrenic psychosis, senile organic psychosis (as far as this condition can be treated on open wards), and with an equally severe degree of illness, probably through the avoidance of hospitalization effects; on the other hand, rehabilitation seems less efficient in the case of patients with neurotic depression.

In the current status of investigation, the social variables employed seem to carry no weight as discriminating factors. Since these results, however, were found exclusively in retrospective studies, the relationships discovered should be checked out in prospective investigations as a next step in the evaluation of day hospital treatment.

CONCLUSIONS

In summary, it seems important to emphasize the following points:

1. No differences between inpatients and day hospital patients as to their physical and psychological impairment were found at the time of admission or transfer to the day hospital.

2. Those admitted primarily as inpatients differed from those admitted primarily as day-hospital inpatients in that their mental and physical impairment was assessed objectively as more serious, whereby the subjective

experience of impairment was often contrary to the objective assessment; there was no difference between the two groups of patients in regard to sociodemographic characteristics.

3. Overall, no difference was found in the average time of stay between the primary (i.e., without pretreatment) and secondary (i.e., following inpatient treatment) patients treated in the day hospital; with diagnostic differentiation, on the other hand, clear advantages of day hospital treatment were shown for specific diagnostic groupings.

4. Virtually all the patients released from the day hospital returned to their accustomed environment in contrast to only three-quarters of the comparable group who received an exclusively inpatient treatment.

5. During the 4 years of observation, no significant difference was found between the readmission rate of patients treated in the day hospital and those treated exclusively as inpatients.

REFERENCES

Barop, H., Kranzhoff, E. U., & Husser, J. (1982). Untersuchungen über Patientenmerkmale einer gerontopsychiatrischen Tagesklinik. In M. Bergener & B. Kark (Eds.), *Tagesklinische Behandlung im Alter*. Darmstadt.

Bergener, M., & Kark, B. (1982). *Tagesklinische Behandlung im Alter*. Darmstadt.

Bierer, J. (1951). The day hospital. An experiment in social psychiatry and synthoanalytic psychotherapy. London.

Bosch, G. & Steinhardt, I. (1983). Entwicklung und gegenwärtiger Stand der tagesklinischen Behandlung in der BRD. In G. Bosch & I. Steinhardt (Eds.), Die Tagesklinik als Teil der psychiatrischen Versorgung. Bonn.

Brocklehurst, J. C. (1982). Survey of geriatric hospitals in Great Britain. In M. Bergener & B. Kark (Eds.), Tagesklinische Behandlung im Alter. Darmstadt.

Cameron, D. E. (1947). The day hospital. An experimental form of hospitalization for psychiatric patients. *Mod. Hosp., 69,* 60–62.

Diehl, J. M., & Kohr, H. U. (1977). *Durchführungsanleitungen fürstatistische Tests*. Weinheim & Basel.

Dzhagarov, M. A. (1937). Experience in organizing a day hospital for mental patients. *Werropathol. Psikhiatr. 6,* 137–147.

Ernst, L., & Wächter, C. (1983). Die gerontopsychiatrische Tagesklinik. In G. Bosch & I. Steinhardt (Eds.), *Die Tagesklinik als Teil der psychiatrischen Versorgung*. Bonn.

Finzen, A. (1977). Die Tagesklinik. München.

Finzen, A. (1981). Modell offener Psychiatrie. *Im Blickpunkt* 8, 7–13.

Kranzhoff, E. U., & Husser, J. (1983). Evaluationsansätze tagesklinischer Behandlung in der Gerontopsychiatrie. *Soz. Präventivmed. 28,* 296–301.

Schulze, G. (1978). Ein Verfahren zur multivariaten Analyse der Bedingungen von Rangvariablen: Hierarchische Rangvarianzanalyse. *Sozialpsychol. 9,* 129 ff.

Thomae, H. & Kranzhoff, E. U. (1979). Erlebte Unveränderlichkeit von gesundh. u. ök. Belastung. Ein Beitrag zur Kognitiven Theorie der Anpassung an das Alter. *Z. Gerontol., 12,* 439 ff.

Wishart, D. (1978). Clustan User Manual. Edinburgh. Churchill Livingstone.

22
Evaluation and Effectiveness of Psychogeriatric Services: An Economic Perspective

Robert G. Jones

In Britain nearly one in every twenty-five members of the workforce is employed by the National Health Service, and just under half of all government spending is disbursed by the Department of Health and Social Security. Much of this expenditure is for the elderly and more than half of all hospital beds are utilized by elderly patients. And yet the British government was recently castigated in the media for spending less per head on health than most other Western countries. Given the chance, any clinician or social worker in Britain will emphasize the problems of dealing with the elderly. They will highlight particularly the elderly who need psychiatric help, and the lack of sufficient resources and facilities. The same song can be heard in every developed country of the world. Clearly it is vital to discuss setting of priorities, planning, evaluation, and effectiveness.

Not long ago I gave a talk on this topic to an international gathering and sadly I had to admit to the audience from the outset that I stood before them naked, as up till then there had been virtually no work on these topics in the field of psychiatry of aging. Unfortunately that lack is still the order of the day, but there can be no doubt of the enormous need for effective services for the elderly (not only for effective psychiatric services) and for their effective planning. The economic imperatives of our time demand cost effectiveness, and in a "sensible" world there would be a planned provision of services to meet the known needs, with built-in programs of ongoing evaluation. In the psychiatry of old age to date every element in this formulation has been sadly deficient, but also, as we will see, this seemingly sensible formulation is a little too simplistic. The aim of this chapter is to introduce some concepts of planning and evaluation to the gerontopsychiatrist. Although there is a dearth of established work in this field there is certainly a dire need for such an information base. Planning decisions are constantly being made which necessarily incorporate judgments about the effectiveness and efficiency of services whether or not they are wisely based. A fuller understanding of issues in planning and evaluation can only help the clinician who needs to get involved in such debates. Are there clinicians who can afford not to be involved? Hopefully this will also help to generate the greater study and attention that this area needs.

In one sense the issues are no different in the psychiatry of old age than elsewhere, but in practice all services for the elderly tend to be forced to address the idea of rationing of resources. A single chapter can only hope to be introductory in nature. The aim is to begin to familiarize the reader with the field and to introduce some ideas of economic evaluation of effectiveness. With an overview of these areas comes also a keener awareness of the difficulties in evaluating psychiatric services for the elderly.

WHY PLAN?

Planning is concerned with looking ahead at the problems we may face when trying to reach our goal. Through foresight we aim to avoid any pitfalls and smoothly achieve success, but unfortunately health problems are frequently complicated. They show great variety, and new problems can pop up unexpectedly. To deal with this complex scenario the organizational framework of a health service needs to be both stable and flexible.

Planning aims to make the future better than it would otherwise be. The National Health Service must plan because there is scarcity of resources with much competition for them, which increasingly leads to demand for the most efficient and economic use of health care. Human resources are also limited. Around one million people are employed by the National Health Service, and their deployment demands careful planning if it is to be effective. Medical technology advances at a fast pace and there is constant change in the pattern of "consumer" demand. Both constantly dictate a flexible response from the Health Service—not only in terms of planning.

Three important basic facets of the planning process begin to emerge from this early discussion: the diagnostic, the implementative, and the evaluative. With the diagnostic process we need first to define the problem, clarify our aim, and lay down a plan for achieving this. The implementative stage involves planning how to actually bring our solution into being. The third stage, so often forgotten, is concerned with evaluating the effectiveness of the plans that have been implemented. This evaluation needs to be fed back into the planning process so that a new diagnosis and/or adjustments of implementation can be made as appropriate. In the real world planning and services have to cope with continual disruption brought by fluctuating availability of cash or other resources and by changing demands.

Thinking more specifically of the planning of services, Wing (1981) suggests that there are three important principles to be borne in mind: responsibility, comprehensiveness, and integration. Responsibility in this context means that the service is responsible to a defined district so that everyone in the district needing treatment, care, or counsel is able to obtain it regardless of their ability to pay. Of necessity, the services must be accessible. Comprehensiveness means that services are set out to be responsive to all those with appropriate needs in their area. Integration demands proper communication between the various agencies involved, ensuring that appropriate services are provided with reasonable continuity of care. The aim with all these principles is to enable a community to deal with social disablement caused by health problems.

WHY EFFECTIVENESS?

Nothing is for nothing and everything has a cost. Though the British National Health Service budget forms a smaller proportion of the gross national product than in most Western countries, it forms a very sizeable proportion of the national economy. Despite a major transfusion of oil wealth, in recent years Britain has suffered its greatest economic slump in decades. There have already been significant cutbacks in many areas in Social Services provision, including for the elderly, and the clear message from government is that there are likely to be even more substantial reductions. For the first time Britain is experiencing real cutbacks in health services in financial terms. This will greatly affect the elderly.

It is essential therefore that the best use is made of available resources, and that the most effective and most beneficial patterns of service are exploited to the fullest.

APPROACHES TO EVALUATION

Work evaluating the effectiveness of psychogeriatric services is lacking. Even more striking is the lack of work with an economic emphasis in evaluation of such services. But there are some effectiveness and economic studies that have been performed either with the elderly in general or in the broader psychiatric field. These studies illustrate the kind of approaches to evaluation that could be used. First, however, it is worth considering some general thoughts on evaluation.

For evaluating services, Wing (1972) has formulated six useful questions:

1. How many people are in contact with the various services that already exist; what patterns of contact do they make, and what are the temporal trends in contact rate?
2. What are the needs of these individuals and their relatives?
3. Are the services presently provided meeting these needs effectively and economically?
4. How many people not in touch with services also have needs and are their needs different from those already in contact?
5. What new services, or modifications of existing services, are likely to cater to unmet needs?
6. When innovations in services are introduced do they in fact help to reduce need?

If we can answer most of these questions we will be making considerable progress. And it is reasonable to add a seventh question to the list: What are the needs of the staff that administer the services, and are these being met?

One tool used to provide answers to some of these questions has been the Psychiatric Case Register (Wing & Hailey, 1972; Wing & Häfner, 1973). These now exist in a number of centers in Great Britain including Salford, Camberwell, and Nottingham. These registers are systems whereby records from a specified set of psychiatric facilities (or indeed perhaps also other facilities) are collected for individual persons from a defined population and accumulated over time. The *Journal of Mental Science* has recorded a description of such a system in operation over 105 years ago in Scottish Mental Hospitals. Great development has occurred with registers in the Scandanavian countries, and psychiatric registers have been kept in several other European countries for many years.

One problem that plagues this kind of enterprise is reliability in diagnosis, with wide variations in the nomenclature and classification of mental disorders. Another problem is comprehensiveness which arises quite acutely in the case of the psychiatry of old age. Psychogeriatric facilities usually exist alongside geriatric facilities, but they may not cooperate with each other. Cases not catered to by the Psychogeriatric Service will probably end up having care provided for them by the Geriatric Service and vice-versa. Clearly, elderly people also make extensive use of other medical facilities which are neither geriatric nor psychogeriatric; and they also make extensive use of a wide range of facilities such as Social Services quite outside the hospital services. Only a comprehensive Geriatric Case Register covering all these services would provide the data base for proper evaluative study. However, such a register would be extremely complicated and expensive to run. To date I know of none in existence.

Nevertheless, we can look at some of the results from the existing purely psychiatric Case Registers and these are instructive. Taking the Camberwell and the Nottingham Case Registers together we find large differences between the two areas in the rate of contact with old people in the respective psychiatric services. The register itself does not tell us why. Almost certainly a comprehensive Geriatric Register would give the answer. A reasonable hypothesis is that old people with dementia were cared for by psychiatric services to a much greater extent in Nottingham than they were in Camberwell during the period. A question arises whether many patients in Camberwell with dementia were being cared for by geriatric services instead, or whether in fact they were not being cared for by any service at all. Considerably greater burdens could have been thrust on families in one area compared to the other.

Continuing a little more with the theme of evaluation and the effects of services on families and communities, it is appropriate here to mention Grad and Sainsbury's study (1968). Their study compared a community oriented service with a more traditional mental hospital based service. It was concerned with psychiatric services to all age groups, but because large numbers of old people were involved useful conclusions could be drawn with regard to the elderly. Their work showed that a community oriented service that tried to keep people at home was able to relieve families of the worst burdens of care for the elderly to an extent comparable with the relief afforded by the hospital-based service. Similar results were suggested by the more limited work of Hoenig and Hamilton in this area (Hoenig, 1968). However, there was still a large load of taxing burdens on families.

NEED

It is necessary at this stage to further define our terms. Our ultimate concern is not the services but the needs of the population that they serve. Can we define need itself? The need for health care could be thought of as endless and limitless. Mathew (1971), in Britain's then Ministry of Health, was one of the first to try to clarify this concept. He argues that the "need for medical care must be distinguished from the demand for care," and both of these should be distinguished from the actual use of services which should be termed "utilization." The need for medical care exists with an illness or disability for which there is an effective and acceptable treatment or cure. Even if this need is present, it is not necessarily followed by utilization, and there can of course be demand and even utilization of services without real need. Nowadays we increasingly find that effective treatment can be horrendously expensive. Newell (1977), for instance, conjures up the image of arthritis being totally curable by injections of dissolved moondust. How then are we to temper our perception of need? Again financial considerations intrude into thoughts of effectiveness.

It is easy to become bewildered when considering effectiveness and need, losing track of what really is important. For an illustration of this Mooney et al. (1980), suggest we think about incontinent people in the community. This is predominantly a population of older women, though not entirely so. Here certainly is a group that has a need, having a medical problem that gives rise to social disability. Perhaps they should all be hospitalized for treatment for their condition—a very expensive way of managing their problem, and not always successful. Some people suffering from incontinence could have their condition permanently cured fairly easily and rapidly, whereas for others there is little hope of a cure. However, much can be done to alleviate the problem; for example, teaching the individual and those around her effective ways of coping with the difficulties so that in effect these difficulties are largely overcome. Thus in the case of incontinence there are different intensities of need for any one treatment, different ranges of severity, and different conditions that give rise to the same disability.

All this discussion avoids the crucial problem of the cost of meeting these needs. Is there a finite amount of sickness that could be removed or an infinite amount of health care that could be supplied to meet an endless degree of need? How do we ration, given that our resources are finite? We cannot meet all needs but we must decide how to spend our money most effectively to meet the needs that we regard as having the highest priority. This discussion also illustrates how we have neatly managed to ignore the wants and the desires of some of those with the needs in the first place. If, for instance, we were to treat all incontinent elderly women in hospitals there would be a large number of very dissatisfied elderly women as the vast majority of the population at any given time are desperate not to be in the hospital. They are most anxious to retain their independence in their own setting. This "need" also has to be very fully considered.

TOOLS FOR ECONOMIC EVALUATION OF HEALTH CARE

We need to look more fully at the economic analysis of health care. What are some of the main tools that have been used for this task? There are three main techniques. First, there is cost-effectiveness, which tries to tell us which way to set about achieving an objective. Secondly, there is cost–benefit analysis which tries to tell us whether achieving an objective is worthwhile. Thirdly, there is marginal analysis which tries to help us decide how far to go in seeking an objective, or what is the best balance of complementary services. We will consider these in more detail.

Cost-Effectiveness Analysis

As doctors our interest is in reducing morbidity and suffering. Perhaps as parents we are also interested in reducing road deaths of children. We are prepared to pay highly for our aims but will not pay any price. Also we wish to spend our money on a variety of aims, and will not concentrate exclusively on only one. Clearly we have a list of priorities. We want to spend our money in the wisest possible way. In other words we wish to obtain the greatest effectiveness for the minimum cost.

Cost-effectiveness analysis is concerned with precisely this sort of issue. It can be useful as a technique to compare two or more programs of action having a similar aim. For example, we may be concerned with reducing deaths from breast cancer. One way might be to increase early detection. To achieve this we might contrast a breast screening clinic set up in one area with a program of active health education on self-examination by health visitors in another area. These slightly differing approaches would have different costs and we would, in a very simple manner, be able to work out the cost per breast cancer detected at a given early stage. The program that had the lowest cost per breast cancer detected would then be indicated as the best by this technique.

In such a cost-effectiveness exercise, what is taken for granted is that our aim is reasonable. The economic analysis only tells us the best way of achieving the aim, not whether it is sensible or economically worthwhile in a broader perspective. This approach is limiting, particularly in the realm of health care, where our aims are rarely simple. The task of the British Health Service is to reduce and contain morbidity, but also to attempt to spread the burden of care and the implications of illness over the whole community rather than allowing them to cause havoc for the individual or his family alone. Within its limits, this sort of cost-effectiveness study can provide us with a great deal of very useful information but it is not adequate to deal with these greater aims.

For psychiatry in general there is a small body of studies, mainly from the United States, where effectiveness and economic aspects have been looked at together. There are also a number of studies that sometimes carry the title of cost-effectiveness studies but that in reality are mere accounting exercises only of interest to a bank manager or budget controller. Unfortunately it is often only this sort of information that is looked at when planning decisions are made. Cost-effectiveness analysis has been applied in the United States quite extensively to approaches to treatment of schizophrenia, but in Britain there are very few studies in the area of psychiatry. In the realm of the psychiatry of old age there are no such studies conducted simply with psychogeriatric services.

The breadth of our aims in psychiatry makes cost-effectiveness studies seem difficult to apply. But there is one approach to overcoming the limitations of these studies. If two alternative treatments are aimed at a specific symptom or set of symptoms it is often reasonable to measure relative effectiveness by mean change scores on these symptoms for each treatment. These mean change scores can then be set against the mean cost of each treatment per patient. This approach has not been used with psychogeriatric patients, but has been applied with geriatric medical patients by Schultz and McGlone (1977) in Denver. They conducted a comparison between treatment of the elderly by a nurse practitioner working together with a physician, versus traditional treatment by a physician working on his own. They studied three groups: ambulatory patients, home bound patients, and those resident in nursing homes. Some of the figures involved in the study are reproduced in Table 22.1 and it will be seen that we are referring to mean goal attainment change score and the mean cost involved per patient to achieve this. For ambulatory patients traditional treatment by the physician only is both more effective and less expensive.

For the patients confined to their own home the study found the reverse, that is, treatment by a physician and a nurse practitioner together was more effective and cost less. In the case of patients living in nursing homes there was a chance of gaining as much of the objective as possible for a fixed cost because for this group the two treatments were around the same in cost, but the combination of the nurse practitioner with the physician was more effective.

TABLE 22.1 A Cost-Effectiveness Study

Patient category	Patients treated by physician only (N = 85)		Patients treated by the physician/nurse practitioner team (N = 82)	
	Improvement (average goal attainment change score)	Average cost per patient	Improvement (average goal attainment change score)	Average cost per patient
Ambulatory	11.31	$448	8.81	$679
Homebound	3.82	$4017	7.70	$2473
Nursing home	2.24	$5813	6.24	$5893

From Schultz and McGlone (1977). Reprinted by permission.

A number of questions immediately arise. What were the goals achieved? Were they worth achieving? Were they the only goals worth achieving, or were there perhaps totally different but highly worthwhile goals that might require a totally different approach? This study does not answer these questions. Cost-effectiveness studies answer some questions but they tend to give rise to many others. At least with this study we gain some useful data for discussion of effectiveness and efficiency of two approaches. This helps us to decide which is best given the cost that we can afford.

Two British studies should be mentioned, though they are less sophisticated than the typical cost-effectiveness approach. First, there is the study by Opit (1978) which is basically a limited costing exercise on elderly sick patients being cared for at home by a home nursing service together with the support of other domiciliary services. Opit's data indicated that with seriously disabled people—basically those bedridden, around 20% of his sample—the cost of home care was equal to or even greater than the average cost associated with residential or hospital care in such patients. Not only that, but there was also evidence that the services provided were inadequate or inappropriate for the need present.

However, there is a limit to how much we can generalize from this approach because it looks at cost in isolation with a fairly circumscribed group of people. It points out an area of great concern but does not help us much with the cost-effectiveness of an overall approach to the care of the elderly. Also, on a point of detail, Opit's study did not take account of capital costs which could have considerably altered the sums.

The other British study was reported by MacFarlane (1979) and earlier by Ross (1976), who looked at "cost benefit" in geriatric day hospitals in Glasgow. Actually the measurement of benefit was fairly crude and it was really another costing exercise. Their conclusion was that day hospital treatment conferred benefit and was considerably cheaper than inpatient care, which they assert would be the alternative treatment in the absence of a day hospital facility. Again, there comes a level of provision of day care at which point, when other services provided into the home are taken into account, the cost becomes prohibitive in comparison with institutional care, especially if the total costs to the whole community are considered.

Cost–Benefit Analysis

The last study mentioned above uses the words "cost benefit" but was not actually a cost–benefit analysis study. Cost–benefit analysis is a much more sophisticated technique and in some modified form probably provides the best tool for comparing the effectiveness of different services and their approaches to treatment. Essentially this type of analysis aims to tell us whether something is really worth doing, the decision being that if the benefits outweigh the cost then it is worthwhile. In a cost–benefit analysis all the possible effects of the program or treatment are measured, at least in principle. Not simply the outcome with symptoms but every conceivable social and financial effect is examined. In a pure cost–benefit analysis these effects are then expressed in monetary terms. Clearly some of the effects of a treatment or program are beneficial to the patients or to the community, but others will constitute a cost. If the total of all the benefits of the treatment exceeds the cost then a cost–benefit analysis would suggest that the program should be carried out. Two or more types of treatment can be compared and the treatment that has the most advantageous cost-benefit ratio will be the one that should be selected.

A necessary aspect of the analysis is to carry out an exhaustive measurement of all the costs and benefits and then to express them, as far as possible, in monetary terms. It is here that the major problem arises with cost–benefit analysis. Treatment programs typically concern themselves with aims that cannot be easily expressed in monetary terms, or perhaps at all. They aim at the relief of symptoms causing distress and at improvements in psychosocial adjustment. How can this be valued? Some researchers have dealt with this problem by simply ignoring the costs and benefits of an intangible nature which they could not measure in financial terms. Some have assigned arbitrary money values to such intangible measures. And some researchers have tried to assign money values derived from compensation damages awarded by courts for injury and disability.

None of these approaches seems to be totally satisfactory and until a better answer is devised it seems best to accept the fact that there are certain things that cannot be measured in monetary terms. But at the same time we must make quite sure they are, in fact, measured and taken into account in any comparison of services.

Again there are no studies of this nature in the field of psychogeriatrics and very few at all in the realm of psychiatry. A study with the elderly which should be mentioned was conducted by Wager (1972) for the Essex County Council. In his study he calculated the comparative cost of residential and domiciliary care, looking at those waiting for residential care. With his study he suggested there would be a greater return for society in the future from a diversion of some resources away from the expansion of residential facilities and toward a selective domiciliary care program for those in substantial need of support. This was a carefully conducted study, but in fact the benefits were not researched and only people on the waiting list were looked at. It is the closest to a cost–benefit analysis study in this area, but in the end it remains very much a costing exercise.

In the absence of a cost-benefit analysis study in the psychiatry of old age it is worth illustrating the approach further by looking at a study from general psychiatry. This approach could be applied with geriatric psychiatry services and many of the issues raised are equally relevant in either area. The study compared two different styles of service dealing with schizophrenia. The two services were a relatively high intensity teaching District General Hospital (DGH) with no designated "chronic beds," versus a traditional Mental Hospital with substantial provision of long-stay beds (Jones, 1980). First-admission schizophrenics were studied four years after their first admission, and longitudinal data were gathered on their four-year experience of employment, income, and consumption of health and social welfare resources. The approach was to carefully measure all the effects of the services. These were assigned as either costs or benefits, and were not restricted to only those that could be detailed in monetary terms. The services were then compared in terms of the monetary cost–benefit outcome, but every effort was also made to look at the so-called "soft costs and benefits" (the intangible costs and benefits) associated with the services as well.

The present State Examination (Wing et al., 1974) was used to measure clinical outcome at follow-up and there were also measures of social performance, of unmet need, and exploration of knowledge and attitudes about the illness and attitudes toward work. A social worker performed an assessment of the burden and other effects on the family, and also obtained a measure of the mental health of the nearest supporter together with more longitudinal outcome measures concerning use of services and income earned after recovery.

Most of these measures were then used to compare the services in terms of psychosocial outcome using the "soft costs and benefits" comparison. This showed the more intensive DGH service was more successful in minimizing chronicity and in a number of other respects, but generally the services achieved a similar outcome. It was then possible to see at what cost the more intensive service achieved its advantages. This meant setting the analysis beside the "hard costs and benefits" economic comparison, which is illustrated in Tables 22.2 and 22.3.

From all the data gathered about the use of various resources, income received, employment record, etc., it was possible to plot all the important monetary costs and benefits to the patients and their families, and to the rest of the community over the four-year follow-up period. Table 22.2 illustrates some of the figures resulting from this calculation and, for example, shows the total psychiatric hospital costs, other health costs, and Local Authority Social Services costs. It was important to take account of income earned (sometimes by other family members being forced out to work) and income lost through work lost. These also had implications in terms of National Insurance contributions, tax and employer contributions to government revenue, as well as more obvious effects on family finances. In fact the economic comparison showed that the DGH service was more economically beneficial to both the patient and family and to the rest of the community.

TABLE 22.2 Annual Costs and Benefits to Rest of the Community

	District general hospital	Mental hospital
Costs		
Psychiatric hospital costs	+£933	+£984
Other health costs	+£28	+£55
Local authority costs	+£85	+£240
Dept. of Employment costs	+£19	+£5
Voluntary agencies	+£53	+£30
Social Security	+£500	+£564
Tax and National Insurance lost	+£66	+£20
Less benefits		
Patient's tax and National Insurance	−£300	−£179
Tax and National Insurance gained	−£7	−£0
Employer's National Insurance contribution	−£96	−£63
Local authority charges	−£0	−£5
Total	£1281	£1651
	Net gain to DGH = £370	

Tables 22.2 and 22.3 indicate the fairly all-inclusive approach employed in this study.

All too often in an evaluation of services the effects on the patient and family outside of the health setting are not considered in any way. Also, the effects of services on other agencies and services in the community, apart from the Health Service, are frequently neglected. In the end it is the effect of the service on both the patient and family, on the one hand, and on the whole of the rest of the community, on the other hand, and therefore its impact on the whole of the community, that is important in its assessment. Tables 22.2 and 22.3 show the costs and benefits split up in this way.

This serves to illustrate how cost–benefit analysis, especially perhaps in this modified form, can be applied appropriately to the evaluation of services in the health and social services field. This kind of approach could be used for assessment of services in the psychiatry of old age. There success is achieved through the value of different services in meeting health and welfare needs in the community, many of which are of an intangible psychosocial nature. Nevertheless there are also hard financial costs and in examining effectiveness it is essential that all the effects of the services be considered together. With this modified form of cost–benefit analysis it is possible to see at what cost one service is more successful than another, in terms of, say, the greater intangible psychosocial benefits it achieves.

TABLE 22.3 Annual Benefits and Costs to the Patient and His Family

	District general hospital	Mental hospital
Benefits		
Patient's earnings	+£700	+£417
Family members forced to work	+£16	+£0
Social Security	+£500	+£564
Money from voluntary agencies	+£0	+£29
Less costs		
Family members prevented from working	−£153	−£47
Special expenses	−£38	−£61
Local authority charges for services	−£0	−£5
Expenditure on patient's food while not in hospital	−£2800	−£260
Total	£745	£637
	Net gain to DGH = £108	

Marginal Analysis

Cost–benefit analysis makes the competing priorities and the costs and benefits involved totally explicit and forces the policy-maker or decision-maker to address the real issues in a detailed way. Marginal analysis brings us again to this fundamental area even more keenly. It aims to tell us how far we should go in trying to benefit from a particular program. Even more usefully, perhaps, it helps to illuminate the situation where two separate but interdependent services work side by side to achieve a common goal. Marginal analysis will help us to decide how to spread our budget between the two services to produce the best mixture and to give rise to the greatest overall benefit. In the United Kingdom the National Health Service and the Social Services work independently but interdependently to provide care and benefit to the elderly. Such a situation may well mean that at any given time resources could usefully be transferred from one to the other to achieve a better overall benefit for a given client group.

To consider this area in more detail we need to think about some key concepts. These are, firstly, marginal benefit and marginal costs and, second, opportunity costs. If we have some kind of service to the community which produces 350 items every day, then the marginal benefit is the benefit derived from the 350th item, the last unit produced. Similarly the marginal cost is the cost of actually producing this last (marginal) unit. A practical example serves to illustrate these terms better.

Britain has the "Meals on Wheels" service whereby, under the auspices of the Social Services and voluntary agencies, hot meals are delivered to disabled elderly people in their own homes. To prepare a similarly nutritious meal regularly would be difficult or impossible for these people. A real need is therefore being met. If we start with the first meal on wheels being supplied, the benefit to the community provided by this is quite large as a meal is being received where before none was provided at all. With two meals on wheels the benefit is still pretty large and perhaps with 100 meals on wheels still the benefit is quite large. But bit by bit as we provide more and more meals on wheels to more and more people the amount of benefit derived by the community decreases as more and more of the need is met. If we continue expanding, eventually there comes a point where we are providing meals to people who do not really need them at all. No real benefit is any longer being obtained. We incur the cost of providing the meal but fail to reap a benefit equal to or greater than the cost. That is the point where the marginal benefit and marginal cost lines intersect. When a service has expanded to the point where the benefit derived from supplying it is exactly equal to the cost of supplying it then that is the point at which we should stop expanding. Supplying more of this service means the cost is greater than the benefit being received (see Figure 22.1).

We are dealing here with the marginal cost and the marginal benefit—the cost and the benefit at the margin associated with supplying the last item of any particular service. It is not the same as the average value of the meal on wheels, for instance, and it is certainly not the same as the value to the

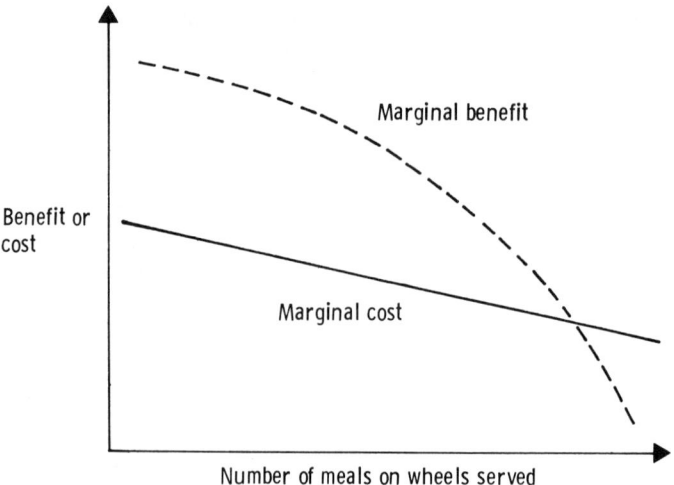

FIGURE 22.1 Marginal cost and marginal benefit with Meals on Wheels Service.

community of the first meal on wheels supplied. There is a law of diminishing returns operating.

The first meal on wheels is very expensive because it requires investment in all the services and equipment necessary to get the service going. Thereafter the meals on wheels will become proportionately less and less costly as more and more are produced. The marginal cost, the cost of producing the last item, is quite different from the average cost. Similarly with the first few meals the benefit will be great as they help those in greatest need but the benefit at the margin declines dramatically as we produce more and more meals. We should not expand a service beyond the point where the marginal benefit and the marginal cost are equal because beyond that point we lose.

Of course, while this all sounds straightforward it presupposes both that we can easily and accurately measure such benefits and costs and that we can convert them appropriately into monetary terms—a difficult undertaking—but thinking in these theoretical terms does help us to observe some underlying principles that are important in planning effective services.

The opportunity cost is an important factor as only a finite amount of money is available. Money spent on one thing cannot then be spent on something else. For the economist the value of something is the amount of money we will forego spending on other things to obtain it. Thus the opportunity cost represents the cost of the opportunity that we forego by spending on Plan A instead of the next best Plan B. Although this concept may not always be explicitly in the minds of planners and decision-makers they are in effect always implicitly making decisions along these sort of lines. It would be preferable for these decisions to be explicit rather than implicit.

In theory we can use these concepts to look at how much emphasis to give to complementary schemes concerned with supporting the elderly at home. For instance a Social Services department may be running a Home Help Service and a Meals on Wheels Service. Both of these aid and support the disabled elderly at home although each focuses on slightly different functions. Having suddenly found more money to spend (probably through increased taxes!) we want to know how to spend the extra money most effectively on both of these programs.

Looking at the Meals on Wheels Service we could build a table of the marginal benefit and the marginal cost for every meal delivered. We could construct a similar table with marginal benefit and marginal cost for every hour of home help delivered. Thus for each service it is possible to derive a ratio of marginal benefit to marginal cost for every level of service delivered. We know we must not expand either service beyond the point where marginal benefit and marginal cost are equal but we would like to know how to divide our spending of extra money on the two services so as to get the best value for money from them in combination.

The answer is to look at the marginal benefit to marginal cost ratios. When we have spent our money most wisely on expanding the services each should be at the maximum possible output level, but with the marginal benefit to marginal cost ratios being the same for both services. Put simply this means getting the same number of £s of benefit for each extra £ spent in both services; see Mooney (1980) for a good illustration of this idea with examples in graphic form. While we mention here only expanding two services, the same applies for our spending of extra money on any number of complementary services.

This example illustrates some of the difficulties as well as some of the benefits of this approach. Once grasped the concepts are fairly simple, but at first sight this is somewhat unfamiliar and difficult territory for most doctors. A more severe problem is the difficulty in defining the monetary value of the marginal benefit associated with, say, the 500th Meal on Wheels served. The ideas are enlightening but there may be great practical difficulty in applying them. These concepts have been applied using the technique of marginal analysis by researchers in Aberdeen (Fordyce et al., 1981). They focused on defining the best "balance of care" for a disabled elderly population (Mooney, 1980). To appreciate their approach we need to think a little more about the theory.

Let us consider the benefit derived by a disabled elderly person being supported in his or her own home. We could take a number of individuals with different levels of disability and place them on a graph where the vertical axis is the benefit achieved by their home support, and the horizontal axis records their increasing levels of dependency (Figure 22.2). For the individual in his or her own home who becomes increasingly dependent, benefit is derived from the supply of increasing services. However, after a certain level of dependency there comes a point when the benefit line flattens out. The individual is so dependent that further services provided to the home no longer help or are perhaps totally inappropriate. If we look at people in residential homes, at low levels of dependency the benefit that they will receive from this service will be small. But as their level of disability and dependency rises so will the benefit they derive from residential care increase until again perhaps we reach a point where dependency is so great that further benefit can no longer be conferred by this service. If we placed both these groups on the same graph we would see that these two benefit lines intersect. At that dependency level we can say that people who are in their own home will now derive greater benefit from being in a residential home. Similarly, below that level of dependency people in a residential home are there inappropriately in the sense that they would derive greater benefit from being in their own home.

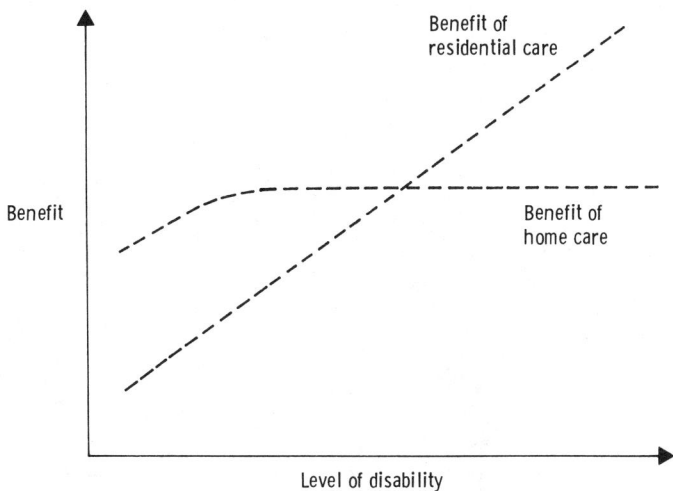

FIGURE 22.2 Benefit derived from residential or home care at different levels of disability.

We can take things a little further and plot on a graph the rising cost of maintaining somebody in their own home as their level of disability and dependency increases. To further complicate things, we can add the benefit line as well (Figure 22.3). There comes a point at a certain level of dependency beyond which the cost of maintaining individuals in their homes will be greater than the benefit that they receive from this. Clearly at that point they should no longer remain at home. Of course in drawing these diagrams we are making the assumption, in a rather ideal way, that it is possible to present in detail the relationships between all the benefits, all the costs, and all the different dependency/disability levels. The reality is not so simple. The costs of living in a residential home can be supplied and the different dependency levels that go with these same costs can also be filled in. Similarly we can measure the costs involved in home support of individuals with various levels of disability. Filling in the benefits is perhaps not possible at this stage, but with this sort of diagram we can at least see the theoretical point at which we should be aiming in order to make the most rational and beneficial use of our limited resources.

These were the kind of ideas used in the marginal analysis study of elderly residents in Aberdeen. Two particular groups were studied: a selected sample of those in their own homes and those in residential homes. Also the costs of those in long-stay geriatric hospitals were examined. What were studied were in fact the marginal groups. Thus residential homes staff, community nursing staff, and social services staff were asked to consider

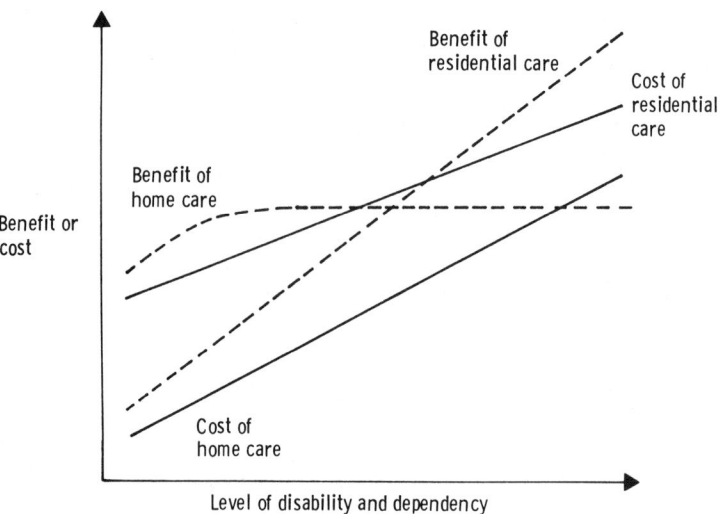

FIGURE 22.3 Costs and benefits associated with residential and home care at different disability levels. (Derived from Fordyce, Mooney, & Russell, 1981.)

their clients in terms of whom they would recommend to move from the community into a residential home if suddenly many more places were made available, and whom they would recommend to be moved from the community into hospital if suddenly more beds became available—in other words those on the margin. The residential homes staff were asked to nominate those whom they would recommend moving back into the community if suddenly some residential homes had to close, and those whom they would recommend to move from the residential homes into hospital if suddenly more hospital beds were made available—again the marginal groups. At the same time descriptions of the dependency and disability levels of these groups and their levels of service consumption were also assembled.

This defined the size and nature of the marginal groups in the community and in residential homes, and the marginal groups among them whom it was felt should appropriately be moved to hospital if this were possible. At the same time information was gathered on the cost of living and the cost of caring services for these individuals in their current placements. Thus overall total figures were derived from the study for differing costs for the different groups in their different settings. This information, together with the dependency and disability levels, gives planners a clear picture of what it would cost to move these marginal groups around between the different compartments of care.

This technique also gives a clear description of the category of people who will or will not be moved if we do or do not spend the money. Decision-makers and planners can then see the costs involved in these different moves together with the disability levels of the people who would be affected by the move. They can then sensibly judge, in terms of moving people, and in terms of the cost involved, whether the balance is about right for the way these services are currently running. Is it necessary to increase one service relative to the other, to make more residential home places relative to those being maintained in their own homes, or to make more hospital places relative to those in residential homes? This enables decision-makers to form judgments about the ratios of marginal benefit to marginal costs.

With this presentation at no time are the issues of met need, unmet need, or setting standards of care discussed. Attention is directed toward resources and implied benefits. Marginal analysis can work with things as they are, given that resources are scarce, as opposed to dealing in the somewhat vague and difficult concept of need. It can help identify the best options in terms of the relative costs.

The concept of marginal analysis, even in circumstances in which monetary values cannot be placed on the benefits, has a use in the sense that it forces decision-makers to think explicitly about the relative weights that they attach to helping this type of person (whose disability is described) as opposed to that type of person (who is also described), having regard for the relevant costs. In other words it encourages explicit consideration of the opportunity costs involved at the margin.

Other Evaluative Approaches

No major studies have examined the effectiveness or the cost-effectiveness of geriatric psychiatry services, but the Aberdeen study illustrates the relevance of more broadly based work with the elderly. There are two other recent important studies that look at the elderly in general.

Challis and Davies have been working in Kent for some years to evaluate support for elderly people in the community by social workers. The social workers coordinate and encourage an informal support system to work in partnership with statutory services in order to keep the elderly person in the community (Challis & Davies, 1980). The social worker manages the case and has to work within a budgeted allowance. Domiciliary and other help can be brought in to maintain the person at home but this has an actual or a "shadow" cost in the budget. This help can be from the Health Services resources, Social Services, or can be voluntary. In their study the budget was two-thirds of the marginal cost of residential care.

Fully detailed results of all this work have not been published, but the indications so far are that the social workers have managed to keep within their budgets and that the mortality of the experimental group has been lowered. The authors intend to conduct a full evaluation of changes in the costs and benefits for matched clients subject to either this experimental approach or to the routine service approach. These early reports are very encouraging, but some observers have commented cynically that perhaps the cost to society of a lower mortality is ultimately greater than the immediate savings.

At the University of York, Wright has extensively examined the problems of "costing care" in the field of the elderly, working with a dependent disabled elderly population (Wright, 1981). The Wright group examined the costs of different settings of care for groups of people in similar dependency categories. They devoted much attention to producing a scale that adequately classified people into useful and meaningful categories of dependency. Their solution was to look at only physical dependency in detail and to apply the Guttman scaling approach. The idea of this is to produce a cumulative, unidimensional scale classifying severity of condition and using only one major judgment; severity or dependency increases as the number of items scored on the scale increases. This approach seems to have been successful, but they were frustrated by having to ignore important factors in their comparisons, such as mental disorder, behavioral characteristics, and prognosis. Nevertheless they examined the major costs in a comprehensive fashion. They looked at capital costs (or housing costs for those living alone), care services costs, general services costs, personal living expenses or personal consumption, and the cost of informal help.

The result is a compilation of extremely useful data about costs in general and the costs of alternative care patterns for patients with similar levels of dependency. The costs of community care were on average less than the costs of residential care, though the differences were often not great in absolute terms. Both were well below the costs of hospital care. A major value of this work is the comprehensive nature of the approach and the frank confrontation of current methodological limitations in this area. The important plea the authors make is for more studies giving information about outcome and quality of care with different levels of dependency, and consideration to be given to the benefits as well as to the costs of alternative patterns of care for the elderly.

The Problem of Effectiveness—The Output of the Service

A basic problem with evaluating the effectiveness of geriatric psychiatry services is deciding what these services are for—what is the "output" we wish to see from the service? In Britain the model is a comprehensive psychiatric service which deals with all elderly people in the community of a defined district. Such a service aims to meet all need for psychiatric assessment, diagnosis, therapy, continuing care, and support. It aims for early ascertainment and strives to aid people to remain in the community, functioning as best possible (Arie & Jolley, 1982). It seeks enthusiastic and fruitful cooperation with the rest of the Health Service, with Social Services, with voluntary agencies and with family and community networks. In Nottingham the model is extended further by actual unification of the medical and the psychiatric services for the elderly into an integrated Department of Health Care of the Elderly. These strategies should yield considerable success in secondary and tertiary prevention, and the service is also alert to possibilities for progress with primary prevention. All this gives a variety of factors on which to judge effectiveness.

Not everyone would agree that this is the business of the ideal psychogeriatric service. Some would emphasize the dichotomy between "cure" and "care" in psychogeriatric services. The ethos of a service for optimum "care" may conflict with the approach needed for greatest effectiveness in "cure."

A useful illustration of the problems in evaluating the "output" of a service is provided by thinking about quality of care for the long-stay psychogeriatric patient and its implications. For such consideration a good frame of reference is Maslow's theory of human motivation which describes five levels of basic needs and goals (Maslow, 1943). We can use these to judge the "effectiveness" (quality of care) of long-stay services. At the first level there are the basic needs for food, rest, shelter, and sex; at the second level the need for protection from threat, danger, and deprivation; at the third level the need for love and social recognition; at the fourth level the need for self-esteem and the esteem of others; and the fifth level the goal of "self-actualization," being oneself, being creative, and inventive.

In theory all these different aspects of "output" could be measured, and great resources expended on achieving "high output" on these ideal objectives for long-stay patients. But such an allocation of resources could be at the expense of the effectiveness of "cure" of the rest of the service. This approach could too easily accept disability and neglect the potential for rehabilitation. In fact, different services, different styles of care, will probably have both advantages and disadvantages. The "best buy" service should result from combining the advantages of different services.

Even with agreement about the aims of an ideal service, there are still great problems defining the relative benefits of different forms of care. Drummond (1980) suggests that we need to be able to (a) specify the main dimensions of benefit, (b) measure the changes along these dimensions induced by particular forms of care, and (c) devise a system of weighting the changes along each dimension to arrive at an overall index of the improvement in health state arising from particular regimens.

Wright (1974) suggests that for evaluating services there is a need for a comprehensive measure of "output" that would include: maintenance of independence; maintenance or improvement of personal health; social integration; physical well-being or nurture; and compensation for disability. While there has been progress with some of these elements, we seem far from such a comprehensive multidimensional measure of benefit and output.

CONCLUDING THOUGHTS

Mooney (1980) described the technique of Programme Budgeting in use in Scotland enabling health authorities to gain an overview of the services they provided and how these matched up against their policy objectives. In his case study the elderly were the major client group in the analysis. The aim was to use readily available utilization statistics (such as bed days or outpatient attendances) to give a general picture of how resources were deployed; how expenditure levels were reached over time; and how plans could be made for future growth or redeployment given the picture of the then current pattern of services. Mooney emphasizes that this is a broad brush approach but gives an example of its practical use in the Scottish Grampian Health Region.

He goes further to suggest that having established with Programme Budgeting the broad strategic outline of a health authority's spending on, for example, the elderly, marginal analysis should be used to examine whether there is the desired balance between the various service components dealing with the elderly. Finally cost-effectiveness analysis or cost–benefit analysis should be used to examine in detail specific service aspects and innovations. They cannot be applied to every service practice as this would be too costly to conduct properly and, of course, would take much time to complete. They should be reserved for crucial questions. In the meantime an effective service of some sort needs to be provided. There is much to recommend this overall approach.

A plea to clinicians and those asking for services would be to formulate plans in terms of the benefits which will flow from a new service set against its cost, rather than emotively assert (often misleadingly) an imperative case of need in order to save lives. Make planners judge whether resources needed to gain these benefits, clearly defined, could really obtain greater benefit elsewhere.

Demographic changes will demand even more major expenditure of health and social service resources on the elderly throughout the Western world. It is certain that increasingly difficult health care choices will have to be faced. The clinician in the psychiatry of old age needs to be a persuasive and effective advocate to press for the right choices to be made. An understanding of evaluative approaches and an awareness of economic concepts of appraisal will add great power to efforts to attain decent and appropriate services for the elderly.

REFERENCES

Arie, T., & Jolley, D. (1982). Making services work: organization and style of psychogeriatric services. In R. Levy & F. Post (Eds.), *The psychiatry of late life.* Oxford: Blackwell Scientific Publications.

Challis, D., & Davies, B. (1980). A new approach to community care for the elderly. *Br. J. Soc. Wk., 10* (No. 1), 1–18.

Drummond, M. F. (1980). *Principles of economic appraisal in health care.* Oxford: Oxford University Press.

Fordyce, J. D., Mooney, G. H., & Russell, E. M. (1981). Economic analysis in health care. *Health Bull., 39,* 29–38.

Grad, J., & Sainsbury, P. (1968). The effects that patients have on their families in a community care and a central psychiatric service—a two year follow-up. *Br. J. Psychiatry, 114,* 265–278.

Hoenig, J. (1968). The desegregation of the psychiatric patient. *Proc. Roy. Soc. Med., 61,* 115–120.

Jones, R. G., Goldberg, D., & Hughes, B. (1980). A comparison of two different services treating schizophrenia: A cost-benefit approach. *Psychol. Med., 10,* 493–505.

MacFarlane, J. P. R., et al. (1979). Day hospitals in modern clinical practise-cost benefit. *Age Ageing, 8 (Suppl.),* 80–86.

Maslow, A. H. (1943). A theory of human motivation. *Psychol. Rev., 50,* 370–396.

Mathew, G. K. (1971). Measuring need and evaluating services. In G. McLachlan (Ed.), *Portfolio for health.* Oxford: Oxford University Press.

Mooney, G. H., Russell, E. M., & Weir, R. D. (1980). *Choices for health care.* London and Basingstoke: Macmillan.

Newell, D. J. (1977). Commentary on environmental factors in dependency. In A. N. Exton-Smith & J. Grimley Evans (Eds.), *Care of the elderly.* London: Academic Press. New York: Grune & Stratton.

Opit, L. J. (1978). Domiciliary care for the elderly sick: Economy or neglect? In V. Carver, & P. Liddiard (Eds.), *An ageing population.* Hodder & Stoughton in association with The Open University Press.

Ross, D. N. (1976). *Age Ageing, 5,* 171.

Schultz, P., & McGlone, T. (1977). Primary health care provided to the elderly by a nurse practitioner. *J. Am. Geriat. Soc., 25,* 443–446.

Wager, R. (1972). *Care of the elderly—An exercise in cost benefit analysis.* Pamphlet by The Institute of Municipal Treasurers and Accountants, London.

Wing, J. K. (1981). Monitoring in the field of psychiatry. In E. M. Goldberg & N. Connelly (Eds.), *Evaluative research in social care.* Policy Studies Institute, Heinermann Education Books.

Wing, J. K., Cooper, J. E., & Sartorius, N. (1974). *The measurement and classification of psychiatric symptoms.* Cambridge: Cambridge University Press.

Wing, J. K., & Häfner, H. (Eds). (1973). *Roots of evaluation: The epidemiological basis for planning psychiatric services*. London: Oxford University Press.
Wing, J. K., & Hailey, A. M. (Eds). (1972). *Evaluating a community psychiatric service: The Camberwell Register 1964–71*. London: Oxford University Press.
Wright, K. G. (1974). Alternative measures of output of social programmes: The elderly. In A. J. Culyer (Ed.), *Economic policies and social goals*. London: Martin Robertson.
Wright, K. G., Cairns, J. A., & Snell, M. C. (1981). *Costing care*. The Joint Unit for Social Services Research at Sheffield University in collaboration with Community Care.

PART VI
Research

23
Innovations in Psychogeriatrics: Interdisciplinary Research*

Ewald W. Busse

The interdisciplinary approach in research and patient care is promoted by some and questioned by others. At a conference in the spring of 1984, the participants in a discussion on models of the teaching nursing home expressed considerable disappointment in their success in developing interdisciplinary approaches both to research and care of the patient (NIA, 1984). Luszki (1958b) expressed certain restrictions regarding the use of the interdisciplinary approach. She said, "Interdisciplinary research is something to be undertaken only when the nature of the research problem demands it." Luszki cites three reasons for developing an interdisciplinary research effort: "(1) When it is necessary to borrow concepts from other fields, particularly when a discipline has pursued a study to the point of diminishing returns, (2) to address a problem that may lie on the border between disciplines, or (3) the problem may require study in a wider context than can be provided by one discipline." It is my belief that all three of these reasons can apply to aging research. Kanowski (1978) stated, "Geriatric research demands a wholistic approach to human existence in a manifold sense. . . . Further, it is by no means clear how the complex problems of the multidisciplinary research should be solved nor that this can be done easily. But from this arises a very stimulating challenge."

*The administrative principles and the rationale described in this chapter are found in the publications, the grant applications, and the required periodic reports to the National Institutes of Health. In addition, much of the research data collected under Duke Longitudinal I and II have been placed in the public domain.

In spite of the discouraging views that have been expressed, the justification for undertaking the interdisciplinary approach is valid. The 1983 Report on Aging Research by the National Advisory Council on Aging of the United States Department of Health and Human Services not only supported interdisciplinary undertakings, but added the following statement: "Research on aging requires more scholars who can bridge the gaps between the biomedical sciences and psychology, sociology, economics, history, and anthropology, and who can apply sophisticated research methods in a multidisciplinary framework appropriate to life perspectives" (p. 8). The recently established Sandoz Prize in Gerontology supports this concept as it includes in its criteria a special emphasis on "multidisciplinary research programs."

This chapter is not a systematic review of multidisciplinary or interdisciplinary research efforts that have succeeded or failed, since pertinent articles or comments are infrequent in the scientific literature. Rather, it will review empirical operating principles that are the result of participation in and close association with interdisciplinary studies for more than 30 years (Busse, 1965).* The majority of the policies and guidelines that will be presented evolved rapidly during the first few years of this experience and were reported twenty years ago. They have continued, with minor modifications, for many years and their usefulness has been demonstrated (Maddox, Busse, & Bentov, 1982).

Luszki and others believe that a major problem of interdisciplinary research is "communication." But of course other major determinants are values, attitudes, etc. These influences will be discussed.

DEFINITION OF TERMS

During the formation of an effective interdisciplinary team, the definition of terms that will be repeatedly used by the team should be agreed upon and written down for further reference and perhaps reconsideration. The following definitions are not universally accepted, and some variations will be mentioned. However, the definitions have endured, probably because they are relatively simple and do not deal with all the conceivable complications.

Group Research. This term describes an assemblage of two or more persons of the same or different disciplines who have some areas of similar interests in their research approaches. It is assumed that they are working in

---

*Permission was granted by *The Journal of Medical Education* to include portions of the original paper in this chapter.

a close proximity to one another which permits some degree of scientific communication. However, there are no formal and specified working relationships. Often large groups of researchers are brought together with the hope that there will be cross-fertilization of ideas from one worker to another and that enthusiasms will cause teams to form spontaneously within the larger group because of such communication and proximity.

Team Research. The participants may be of the same or different disciplines, and it is assumed that they are in close proximity, but the working relationship is explicit yet informal. (A team will be most effective if participants are working in the same facility and have informal contacts several times a week.) These people are working together to achieve a goal by following a predetermined plan. Each member of the research team has an assigned task of data collection and integration and analysis. The team is highly dependent upon all members to center their major efforts around the team goals and to keep their individual work timed according to the team's overall plans. In addition to being responsible for his assigned task, each member of a team must communicate the cross-correlate data. The team is highly dependent upon these fundamentals if it is to achieve the prescribed goal.

Multidisciplinary (Group) Research. Multidisciplinary research is a type of group research involving several distinct scientific disciplines. The investigators are identified as a group because they are working in proximity and have interests in a common research topic. It is hoped and assumed that there is a maximum of communication between the investigators and, therefore, that the potential of their work is increased.

A Research Group. A research group may include in its composition one or more disciplinary or interdisciplinary research teams.

Interdisciplinary (Team) Research. Interdisciplinary research is a team effort. The team is composed of two or more individuals representing distinct scientific disciplines who, because of their particular skills and interest, will accept certain responsibilities and will cooperate and collaborate with other members of the team to achieve their goal. The meaning of the prefix "inter" is "mutual" rather than just "among" or "between."

Individual Research and Coinvestigation. In individual research a single scientist, by his own efforts or by directing the efforts of others, is solely responsible for the research. Coinvestigation implies that the research activity is being conducted by equally responsible partners. Their job responsibilities may not be identical, but they are balanced with each investigator having clear responsibility for certain tasks.

Other Definitions

Piaget (1970) believed that interdisciplinary collaboration had three levels of interaction. The "multidisciplinary" level was the first and lowest level of Piaget's interactions. This level occurs when the solution to a problem makes it necessary to obtain information from two or more scientists without change or enrichment to any of them. The disciplines are merely juxtaposed. This level is frequently seen when research teams are first formed. Its members exchange information, but have no real interactions. Piaget's second level is that of true interdisciplinary collaboration. At this level, cooperation among various disciplines results in reciprocal exchanges with integration and enrichment which permits problem solving beyond that usually found within the boundaries of disciplinary or professional areas of knowledge and competence. The third level of Piaget's model is transdisciplinary. This level is an ideal and rarely, if ever, develops. Piaget describes this level as one in which each person possesses various knowledge and does not represent any discipline. Knowledge is truly synthesized.

The term "group," when used in conjunction with therapy, takes on considerably more structure than was utilized in the "Duke" definition of group research. Consequently, "group therapy" resembles team research. Most members of a successful research team are aware of many of the principles of group dynamics. Members of a team understand the positive and negative features of the pressure to conform and appreciate the support that a group can provide including the realization that identifying with a team of successful scientists adds to their own self-esteem. To discuss these similarities and differences would require considerable time and effort, as there are numerous techniques included in the rubric of group psychotherapy (Rosenbaum, 1976). It is my opinion that a successful therapeutic group must gradually take on many of the features of a successful research team.

DEVELOPMENT OF AN INTERDISCIPLINARY TEAM

Considerable time and effort is required to develop an effective interdisciplinary team.

Selection of Participants

Unfortunately there is a limited number of scientists and scholars who have had a satisfactory experience in participating in interdisciplinary research. Not all professional persons are suited for work in an interdisciplinary setting. Many scientists are resistant to any attempt to involve them in a genuine interdisciplinary effort. Such resistance may stem from a number of factors, but when it is strong, any coercive pressures may result in a serious disruption of the team effort. However, bias and prejudice exist in almost all people and some resistance can be expected in any member of a team. Fortunately, there is an increasing number of young scientists who appreciate the limitations of their own discipline and welcome the added knowledge and skill that can be derived from working with other investigators.

There are parallels between development and maintenance of an effective interdisciplinary research team, and the composition and success of an athletic team. Members of an athletic team are selected because of demonstrated individual skills, but the success of the team requires that each member of the team contribute to and maximize the skills of others (Shivers, 1980). The ultimate success of a team is related to keeping the goals in focus and maintaining balance, motivation, and morale among its members. In addition, a team must establish procedures and have adequate substitutes for absent members.

When discussing with an individual possible participation in an interdisciplinary effort, special attention should be given the candidate's attitude toward his or her own profession and the satisfactions he or she receives from the work. The candidate must be content with his or her learning experience and professional choice. A candidate who has serious doubts about his or her professional choice does not possess sufficient security and identity to function within an interdisciplinary group. The insecure professional is extremely vulnerable to the criticism of other disciplines (Kubie, 1953). A good member of a team should be able to succinctly express views and opinions and to explain the process of problem solving.

Disciplinary Influence and Interactions

In addition to personality differences among members of a discipline there are behavioral and attitudinal characteristics associated with a professional discipline. Such characteristics result from basic differences in interests and skills which originally determined vocational choices. Additionally, there are processes of professionalization within each discipline. The process of professionalization includes the rules of entry, the inculcation of attitudes, values, and loyalty, and the acquisition of patterns and standards of behavior. Furthermore, within established disciplines, members learn both specific research techniques and approaches, as well as patterns of inquiry and problem solving. These differences, some of which have a positive influence and some a negative influence on the interdisciplinary approach to research, are significantly influenced by the overall graduate program which produces the various doctor of philosophy and doctor of medicine specialists, and by the particular periods of time during which these studies are pursued.

At the outset of the development of a research team, there is an assumed status hierarchy (Luszki, 1958a). This hierarchy, as perceived by the various members of the team, is not a consistent one but is related to the current status system that exists within the academic structure and within society as a whole. As a team works together, the hierarchy undergoes considerable change. The skillful, creative, and industrious investigator assumes a higher place in the group. A special hierarchy is developed within the team, and shifts occur that are related to many factors. This is not appreciated or understood by a guest attending a team meeting. In fact, a visitor can be upset to find his discipline is not the highest in the "pecking order." The leadership in an interdisciplinary effort must make certain that team meetings are not utilized as a dueling ground or as a forum for debating the conflicts and power struggles between scientific disciplines. The work of an interdisciplinary team should be sufficiently challenging and exciting so that attention of the team is focused solely upon the interdisciplinary project and related material. It is the author's observation, however, that the respect and understanding that develop between disciplines within such a team often promote goodwill and reduce rivalries. This experience of developing tolerance for divergent techniques and appreciation of the training and capacities of others is one of the major positive side effects that result from projects that are well conceived and well carried out.

Team and Individual Research

It is prudent for an individual to establish a balance between the research team commitment and independent investigation. An investigator whose research activity is limited to participation in an interdisciplinary team is likely to encounter certain difficulties that reduce his effectiveness as a team member. An administrator or a member of a service profession may take the position that he is heavily burdened with other work responsibility, and, therefore, he can do only team research because he must carefully allocate his research time. This decision may also be influenced by other motivations such as a safer or easier way to conduct research since the physician will receive the help of members with more knowledge of investigational procedures. Such a decision to participate in team activity and not to pursue individual but related research may appear to be based upon good reasons. Unfortunately, such team members are more vulnerable to loss of self-esteem than those who have both team and individual research interests. If the contribution of such an investigator to the team is criticized or doubted, this source of maintaining self-esteem is disrupted. He may feel uncomfortable, yet he is too dependent on the team for research prestige and publications to deal effectively with the situation. Some of these persons will terminate their relationship with the team, and others will attempt to hold on. Either pathway is marred by unpleasant reactions which sooner or later cause difficulty for the individual and the team. The leader of an interdisciplinary team must be alert to this type of complication, for prevention is better than attempts to correct the problem.

PROCEDURES

Hypotheses, Questions, and Research Methods

The formulation of hypotheses and questions to be answered are the prerequisites of well planned research. The development of both hypotheses and questions by an interdisciplinary team often requires a prolonged period of discussion but is an excellent learning experience. Sound interdisciplinary research projects will be developed by groups who are willing to make the necessary sacrifices and who have resources for covering the planning period.

New Members and Dissatisfaction

It should also be anticipated that new members of an interdisciplinary team who are not present at the origin of the project usually are to varying degrees dissatisfied with the original aims and design of the project. New members include both those who are hired when the project is first funded but who did not participate in the original formulation, and those investigators brought in as replacements. The degree of dissatisfaction affects the usefulness of the new member to the team. When it is minimal, even though it cannot be completely resolved, dissatisfaction can be converted to a strength by the promotion of satellite projects that have a rational relationship to the main project.

Changes and New Observations

It is important that the original team unanimously consent to and agree to support the aims of the project as well as the research methodology. If a responsible member of the team wishes to change his methods of observation or procedures, he should be asked to present his views to the team and have the team agree to the change. An unauthorized change by one person can invalidate the observations of other members of the team and hence render a segment of the work useless.

Once a research procedure has been adopted, it undoubtedly will be under periodic review, and investigators will want to introduce new observations and alter procedures. In an interdisciplinary team this must be accomplished by an established process. The investigator should present with an adequate explanation the work that he wishes to do. The team discussion frequently sharpens the proposal. This is an important ingredient in a scientific process and should not be minimized as it is one of the great strengths in interdisciplinary research.

Core and Special Data

One of the values of an interdisciplinary research effort is that time and effort are saved by having necessary central or "core" data that include control ("core") measures and identifying characteristics used by all members of the team. Such data must be carefully planned and collected and, without reservation, be available to each member of the team. There are times when the individual investigator believes he needs control (core) or identifying data not clearly useful to the entire group. When this occurs, the investigator must have the responsibility for programming it and properly fitting it into the entire procedure. It also must meet the criteria for acceptance which have been spelled out. Special data are those observations and procedures that are a fundamental part of the experimental design of the core project, and the result of ideas generated or accepted by the assigned investigator, which reflect the area of his or her professional competency. In a previous section the desirability of combining team research with individual research was pointed out. However, within the design of the team, the investigator who confines his interest to the data resulting from his narrow field of professional interest will find that he is unlikely to remain a contented and effective member of the team.

Satellite Projects

Satellite projects are not the direct concern of the team but are very important for the continuing success and effectiveness of the individual investigator. Satellite projects, if encouraged, will easily develop from the team project. Research ideas are generated that cannot be carried out within the team framework. However, these relatively independent satellite projects often have tremendous feedback into the team project and provide a source of new stimuli.

Satellite projects, when combined with interdisciplinary longitudinal study, produce certain problems. For example, if an individual investigator wants to utilize the longitudinal subjects because of the advantage afforded by control or baseline data that have already been established, he cannot be permitted to do so without the advice and consent of the interdisciplinary team. Unrestricted access to the subjects and the collected data without proper review could lose the subjects, invalidate the research, and destroy the morale of the team. A satellite project that is painful physically or psychologically could result in the loss of volunteer subjects.

Utilization Data for Publication

The large number of observations collected by an interdisciplinary team require complex methods of cross-correlation and statistical analyses (Maddox, Busse, & Bentov, 1982). The disputes over jurisdictional control and rights of publication can produce dissension in an interdisciplinary team; therefore, the possibility of such difficulties should be anticipated and reduced by establishment of ground rules. "Core" data must be available to every member of the team. "Special" data is the assigned responsibility of an individual investigator, so when the observations, analyses, or conclusions are utilized by another investigator for publication, the person whose work is incorporated should participate as a coauthor or a reviewer and a footnote should mention the contribution to the article. Although at times there are reasons for deviating from the rule, in general the individual who assumes major responsibility for writing the article should be the first author. With continuing proper communication there should be few problems that cannot be amiably resolved.

Meetings and Minutes

Regularly scheduled meetings are necessary to any team effort to establish and maintain communication, coordination, and cooperation. The frequency and the length of the meetings must be planned. Once a month is not sufficient. The meeting should be an exciting opportunity for learning, for maintaining interest and motivation, and for generating new research ideas and opportunities for interdisciplinary work. Agendas for the meeting should be prepared and should include time for clarification of administrative procedures, budgetary explanation and reviews, review of research progress, clarification of research techniques, reports from the current literature, and an opportunity to present preliminary drafts of scientific papers resulting from the interdisciplinary research.

The administrative portion of the meeting usually follows the scientific period. All decisions that relate to the functioning of the team must be carefully recorded and the reasons for arriving at that decision clearly elucidated. Perhaps the reason for this can best be understood by the use of an example. After the team has discussed alternative laboratory procedures and has selected one to be included in the central observations, the reason why procedure "A" was selected rather than procedure "B" should be recorded. Months later, the question might arise, "How did it happen that we selected procedure 'A' when procedure 'B' seems to be just as good or better?" If a debate develops, it is often evident that group recall is incomplete and distorted, and the only reliable resource is the accurate minutes of the meeting when the original decision was made.

Personnel Losses and New Personnel

A successful interdisciplinary research team will probably function for two or more years. Members of the team may be offered attractive positions because of the experience and reputation that they have developed while part of a successful team. Consequently, there are rights and privileges of a departing team member which must be understood. He or she cannot take the data with him, and he cannot insist that because he was responsible for the collection of this data that he will remain a member of the team even though he is remotely located for the duration of the project. Obviously, he must be replaced, and an individual who replaces him must feel he is not a second-rate citizen. Although there are no absolute rules, a member who leaves the team should complete data analyses but not necessarily the writing of papers prior to departure. When he publishes the papers, he must adhere to all of the previously established rules and courtesies developed by the interdisciplinary team.

If the replacement of a resigned member causes a distortion in the data collection, the value of that particular effort can be destroyed. For this reason the new member should fully understand the methods, the observations, and the recording techniques. It is also essential that the new member appreciate why certain approaches were adopted so that he or she can work comfortably within that structure.

LONG-TERM RESEARCH

In another part of this chapter reference was made to the advisability of individual investigators participating in individual as well as interdisciplinary research. A long-term study increases the period of data collection and is apt to slow down publications. In addition, papers are likely to be reviewed at the team meetings before they are presented at conferences or submitted for publication; therefore, they may require greater time and effort. Investigators, particularly young ones who are in the process of establishing their scientific reputations, cannot afford to wait a long period of time before publishing. Perhaps the "publish or perish" rule is unfortunate, but it is a reality and it must be given proper consideration. Therefore, it is wise for the individual members of the team to participate in satellite or peripheral projects. The investigator is wise to plan such short-term studies so that they can be brought to a point where they are publishable and are not dependent on the results of a long-term project.

COMMENTS

The policies, guidelines, and operating principles that are represented in this chapter are not intended to be an exhaustive review of the merits, limitations, application, and administration of interdisciplinary research. There are other important considerations such as the setting (Rioch, 1958), and the problems of cross-discipline communication are not covered in detail. It is possible that interdisciplinary research will flourish in one facility or community but die in another. The factors presented here should be given consideration. Of major concern is the problem of communication, as good communication is a source of stimulation and learning for all (Luszki, 1958a). It is believed that particular types of team structure are needed to accommodate the specific demands and working environment of the research team. No attempt has been made in this chapter to treat this subject.

The interdisciplinary research approach, particularly in the study of problems of aging and the aged, is likely to be involved with rather large numbers of subjects or patients and with methods and possible conclusions of a social, economic, and political nature that can produce adverse reactions and criticisms (Woolman, 1964). Again, no effort is made in this chapter to offer any helpful suggestions or specific solutions to this vexing complication.

NEW SCIENTIFIC DISCIPLINES

Marcel Boist (quoted by Pennington, 1981) says that true interdisciplinary collaboration can have two results—either a new discipline is born, for example gerontology, or established disciplines expand toward each other and overlap (geriatric psychiatry). Both results exist and contribute to the advancement of science and education.

It is my belief that established disciplines can merge or fragment as the result of many factors including the overlap of expanding knowledge and the mutual use of research techniques. Fragmentation or splitting takes place when one component of an established discipline insists on departing from the traditional professional roles and values. I believe that neuroscience is taking on many aspects of an emerging new scientific discipline.

SUMMARY

This chapter attempts to review practices and policies that should be considered in the development of an interdisciplinary team and that are usually required for its successful functioning. Interdisciplinary research can be distinguished from multidisciplinary research. The selection of capable participants for interdisciplinary work is limited, as all competent scientists and scholars are not able to work effectively as members of a team. In order to maintain the morale and efficiency of an interdisciplinary team, it is necessary to provide a research climate that is exciting and rewarding. Such a favorable research climate must be planned and maintained. These factors and conditions are of utmost importance to the research administrator.

Participation in interdisciplinary research is a unique learning experience. Participants expand scientific knowledge, acquire new skills, and gain an understanding of behavior, motivation, and values of themselves and of colleagues.

REFERENCES

Busse, E. W. (1965). Administration of the interdisciplinary research team. *The Journal of Medical Education, 40*(9, Pt 1), 832–839.

Kanowski, S. (1978). The academic tasks in gerontopsychiatry. In A. D. Isaacs & F. Post (Eds.), *Studies in geriatric psychiatry.* New York: Wiley.

Kubie, L. S. (1952). The problems of maturity in psychiatric research. *Journal of Medical Education, 28,* 11–27.

Luszki, M. B. (1958a). *Interdisciplinary team research methods and problems.* New York: NYU Press.

Luszki, M. B. (1958b). The challenge of the interdisciplinary team approach in research. *Proceedings of Seminars, 1957–1969,* Duke University Council on Aging.

Maddox, G., Busse, E., & Bentov, M. (1982). The Duke Multidisciplinary Longitudinal Studies of Normal Aging. *Center Reports on Advances in Research, 6*(1).

Maddox, G., Busse, E., & Bentov, M. (1982). Data management and strategies of analyses. *Center Reports on Advances in Research, 6*(1), 4–5.

National Institute on Aging. (1983). Report of the National Advisory Council on Aging: For a national plan of research on aging. Washington D.C.: Department of Health and Human Services.

National Institute on Aging and The Beverly Foundation. (1984). Conference on: The teaching nursing home: A new approach to geriatric research, education and clinical care, March 25–27, 1984, Washington D.C., E. Schneider (Ed.), *The teaching nursing home.* New York: Raven Press, 1985.

Pennington, E. A. (1981). *Interdisciplinary education in nursing* (pp. 2–5). New York: National League for Nursing, Pub. No. 15–1877.

Piaget, Jean. (1970). The epistemology of interdisciplinary relations in interdisciplinarity. In Leo Apostel (Ed.), *Problems of teaching and research in universities* (pp. 127–139). French Organization for Economic Cooperation and Development.

Rioch, D. K. (1958). Multidisciplinary methods of psychiatric research. *Journal of Orthopsychiatry, 28,* 467–482.

Rosenbaum, M. (1976). Group psychotherapeutics. In B. B. Wolman (Ed.), *The Therapists' Handbook,* (pp. 163–181). New York: Van Nostrand Reinhold.

Shivers, J. S. (1980). *Recreational leadership: Group dynamics and interpersonal behavior.* Princeton: Princeton Book Company.

Woolman, M. (1964). Beureaucratic structure and research restriction. Presented at the meeting of the American Orthopsychiatric Association, Chicago, Illinois, March 1964. Washington DC: Institute of Education Research, Inc., special publication.

24
Current Developments in Psychogeriatrics in the United States

Sanford I. Finkel

In preparation for the United Nations World Assembly on Aging, held in Vienna in 1982, the United Nations Division for Economic and Social Information released the following statement:

> Aging has long been of concern to the developed countries. In the developing countries, that concern is only just beginning to emerge, however. Declines in both the birth and death rates due to improved medical care has meant that a portion of old people in the population of these countries is rising. By the year 2000, it is estimated that half of the total of the aged population in the world will reside in Asia and the Pacific, with the developing countries of the region having the greatest proportion. (UNDESI, 1982c)

Similarly, in Latin America "economic growth and social progress has influenced fertility, mortality, and some types of migration, and has resulted in a continuing increase in the numbers and proportional percentages of older people. By 2025 the over-60 population will rise 3 to 5 times, from approximately 21 million now to 73 million or more. During the same period the economically active population aged 15 to 59 and the child population will grow much more slowly" (UNDESI, 1982b).

As for Africa, according to United Nations demographers, "the segment of the population 60 years and older will increase by a factor of 5 between 1975 and 2025, shifting from 20 million to 102 million persons. In the next 20 years alone, a 40% increase in the population 60 years and older is expected in West Africa, approximately 38% in North Africa, 36% in East Africa, and 33% in Central and Southern Africa" (UNDESI, 1982a).

With this clear evidence of an aging pattern worldwide, we must all be aware of information and policies that affect the elderly within our national borders. We must be quick to share this information with our colleagues, to discuss it, and to arrive at a clear understanding of the problems and opportunities that present themselves to us.

It is with this thought in mind that I share the following recent developments in the United States. Of course, this is a partial list but it will serve as an indication of the richness of recent developments within America and their potential application for other countries.

COMPUTERS, ELECTRONICS, AND COMMUNICATIONS TECHNOLOGY

The revolution in computers, communications technology, and electronics is beginning to have an impact on the mental health and psychiatric illnesses of elder people. With the acceleration of technological advances, we can anticipate dramatic opportunities in the near future. These would include the following examples:

1. The availability of a small computer that will provide the older person with information on when and how to take his/her medication (Finkel, 1980). For example, a computer carried in a purse or pocket can give off a signal and even a printout advising the person that it is time to take specific medications. This signal could then continue to provide such information throughout a 24-hour period. This could well increase patient compliance, decrease the possibility of accidental overdosage because the patient "forgot" that he/she had already taken the medication, and reduce the person's anxiety about remembering when to take medications. In fact, Advanced Professional Training services has developed a small medication device holding a two-week supply of medication that is dispensed automatically according to a preset schedule. Incorporating solid state electronics and microprocessor circuitry, the lock device ($3 \times 5 \times 1.5$) uses a buzzer and a multiple-timing mechanism. By muting the sound, the patient releases and can remove one prescribed item; the action of removing the item resets the device, automatically relocking it until the next prescribed time and buzzer sound.

2. The development of communication between patient's residences and emergency rooms provides a mental health function for many elderly, diminishing the anxiety that accompanies being alone and incurring a medical emergency. It is conceivable that in the near future, urban areas will have a specialized program for geropsychiatric emergencies, located in an emergency room setting. Such arrangement, using specially trained staff,

could conceivably reduce the need for psychiatric hospitalizations or even long-term care placement for elderly with high risk psychiatric problems.

3. We now have the technology for people to communicate with each other via television. Columbus, Ohio, has had a variety show that allows two-way conversations with viewers. For some lonely elderly, such as those who are homebound, such technology could provide important interpersonal contact. Although not as effective as human presence, such communication could provide stimulation and decrease the sense of isolation. It is possible that we could develop computer centers to match people with similar interests and ethnic backgrounds, perhaps even in different parts of the country. It is also conceivable that some psychiatric visits could be conducted via television. In northern winters, when mobility may be extremely limited, the opportunity for doctor and patient to "see" each other would have special value.

4. For those who have difficulty seeing, many new computers have the size of letters increased, thus facilitating reading.

5. Many elderly need services, yet coordinating an available service to the person in need is often difficult. The "bureaucratic maze" (Lieff, 1984) creates many difficulties. Appropriate computerization would facilitate helpful referrals.

6. Software could be developed to provide medically and socially relevant subjects to older people.

7. Technology can be made available to provide physiological monitoring of blood pressure and pulse at home via television or telephone.

The elderly are the logical group on whom to focus for the following reasons:

1. The cost of medical services is skyrocketing.
2. Most American elderly have televisions and telephones. Much of our current technology can be adapted to and coordinated with telephones and television. It should also be noted that people with telephones have lower mortality rates.
3. The cost of technology—home computers, TV's, and telephones—has come down to the extent that often these devices are less expensive than an emergency room visit. They could be utilized to decrease expensive emergency room visits and institutionalization and increase efficient use of agency and hospital time.
4. Psychogeriatrics is an area of medicine where there is a true shortage of physicians and thus early evaluation and monitoring, appropriate referral, and ancillary help for the physician is vital.
5. Psychogeriatrics is a complex area of medicine, needing a large knowledge base. For example, an inpatient may utilize 5 to 10 medications,

which can lead to potentially detrimental drug interactions. Proper computerization would allow information to be automatically available for every prescription.

It should also be emphasized that great advances have been made in communication devices for visually and auditorily handicapped individuals, which would also allow many homebound elderly to use these systems in the face of diminished vision or hearing. Computerized cognitive assessment has been used to evaluate the acute effects of amitriptyline and memory in the elderly (Branconnier, 1981).

Advances in the United States will certainly be available and exported to other countries. Of course, several other countries are working on similar technology and the mutual sharing of ideas should be universally beneficial.

DEVELOPMENT OF NEW ORGANIZATIONS

The Alzheimer's Disease and Related Disorders Association

The ADRDA has become a major force in the furthering of understanding of dementia. Remarkably, this organization is only seven years old. A local group in Seattle, Washington calls itself project ASIST (Alzheimer's Support, Information, Service Team). Since its inception in 1978, chapters have been established throughout the country and number in the hundreds.

ADRDA's goals are:

1. To support research into diagnosis, therapies, causes, and cures for Alzheimer's disease.
2. To aid in organizing family support groups in their own localities so as to give assistance, encouragement, and education to afflicted families.
3. To sponsor educational forums.
4. To dispense information to both lay and professional people regarding Alzheimer's disease.
5. To advise government agencies (federal and state) of the needs of afflicted families as well as the need for extensive research on a nationwide scale.
6. Most importantly, to offer assistance in any manner whatsoever when needed by those afflicted and their loved ones.

Attempts are also made to educate the public and to establish legal and psychiatric referral networks for afflicted families.

By eliciting the support of family members who have beloved spouses and parents with this condition, the organization and its cause have established an enormous base of support. In 1982 approximately $4 million was spent on research for dementia. The total increased to $50 million by 1985. In 1984, five centers were established to intensively study this condition. Five more were added in 1986.

A former U.S. Secretary of Health and Human Services, Margaret Heckler, defined this problem as her highest priority and was at the forefront in facilitating the funding and expanding of services to this afflicted group. The organization has had major input into several publications, including *The 36 Hour Day* (Mace & Rabins, 1981).

The remarkable breakthroughs which have been initiated or catalyzed by this group can be an inspiration to individuals all over the world who wish for greater attention from the public and government for this illness.

Foundation for Grandparenting

A second group which has had a growing impact on the American scene is the Foundation for Grandparenting. This group has emphasized the relationship between grandparent and grandchild as a meaningful, healthy, and positive relationship. Grandparents are family historians, story tellers, sources of wisdom, and loving "best friends and companions."

Because divorce creates separation and pain for grandparents and grandchildren, the foundation has facilitated the initiation of legislation to establish the legal rights of grandparents to maintain contact with their grandchildren.

Arthur Kornhaber and Kenneth Woodward in their book, *Grandparents and Grandchildren: The Vital Connection* (1981), have studied this interrelationship and find that only five percent of children in the United States enjoy close and regular contact with at least one grandparent. When a child is born, the relationship with grandparents is usually not discussed. With sharp increases in broken families and working mothers, grandparents are needed more than ever. The authors warn that "much of the caretaking responsibilities formerly exercised by grandparents as well as by parents have now been turned over to impersonal outsiders: daycare centers, schools, peers, and the omnipresent television set. Ours is becoming a society of surrogates; surrogate families, surrogate parents, and surrogate grandparents." The studies in this book demonstrate how emotional attachments between grandparents and grandchildren are unique: "Grandparents and grandchildren are naturally at ease with each other while both have intense emotional relationships with the middle generation. In short, grandparents and grandchildren do not have to do anything to make each other happy! Their happiness comes from being together."

This problem may exist in the United States to a greater degree than in other countries. In many developing countries perhaps this problem exists only to a minor degree. However, effects of urbanization, dissolution of marriage, and fiscal pressures may intensify this problem even in developing countries. Awareness of this problem and the determination to maintain grandparents as a resource for grandchildren and vice-versa benefits all countries.

American Association for Geriatric Psychiatry

The AAGP, organization with approximately 800 dues-paying psychiatrists, represents but 16% of the over 5,000 psychiatrists who identify themselves as having a significant interest in aging. AAGP publishes a newsletter six times a year and provides information about research, meetings, new books, educational aids, government policy, psychogeriatrics in recent literature, and pharmaceutical developments. This permits a broad sharing of information and the development of many collegial relationships. Not uncommonly, researchers in different parts of the country contact each other to collaborate and develop a better understanding of the work of others.

Further, AAGP puts out a membership directory of all its member psychiatrists, including their location, special areas of interest, and phone numbers. It therefore serves as a wide referral source which facilitates the successful finding of the appropriate specialist in psychogeriatrics.

The International Psychogeriatric Association (IPA) is partly patterned on this foundation and has adopted parts of its format to enhance sharing of information. Of course, IPA has also begun to have annual didactic meetings which permit professionals from all parts of the world to participate and learn together.

RATING SCALES

The authors have used the Global Deterioration Scale (Reisberg et al., 1982) scale successfully for the past seven years and have validated it against behavioral and neurophysiological measures in patients with primary degenerative dementia. The authors describe seven stages:

1. *No cognitive decline.* Here patients have no complaints of memory deficit and the clinical interview elicits no evidence of such.
2. *Very mild cognitive decline.* This is the phase of forgetfulness. Patients complain of memory deficit, usually of forgetting where familiar objects have been placed or names that they formerly knew well. No objective evidence of memory deficit is obtained in the clinical interview or in employment or social situations.

3. *Mild cognitive decline.* This is the earliest stage of definite clinical deficit. However, often intensive interviews are necessary to obtain evidence of such. Read material may be poorly retained and names are quickly forgotten. Decreased performance in employment and social situations become manifest and difficulties in word finding become evident to intimates. Patients may get seriously lost in an unfamiliar situation. Mild to moderate anxiety with denial accompanies this stage.

4. *Moderate cognitive decline.* This is the late confusional phase and clear-cut deficit is apparent in the clinical interview. Concentration deficit is evident as is decreased knowledge of recent events in their own lives or current events in the world. Details of personal history may be forgotten, and ability to travel alone is curtailed. Though certain complex tasks can no longer be performed, patients usually remain oriented to time, place, and person, and may still navigate well in familiar locations. Denial becomes a dominant defense mechanism because acknowledgement of the intellectual loss is often too overwhelming for conscious acceptance and recognition. Flattening of affect and withdrawal may also be noted during this period.

5. *Moderately severe cognitive decline.* This is the phase of early dementia. In this stage patients need assistance in order to survive, and may have difficulty recalling their address and phone number, names of close family members or of schools from which they graduated. Disorientation to time and place may occur and even a well educated person may find it difficult to count backward from 20 by 2's. Nevertheless, patients may retain knowledge of major facts about themselves. They know their own names and generally the names of spouse and children. They handle their toileting and eating satisfactorily but may need help choosing clothes or getting dressed.

6. *The stage of severe cognitive decline.* This is the middle phase of dementia. Here patients may even forget the name of their spouse, on whom they may depend entirely for survival. They are unaware of all recent events and experiences in their life. They have sketchy knowledge of their past life but are generally unaware of their surroundings. They have difficulty counting backwards from 10.

These people require a great deal of assistance with activities of daily living. They may become incontinent. Though they still may be able to travel to familiar locations, increasingly they need assistance.

At this stage one may find delusional behavior, obsessive symptoms, anxiety, and agitation.

7. *Very severe cognitive decline.* Here all verbal abilities are lost. There is no speech at all, only grunting. Patients are incontinent and require assistance in eating and toileting. They lose psychomotor skills, including the ability to walk. Generalized focal and abnormal neurological signs and symptoms are frequently present.

The Global Deterioration Scale provides us with an opportunity to delineate stages of dementia the world over. It provides us with a common language and a frame of reference to discuss our patients and their conditions. The universal acceptance of rating scales such as the Global Deterioration Scale will provide us with a stronger base for our discussion and understanding.

THE TEACHING NURSING HOME

One of the more remarkable developments of the past few years has been the increasing importance of the nursing home as a base of training and research in geriatric medicine. Traditionally nursing homes have been associated with poor care, minimal education, and no research.

There are now more nursing home beds than acute hospital beds in the United States: 1.4 million versus 1 million. Approximately $30 billion dollars a year is now spent on nursing homes. Because the over-age-85 group is the fastest growing segment of the American population and 20 to 25% require nursing home placement, we anticipate a significant increase in nursing home beds over the next few decades. Home health care and better community services will not obviate the need for round-the-clock institutional care.

In an exciting article Leslie Libow (Rubin, 1982) points out that the initial residency-fellowship programs in geriatrics in the United States, which provide physicians with formalized and approved geriatric training, began with the nursing home in 1972. The focus is on lifelong care, as well as rehabilitation. Fellowship training programs linked to nursing homes have been established in New York, California, Massachusetts, Wisconsin, Washington, Arkansas, and other states. The National Institute on Aging established a Geriatriac Medicine Academic Award. The NIA and The Robert Wood Johnson Foundation currently support five and eleven teaching nursing home programs, respectively. Clinical and educational programs in geriatric medicine include ambulatory care (assessment of the frail elderly and special emphasis clinics in osteoporosis, memory loss, falls, incontinence, and menopause); geriatric consultation services; inpatient assessment and management; home care; rehabilitation units; and day services.

Research programs in geriatrics at the Mt. Sinai Medical Center and the Jewish Home and Hospital for the Aged in New York include basic aging (immunology and biology, homeostasis and physiology, and neurosciences) and clinical geriatrics (pharmacology, memory, incontinence, osteoporosis, falls, hypertension, cardiovascular disease, house care delivery, immunology and infection, ethics, and assessment).

Dr. Libow suggests that there will be one academic nursing home per medical school (approximately 127) and one per teaching hospital (over 400) and that they will become major geriatric medical centers or geriatric health centers. Many elderly patients will be admitted to the geriatric health center which will cost less than hospital care and will allow age-specific treatment. A geriatric interdisciplinary team to provide evaluation and ambulatory care programs geared to the frail elderly will be located at these centers. Rather than specialists found at acute hospital centers such as transplant teams and cardiac cather experts, specialists in problems for the elderly will render evaluations and opinions on dementia, memory problems, urinary incontinence, falls, osteoporosis, family crisis, and nutrition. All medical and allied health students and postgraduates must receive training at the nursing home and geriatric center. Thus the nursing home will be a central part of each community's health care service for the elderly.

With this new coordination and influx of energy, the nursing home will no longer be a place to avoid. Large numbers of physicians will work at nursing homes, attending to patients at geriatric centers, making house calls, and dealing with frail elderly. The significantly increasing numbers of physicians in the United States make this more likely, as does the prospect of the potential enjoyment of this work.

Funding for patients in nursing homes, however, remains a serious problem. The annual $30 billion bill will increase to $75 billion by 1990. Approximately half these costs are paid for through personal savings. Government, individuals, and their families will be unable to support such care without innovative insurance planning.

It is conceivable that diagnostic related groups will be extended to nursing homes in order to place a limit on dollars available for care of a patient with a particular diagnosis. This will likely allow a person to be in a nursing home for a period of time, and then the patient and family must determine whether a person should continue in the nursing home or return home.

As nursing homes grow in number, particularly in developing countries, they can avoid the negative stigma that they have achieved in the United States. This can be done by utilizing the nursing home as a teaching facility, as a research facility, and as an example of innovative and superior geriatric medical care.

PREVENTION AND TELEVISION

Little attention is paid to prevention, the process of keeping mental illness from happening. There are many factors that contribute to mental illness in late life—financial problems, physical problems, poor living situations, poor nutrition, lack of social services, poor access to services, lack of transportation, to name a few.

In recent years more attention has been paid to television and the image of the older person depicted to the elderly themselves and to other age groups. It has been determined in a number of studies (e.g., Rubin, 1982) that older people are grossly underrepresented on television and that their characterizations are often inaccurate and negative. They are often presented as hapless, helpless, and confused. Although they represent over 11% of the American population, they represent about 2% of the characters on television (Gerbner et al., 1980).

Their characterization is also negative. Males are increasingly "bad guys" as they age and are seen as ineffectual, while women are failures. "In a world of generally positive portrayals and happy endings, only 40% of older male and even fewer older female characters were presented as successful, happy, and good" (Arnoff, 1974). Whereas younger people, especially children and adolescents are portrayed with positive personality traits, older people have significantly more negative traits. Older women are more apt to be viewed as victims of violence, whereas men are "ineffectual" (Signorielli, 1982).

A more recent study (Signorielli, 1983), indicated that older people made up only 2.3% of characters on prime-time network dramatic television. People over 70 comprised less than 1%. Women were casted in few romantic situations. Though younger women are available for older men, younger men are not available for older women. In this way, television perpetuates the negative stereotyping of older women. Older women are unsuccessful more often than they are successful, something seen in this group only. Older men are the only group more apt to commit violent acts than to be victims of them. Older women are six times more likely to be hurt or killed than to hurt or kill others.

This study further determined that few characters are in need of medical help. Although prime-time programs include 12 doctors and 6 nurses a week, older people rarely have visual impairment and they are almost always ambulatory. Characters frequently snack and drink alcoholic beverages. Yet obesity, which inflicts 25 to 45% of all Americans, is rarely depicted; only 6% of men and 2% of women on television are obese.

Signoriella asks how these images affect viewers: "For heavy viewers, television virtually monopolizes and subsumes other sources of information, ideas, and consciousness. Thus, we have suggested that the more time one spends 'living' in the world of television, the more likely one is to report perceptions of social reality which can be traced to television's most persistent representations of life and society." In fact, she determines that the more people watch television, the more they perceive older people in negative and unfavorable terms. Further, heavy viewers also believe that older people are diminishing in ranks in our society. This appears to be a reflection of the infrequency with which they are depicted.

It may be that these inaccuracies persist in order to aggrandize the middle age group which are more apt to have expendable consumer income. In any event, the impact of television on perceptions of older people, including older peoples perception of themselves, can be profound and can contribute to low self-esteem, social withdrawal, and depression. In each country researchers need to spend time exploring the role of older people on television and the impact of this on the perception of older people. With those countries currently undergoing growth in television production or imports such considerations can be utilized in planning programs so as not to evolve the same problems that have developed in the United States.

SLEEP DISORDERS IN LATE LIFE

Older people are more apt to complain of difficulty in falling asleep, in staying asleep, and in feeling rested during the day. They are also more apt to need frequent naps during the day. The complaints of insomnia appear to be age related (Miles & Dement, 1980). Insomnia is more apt to be a complaint of people over 60 (up to 90%) whereas it is virtually absent between the ages of 8 and 10.

It has been well determined that REM slow-wave sleep (stages 3 and 4) is reduced in older people. Further, awakening after sleep onsets is more frequent, as is a longer adjustment to alterations in the sleep–wake schedule.

In order to assess sleep, an older person (Reynolds et al., 1984) should keep a sleep–wake diary for two weeks. A physical examination, an audio cassette tape of the breathing pattern during sleep, and temperature measures to document circadian rhythm abnormalities are also indicated. A complaint of insomnia of less than three weeks duration is considered transient, whereas insomnia for over three weeks mandates further evaluation. Evening use of caffeine, nicotine, and alcohol have all been implicated in irregular sleep–wake schedules, as have excessive environmental noise or temperature. Other causes of insomnia include dependency on central nervous system depressants, sleep apnea (heavy snoring or labored breathing which affects over 35% of older people), nocturnal myoclonus, dementia, depression, chronic pain, gastroesophageal reflux, institutionalization, and poor nutrition.

Reynolds et al. give a number of suggestions for treatment including the omission of alcohol and caffeine, the use of the bedroom for sleeping only, the elimination of medication that might interfere with sleep, the treatment of depression with antidepressive medications, and a comfortable bed and surroundings. They point out that 25 to 40% of hypnotics were used by the elderly, and that there are many problems associated with sleeping medication, including drug tolerance, daytime hangover, rebound insomnia, exacerbation of sleep-disordered breathing, and impairment of cortical functioning. Nevertheless, medication may be helpful for many older people with insomnia. Contrary indications include kidney, liver, or lung disease with potentially dangerous interactions, suicide risk, risk of injury on the job, tendency to abuse drugs, and heavy snoring. Prescribe the lowest effective dose to be taken 30 minutes before bedtime and limit use to fewer than 20 doses per month for not more than three months.

It must be emphasized that older people do not need less sleep, but have a diminished ability to sleep with shallower and more fragmented sleep patterns than a young adult. Practically, an older person is advised to go to bed only when sleepy and to work toward the goal of going to bed at the same time each night and getting up at the same time each morning, with the elimination of medication. Avoiding the use of the bedrooms for nonsleep activities such as reading or watching television may enhance the image of the bed as a powerful stimulus to sleep.

CONCLUSION

This chapter has included several examples of innovative developments in the United States: computers and communication technology, the development of new organizations with special interests in aging, the development of new rating scales, the utilization of the teaching nursing home, an example of primary prevention through better utilization of television, and management of late-life sleep disorders. The ideas contained herein have application to both developing and developed countries and serve as an example of our opportunities to share information in the exciting arena of psychogeriatrics.

REFERENCES

Arnoff, C. (1974). Old age in prime time. *Journal of Communication,* number 4, 86–87.
Branconnier, R. J. (1981). Evaluation of drug efficacy in dementia: A computerized cognitive assessment system. *Psychopharmacology Bulletin, 17*(1), 4–6.
Finkel, S. (1980). President's Page. *American Association for Geriatric Psychiatry,* number 4, 18.
Gerbner, G., Gross, L., Signorielli, N., & Morgan, M. (1980). Aging with television: Images on television drama and conceptions of social reality. *Journal of Communication,* number 1, 37–47.

Libow, L. S., (1984). The teaching nursing home: Past, present and future. *Journal of the American Geriatric Society, 32*(8), 598–603.

Lieff, J. D. (1984). Communications techonology in geriatrics. *International Psychogeriatric Association Newsletter, 2*(1).

Mace, N., & Rabins, P. (1981). *The 36 hour day: A family guide to caring for persons with Alzheimer's disease, related demented illnesses, and memory loss in later life.* Baltimore, MD: Johns Hopkins University Press.

Miles, L., & Dement, W. (1980). Sleep and aging. *Sleep, 3,* 119–220.

Reisberg, B., Ferris, S. H., DeLeon, M. J., & Crook, T. (1982). The Global Deterioration Scale for assessment of primary degenerative dementia. *The American Journal of Psychiatry, 139*(9), 1136–1139.

Reynolds, C., Cupfer, D., & Sewitch, D. (1984). Practical geriatrics: Diagnoses and management of sleep disorgers in the elderly. *Hospital and Community Psychiatry, 35*(8), 779–781

Rubin, A. M. (1982). Directions in television and aging research. *Journal of Broadcasting, 526*(2), 537–551.

Signorielli, N. (1982). Marital status and T.V. Drama: A case of reduced options. *Journal of Broadcasting, 526*(2), 585–598.

Signorielli, N. (1983). Health, prevention and television: Images of the elderly and perceptions of social reality. In S. Simson, L. Wilson, J. Hermalin, & R. Hess (Eds.), *Aging and prevention: New approaches for preventing health and mental problems in older adults.* New York: Hayworth.

United Nations Division for Economic and Social Information (UNDESI) (1982a, June). *Member states in Africa take action on aging.* New York: United Nations Department of Public Information.

United Nations Division for Economic and Social Information (1982b, June). *Planning ahead for Asia and Latin America* (DPI/DESI NOTE WAA/5 22). New York: United Nations Department of Public Information.

United Nations Division for Economic and Social Information (1982c, March). *Programme on Action for Asia and the Pacific on Aging* (DPI/DESI NOTE WAA/4 15). New York: United Nations Department of Public Information.

Woodward, K. L., & Kornhaber, A. (1981). *Grandparents/grandchildren: The vital connection.* Garden City, New York: Doubleday (Anchor Press).

PART VII
Humanistic Perspectives

25
Education for Death

Robert Kastenbaum and Reinhard Schmitz-Scherzer

"When there is something wrong with dying, then there is also something wrong with living." This statement by a geriatric nurse reminds us that one cannot really separate care of the dying person from its overall biographical and situational context. Attention must be given both to the long life that has been experienced and to the short time remaining. Furthermore, the skills, motives, and philosophy of the caring person must also be taken into account. As Erlemeier (1972) and many others have observed, discomfort with their own mortality has led many clinicians to avoid the aged and the dying. Confrontations with suffering and death remain an everyday threat in much of the world, but are excluded from general view in modern industrialized societies. The sense of helplessness engendered by encounters with pain and physical deterioration is as disturbing to scientists and mental health experts as it is to the public at large. The increasing popularity of terms such as "death with dignity" and the resurgence of interest in a "happy afterlife" represent an increased willingness to discuss the topic, but do not necessarily address the realities of dying or assuage the anxieties of family and caregivers.

This chapter explores some of the positive steps that have been taken toward education and effective care, as well as the barriers that remain to be overcome. Our approach is interdisciplinary, in keeping with the character of the overlapping fields of thanatology and gerontology. These areas of scholarly and applied endeavor were first envisioned by the biologist Elie Metchnikoff who in 1903 called for "the scientific study of old age and of death, two branches of science that may be called *gerontology* and *thanatology,* (and) will bring about great modifications in the course of the last period of life." Both fields call upon the contributions of biologists, physicians, nurses, sociologists, philosophers, psychologists, historians, and many others (Schmitz-Scherzer & Becker, 1982). It is generally recognized that no one field has the monopoly or *the* answer, but that all can offer useful knowledge, techniques, and perspectives.

Succinct reviews of behavioral thanatology are available elsewhere (e.g., Kastenbaum & Costa, 1977; Wittkowski, 1978) with a variety of new European contributions recently made available (Howe & Ochsmann, 1984). Explorations of therapy have been made by Feigenberg (1977), Sobel (1981), and Spiegel-Rosing & Petzold (1984), among others. The interface between thanatology and gerontology has recently been reviewed and discussed by Kalish (1985) and Kastenbaum (1985). Our focus here is more specific to the relationship between the clinician and educator on the one hand, and the dying older person and his or her family on the other. We begin with a consideration of what the dying older person wants and needs, taking into account, however, the great diversity of individuals and situations. This is followed by an exploration of educational needs for personnel working with terminally ill elders and their families.

WHAT DOES THE DYING OLDER PERSON WANT AND NEED?

The older person whose death is in near prospect may express a variety of needs through verbal and nonverbal behavior. Two of the most common and pressing needs are discussed here to illustrate the larger set of concerns that can be found among those facing death after a long and active life.

Maintaining Vital Interpersonal Relationships

The dying person is threatened with total loss: of worldly possessions, physical functioning, mental life, and human relationships. The religious person may believe there is compensation in the form of everlasting bliss. Nevertheless, even those with a strong faith in an afterlife must cope with the palpable separation from loved ones here and now. Of all forms of actual and potential loss in the dying process, it is the fear of abandonment by a crucial person that often takes precedent.

The importance of vital interpersonal relationships has been observed repeatedly (e.g., Rest, 1978; Koch & Schmeling, 1982). This is by no means unique to the dying older person. Harry Stack Sullivan's recognition of loneliness as a major cause of anxiety and depression (Sullivan, 1953) has been amply documented by recent studies (Perlman & Peplau, 1984). Nevertheless, the need for human contact is intensified by life-threatening illness (Rest, 1978; Koch & Schmeling, 1982). Those without satisfactory personal relationships appear to be at greater emotional and perhaps even at greater physical risk during their final illness (Weisman & Worden, 1975).

It is not unusual for the patient to experience greater concern over disruption of a relationship than over the prospect of death itself. As one 87-year-old man said, "I have gotten used to death. Hell, I used to go to ball games and weddings. Now it's only funerals. The only thing (is), I don't want them to bury me until I'm dead. It's hell on earth, being left alone." This man, like many others, had definite ideas about the kind of companionship he needed. "I want my own people. I brought wine and bread to my grandfather before he croaked. Where are my kids now?"

The recently completed National Hospice Demonstration Study (USA), the most extensive investigation of terminal care ever conducted, has again affirmed the significance of personal relationships (although much of the project focused on cost and organization of care). Most of the patients, whether cared for by hospices or hospitals, were elderly, and almost all were afflicted with terminal cancer (Mor, Greer, & Kastenbaum, 1986). The desire to remain in close contact with loved ones emerged as a critical component of the self-perceived quality of life. Even more frequently mentioned than control of pain and other physical symptoms was the wish to have the companionship of those few people who meant the most to the patient.

There are many implications here for the professional caregiver. From the standpoint of case management, for example, one would be advised to refrain from actions that strain or endanger existing personal support systems. To cite but one common situation, physicians have sometimes overlooked the role and needs of the patient's elderly spouse. The professionals move in and take over. Little information is given to the spouse, nor is that person's opinions and feelings explored. Consequently, the spouse who had been closely involved in the well-being of the patient for many years is abruptly pushed aside. Feeling frightened and useless, the spouse's own problems become intensified and he or she is in a less favorable position to comfort the patient. Whatever undermines or disrupts primary interpersonal relationships is a questionable intervention, no matter what might be its justification from a strictly medical or technical standpoint. From the standpoint of education (to be discussed further below), there is the opportunity to help both family members and professional caregivers develop a more effective orientation toward the dying person.

Counselling and psychotherapy may also have a place. Even when the relationship with the therapist itself becomes very important, the goal is not to replace but to clarify, strengthen, and renew existing relationships. The older person facing death might be emotionally isolated from or in conflict with the spouse, an adult child, or some other highly significant individual. This can either be a problem of long duration or a relatively new situation that has arisen in connection with the final illness. Obviously, some type of brief therapy (e.g., Beck & Emery, 1985; Gallagher, 1985) is most appropriate. It is usually most effective to set limited and specific goals for the therapeutic intervention. In one instance, for example, the dying person may be withdrawing from a family member because he fears that person's anger and rejection. Successful short-term therapy might consist of reducing this apprehension and placing past episodes of antagonism and injustice into a new perspective to promote supportive intimacy in the present. An older woman not far from death was able to admit to her son that she had been "sneaky" in breaking up one of his love affairs many years ago. "You have a right to be mad at me, and I might have been wrong, but I just felt very strongly that woman was wrong for you. I would have hated it if somebody had done that to me. But I did it for you, for your happiness. I hope you can forgive me now." He could and did. The specific problems that interfere with a key interpersonal relationship can take many different forms. Nevertheless, the therapeutic goal is often the same: Help these two people to accept and comfort each other during this critical period in their lives.

Remaining Useful and in Control

Older people all too often are perceived as neither useful to others nor in control of their own lives. It is also common to assume that the dying person, regardless of age, must be only a recipient, not a provider of services. The expectation of disutility and lack of control is even greater when the person is both old and dying. In the presence of an aged, frail, and physically deteriorating person it is easy to assume that all claims for running one's own life and helping other people have been relinquished. This is not necessarily the case, however. Despite severe physical restrictions, the afflicted individual may have not only the need but also some remaining capacity to function in a competent manner. How much the person can still accomplish in an objective sense is less important than the satisfaction derived from being able to do *something* for one's self and for others, to avoid complete passivity and helplessness.

The desire to "still be useful" and to retain some control over one's life was often expressed by patients included in the National Hospice Demonstration Study. Our own clinical observations suggest that most people nearing the end of a long, debilitating illness do recognize the limits of their strength, endurance, and mobility. They understand that they must accept some realistic dependency upon others, and that many previous areas of activity are now beyond their grasp. Nevertheless, they still prize their remaining abilities, including ways in which they can be valuable and useful to others. Confined to bed and chair, one woman continued to embroider a pillow cover for her grandchild, who visited daily to say hello and see the progress. Another woman managed to prepare tea for her husband and the hospice volunteer until two days before her death. These exemplify acts that are "small" from an objective standpoint, but that convey meaning. Anybody who has had a period of physical incapacity should be able to recall the satisfaction of again being able to do little things for one's self. The old person approaching death has usually had a long and responsible life. Continuing at least a few symbolic activities can provide a valuable and well-earned sense of competence despite all the losses and restrictions.

Social psychological experiments such as Langer and Rodin's (1975) have demonstrated that the institutionalized elderly develop improved morale and self-esteem when given the opportunity to take an active role in their own affairs, as contrasted with simply obeying rules and receiving services. The majority of terminally ill elders have never been long-term institutional residents, and therefore bring with them an even greater reserve of competence and independence. They will find ways of maintaining some degree of competence, control, and interpersonal mutuality if the social and physical environment supports these actions (Kastenbaum et al., 1980). Medication that either fails to alleviate pain and other symptoms or that compromises intellectual functioning can undermine the dying person's ability to retain some measure of control. Treating the aged patient like a child instead of a mature adult also makes it difficult for the person to function competently. Even those caregivers who avoid medication errors and infantilization, however, may not be sensitive enough to the patient's expressions of need to give something back in return and to keep control over some areas of daily life.

It may seem more efficient to do things for the patient, rather than provide the opportunity for the patient to do things for him or herself. The caregiver may keep busy in order to keep his or her own anxiety under control, and thereby reduce the opportunities for the patient to do likewise. It is an exceptionally valuable nurse, volunteer, physician, or case manager who can identify with the patient, who can appreciate to some extent how the situation looks to a person with severe physical impairment but the desire to remain part of the human community. "I would want to be asked, rather than told," such a caregiver will think. "Today I might want to give you good advice about planting your strawberries, rather than hear the same old questions about my bowel movements from you."

Mental health consultants can help with planning and monitoring an entire case management system that affords the patient the best opportunity to remain in control (Kastenbaum, 1978). Such a plan would reduce the number of unnecessary intrusions into the patient's own sphere of control, and enlist the patient's active collaboration into the management of care from the very beginning. Much attention would be given to behavioral options so that the patient would almost always have some degree of freedom (including, of course, the freedom to let others decide). Active collaboration of this kind among patient, family, and professional caregivers reduces the likelihood of the extreme mental devices that are sometimes employed in the desperate impulse to stay in control. Psychotic flights from reality, sudden lapses into "senility," and suicidal attempts exemplify some of the actions that may be taken in an effort to assert control over one's rapidly disintegrating life. Helping the patient to exercise behavioral options from the very beginning of treatment and maintaining the spirit of collaboration and mutual respect can sharply reduce the need to resort to such extreme actions. "What might this person still do for him or her self? What decisions might still be important to him or her?" These questions should never be far from the thoughts of the clinician.

Freedom from Unbearable Physical or Emotional Pain

Older adults in general have at least, if not more than, their share of mental and emotional difficulties (e.g., Kahn, 1975). Physical problems also increase with age. Both physical and emotional distress are likely to become intensified as the older adult faces death. One approaches this subject, then, in the recognition that reality often is harsh. A lifelong hypochondriac, for example, may be experiencing "real" distress of frightening intensity. A person who brought depressive tendencies into the brightest situations now faces actual loss of great magnitude. The ebullient man whose vigor and good nature helped many others through the years suddenly finds himself too weak to continue this role. The woman who once could bear pain and sacrifice her needs for her loved ones now can find little reason to endure suffering or even to endure life. Nothing could be more inappropriate and counterproductive than entering such situations with the stale psychiatric attitude that emotional problems are "all in the mind." Individual personality dynamics remain crucial, but one must appreciate and respect the altered reality that comes with being old and terminally ill. Equally useless is the assumption that nothing can be done to bring comfort and renew the will to live.

The hospice approach to terminal care has made it clear that comfort is possible for many elderly (as well as younger) adults in their last phase of life. The basic principles and techniques of hospice care have been described in detail elsewhere (Kastenbaum, 1986; Stoddard, 1978). Some goals, such as continuation of the care pattern through time and place, are difficult to achieve outside of hospice or equivalent systems. Nevertheless, the core philosophy and many of the techniques can be actualized in a variety of clinical situations if there are the people and the desire to do so.

From a psychosocial standpoint, one of the most valuable contributions that can be made is to reduce the fear of unbearable distress. Terminally ill patients and their families sometimes express more concern about the suffering that might yet occur than about the symptoms currently being experienced. "How much more will I have to bear?" becomes a vital concern. Family members may become demoralized from thinking about scenes of agony that have not yet happened. Useful interventions can include permission to express one's concerns openly, accurate information that can reduce some of the apprehension, and teaching patients and/or family techniques by which they themselves can reduce or cope more easily with distress. A forward-looking physician might be persuaded to set up a pain control regime in which the patient selects and administers his or her own medications. A spouse might be taught how to provide skin care, and the patient might learn breathing exercises that reduce discomfort.

Additionally, therapists skillful in relaxation techniques and guided imagery might find these procedures of value to both patients and family. At the very least, these procedures are noninvasive, have no obnoxious medical side effects, and give people something constructive to try. Some patients do derive significant benefit from relaxation and guided imagery procedures, reducing some of the dependency on medication and alleviating apprehension about the prospect of suffering more than one can endure.

Providing support to the caregivers (including family and volunteers, if any) can also be an effective, if indirect, way to reduce the patient's distress. One listens; one promotes clear communication; and one assists in the search for alternative solutions. Above all, one works toward building and maintaining a sense of "basic security" (Sullivan, 1953) in the situation. When everybody involved has come to be seen as "dependable," "predictable," and "good willed," and the situation itself has come to be seen as "under control," then the patient can relax a little. Medication can be more effective because it has only the pain or other physical symptoms to control, instead of also struggling against the perception that anything might go wrong at any moment. What presents itself as pain, nausea, or fatigue may also have a component of anxiety or even despair arising from a sense of insecurity in the general situation. The skillful therapist or other support person can do much to "relax the situation" in a relatively unobtrusive way.

PREPARING PEOPLE TO WORK WITH THE DYING

Those who attempt to provide humane and effective care for the dying person have their own needs as well. Among the most obvious is the need for a sense of competency and perspective in approaching the terminally ill and their families. Pioneers such as Cicely Saunders, founder of St. Christopher's Hospice, had to develop their own skills and philosophies as they went along. Even today, many physicians (Koch & Schmeling, 1982), hospital pastors (Schmitz-Scherzer & Becker, 1982) and others receive little or no academic preparation for the challenge of working with the dying. Progress has been made, however, in the development of experiential and professional education in this sphere. Several representative studies and programs are reviewed here.

The Caregiver's Distress

First, it has become clear that caregivers often do experience distress that is associated to some extent with their lack of professional preparation to cope with their challenging responsibilities. A series of studies in West Germany reveals that the first experiences with dying people often are marked by feelings of helplessness, inadequacy, and uncertainty (Buchholz-Engels, 1978; Hoffman, 1978; Alexa, 1978; Weissbrodt, 1978; Linke, 1978). The respondents, whether nurses, chaplains, or physicians, emphasized their lack of adequate professional education in thanatology as a major cause of the distress they experienced when encountering either a dying person or an unexpected corpse. Colleagues were seldom of much help either, having had little training of their own and displaying the usual tendency to avoid contacts with the dying. Clinical supervisors were often reported as perfunctory and ineffective in helping new staff understand and cope with the stress they experienced.

Typically, the reaction to one's disturbing first experience was to fall back on earlier and not very adaptive behavior patterns, essentially, private and personal rituals that attempted to protect the caregiver without providing much comfort to the patient. The dismay reported by a diversity of caregivers in West Germany parallels experiences often noted in the United States (Kastenbaum, 1986). Until the recent implementation of "death education" programs in some professional schools and liberal arts curricula, it has been unusual for American physicians, nurses, ministers, psychologists, and others to bring knowledge and personal security to their early efforts with the dying.

Research and clinical experiences in both nations reveal many common sources of distress. These include the frustration experienced because one feels almost as helpless—if not more helpless—than the patient himself. Young professionals today are trained to "take charge" and feel "in control," orientations that can be defeated quickly by the realities of terminal illness. Shock reactions to sudden, unexpected death, feelings of guilt that one should have done something more or different, fear of responding to "catch questions" from patients or families, and a strong sense of identification with the dying person are among the problems that are often experienced by caregivers unprepared for their responsibilities in death situations.

The list of difficulties encountered by caregivers is quite extensive. Some reported feeling at a loss because they knew so little about the dying person prior to his or her final illness. Others had known the individual previously and were concerned because they had never cared much for him or her. Problems in communicating with fatigued and withdrawn patients were often mentioned, as was the fear that one would be asked to "work miracles." The sights, sounds, and odors that sometimes accompany advanced physical deterioration also disturbed and even disgusted some caregivers. One is tempted to observe tartly that the dying person has even more right to be upset by all these problems because they are all happening to him or her! Nevertheless, the caregivers' reactions are also important and the problems they report help to provide an agenda for death education programs.

Types of Death Education and Some Outcomes

A wide variety of educational and training efforts have been mounted in recent years. These have made use of a rapidly increasing number of publications, bibliographies, and audiovisual aids (Wass et al., 1980). Programs have been directed to students at various levels from elementary school to postdoctoral institutes. They have varied in focus from general explorations of death and its meanings to specific problem areas (e.g., symptom control in terminal cancer, prediction of pathological grief reactions, suicide prevention, etc.). Some programs have been built upon scholarly books and articles; others have directed attention to the participants' own attitudes, feelings, and motives. Many colleges and universities offer semester-long courses on death as part of their regular curriculum. Among these courses themselves there is marked variation in topics covered. Suicide, for example, may be given systematic attention in one course and barely mentioned in another. One course will focus almost entirely upon terminal care and grief, while another includes consideration of religious values, the threat of nuclear war, and many other topics. Church and community agencies occasionally sponsor two or three day "intensives" that involve experiential exercises and encounters as well as lectures. The training programs conducted for volunteers by hospice organizations are often among the most carefully planned and supervised types of death education available, if more limited in scope than an academic course.

The faculty for the various types of death education programs also represent a great diversity of disciplines and approaches. The list includes but is not limited to psychologists, psychiatrists, oncologists, nurses, ministers, social workers, and music therapists. It must also be said that the level of expertise and overall quality also differs appreciably. One training program may be directed by a person with years of direct experience in caring for dying people and their families; another may be organized by somebody who has only read a book or two on the subject.

Examination of the death education process and its outcomes has only recently started to attract research attention, not surprising since most of the programs themselves are still rather new. In an Australian study, Channon (1984–1985) found that few medical students had known somebody from their own generation who had died. Their prior experiences with death had usually involved grandparents or distant relatives. The most typical experience with death was in the cadaver room as part of their medical training. Those about to embark upon a career intimately associated with the struggle against death had brought with them relatively little personal experience. The results of this study appears to be consistent with what many faculty in medical and other professional schools have observed: Today's youth enter professional life from a background involving very little direct encounter with death. A somewhat different picture emerges, however, when one analyzes the personal experiences of those who enroll in optional death education courses and workshops (Doka, 1981–1982). Voluntary participants are more likely to have experienced the death of people close to them than are those who take part because they are required to as part of a systematic exposure for all nursing, medical, or pastoral students.

Reduction of death-related anxiety is sometimes a goal of courses and workshops. This is regarded as an appropriate goal because of the high level of apprehension and stress that has often been reported by caregivers (as noted earlier). There have been a few limited confirmations that experience in a death education program can lower anxiety levels (e.g., Cook et al., 1984–1985; Waldman & Davidshofer, 1983–1984). Additional studies are needed, however, especially in the duration of such effects and their relationship to actual behavior in death-related situations. Whether or not reduction of death-related anxiety should be a primary goal is a question that should be asked more often. Although very high levels of anxiety produce subjective distress and interfere with personal and professional functioning, the overall relationship among anxiety, subjective experience, and objective performance is far from clear. Note for example, that women in general score higher than men on psychometric measures of death anxiety (Pollak, 1979–1980; Da Silva & Schork, 1984–1985), and yet many more women than men actually provide direct care to the terminally ill. The ability to feel and recognize anxiety may represent a valuable sensitivity and openness to experience. Considering also the fact that anxiety has a general function as an alarm signal, one might be premature in concluding that thanatological education should have the primary purpose of reducing anxiety associated with death. There are times when it is appropriate to be anxiously alert, although not to the point of disorganization and panic.

Where reduction of death-related anxiety is a relevant and appropriate goal, however, open discussion within a mutually supportive learning environment appears to be a simple and effective technique for many students. One discovers that talking about death does little harm and, in fact, can release long-suppressed tensions.

A related and broader goal sometimes implemented through death education is to help the learner understand his or her own feelings about death more fully and to review and perhaps revise long-standing attitudes. This approach does not attempt to dictate a particular set of new attitudes and values to the learner, but, rather, provides an opportunity to achieve new personal integrations of thought and feeling. Students often report that they have never before had an occasion to share their death thoughts and experiences with other people. Sharing experiences within the supportive context of a death education program can have a therapeutic effect. For the first time in her life a graduate student of social work may realize that she was not "wicked" or even very unusual in becoming angry with her husband when he died suddenly, leaving her with a house full of children to raise. A doctoral candidate in counseling psychology may recognize that his sleep disturbances started when, in late childhood, he was forced to use the bed in which his grandfather had recently died. Individuals can make their own discoveries through a combination of readings, lectures, and explorations of personal experiences. Obviously, instructors in such courses must be good listeners as well as competent in their subject matter.

In graduate seminars, especially in medical and other professional settings, it can be useful to provide extensive role playing and other active learning procedures. By testing out in advance situations that they might encounter later in their careers, the students have the opportunity to develop new skills and dissipate apprehension. They can be exposed to "catch questions" in these practice sessions, placed in conflict between the wishes of patient and family, or confronted by "impossible demands" or "unrealistic responses." Almost all experiences reported as stressful by caregivers working with their first dying patient can be simulated effectively with the help of skilled faculty.

Although emotional factors (such as overidentification with the clients, guilt over not being able to "cure death," etc.) deserve much attention, one should not overlook the importance of helping students, volunteers, and newly minted professionals to appreciate technical, administrative, and strategic factors as well. A few examples will be cited:

1. *Recognizing and respecting the way that others in the situation are inclined to function.* The nurse and the social worker, for example, bring different skills and different sets of expectations to the client and family. Although they may be equally competent and dedicated and working

toward the same general goals, there is also the potential for mutual misunderstanding and even antagonism. The terminally ill client and his or her family may be caught between a nurse who has waited until the last moment to recognize the need for a social worker's intervention, or a social worker who has initiated financial and administrative paperwork without understanding some important particulars of the patient's condition that are obvious to the nurse. Similar situations can arise among all those involved in terminal care, not excluding the physician or the minister, the dietician or the attorney. Successful terminal care programs usually involve educational efforts that help all the caregivers to understand and respect each other's knowledge, skills, roles, and responsibilities.

2. *Learning how to adjust the situation so that the "incentives" favor the patient and the family and do not introduce conflict among caregivers.* It is necessary but not sufficient that the caregiver, whether a professional or a volunteer, develop a basic understanding of reciprocal role relationships. Each participant has the further responsibility of contributing to a situation in which all can work coherently toward the same goal. In the United States, for example, financial incentives may tempt the physician to hospitalize an elderly cancer patient, despite the client and family's preference for staying at home. Resentment, antagonisms, and reprisals can occur under circumstances such as these. By recognizing problems with priorities and incentives that are structural, that are inherent to the situation, the participants have the opportunity to resolve the difficulties before they prove harmful to the client or disruptive to themselves. Some hospices, for example, have been able to make the option of staying at home more attractive to physicians because of the quality of supplementary care provided, thereby overriding the financial disincentive.

3. *Acquiring specific skills related to terminal care that are not usually imparted in general professional training.* Reference was made earlier to extreme and unadaptive behaviors that might be shown by patients who fear they have lost control of the situation. Physicians, nurses, and other professionals are not exempt from this difficulty either. And sometimes it is not primarily a motivational or emotional difficulty on the part of the caregiver that is responsible for the difficulty. It may simply be that one does not know what to do in the situation! A physician quickly leaves the bedside of a terminally ill old man because he has not learned that there are a variety of comfort-giving actions he could provide, both at the scene and through his orders and recommendations. An occupational therapist assumes there is nothing to be done for a frail old person with not long to live, and therefore does not make a serious therapeutic assessment, missing an opportunity that would have been recognized by those in the profession who have received special training in geriatrics. A psychiatrist or psychologist hastily concludes that the patient is out of contact and not a candidate for therapy.

A different and more hopeful conclusion would have been drawn by a colleague with better training in geriatrics and a more subtle grasp of the fluctuating levels of awareness and resistance often found. Geriatrics and, to a lesser but still valuable extent, thanatology have a variety of specific lessons to offer. The caregiver does not have to begin—or remain—unprepared and therefore especially vulnerable to anxiety and error.

CONCLUDING NOTE

Care of the older person who is facing death after a long life might be considered a moral responsibility as well as a clinical challenge. Lack of professional training, personal anxieties, and a general aversion from death-related topics in technologically advanced societies are among the factors that have delayed the advent of humane and effective terminal care. Sufficient progress has been made on all fronts to dispel the assumption that nothing can be done for the older person with a terminal illness. This chapter has simply explored a few of the major needs expressed by dying elders and a few of the techniques that have been found useful in meeting these needs. It is likely that a new generation of caregivers, researchers, and educators will make significant contributions that go well beyond what could be reported here. Certainly, the need for enlightened care will continue so long as people grow up, grow old, and, finally, confront the death that is within us.

REFERENCES

Alexa, M. (1978). Verhaltens- und Erlebensaspekte in der berufsbedingten Konfrontation mit Tod und Sterben bei Ärzten. Diplomarbeit, Psychologisches Institut der Universität Bonn.

Beck, A. T., & Emergy, G. (1985). *Anxiety disorders and phobias.* New York: Basic Books.

Buchholz-Engels, (1978).

Channon, L. D. (1984). Death and the preclinical medical student: Part 1. Experiences with death. *Death Education, 8,* 231–236.

Cook, A. S., Oltjenbruns, K. A., & Lagoni, L. (1984–1985). The "ripple effect" of a university sponsored death and dying symposium. *Omega, Journal of Death and Dying, 15,* 185–190.

DaSilva, A., & Schork, M. S. (1984–1985). Gender differences in attitudes to death among a group of public health students. *Omega, Journal of Death and Dying, 15,* 77–84.

Doka, K. J. (1980–1981). Recent bereavement and registration for death studies courses. *Omega, Journal of Death and Dying, 12,* 51–60.

Feigenberg, L. (1977). *Terminalvard.* Lund: Liber Laromedel.

Gallagher, D. (1985). *Socializing the elder patient in cognitive/behavioral therapy.* Paper presented at the annual meetings of the American Psychological Association, Los Angeles.
Hoffmann, K. (1978). Verhaltens- und Erlebensaspekte evangelischer Krankenhausseelsorger bei ihrer Begegnung mit sterbenden Patienten. Diplomarbeit, Psychologisches Institut der Universität Bonn.
Howe, J., & Ochsmann, R. (Eds.) (1984). *Tod- Sterben- Trauer.* Frankfurt am Main: Fachbuchhandlung for Psychologie Verlagsabteilung.
Kahn, R. L. (1975). The mental health system and the future aged. *The Gerontologist, 15,* 24–31.
Kalish, R. A. (1985). The social context of death and dying. In R. H. Binstock & E. Shanas (Eds.), *Handbook of aging and the social sciences* (2nd ed.) (pp. 149–172). New York: Van Nostrand Reinhold.
Kastenbaum, R. (1978). In control. In C. A. Garfield (Ed.), *Psychosocial care of the dying patient* (pp. 227–244). New York: McGraw-Hill.
Kastenbaum, R. (1985). Dying and death: A life-span approach. In J. E. Birren & K. W. Schaie (Eds.), *Handbook of the psychology of aging* (pp. 619–646). New York: Van Nostrand Reinhold.
Kastenbaum, R. (1986). *Death, society and human experience* (3rd ed.). Westerville, OH: Merrill.
Kastenbaum, R., Barber, T. X., Wilson, C., Ryder, B. L., & Hathaway, L. B. (1980). *Old, sick and helpless: Where therapy begins.* Cambridge, MA: Ballinger.
Kastenbaum, R., & Costa, P. T. (1977). Psychological perspectives on death. In M. R. Rosenzweig & L. W. Porter (Eds.), *Annual review of psychology* (Vol. 28, pp. 225–250). Palo Alto: Stanford University Press.
Koch, U. & Schmeling, C. (1982). *Betreuung von Schwer- und Todkranken.* München: Urban & Schwarzenberg.
Langer, E., & Rodin, J. (1976). The effects of choice and enhanced personal responsibility for the aged: A field experiment in an institutional setting. *Journal of Personality and Social Psychology, 34,* 191–198.
Linke, B. (1978). Dererminanten der Erlebens- und Verhaltenweisen von Krankenschwestern bei der Konfrontation mit Tod und Sterben. Diplomarbeit, Psychologisches Institut der Universität Bonn.
Metchnikoff, E. (1903). *The nature of man.* New York: Putnam.
Mor., V., Greer, D., & Kastenbaum, R. (Eds.) (1986). *The hospice experiment: Is it working?* Baltimore, MD: Johns Hopkins University Press.
Perlman, D. & Peplau, L. A. (1978). Loneliness research: A survey of empirical findings. In L. A. Peplau & S. E. Goldston (Eds.), *Preventing the harmful consequences of severe and persistent loneliness* (pp. 13–46). Rockville, MD: U.S. Department of Health and Human Services.
Pollak, J. M. (1979–1980). Correlates of death anxiety: A review of empirical studies. *Omega, Journal of Death and Dying, 10,* 97–122.
Rest, F. (1977–1978). *Praktische Orthothanasie im Arbeitsfeld sozialer Praxis.* Bd. I und II. Opladen: Westdeutscher Verlag.
Schmitz-Scherzer, R. & Becker, K. F. (1982). *Einsam sterben - warum?* Hannover: Vincentz Verlag.
Sobel, H. J. (Ed.) (1981). *Behavior therapy in terminal care.* Cambridge, MA: Ballinger.
Spiegel-Rosing, I. & Petzold, H. (1984). *Die Begleitung Sterbender.* Paderborn: Junfermann.
Stoddard, S. (1978). *The hospice movement.* New York: Stein & Day.

Sullivan, H. S. (1953). *The interpersonal theory of psychiatry.* New York: Norton.

Waldman, D. A., & Davidshofer, C. (1983–1984). Death anxiety reduction as the result of exposure to a death and dying symposium. *Omega, Journal of Death and Dying, 14,* 323–328.

Weisman, A. D., & Worden, J. W. (1975). Psychosocial analysis of cancer deaths. *Omega, Journal of Death and Dying, 6,* 61–65.

Wass, H., Corr, A. A., Pacholski, R. A., & Sanders, C. M. (1980). *Death education: An annotated resource guide.* Washington, DC: Hemisphere.

Wittkowski, J. (1978). Tod und Sterben. *Ergebnisse der Thanatopsychologie.* Heidelberg: Quelle & Meyer.

26
Learning to Accept Death: Dealing with Terminally Ill and Dying Patients

Manfred Bergener

In 1980, von Soest carried out a remarkable, thought-provoking study. He found that doctors' calls on the elderly and chronically ill were significantly shorter than visits to other patients; in the case of persons who were terminally ill or dying, they were the shortest of all. The findings of this study show that such neglect is more than the question of a difficult burden from the doctor's point of view: it is rather the matter of an unfulfilled obligation which is not to be explained away alone through the excuses of overwork and lack of time, although these factors all too often determine a doctor's actions. Perhaps we are too much medical practitioners to be capable of acting as physicians, too. Practiced in the techniques of examination and exploration rather than counseling, we cannot seem to find the words of compassion for the suffering of the patient whose illness is irreversible or who is going to die soon.

The ability to speak and listen to the patient, and have time for him, is and will remain, in spite of ever more advanced psychological techniques and "styles of approach," the most important prerequisite in dealing with terminally ill and dying patients. This method of approach does not mean that the doctor instructs, prescribes, and leads the way while the patient follows; on the contrary, this procedure consists in mutual recognition, in reciprocal give and take, in dialogue. It involves the facility of two people to open themselves to each other and is based on mutual trust, on reliability.

The familiar form "Du" in German (as if speaking to a minor), which is still used much too often in dealing with patients, conveys aloofness rather than trust. And the sham plural "we" (also shamefully overused in the medical profession) as in, "How are *we* feeling today?" fails to overcome existing barriers. (Why shouldn't this also be considered a form of "malpractice?") In looking for a comparison in order to show what is important in dealing with the terminally ill and dying, there comes to mind the image of mountain climbers roped together: a relationship that is based on mutual understanding and is a reciprocal affair. Instead of the one always following the other, they follow each other, head and heart acting together, never one without the other, but also never one *instead* of the other; medical competence without excluding compassion and mutual trust: here, too, not one instead of the other and never "head over heels"—much rather, when in doubt, "heart over head," as Ulla Hahn entitled her first book of poems. The behavior of a doctor in dealing with the terminally ill and dying can only be effective if an awareness is maintained of the fixed limits of a human life, something that torments the physician too. Only a person who is aware of his own fears and despair is really free to devote himself to others. The true point of departure here lies in the recognition of our imperfection. The finality of life as the paramount reality forms the basic theme of this relationship, a discussion leading to the recognition that suffering—and also death—does not constitute the irrevocable end, but rather "a passing over to the other shore."

Dealing with terminally ill and dying patients, in much greater measure than with the acutely ill (where the mastery and performance of technical, often highly complicated tasks dominate) requires a compassionate maturity, along with the ability to identify the therapeutic reasoning in seemingly insignificant, minor and simple assistance. This leads us away from the misunderstanding that theoretical knowledge about illnesses, their cause and treatment, constitutes the essential element for the actions of a doctor. Actually, perseverance and patience as well as mental and physical strength are required when the situation calls for giving the patient the feeling that "you are there for him." Terminally ill and dying patients have need of someone to keep them company, and they are afraid that the counseling offered them is not intended to be taken seriously; they are disappointed when the closeness they hoped for does not materialize. How often the bustle and activities, as well as the administering of medical, technical, and nursing services, especially in modern hospitals, stand in the way of this genuinely human experience, this dedication of ourselves to each other.

CONTACTS WITH INDIVIDUALS CANNOT TAKE THE PLACE OF FACE-TO-FACE MEETINGS

Here we have a paradoxical development: the multiprofessional team in the hospital makes possible a wealth of individual contacts. Doctors, attendants, nurses, psychologists, social workers, and occupational and physical therapists are all involved. Nevertheless, this does not mean that, because we have "individual contacts," we can dispense with the tête-à-tête. These fleeting contacts with individuals expose the neglect of psychic, social, and emotional needs; they reveal our paucity of feeling, our inability to empathize. Frequently remarks and counsel, consisting of appeasement and generalization, utterances that moralize, rebuff, and hide needs, serve to evade and resist the true concerns of the other person, in fact serve to maintain "distance." Where conversations are anticipated, where hope and expectations are associated with this discourse, the individual withdraws into the anonymity of the therapeutic team, begins to search for words and, with these words, to evade the conversation.

Whoever must deal with patients who are terminally ill and those who are dying should never try "to find solutions," but in giving answers should see the patient as a person, in his entirety, and not lose sight of the fact that he is a human being. It is our job to give the other person a chance to know himself, to formulate his ideas and express himself. Nothing is more important than to take his fears seriously, to listen to his problems and to endure his questions. Here is a demand that pushes us to the limits of what we can bear, and often beyond. Thus, in dealing with the psychic guidance of patients who are terminally ill or dying, a constant aura of tension is generated; the more medical and human abilities are demanded, the less medicine, in spite of all technical advances and modern achievements, is able to accomplish. When we are confronted with the question of what we are actually doing when the patient is at the mercy of medical life support systems, we face the challenge of opening a way for the patient to come to terms with himself, to attain that for which our judgment is no longer sufficient.

There are no general, mandatory rules in the sense of established formulas, either in psychic guidance or for dealing with terminally ill patients and those who are dying. The doctor, in these cases faces a task that requires, in addition to professional competence, humaneness and charitableness as well. (These are terms which sound almost antiquated, old-fashioned, and out of date. For just this reason they were chosen and consciously used in this context.) Crucial, however, is the matter of presenting such a situation in a way that makes it possible for patients to gain an insight into its inevitability: not to shy away from urgent thoughts about its irreversibility and finality; to stand firm in the inevitability of his fate.

SPECIAL DEMANDS ON THE PSYCHOTHERAPEUTIC COMPETENCE OF THE DOCTOR

How often the doctor faces people who withdraw in panic because of emotional barrenness, fear, loneliness—in search of security, warmth, and protection—and how often he senses his inability to provide help; how often everything goes wrong because the first sentence won't come, and he remains unable to hold a conversation. In a similar manner, this applies to every situation involving examination. What matters is not only this or that technique in the performance of a more or less specialized method of examination, but rather an ability to adapt oneself to the varied situations involving individual examination, and thereby to respect all the personal idiosyncracies of the patient. This is valid also for the dialogue between doctor and patient. What persons who are terminally ill or dying expect from this contact is to be listened to patiently–above all, to have an interest shown in their needs and complaints.

Let us ask how patients deal with the actual or presumed experience of illnesses which threaten their lives, in what psychic conflicts they become involved as a result, and what must be done to manage the psychic crises which develop from this situation. Without a doubt, an illness that threatens existence represents an especially tumultuous event in the life of a human being—an existential challenge. Because of this, extraordinary demands are made on his ability to deal with this situation, to adjust to it, and to resign or reconcile himself to it.

In varying degrees, a serious illness often means several threats at once. If we try, in our own minds, to clarify the mental processes that serve to ward off the dangers of such a serious threat, it is useful to consider the variety of strategies people use in order to stand up to a reality that cannot be dealt with in any other way, to bear the unbearable burden of this reality, an incurable illness that threatens life itself. Then again, this experience, the awareness of one's own illness, that one is truly stricken, that his life will come to an end, can cause depression. Associated with this may be feelings of guilt and a presentiment of death which often cannot be explained.

Often, in the presence of a threat, the processes of coping and defense emerge simultaneously in the behavior of persons who are seriously ill. How this happens in individual cases depends on several factors which are determined by particularities of the underlying illness itself, on the structure of the patient's personality, and finally on the total situation, including the social background, the available social contacts, the doctor–patient relationship, the particulars of hospitalization, and, last but not least, on the structural realities of the hospital itself.

Threatening life experiences constitute an existential stress. They can cause crises in which a person becomes critically aware of his own insufficiencies and mortality, of his own futility, accompanied as well by a feeling of uneasiness, of not being able to cope, of a sense of inferiority. At the same time, however, these situations include the possibilities of disengagement and of overcoming. On the other hand, they can set in motion aggressive/protective mechanisms, whose persistence can ultimately lead to seriously aberrant behavior; likewise to attempted or completed suicide.

THE WILLINGNESS TO ENDURE AND THE ABILITY TO SYMPATHIZE

There are situations in which the composure, even the optimism of a person whose life is threatened, seems incomprehensible and even inconceivable. Here are situations in which optimism, an interest in life, and vital behavior are in striking contrast to the findings of medical research. In particular, it cannot always be determined for certain whether it is a case of euphoria (e.g., related to toxic or other influences on the brain) or just the opposite—a question of psychodynamically explainable processes. That burdensome aspects of life can undergo an overcompensation or distortion is clearly recognizable to the extent that psychodynamic processes are phenomenologically involved in very different adaptive and defensive mechanisms. According to Freud, among the most important of these are repression, rationalization, displacement, formation of response, projection, regression, avoidance, and denial. We learn from the philosopher, Karl Popper, that one of the fundamental effects of avoidance consists in its ability to bring about perhaps exactly that which should be avoided.

With patients who are critically ill, denial is a defense mechanism which is seen especially often. In other cases, as a result of a selectively altered relation to environment, massive psychotic crises can develop; and these, too, are an attempt to facilitate or actually make possible a coping with a particular experience or mode of existence.

In many cases, primitive introjection and projection mechanisms are associated with denial while another form of defense, repression, according to Freud, is usually accompanied by differentiated projection and identification. The knowledge or the dynamics of this kind of defense mechanism is of special importance for terminally ill patients because it can determine the adjustment of those involved with each other. Kübler-Ross, in her book "Verstehen was Sterbende sagen wollen," has described this graphically. If a patient is encouraged in what for him is a life-threatening situation, supported in an unrealistic attitude, he will thus often take over this interpretation as his own, out of the fear that the admission of the inevitability of his situation would lead to a loss of contacts and human relationships which are vital for him—family, doctors, nurses, and attendants. How we should therapeutically handle mechanisms such as defense, depression, and denial poses a difficult question that cannot be answered generally. How we answer this question in individual cases depends on whether and on how far the patient is accessible to us, on how far his experience of us can be assimilated, and on how much of our practical knowledge can be conveyed to him. This assumes not only a willingness to endure suffering but also the ability to sympathize.

If a person who is terminally ill or dying is at all able to comprehend his situation, or if he is unable to interpret his situation for himself, is he, as a result, dependent on the information and interpretation of a doctor? The validity of this assumption, according to which a terminally ill or dying patient is not able to understand his situation, cannot be substantiated by empirical research. The question, therefore, is not: to enlighten or not to enlighten; neither is it to reveal the diagnosis or not. It is rather a question of dealing with patients who are already aware of their fate through their own understanding or individual, particular foreknowledge.

THE CRUCIAL FIRST CONVERSATION

If a first conversation does not collapse into mere words, the biographical anamnesis forms the bridge over which a connection between the inner and outer life story of the patient becomes recognizable. A psychotherapeutic conversation should become a dialogue between two persons, not a conversation about some mere thing. To have trust, to want trust, and to be able to trust are the three indispensable pillars that support this relationship. At the same time, this dialogue constitutes the prerequisite for further psychotherapeutic steps. These elements of trust sustain the independence and autonomy of the patient and, at the same time, contribute to the relief of dependence. In the dialogue with his doctor, the patient, in spite of his terminal illness, should feel that he is being taken seriously. He should feel accepted and challenged to accept himself and his fate, whereby he is able to find and to realize himself. On the other hand, this can be made substantially more difficult or blocked altogether by defensive behavior on the part of doctors, nurses, and attendants. Defensive behavior, as can be observed day in, day out in routine clinical practice, dominates the ward atmosphere today more than ever before. The expression of guilt feelings vis-à-vis the patient in the form of overactivity, as well as overidentification or overengagement, can mobilize and strengthen fears on both sides.

THE PSYCHIC AFFLICTION

More than ever all colleagues who deal therapeutically with terminally ill and dying patients must be made aware that physical and mental illness always involve a patient's psychic bewilderment; the psychic and physical components enter into an inseparable relationship. The physical element, therefore, also expresses what we feel and experience: conflicts and crises, fears and needs, capitulation and failure all project themselves physically. Doctor Benn Kline writes as follows about his dying Gramp:

The last time that I examined him it was pretty obvious that he didn't want to live any longer. Certainly this is not especially unusual. On the other hand, it was really remarkable that he took out his dentures and declared: "There you are, I don't need them any more." That was something which I had not experienced before with any human being. It was not uncommon either for him to see clearly that the time had come for him to die. I am convinced that human dignity must not be lost in dying either. And since he had now decided that he no longer wanted to suffer the indignity of remaining alive, it was no longer our task to prolong his life. It would have been, I believe, cruel, for a person has a right to his dignity—not only in life but also in death. As he took out his dentures and said: "I don't want to live any longer," there was no longer any question in my mind—an artificial nourishment and the extention of life through medication was no longer to be considered. I wanted him to be allowed to die in dignity.

As doctors we should allow ourselves to be guided by the conviction that human dignity should not be lost, even in dying. How often, however, this dignity is sacrificed when terminally ill and dying persons are subjected to the dehumanizing practices of clinics and institutes. In our times, the process of dying has been shifted more and more to the hospital. Here a change in awareness should finally lead to a return to traditional practice. A precondition for this change, however, is a radical change in the thinking and methods of doctors which recognizes suffering, dying, and death as the fundamental categories related to an anthropologically oriented medicine.

In medical practice, a basically realistic view of death should be developed, as Peter Sloterdijk has expressed it: "a way of thinking about death which, in a technically more intimate way than any other, makes us aware of the fragility of the body, the progress of our organism towards death—whether this be in health, illness or growing older."

We must rid medicine of the delusion that everything should be done that it is possible to do and ask ourselves what our successes in medicine amount to, measured against our inability to relieve suffering and walk hand in hand with those who are dying.

REFERENCES

Kübler-Ross, E. (1982). *Verstehen was Sterbende sagen wollen*. Stuttgart: Kreuz Verlag.
Jury, M. & Jury, D. (1982). *GRAMP—Ein Mann altert und stirbt*. Berlin/Bonn: Verlag J.H.W. Dietz Nachf.
van Soest, A. H. (1980). Ärztliche Bemühungen bei sterbenden Menschen. *Akt. geront.* 10, 161.
Sloterdijk, P. (1983). *Kritik der zynischen Vernunft*, Vol. 2. Frankfurt/Main: Suhrkamp.

27
Outlook

Manfred Bergener

The contributions to this volume demonstrate the wealth of findings and insights that has accumulated over the past decade in the field of aging and its related diseases. Our priority now is to strengthen the status of geriatrics and especially of psychogeriatrics as an independent medical discipline while at the same time further integrating it into the practice of general medicine.

In order to prepare the way for the interdisciplinary approach necessary to geriatrics and psychogeriatrics, it is imperative to construct a suitable methodological framework. Such a framework, in turn, requires the development of a novel logic of research that does away with the traditional generally prevalent thinking in terms of separate and distinct disciplines. Universities to this day have not done nearly enough to reaffirm an interdisciplinary orientation. Establishing gerontological research institutes and increasing the number of geriatric hospitals will contribute much to support this endeavor. The most important requirement, however, for the realization and legitimation of the approach advocated here is the formulation of a coherent scientific theory that not only states the *raison d'être* but also deals concretely with the possibility of theoretical refutations from different sectors. Thus, the prerequisites for geriatrics and psychogeriatrics are both practical and theoretical in nature: on the one hand, a suitable methodological framework, on the other hand, a scientific theory of legitimation.

In the editor's view, psychogeriatrics today is to be understood as a model of a broadly conceived psychosomatic pathology. It goes beyond the claim of an independent, separate medical discipline, however. Defining itself through the basic principles of the holistic paradigm, psychogeriatrics represents a unique concept of medical thought and action. Within the holistic paradigm, health and illness are not mutually exclusive static conditions, but complementary elements of a totally unified process. In this sense, psychogeriatrics may be seen as the heir to a more than 2000-year-old medical tradition, whose founder Hippocrates countered the trend of fragmentation and classification of organic disorders with the idea of holism. Only in the past two hundred years has the emphasis on natural science, which dominated the conceptualization of disease, pushed into the background the view of health and illness as integral components of the total life experience.

In psychogeriatrics as in medicine in general, it is now a matter of retrieving and reaffirming this holistic, psychosomatic conception of disease. Psychosomatics has become a discipline devoted to overcoming the dualistic conception of human beings. Presently, the emphasis is on establishing the connections among the presence of specific disease symptoms, the life style of the individual, and the psychological reactions of the individual to particular life events. The actual, experienced conflict situation is not the exclusive determining factor. More important usually are the resulting responses to the conflict situation, which themselves are considerably influenced by the individual personality structure. Thus, psychological reaction as affected by personality structure, not the disease itself, is an indicator. A variety of psychodynamic constellations may be obfuscated by the tangible and distinct symptoms of both functional and organic syndromes. These psychodynamic constellations are in turn molded by the personal fate of the individual as well as by his or her social and cultural environment.

Thus, the principle that "age-based" organic disorders alway represent irreversible defects and deterioration, in the process having a leveling effect on the individuality of the ill person, has justifiably been abandoned by psychogeriatrics. This deficit model of aging was an outgrowth of a medical concept that in the past distanced itself further and further from the patient. In the future following an individualized approach and a comprehensive psychiatric pathology, the symptomatology and the disease processes of the aged will gain a new dimension: the spiritual, emotional, and psychological realm. Many demonstrable symptoms of psychogeriatric diseases develop as the result of the dialectic between the internal and the external life courses of the individual. This applies to organic processes as well as functional syndromes. Drug therapy alone can never fulfill the demand for a comprehensive treatment strategy. New treatment insights will result from a focus on the life history of the individual in question. The formal reductionistic objectification of physics, chemistry, morphology, etc., will be negated in order to put these disciplines back on a patient-oriented track. The fundamental prerequisite for diagnosis, treatment, and rehabilitation of all aging-related diseases, both organic and functional, is a holistic approach that presumes a strong ecological consciousness and relies on a strong spiritual consciousness. Not only when dealing with depression and anxiety syndromes but also in psychosomatic disorders and dementia, and above all when dealing with the incurably ill and dying, such an approach becomes more and more self-evident.

Multidimensional diagnostics and effective treatment concepts presuppose not only an interdisciplinary orientation, but also the further development of multiprofessional cooperative strategies. The creation of a structural framework for these strategies is a challenge that has yet to be tackled in research, in hospitals, and in private practice. Finally, we must emphasize that the realization of this goal depends upon fundamental changes in the structure and organization of medical education itself. What is urgently needed in our universities is the development of a new medical education system that, in addition to ensuring professional competence, passes on and promotes competence in interdisciplinary and comprehensive thinking and cooperation.

Psychogeriatrics represents the discovery of the greater whole, the overall picture, the totality composed of a vast variety of perspectives. Many experts have in the past excelled in researching one specific perspective. No doubt this will and must continue: further research creates new specialties and new specialists. Understanding the whole, however, is a greater and more rewarding challenge.

And now a word on the situation of clinical pharmacology and pharmacotherapy within psychogeriatrics. There is no doubt that both in the areas of basic research and clinical application much has been set into motion. At the same time, neither the experimental research nor the clinical-pharmacological research has fulfilled the expectations they had created. Particular difficulties arise in the application of psychometric methods, which are the products of the reciprocal relationship between psychological and somatic phenomena. Resolving these difficulties in the future will not mean creating new measurement methods for each new case. Rather, a new research area, clinical psychophysiology, will gain in prominence: a multidimensional science whose goal it is to comprehend multivariate relationships between physiological data on the one hand and psychological processes on the other.

The gathering of population samples with homogeneous symptoms to be used in treatment research is a further important problematical area. The carrying out of large-scale methodologically complicated longitudinal studies requires in the light of multimorbidity and polysymptomatology in the aged, international cooperation in the form of joint research. Such studies to this day have not taken place. Studies on a much smaller scale will still be carried out in many places. Meanwhile the mistrust regarding the use of an ever increasing number of drugs among the aged will continue to exist.

Not even the sizable number of so-called double-blind studies could change matters. Because of the many methodological deficiencies, they produce only an apparent accuracy which actually does not exist. That which is measured is often too far removed from that which should be measured.

Further advances will only be possible when strategies have been developed that take biological, psychological, and psychophysiological elements equally into consideration. Along these lines, also, treatment research could serve as an example of interdisciplinary strategies, since these strategies should include basic research as well as practice. Perhaps it is too early to speak of an independent gerontopharmacology; however, there can be no doubt that the principles of general pharmacology must undergo modification when applied to the aged. Only when the basic guidelines for this up-and-coming discipline are in place will the degree of treatment safety and control satisfy the clinical requirements. The side-effects and dangers of treatments are not always sufficiently weighed against the expected benefits. This is still true even if taking into account that further advances always bring new dangers, dangers resulting from the steadily rising dominance of technology in medicine as well as from more effective drugs. The risk/benefit ratio is therefore problematic: the correctness of a medical fact cannot be implied alone by its success. The fact that a cure was predicted in no way means that the diagnosis or treatment was correct. An ill individual could have been cured because or in spite of the treatment or coincidentally, or because of his belief in getting cured. Therefore, pharmacotherapy among the aged should maintain especially high methodological and ethical standards. It is not to be practiced in isolation: psychological and sociological treatment standards are becoming important integral elements of psychogeriatric therapy.

Another basic problem is the early detection of mental disorders in the aged. Not only functional disorders can be treated and reversed if they are detected early enough. The urgent task of future psychogeriatric research is to detect and diagnose the disease in its early stages.

Yet another issue needing resolution is the still prevalent separation of treatment and care, both conceptually and organizationally. Because of this situation, the necessary cooperation and coordination between treatment and rehabilitative measures in geriatrics and especially in psychogeriatrics fails to materialize. All rehabilitation measures should be considered integral components of psychogeriatric treatment.

The guaranteed provision of necessary geriatric care depends upon the presence of many varied "lines of defense." The geriatric hospital, the last line of defense in this string of structures, should not be used for long-term purposes. Preferable for long-term care are the ambulatory clinics and day hospitals which must be further developed. Assessment units could serve as connecting links between institutions providing more comprehensive care. All medical and social services must maintain effective cooperation.

The provision of adequate care for the demented and those severely in need of nursing care will take precedence in the future. Developing the adequate bases for this task is one of the greatest challenges that gerontological and geriatric research is facing today.

INDEX

A

Abnormal brain aging
  cortical flow and global metabolic measures in, 152–153
  etiology of, 149–150
Abrams, M., 221
Acalculia, 323
Accidents, mortality by age from, 98, 99
Acetylcholinesterase, *see also* CSF acetylcholinesterase
Active physiotherapy
  in elderly, 418–419
  prerequisites for, 419
Activities of daily living (ADL)
  in FAST stages, 315–317
  index, 426, 427
  in senile dementia, 273, 274
Acute cerebral hemorrhage, treatment of, 301
Acute confusion, mortality in, 114–115
Adaptation, to distress, 510
Adaptive mechanisms, in critically ill, 522–523
Adjustment
  aging and, 78–79
  disorders, 91–92
Admission, to geriatric psychiatry unit, 138–143
Affective disorders
  cerebral pathology, 234
  diagnostic protocol, 143
  in elderly, 113
  outcome over time, 114
  somatic illness and, 116
  symptoms, AD, 329
  treatment and management, 145
African culture
  initiation processes in, 61
  role of old in, 59
Age-related cerebral disorders
  biochemical markers, 174–180
  direct study, 180–186
  problems in diagnosis, 173
  techniques to study, 172–193
Age structure in Europe, development of, 216
"Ageism," 377, 394–395
Age-related disorders, holistic approach to, 526–527
Aging
  basic problems of, 82
  biopsychosocial stresses of, 82–83
  brain CT, 180–181
  CNS, 148
  definition, 49
  in Japan, 251
  major characteristics, 34
  mental health problems, 215; *see also* Depression in late life, Neuroses in late life
  molecular biologic aspects, 12–42
  personality and, 223–226
  process, 220
  psychological adaptation, 393
  real pathology of, 220
  sleep and, 205–207
  sociocultural conditioning, 50–51
  sociologic definition, 47
Aging population, worldwide, 488–489
AGP system, 440, 441

531

Agitation, in AD, 317, 329
Alcohol abuse
  in later life, 224–225
  U.S. lifetime incidence, 87
Alcoholic dementia, 268–269
Alcohol Dependence Scale, 144
Alexander, F., 101
Alexander's psychodynamic theory, 101
Allelochemicals, cancer and aging, 15–16
Alterations, random and nonrandom, 30
Altered brain function, neurochemical markers of, 174–179
Alternative care patterns, costs of, 466–468
Alzheimer, A., 118, 309
Alzheimer's dementia
  depression in, 236
  neuroepidemiology, 217
Alzheimer's disease (AD)
  affective symptoms, 327
  care needs, 327–328
  characteristics and course, 267, 311
  early and late-life, 119
  FAST stages, 312–322
  GABA levels, 178
  immunological function, 178–179
  mortality rate, 321
  multiaxial diagnosis of, 126
  multiinfarct dementia and, 119–121
  pathological changes in, 118–119
  PET study, 161
  philothermal response, 179
  relationship of functional hierarchy to human development, 320
  serum somatomedin in, 178
  somatostatin levels, 178
  vascular factors, 309
  Xenon-133 inhalation test, 156
Alzheimer's Disease and Related Disorders Association (ADRDA), 491–492
Alzheimer's disease support groups, 307, 491–492; see also under specific group
Alzheimer's presenile dementia, diagnosis, 323
Ambulatory ability, in AD patients, 318–319, 325

American Association for Geriatric Psychiatry (AAGP), 493
Aminoacylation, age-related changes, 34
Amnestic syndrome, 276–277
Aneurysm formation, in hypertension, 292
Ancestor worship
  in African societies, 62–63
  aging family and, 61–63
  in Christian denominations, 62
  distinctions in, 63
  in Eastern nations, 62
  original model for, 62
Audiologist, role in geriatric psychiatry unit, 142–143
Anger, in AD, 329
Angiotensin-induced hypertension, in intestinal vessels of rats, 289–290
Animal behavior studies, 52–53
Animal sociology, system social effects, 44
Animation, 422–424
Anticipation of irreversibility, 440
Antidepressant drugs
  affective disorders, 145
  effectiveness, 117
  in elderly, 370–372
  response to, 129–130
Antihypertensive therapy
  animal studies, 300
  cardiovascular complications, 300
  human studies, 300–301
Autoregulation, see also Cerebral blood flow autoregulation
  disturbed, 289
  in hypertensives, 290
  in normotensives, 290
Anxiety
  etiology in elderly, 89–90
  pain and, 509
Anxiety disorders
  characteristics of, 89
  substance abuse and, 89
  types of, 89–90
Anxiety neurosis, in elderly, 86–87
Aretaeus of Cappadocia, 308
Aristotle, 66
Art therapy, 425
Arteriosclerosis, mortality by age, 98, 99

Index

Arteriosclerosis of brain vessels, CBF and energy metabolism, 152
Arteriosclerotic dementia, diagnosis, 267
Ascorbate, oxygen detoxification by, 15, 16
Ascorbic acid reqirements, in elderly, 351
"Aspiration framework," 69
Assertiveness training, in elderly, 381
Associations, *see under specific association*
Attending personnel, psychology of, 414–415
Attitudes toward health, factors, 412
Awake-confused state, 264
Awareness, coherent thought and, 263

B

Ba, A. H., 61
Baboons, social organization, 52
Balance of care, 464
Barbiturates
  side effects, 368
  use of, 369
Bartlett, 220
Bathing and toileting, in AD, 316, 317
Bedsore prevention, 418
Behavior therapy, 381–383
  assertiveness training, 381
  in chronic hospitalized patients, 388
  cognitive approach, 381–382
  of depression, 385
  desensitizing, 381
  of elderly, 395
  environmental changes in, 382–383
  operant techniques, 381
"Being moved," 101
Benefit of care, definition, 469
Benzodiazepines, pharmacokinetics, 369–370
Bereavement, depression and, 230
Bierer, J., 433
Binswanger's disease, 268
Biogerontology, study of life-span and, 10
Biological aging
  characteristics, 47, 363–364
  equilibrium, 47

life expectancy and, 9
Biosocial organization
  of baboons, 52
  survival and, 51–52
  of wild fowl, 653
Bipolar affective illness, in old age, 242–243
Blessed, G., 112–114
Bleuler, M., 115, 218
Blindness, in elderly, 390
Blood–brain barrier (BBB), hypertension and, 290, 291
Blood flow in the brain
  blood pressure and, 287
  schematic representation, 286–287
Blood pressure, brain blood flow and, 286–287
Blood sedimentation rate (BSR), CBFR autoregulation and, 299
Bobath's techniques, 419
Body composition, in elderly, 355–356
Body mass, aging and, 355
"Body preoccupation," psychosomatic effects, 97–98
Body water composition
  age-related changes, 363
  body weight and, 356
Body weight, age-related changes, 363
Boist, M., 485
Brain biopsy, for AD, 165
Brain changes, structural aging, 149
Brain circulation, factors in, 285
Brain damage, depression and, 234–236
Brain failure, as medical problem, 339
Brain function, *see also* Altered brain function
  tests of, 338
Brain pathology, mental functioning and, 112
"Breakthrough," 289, 290
Brief Cognitive Rating Scale (BCRS), 311–312
Brief therapy, for dying, 506
Buddhism, foundations of, 65

C

Calcium requirements, in elderly, 351–352

Cameron, D. E., 433
Cancer, elimination, life-span effects, 8–10
Capping, hnRNA, 23
Carbon dioxide baths, 419
Cardiac illnesses, mental deterioration in, 345
Cardiovascular diseases
 delirium and, 256
 elimination of, life-span effects, 8–10
Caregiver's distress, 510–511
"Catego" diagnosis, 122
Catego program, 131
Cause of death, in different age groups, 98, 99
Cell transplants, survival of, 4, 6
Central nervous system (CNS)
 in aging, 148
 delirium and, 256
Cerebral aging, definition, 149–150
Cerebral blood flow
 autoregulation, see Cerebral blood flow autoregulation
 in CVD, 295–297
 defects, 166
 determinants, 285
 in healthy adults, 285
 measures, 154, 156
 patterns, 150, 151
Cerebral blood flow autoregulation
 in animals, 289–290
 brain damage and, 296
 determinants, 289
 in hypertension, 288–289
 impairment, 289
 mechanisms, 287–288
Cerebral circulation, blood pressure and, 285–288
Cerebral disease, paraphrenia and, 118
Cerebral function, diet and, 356
Cerebral ischemia, in elderly, 148
Cerebral glucose consumption (CMRglc), in normal aging, 150–152
Cerebral glucose flow, PET studies, 159–160
Cerebral hemisphere diseases, impairment categories, 260
Cerebral hemorrhage, in hypertensives and normotensives, 292, 295

Cerebral imaging techniques
 cognitive function and, 182
 direct study of brain, 180–186
Cerebral infarction
 differential diagnosis, 325
 dysautoregulation index and, 296, 298
Cerebral metabolic rate, PET study, 159
Cerebral metabolic rate for glucose (CMRglc), PET study, 184
Cerebral metabolic rate for oxygen (CMR_{O_2})
 early study, 183
 in normal aging, 150
 PET study, 183
Cerebral metabolism
 age and, 166
 delirium and, 257
Cerebral oxygen flow, PET study, 160–161
Cerebrospinal fluid (SCF), neurochemical markers of altered brain function in, 174–179
Cerebrospinal fluid acetylcholinesterase
 in AD, 175, 176
 dementia and, 175–176
 electrical stimulation effects on, 175
 in normal subjects, 175
Cerebrotoxic substances, 234–235
Cerebrovascular dementia, Xenon-133 inhalation study of, 156
Cerebrovascular disease (CVD)
 blood pressure and, 293–294
 chronic stage, treatment, 301–302
 hypertension in, 285
 in manic depressives, 115–116
 mortality, by age, 98–99
Change, capacity for, 48–49
Character changes, in elderly, 224
Child–parent support, 68
Choline acetyltransferase, in AD, 176
Cholinesterases
 in AD, 175
 types and distinction, 174
Christianity, view of elderly in, 66–67
Chronic brain syndrome, depression and, 236
Chronic drug intoxication, dementia and, 265, 266

Chronic hospitalized patients, therapy for, 387–389
Chronic ischemia, in dementia, 160–162
Chronic respiratory diseases, mortality by age, 99
Chronicity, rehabilitation and, 411
Cicero, 66
Clans, role of elderly in, 59
Classical psychosomatics, principle of, 96
Classification of psychiatric disorders in later life, 109–135
Classification systems
 in geriatric psychiatry, 121–126
 multiaxial, 122–123
Clustan Program, 442
Clinical diagnosis, reference diagnosis and, 130–132
Clinical epidemiology, 218–219
Clomethiazole, pharmacokinetics of, 369
"Closed-to-self" personality, 103
Clouding of consciousness, 253–254
Codex Hammurabi, 56
Condon Restriction Theory, 33–34
Cognitive decline in dementia
 characteristics of, 261, 262
 degree of, 493–494
 rating, 493–494
Cognitive functioning
 in AD, 314–317
 tests, 264
"Cognitive restructuration," 79
Cognitive Theory of Aging, 389–390
Cohen, M., 420
Coinvestigation, definition, 477
Comatose state, in AD, 326
Communications technology, elderly and, 489–490
Complex adaptive systems, aging and, 49
Compliance
 of elderly, 368
 factors in, 372–373
 improvement, 372
Computed tomography (CT) brain scan
 CBF measures, 156
 cerebral atrophy and, 181–182

in demented and control patients, 182
 description of, 180
 in normal aging, 180–181
 use, 143, 325
Computed tomography-derived brain atrophy index, 181
Computers, implications for elderly, 489–490
Confusional states
 factors affecting, 343–344
 management, 343
 in physical illness, 342–343
 somatic causes, 129
Consciousness, definition, 253
Constructional apraxia, in dementia, 262
Continence, in AD, 316–318; see also Incontinence, Bathing and toileting
Continuity of treatment, in day hospital, 435
Control, dying patient's need for, 507–508
Coping
 health and, 102
 mechanisms, 102
 style, 104
Core data, description, 482
Cortical flow
 in abnormal aging, 152–153
 blood pressure and, 296, 297
 in normal aging, 150–152
 studies, 153–155
Cortical sulcal width, during senescence, 181
Cosmological cycle, 59–61
Cost-benefit analysis
 description, 457–458
 in geriatric day hospital, 457
 of health services, 470
Cost-effectiveness analysis
 in day hospital, 438–439
 description, 455
 of health services, 470
 studies, 455–456
"Costing care," problems of, 468
Creutzfeldt-Jakob disease (CJD)
 CBF in, 152
 dementia and, 269
 differential diagnosis, 345

occurrence and presentation, 326
PET in, 162, 164
signs and symptoms, 326
Criminal tendencies, in later life, 224
Crisis intervention, in day hospital, 434
Critical Flicker Fusion Test, 238
Cross-discipline research, 485
Cross-links, 31
Cryogenic cell storage, cell viability and, 5
Cultural leadership function, of elderly in nonliterate society, 58–59
Culture, social organization and, 56
Cyclothymia, day hospital care, 436, 437

D

Darwin, C., 52
Day Hospital of the Rheinische Landesklinik Köln, 434–435
Day hospital care, 438–447
Deafness
affective disorders and, 117
paraphrenia, and, 117, 245
de Ajuriaguerra, J., 420
Death
causes of, 7–9
counseling and psychotherapy in, 505–506
learning to accept, 518–524
medical view of, 524
separation and, 504
Death with dignity, 523–524
Death-related anxiety
in men and women, 512
reduction of, 512–513
Defense mechanisms
in critically ill, 522–523
physiologic response, 102
Degenerative brain conditions, dementia in, 269
Dehydration
confusional disorders and, 343–344
in elderly, 352
Delirium in the aged
clinical course, 255
clinical features, 254
disorders causing, 256

DSM-III definition, 253
etiology, 253–254, 258
medications in, 258
occurrence, 251
pathogenesis, 255
subtypes, 254
treatment, 257–259
Deluded psychotic depressives, management, 241
Dementia, see also Senile dementia
care for, 339, 528–529
cerebral degeneration in, 261
clinical course, 260–263
clinical features, 259–260
cognitive changes, 261, 262
definition, 307
delirium in, 261
depression and, 262, 263
diagnosis of, 131, 307, 345
DSM-III definition, 259
early features, 261
in elderly, 113
ergotherapy in, 422
etiology, 265–269
head trauma and, 268
hemodynamic and metabolic approaches to, 148–171
MSE in, 263–264
normal pressure hydrocephalus and, 266–267
onset, 260
personality changes, 262–263
psychopharmacological approaches in, 275–276
psychotropic management, 276
remedial causes, 265–266
reversibility, 259
somatic causes, 129
stages, 261–263
treatment and management, 145, 275–276
unusual case, 268
Dementia syndrome, psychiatric disorders with, 269–271
Dementia syndrome of depression
in AD, 234
diagnosis, 233
presentation, 233
Dementia protocol, 143
Demography, health care resources and, 470–471

Dental state, diet and, 356
[18] F-2 Deoxy-D-glucose (FDG) positron emission tomography study, 184–185
Dependency
  caretaker and, 414–415
  on therapist, 378
"Depletion anxiety," 78
Depression, *see also* Unipolar depression
  age of onset, 232
  brain damage and, 234–236
  cerebral changes, 232
  cognitive impairment, 238
  differential diagnosis, 325
  in elderly, *see* Depression in late life
  hypochondriasis and, 90
  in Japan, 237
  learning and acquisition in, 234
  life events and, 237–238
  MAO activity and, 238
  multiinfarct dementia, 121
  predisposition, 236
  prognosis, 239–240, 242
  pseudodementia in, 270
  psychotherapy versus pharmacotherapy in, 241
  rehabilitation, 412–413
  sleep analysis in, 201, 203
Depression in late life
  diagnosis, 229
  occurrence, 84–86, 115–116, 228–232, 370
Depression scales, 236; *see also under specific scale*
Depressive neurosis, *see* Dysthymic disorder
Depressive pseudodementia
  occurrence of, 116–117
  organic-functional continuum of, 232–233
  use of term, 232
Depressive syndromes, therapy, 384–386
Descartes, 96
Desensitization, in elderly, 381, 392
Devaluation, of elderly, 70, 71
Development, sociocultural, 50–51
Developmental tasks, of late life, 79–80

Deviant personality, age-related changes, 223–224
Deoxyglucose PET scan, 162–164
Dexamethasone Suppression Test (DST), 143, 233
Diabetes
  mortality by age, 99, 100
  in psychogeriatric patients, 344
Diagnosis
  day hospital care and, 436
  reliability of, 452
Diagnostic Interview Schedule (DIS), 87, 138
Diagnostic laboratory tests, 342
Diagnostic process, steps in, 450–451
Diagnostic protocols, in geriatric psychiatry, 143–144
Diagnostic Related Groups (DRG), 496
Diagnostic and Statistical Manual of Mental Disorders, Third Edition (DSM-III)
  neurotic disease diagnosis, 127
  OBS classification, 252–253
  operational definition, 87–90
  use of, 130, 132
Dialysis dementia, 268
Diastolic hypertension, stroke and, 294
Diazepam, pharmacokinetics, 370
Diet, elderly, 349
Dietary fiber requirement, elderly, 352
Dietary habits, 352–353
Dietary surveys, 353
Differentiation, of multicellular organisms, 122
Digoxin, pharmacokinetics in elderly, 366
Disability, rehabilitation and, 415
Disablement of the senses, 390
Discharge, of geriatric patients, 146
Disease elimination, life-span effects, 12
Disease staging, purpose, 311
Disorders of initiating and maintaining sleep (DIMS), 194
Dissatisfaction, among interdisciplinary team members, 481
Distress, caregiver, 510–511

Disturbed states of wakefulness, 263–264
Division of labor, in human society, 56
DNA
  age-dependent changes in, 17–19
  injury to, 15–16
  organization of, 18
  repair systems, 15, 17
DNA damage
  aging and, 32
  gene realization effects, 14, 15
  oxygen radicals in, 14–15
  protective mechanisms against, 35–36
DNA lesions, consequences, 17
DNA polymerases, age-dependent changes, 18
DNA sequence, of cells, 13–14
Dominance orders, 53
Dopamine-β-hydroxylase levels
  in AD, 176–177
  in aging, 176
Down's syndrome of middle age, 323
Dressing, in AD, 316
Drug absorption, in elderly, 364
Drug Abuse Screening Test, 144
Drug elimination, in elderly, 365–366
Drug epidemiology, 219
"Drug holidays," 344
Drug intoxication, paraphrenia and, 118
Drug metabolism, in elderly, 365–366
Drug therapy, in geriatric medicine, 362–376, 526–527
Drug volume distribution, in elderly, 364
Dyads, research on, 45–46
Dying patient
  contact and conversation with, 519–520
Dysautoregulation index
  in cerebral infarction and controls, 296, 298
  and duration after cerebral infarction, 296, 298
  multivariate analysis of factors, 299
Dysthymic disorder
  in elderly, 88–89
  features, 88
  presentation, 88
  U.S. lifetime incidence, 81
control in, 507–508
doctor's role, 520–521
neglect of, 518
needs and wants, 504–508
preparing people to work with, 509–515
spouse's role, 505

E

Early-onset depression, 239–240
Economic evaluation of health care, 454–470
Education for death, 503–517
Effectiveness, need for study of, 451
Elderly, see also Aging
  adjustment disorders in, 91–92
  common characteristics, 373, 408
  diversity in, 75
  neuroses and, 85–90; see also Neuroses in late life
  self-image, 43
  sleep disorders in, 498–499
  somatoform disorders in, 90–91
  television characterization, 497
"Eldership complex," 62
Electroconvulsive therapy (ECT)
  for depression, 128, 240
  effectiveness, 241–242
  use, 145
Electroencephalogram (EEG), use of, 195–196
Electroencephalogram sleep variables, 201
Electrolyte imbalance, in confusional states, 344
Electromyogram (EMG), use of, 195–197
Electrooculogram (EOG), 195–197
Emotional factors, in death, 513
Emotional lability, in AD, 316, 329
Emotional pain, in terminally ill, 508–509
Endoribonuclease VII, development and characteristics, 25–26
Energy requirements
  of elderly, 349–350
  in healthy males aged 30–80, 350
  protein metabolism and, 350–351
Energy transduction
  nucleoside triphosphatase in, 27–28

Index

poly A (+) mRNA molecule effects on, 27–28
Environmental change, and behavior therapy of aged, 382–383
"Environmental docility," 220, 413
Environmental support, in delirium management, 257
Enzymes, age-related changes in, 30, 33, 363
Epidemiology
  description, 219–220
  of neuroses in later life, 86–87
Ergotherapy, 421–422
Erikson, E., 79–80
Error Catastrophe Theory, 17, 32–33
Essen-Moller, 122, 123
Esquirol, J. E. D., 309, 310
Estrogen, NTPase activity and, 28
Eukaryotic cells, development and aging in, 13
Evaluation of psychiatric services, 451–453
"Exchange," as social gerontology concept, 67–69, 71
Exclusion of stimuli, 78
Exogenous toxins, delirium and, 255–257
Experience
  memory and, 58
  survival and, 53–54
Extended life course initiation model, 61

F

Factor X, 101
Falling, fear in elderly, 392
Family history, in depression, 117
Family therapy, 380
Fasting blood sugar (FBS), CBF autoregulation and, 299
Fecal incontinence, in AD, 316–317, 325
Feighner criteria, 130, 132
First night effect (FNE), 204
Fertility-mortality system, 51
Flooding, use of, 381
Foundation for Grandparenting, 492–493
Fragmentation, of disciplines, 485
Freese, A. S., 308

Freud, S., 377, 522
Fulfillment, conditioning of, 50–51
Functional assessment staging
  for AD, 312–313, 321–322
  deficits in, 320
  in dementia differential diagnosis, 323–326
  items in, 313
  nonordinality, 324
  in normal aging, 313, 321, 322
  in severe dementia staging, 322–323
  stage 1, 314
  stage 2, 314
  stage 3, 314–315
  stage 4, 315
  stage 5, 316
  stage 6, 316–317
  stage 7, 317–320
  use, 312, 323
Functional ergotherapy, 421–422
Functional measure of rehabilitation, 426
Functional mental illness, 110–111
Fungal meningitis, dementia and, 265, 266
Functional psychiatric disorders in old age, 223–250

G

Gait, in AD, 318
Gajdusek, C., 217
Galen, 308
Gamma amino butyric acid (GABA) levels, 178
Gene expression
  control of, 31
  in multicellular eukaryotes, 29
Gene realization, DNA damage, 14, 15
General psychiatry, cost-benefit study of, 458–459
"Geriatric" drugs
  clinical studies, 367
  definition, 362
  use, 366–367
Geriatric medicine
  objectives, 342
  problems, 408
Geriatric psychiatry
  home visits, 137–138

multidimensional assessment, 136–147
nursing care, 139–140
setting for, 137
team approach, 136–137
Geriatric psychiatry unit
admission to, 138–143
audiologist's role, 142–143
discharge and follow up, 146
efficiency and efficacy, 146–147
nutritionist's role, 142
occupational therapist's role, 141
pharmacist's role, 141–142
preadmission assessment, 137–138
psychologist's role, 141
physiotherapists role, 142
size of, 138
social worker's role, 140–141
Geriatrics
research, 475, 495
resident-fellowship programs, 495
self-theory and, 69–70
Germ cells, aging, 12–13
Gerontological research, 525
Gerontology
research directions, 8–9
social dimensions, 43–74
Gerosociology
description, 44
systems approach, 48–49
theoretical elements, 45–48
Global Deterioration Scale, 311, 329, 493–495
Global metabolic measurements
in abnormal aging, 152–153
in normal aging, 150–152
Global rehabilitation
aim, 409–410
efficacy, measures, 426
techniques, 416
Grandparents, role, 492
"Granny-proof" packages, 372
Grasp reflex, in AD, 319
Great Britain, expenditures on elderly, 449
Group research, definition, 476–478
Group therapy
in aged, 228, 379–380
for depressive syndrome, 385
in OBS, 386
in senile psychotics, 380
in stroke patients, 392
Guilt, in relatives of disabled, 393

H

Haan, N., 103
Haber-Weiss reaction, 15
Hahn, U., 519
Hallucinations, 254
Hamilton Depression Scale, 236
Happiness, human development and, 49
Hasegawa's Dementia Scale
description, 265, 272
validity and reliability, 264
Head trauma, dementia and, 268
Health care, over life-span, 5–6
Health self-evaluation, 389
Hearing aids, use of, 426
Hearing impairment
of elderly, 390
management, 142–143
Heart disease, see also Cardiovascular disease
mortality by age, 98, 99
Heckler, M. M., 308
Hepatic/renal failure, dementia and 265, 266
Heterogeneous nuclear RNA (hnRNA)
capping, 23
particles, 22–23
polyadenylation of, 21
Higher cortical function impairment, in dementia, 260
Hill, T., 27
Histones, age-related changes in, 18
Holter, N. J., 195, 197
Holter recording technology
development, 197–199
playback analysis, 198–199
in sleep, 198
Home care
benefit of, 395, 465–466
costs, 456–457, 465–466
Home visits, in geriatric psychiatry, 138–139
Homovanillic acid, in CSF of AD patients, 177
Hospice care, of terminally ill, 508–509

Index

Hospital care, cost-benefit study of, 459–461
Hospital malnutrition, in elderly, 354
Hospitalization, health risk, 413–414
Human longevity, 3–11
Human personality, society and, 50
Human survival curves
  by country, 4
  rectangularization, 3, 5–8
5-Hydroxyindoleacetic acid, in CSF of AD patients, 177
Hypnotic medication, use in elderly, 368–369
Hypercapnia, vasodilator response in aging, 154, 155
Hyperlipidemic dementia, 268
Hyperparathyroidism, symptoms, 345
Hypertension
  cardiac function and, 293
  CBF autoregulation in, 288–289
  in CVD, CBF effects, 295–299
  lacunar state of brain in, 292–293
  pathological cerebral vessel, changes, 293, 294
  as a risk factor, 293–295
  stroke and, 285–305
  treatment, 300–302
  vascular arteriosclerotic changes, 292
Hypertensive encephalopathy
  blood–brain barrier damage, 291
  clinical symptoms, 291–292
  description, 290
  development, mechanism, 290–291
  treatment, 301
Hypochondriasis
  characteristics, 90–91
  depression and, 90, 232
  in elderly, 90–91
Hypotensive drugs
  for acute stage cerebral hemorrhage or infarction, 302
  for chronic stage of stroke, 301–302
  for hypertensive encephalopathy, 301
Hypothesis of aging and life maintenance processes, 34–36
Hypothyroidism, dementia and, 265, 266
Hysterics, symptomatology in later life, 227

I

Iatrogenic effects, of drugs, 219
Illness, psychological effects, 83
Immobilization syndrome, symptoms, 410
Immunologic function, in AD, 178–179
Impairment, rehabilitation and, 415
Incest, 55–57
Incontinence, *see also* Bathing and toileting, fecal incontinence
  management, 417
  therapy, 391
Individual psychotherapy
  in aged, 379
  in depression, 385
  poststroke, 392
Individual research, 477, 480–481
Infanticide, 65
Influenza and pneumonia, mortality by age for, 99
Inferior orbitomeatal line, PET scans and regions of interest above, 158
Information transfer, elderly and, 53–55
Ingratitude, in modern society, 68
Initiation processes, in African culture, 61
Insomnia
  age-related, 498
  etiology, 498
  evaluation, 207–208
  occurrence, 194
  treatment, 498–499
Institutions, for elderly care, 408–409
Instrumental activities of daily living, 426, 427
Interdisciplinary collaboration
  definition, 477
  levels, 478
  research and, 475
  results, 485
  team development, 479–480
Internal medicine, psychogeriatrics and, 337–348
International Classification of Disease-9, 125
International Classification of Disease-10, 125

International Psychogeriatric Association (IPA), 493
Interpersonal relationships, of dying person, 504
Interpersonal therapy, in depression, 241
Intervening sequence (intron), 22, 25
Intracellular compartmentalization, description, 13
Introversion, aging and, 77–78
Involution depression, day hospital care for, 436–438
Iron requirement, in elderly, 352
Irritability, in AD, 329
Isolation, depression and, 231

J

Jakob-Creutzfeldt disease, see Creutzfeldt-Jakob disease
Judaism, view of elderly in, 66–67

K

Kinesitherapy, 418
Kinship system, ancestor worship and, 63
Kline, B., 523–524
Kohut, H., 80–82
Kornhaber, A., 492
Korsakov's disease, 268, 276–277
Kraeplin, 309
Kraepelinian system, 122
Kramer, M., 216
Kübler-Ross, E., 522

L

Lacunar state of brain, 292–293
Language therapy, 424–425
Late life
  developmental tasks, 79–80
  normal psychology, 77–79
  psychological disorders in, 84–85
Late-onset depression, 239; see also Depression
Late paraphrenia, see also Paraphrenia
  predisposing factors, 243–244
  schizophrenia and, 117, 118
Lazarus, R. S., 102
Lean body mass, calculation/definition, 355
Learned helplessness, 412
Levine, M., 417
Libow, L., 495–496
Life expectancy, changes in, 8–9
Life phases, social evaluation, 43
Life satisfaction, depression and, 230
Life Satisfaction Index (LSI), 440
Life-span
  factors affecting, 3–6
  morbidity and, 98–100
  schizophrenia over, 127–128
Lifetime Drinking History, 144
Lithium
  for depression, 242
  for manic disorders, 243
  response to, 130
  use, 145
Lipofuscin, development, 30–31
Living situation, analysis of, 437, 438
Living will, 341
Locomotor behavior, increasing, 384
London Psychogeriatric Scale (LPGS), 140
Longevity, in human culture, 57–58
Long-stay geriatric hospitals, relative costs, 465–466
Long-term care
  elderly in, 75
  psychogeriatric rehabilitation and, 429
Long-term research, 484–485
Loneliness
  in aged, 394
  anxiety and depression, 504
Loss, sociopsychological definition, 47
Ludotherapy, 420
Luszki, M. B., 475, 476

M

Major depressive disorder, U.S. lifetime incidence of, 87
Major tranquilizers, in late paraphrenia management, 245
Malignant neoplasms, mortality by age for, 98, 99

Malnutrition, in elderly, 353–354, 357
Manic depression, in late life, 115–116
Manic disorders, 242–243
Maprotaline, pharmacokinetics, 371
Marginal analysis, description, 461–467
Marginal benefit
  description, 461
  of social services, 462–463
Marginal cost
  description, 461
  of social services, 462–464
Marital relationships, in later life, 46
Martin, L. J., 379
Mass lesions, dementia and, 265, 266
Massage, precautions, 19
Mattis Dementia Rating Score, 185
Maturity
  biosocial function and, 54
  definition, 48
Maximum life-span potential (MLP), 34–35
Meals-on-Wheels, marginal costs and benefit of, 462–464
Mean arterial blood pressure (MABP)
  CBF and, 286–289, 290, 299
  mean cortical blood flow and, 297
Medical admission protocol, for geriatric psychiatry patients, 139
Medical care, computer-assisted, 490
Medical treatment of psychogeriatric patients
  ethical/moral issues, 340–341
  family decisions in, 341
Medication, *see also under specific drug and drug type*
  causing delirium, 257, 258
  in dementia management, 259
Memory
  in dementia, 234, 260
  readaptation, 425
Mental disorders in aged
  diagnosis and management, 528–529
  factors contributing to, 496–497
  with medical/surgical conditions, 251
  natural history, 110–112, 128–129
  occurrence, 109–112
  outcome, 111, 112, 218
  potentially reversible, 343
Mental State Questionnaire (MSQ), 140
Mental Status Examination, in dementia, 263–264
Messenger RNA (mRNA)
  intranuclear and intracytoplasmic transport and metabolism, 19–20
  transcription, 21
Metabolic disorders, organic affective syndrome, 277, 278
Metchnikoff, E., 503
Milieu therapy, 380
Mind–body interaction, 338–342
Mini Mental State Examination (MMSE), 140
Mixed function oxidases, in elderly, 365–366
Mobility, of elderly, 390–391
Model of Hierarchical Rank-Variance Analysis, 441
Molecular biology of aging, 12–42
Monoamine oxidase activity, depression and, 230
Monoamine oxidase inhibitors (MAOI), use, 145
Morbidity, life-span and, 98–100
Mortality
  in AD, 321
  mental disorders in old age and, 85, 111–115
Mosaic Decalogue, 56
Motivation, rehabilitation and, 413
Motor animation, 420
Movement therapy, 420
Multiaxial diagnosis
  "classification," 125–126
  correlation and validity, 126
  DSM-III, 123–126
Multidimentional assessment, in geriatric psychiatry, 136–147
Multidimensional diagnostics, 527
Multidimensional Observation Scale for Elderly Subjects (MOSES), 140
Multidisciplinary research, 477
Multiinfarct dementia
  with AD, 120
  atypical cases, 120–121
  CBF in, 152

in cerebral aging, 149–150
depression with, 121, 235
diagnosis, 267–268
diagnostic criteria, 120
differential diagnosis, 119
global metabolism in, 153
hypertension and, 119
PET scan of, 161, 163, 164
Multimorbid patients, management, 338
Musculoskeletal control, in AD, 319
Music therapy, for aged, 384, 425
Myocardial infarction, therapy in, 391

N

Narcissistic investment, self-psychology and, 82
National Hospice Demonstration Study, 505
Natural death, 7–8
Need for health care, 453–454
Needs, of dying patients, 520–521
Neuroepidemiology, 217–218
Neuroleptic drugs
  effects, 114
  response, 130
  for schizophrenia, 127
  use, 146
Neurologic disorders
  differential diagnosis, 345–346
  organic affective syndrome and, 277, 278
Neuropharmacology, of AD brain, 329
Neuroses
  diagnostic protocols, 144
  treatment and management, 146
Neuroses in late life
  characteristics, 85
  concomitant disorders, 85–86
  diagnosis, 87–90
  vs. early life, 226–227
  epidemiologic considerations, 86–87
  etiologic factors, 84–85
  presentation, 85–86, 92
  psychodynamic factors, 84
Neurosurgical shunt, for normal pressure hydrocephalus, 267

Neurotic depression in elderly
  atypical presentation, 85–86
  endogenous vs. reactive, 231
  occurrence of, 86–87
Neurotransmitter deficiency, in dementia, 150
Neurotransmitter levels, in AD brain, 176
New scientific disciplines, 485
Nomifensine, 238
Nonanalytical psychotherapies, 386
Noncompliance
  adverse drug effects and, 373
  causes, 372
Nonhistone chromatin proteins, age-related changes in, 18
Nonhistone mRNA biosynthesis, processing steps in, 21, 22
Noninvasive CBF measurements, 153–164
Nonparametric U-test, 440
Nonrandom alterations, causes, 30–31
NonREM sleep, 195, 206
"Nootropic" drugs, use, 367–368
Noradrenergic neuronal systems, in AD, 177
Normal aging
  cortical flow and global metabolic measurement, 150–152
  defining, 75
  models, 75
Normal human development, FAST stage deficits and, 320
Normal neuroticism of old age, 394
Normal pressure hydrocephalus
  dementia with, 265–267
  diagnosis and management, 267
Normal psychology of late life, 77–79
Nortriptyline, pharmacokinetics, 371
Nuclear magnetic resonance imaging (NMRI) of brain
  in AD, 180, 183
  use, 325
Nuclear pore complexes, 26
Nucleoside triphosphatase (NTPase)
  activity, 28
  energy transduction, 27
Nursing care
  in delirium management, 258
  for geriatric psychiatry patients, 139–140

rehabilitation and, 416–418
Nursing homes
  funding, 496
  as training and research centers, 495–496
Nutrition and the elderly, 349–361; see also Diet
  diet and, 349–356
  public health aspects, 356–357
  social factors, 357
  specific aspects, 358
Nutrition-immunity interactions, 356
Nutritionist, role in geriatric psychiatry unit, 142

O

Obesity in elderly
  etiologic and pathological factors, 354–355
  mortality and, 354
  social factors, 355
  treatment, 355
Obsessional symptoms, in old age, 227
Occupational therapist, role in geriatric psychiatry unit, 141
Old age, Western attitudes toward, 66–67
Old-old, definition, 75
"Open-to-self" personality, 103
Operant techniques, use, 381
Opportunity costs, 461
Organic affective syndrome, 277–278
Organic brain dysfunction, in medically ill, 342
Organic brain syndrome (OBS), 251–284
  classification, 252–253
  definition, 252
  subcategories, 253–277
  therapy, 386–387
Organic disorders, age-based, 526
Organic mental disorders
  day hospital care, 436
  dementias and, 260, 338
  diagnostic criteria, 128–130
  early causes, 128
  mortality, 111
  in old age, 110

Orgel, L. E., 17
Orthostatic hypertension (OH), CBF autoregulation and, 299
Osteomalacia, in elderly, 351
Output of service, evaluation and measurement, 468–470
"Overbalance," 67–69
Oxygen detoxification, 15–16
Oxygen radicals, DNA damage by, 14–15
^{15}Oxygen steady state technique, 183

P

Pacing, in AD, 329
Paranoid illness
  definition, 244
  of later life, 224
Paranoid psychoses
  day hospital care, 436, 437
  diagnostic protocol, 144
  etiology, 244–245
  symptomatology, 243–244
  treatment, 245
Paraphrenia
  diagnostic protocol, 144
  somatic association, 117–118
  treatment and management, 145–146
Parkinson's disease
  AD and, 329
  CSF markers, 174
  dementia in, 174
Passive psychotherapy, 419
Pathological grief, therapy for, 385–386
Patient associations, 393
Patient-care personnel, attitudes of, 414–415
Patient care plan, nurse's role, 417
Pearl, R., 5
Perfusin pressure of the brain, factors in, 286
Personality
  aging and, 77
  dementia and, 260, 262, 263
  deviations in, 223–226
  rehabilitation and, 413
  in team research, 479–480
  view of, 70

Personality disorders
　diagnostic protocol, 144
　treatment and management, 146
Personality organization
　development, 104
　of Haan, 103
　in men and women, 103
　stability over time, 103
　types of, 103–104
Personality style, aging and, 77
Personality typology
　empirical support for, 102–103
　health and, 100
Personnel issues, in interdisciplinary team, 484
Pharmacist, role in geriatric psychiatry unit, 141–142
Pharmacodynamic factors, age-related changes, 363–364
Pharmacotherapy
　delirium and, 257, 258
　in geriatrics, 527
Philothermal response, in AD, 179
Phobic disorder
　development, 227
　therapy, 386
　treatment, 228
　U.S. lifetime incidence, 87
Phosphofructokinase (PFK), sudden death and, 152, 153
Physical decline, and mental health in aging, 85
Physical disability
　differential diagnosis, 325
　in elderly, 389
　management, 390
Physical exercise
　calcium requirements, 351–352
　energy metabolism, 350
Physical health, geriatric problems, 139
Physical pain, in terminal illness, 508–509
Physical/spiritual aspects of life, 61
Physical therapy
　approach to, 418
　in cardiac patients, 391
　with psychotherapeutic elements, 420–421
Physiological support, in delirium management, 257
Physiotherapist, in geriatric care, 142

Physiotherapy
　active, 418–419
　desensitization, 392
　passive, 419
　psychotherapeutic elements, 420–421
Piaget, J., 478
Pick's disease
　CBF in, 152
　PET study of, 161–162, 164
　Xenon-133 inhalation study, 156
Planning of services, 450–451
Plasma protein binding, in elderly, 364–365
Plasticity, in life course, 56, 57
Plum, F., 217
Polyadenylic acid sequence addition of mRNA, characteristics and age-related changes in, 23–25
Polydrug therapy, in elderly patients, 344, 364–365
Polygraphic recordings
　analysis of, 198–199
　conditions for, 197
Polymorbidity, rehabilitation and, 411
Positron emission tomography (PET) study
　in abnormal aging, 160
　of AD, 161
　and cerebral metabolic rate in different hemispheres, 159
　compounds in, 157
　in dementia, 160
　description, 180
　with 18-fluorodeoxyglucose techniques, 160
　^{11}C-L-methionine, 186
　in normal aging, 157–159
　performance scores on, 185
　in Pick's disease, 161
　for regional blood flow and metabolism, 157–164
　variations in, 157
Poststroke depression, 235–236
Poststroke psychosocial disorders, interventions, 392
Posttranscription, DNA, 21–30
Potassium requirements, in elderly, 352
Preadmission assessment to geriatric psychiatry unit, 137–138
　social worker's role, 140

Present State Examination, 122, 130, 131, 459
Prestige, function of, 54
Preventive medicine, 345
Preventive rehabilitation
 aim, 409
 techniques, 416
Prichard, J. C., 309
Primary degenerative dementia, stages, 493–494
"Principle of self-interest," 67
Problem behaviors, in senile dementia, 275
Problem-centered psychoanalytic therapy, 385
Professionalism, in team research, 479–480
Progesterone, NTPase activity, 28
Prosthetic devices, for elderly, 425–426
Protection
 in biosocial organization, 52–59
 in delirium management, 259
Protective mechanisms, against gene damage, 35–36
Protein fractions, levels in elderly, 363
Protein metabolism, in elderly, 350
Protein requirements, in elderly, 350–351
Protein synthesis, age-related changes, 31
Pseudodementia
 in aging, 232
 depression and, 233, 270
 diagnostic criteria, 269, 271
 features, 270
 frequency, 270
 neuroendocrinological testing, 270
 neuropsychological testing, 270–271
 terminology, 269
Psychiatric Case Register, use of, 452–453
Psychiatric diagnosis
 in late life, 87–90
 operational criteria and, 130
Psychiatric ergotherapy, 421–422
Psychiatric services, impact of, 453
Psychic factors, in physiologic responses, 101
Psychoanalytic therapy, 379–380, 388
"Psychodynamic constellation," 101

Psychogeriatric day hospital
 admission criteria, 441
 advantages, 447
 cluster characteristics, 444, 445
 definition, 432
 description, 436–438
 future of, 433–434
 history, 432–433
 organization and therapy in, 434–435
 patient comparisons, 447, 448
 social variables, 442, 445
 treatment criteria, 434
 treatment evaluation, 438–447
 treatment function, 433–434
Psychogeriatric disorders, epidemiology, 215–222
Psychogeriatric rehabilitation
 medicosocial organization and, 428–429
 origins, 409
Psychogeriatric services, evaluation and effectiveness, 449–472
Psychogeriatrics
 cost-benefit studies, 458
 cost-effectiveness studies, 457
 current developments, 488–500
 decision to treat in, 341–342
 ethical issues 339–340
 interdisciplinary research, 475–487
 in medicine, 337–348, 526
 priority problems, 340–341
Psychological aspects of aging, 75–95
Psychological crises, treatment and management of, 141
Psychological disorders, of later life, 84–85
Psychological problems, and sickness in elderly, 412–415
Psychological regression, cause of, 410–411
Psychological tests, 111, 260; see also under specific test
Psychologist, in geriatric psychiatry unit, 141
Psychometric tests
 in AD, 322
 use, 338–339
Psycho-organic reactions, of psychiatric disorders, 218
Psychopathology
 development of, 81–82

in elderly, 82, 227
Psychosis, early use of term, 113
Psychosocial crises, diagnostic protocol, 144
Psychosocial epidemiology, 219–221
Psychosomatic diseases
  dementia and, 338
  in elderly, 96–105, 226, 526
  over life-span, 97–98
  WHO classification, 97–98
Psychosomatics and geriatrics, common characteristics, 96–97
Psychotherapy
  with aged, 227–228, 277–403
  aims, 378
  for chronic hospitalized patients, 388
  in depression, 241
  doctor competence in, 520–521
  for family, 424
  forms of, 378
  indications, 378
  in rehabilitation, 424
  therapist–patient relationship in, 378–379
Psychotic symptoms
  in AD, 317, 329
  in delirium, 254
  in senile dementia in Japan, 274
Psychotropic drug use
  in dementia, 276
  in elderly, 219

Q

Quail oviduct system, postranscriptional modification process in, 28–29
Quality of care, 469
Quality of life, 339, 342

R

Random alterations, causes, 30
Rapid eye movement (REM)
  definition, 195
  EEG patterns, 200
  sleep, age and, 206
Rating scales, *see under specific scale*

Reactive depression, day hospital care for, 436–437
Reading, computer-assisted, 490
Readmission, of day hospital patients, 446–447
Reality orientation
  for OBS patients, 386–387
  use of, 383
Rechtschaffen und Kales manual, 199
Reciprocity, exchange and, 68
Redlich, E., 309
Reflexiveness, in aging, 49
Regional cerebral flow, of blood and oxygen in gray matter, 162
Regional superficial CBF, 153–154
Rehabilitation
  definition, 407–408
  efficacy, evaluation, 426–427
  external factors, 413–414
  factors, 410–411
  general characteristics, 409–411
  institutions for development, 428–429
  instruments of, 416–426
  interdisciplinary team, 427
  patient and, 415
  personality and motivation in, 412–413
  personalization, 416
  philosophy, 411
  strategy, 415–416
  timing and duration, 411
Reisberg, 115
Relatives, groups for, 393
Relaxation
  techniques, 420
  therapy, 391
Relocation, of paranoid patients, 245
Reminiscing, function of, 83
Remotivation, 383
Renal clearance, drug excretion effects, 365
Reorganization of values, in aging, 78
Replication, 13–19
Research Diagnostic Criteria, 130
Research group, definition, 477
Research methodology, changing, 481–482
Resensitization, in OBS, 387
Resignation, in aging, 412
Retirement, stress and, 97–98

Revitalization, for chronic hospitalized patients, 388
Ritalin Challenge Test, 143
Ritual ambivalence, in traditional societies, 64–65
Reward system, use, 382–383
RNA
  age-dependent changes, 19–21
  damage, protection from, 35–36
  methylation, 23
  polymerases, transcription and, 19
  splicing, 25–30
Roach, M., 308
Role of old
  in animal world, 51–53
  in cosmological society, 59–61
  in human society, 54
  in modernized societies, 63
  in nonliterate societies, 58–59
  in religions, 71
  in traditional societies, 64–65
Role-playing, in death education, 513

S

Sampling overview, of day hospital patients, 439
"Sanyasin," 65
Satellite projects, development and undertaking, 482–483
Saunders, C., 509
Schildkraut hypothesis, 370
Schizophrenia
  age-related changes, 218
  classification, 127
  day hospital care, 436–439
  diagnostic criteria, 127–128
  as paraphrenia precursor, 117
  psychiatric care, costs, 459
Schultz's autogenic training, 420
Scoring criteria, for sleep, 200
Secondary behavioral features of dementia, 275
Seizure states, dementia and, 265–266
Self
  definition, 80
  development, 80–81
Self-actualization, in health care, 469
Self-care
  training, 384
  two-phase plan, 417
Self-esteem
  building, 384, 392–393
  factors in, 390
Self-expression, 70
Self-help, teaching, 418
Self-image
  aging and, 43, 77
  changes, 69–70
  development, 69
Self-induced support for elderly, 69
Self-psychology, aging and, 80–83
Self-reflexiveness, 50–51
Self theory, 69–70
Senescent population, characterization, 217
Senile dementia
  in Japan, *see* Senile dementia in Japan
  mortality in, 114
Senile dementia of the Alzheimer's type (SDAT)
  APA definition, 310
  CBF in, 152
  in cerebral aging, 149–158
  current beliefs on, 309–310
  diagnosis, 323
  global metabolism in, 153
  medical awareness, 306–308
  occurrence of, 267
  phases of, 310
  public awareness, 308–311
  staging, 311–320
Senile dementia in Japan
  ADL and, 272, 274
  epidemiologic study, 271–275
  level of care, 274–275
  prevalence of, 272
  problem behaviors, 275
  psychotic symptoms, 274
Senile dysthymia (or dysphoria)
  diagnostic criteria, 228–229
  etiology, 229–231
  prevalence, 228–229
  treatment, 231
Senile incoherence, 309
Senile paraphrenia, symptomatology, 244
Senile seclusion
  characteristics, 225–226
  mental illness in, 226

Senilicide, 64–65
Senility, definition, 307
Sensorimotor deficits, in dementia, 262–263
Sensory deficits
 geriatric, assessment, 138–139
 in paraphrenia, 117–118
Sensory deprivation, delirium and, 255, 256
Serious illness, threat of, 521
Serum somatomedin level, in AD and normal subjects, 178
Sex, living conditions and diagnosis of day hospital patients, analysis, 437–438
Sexual maladjustment, in late life, 224
Severe hypertension, effect on cerebral vessels and BBB, 289–290
Sharing, in death education, 513
Short-term studies, 485
Simple homeostatic systems, aging and, 49
Sloterdijk, P., 524
Sleep, *see also* NonREM sleep, REM sleep, Insomnia
 in AD, 329
 aging and, 205–207, 368
 analysis, in depression, 201, 203
 assessment, 498
 disorders, 498–499
 distribution, 24-hour, 207
 electrophysiology of, 194–211
 environmental influences, 204
 latency, 205
 measurement, standards and methodology, 202–204
 parameters, 205–207
 polygraphic characteristics, 202, 206
 polygraphic recording, 195–199, 203–204
 quality, in elderly, 498–499
 slow-wave, aging and, 206–207
 stages, 206
Smith, E., 165
Social exclusion, 64–65
Social gerontology, 67–70
Social intimacy, depression and, 237, 238
Social order, species survival and, 56
Social organization, impact of, 44
Social therapy, 383

Social worker, role in geriatric psychiatry unit, 140–141
"Society of surrogates," 492
Sociobiological gerontology, elements of, 51–53
Sociocultural conditioning, 50–51
Socioeconomic status, depression and, 231, 236–237
Somatic cells, aging, 12–13
Somatic disease
 affective disease and, 116
 in elderly, 90–92
 in mental illness, 121–122
 psychotherapy in, 389–390
Somatic Mutation Theory, 32
Somatic and psychiatric geriatrics, 408–409
Somatization, in AD, 329
Somatostatin levels, in AD and other diseases, 178
Special data, description and assignment of, 482–483
Specific rehabilitation
 aim, 410
 techniques, 416
Speech therapy, 424
Speech and vocabulary, in AD, 318, 325
Spiritual leadership, elderly's role in, 59
SPREAD, 410
Stress
 adjustment disorders and, 91–92
 illness and, 521
Stroke
 hypertension and, 293–295
 therapeutic intervention, 391–392
 treatment, 301–302
Structural overbalancing, description, 48
Structured program remotivation therapy, 389
Substance abuse, *see also* Alcohol abuse
 day hospital care, 436, 437
 diagnostic protocol, 144
Suicide
 death education and, 511
 in elderly depression, 246
 mortality, by age, 99
Sullivan, H. S., 504

Index

Superoxide catalase, oxygen detoxification by, 15, 16
Superoxide dismutase, oxygen detoxification by, 15, 16
Superoxide peroxidase, oxygen detoxification by, 15, 16
Swift, J., 215
Symptom Check List (SCL-90), 440, 441
Systemic illness, organic affective syndrome and, 277, 278
Systems approach
  to human society, 46–47
  to gerosociology, 48–49
Systolic blood pressure, stroke risk and, 294

T

Technology, elderly and, 490–491
Temperature
  cell duplication and, 5
  regulation, delirium and, 256
Terminal care
  factors in, 513–515
  skill acquisition, 514–515
Terminally ill patients
  dealing with, 518–519
  neglect of, 518
Tertiary syphilis, dementia and, 265, 266
Tetracyclic antidepressants, pharmacokinetics, 366, 371–372
Thanatology, gerontology and, 503–504
Thiamin requirements, in elderly, 351
Thought impairment, in dementia, 260
Thyroid releasing hormone (TRH), 345
Thyroid-stimulating hormone (TSH), 345
Time in bed, aging and, 205
Token Economy System, 381, 388–389
Total approach to elderly, 408
Total sleep time, in different aged patients, 205
Toxic chemicals, in diet, 16
Toxicity, organic affective syndrome and, 277, 278

Transference, in psychotherapy of aged, 378–379
Transient amnestic syndrome, 276
Transient situational disturbances, see Adjustment disorders
Transplanted tissue, behavior of, 5
Trauma, delirium and, 256
Treatment modalities
  decision to assign, factors in, 443–447
  for mental illness, controlled trials, 130–131
  pharmacogeriatric research, 528
Tricyclic antidepressants
  for depression, 240
  pharmacokinetics of, 371–372
Triplet nucleotides, translation, 33
True amnesia, 276
Trust, doctor–patient, 523
Tuberculosis, elimination, life-span effects, 10
Type A personality, 100, 103
Type B personality, 100

U

Unipolar depressions
  causes, 236–239
  conditions associated with, 232–236
  symptomatology, 231–232
  treatment, 240–242
Urate, oxygen detoxification by, 15, 16
Uremia, in psychogeriatric patients, 344
Urinary retention, in acute confusional states, 344
Urine, drug excretion, 365
Ursin, 96, 102, 104

V

"Value history," 341
Vascular arteriosclerotic changes, in hypertension, 292
Vascular dementia, in Japan, 272
Ventricular size, aging and, 181
Visual deficits, in paraphrenia, 118
Visual illusions, in delirium, 254

Vitamin deficiency, dementia and, 265, 266
Vitamin D requirements, in aged, 351
von Soest, 518

W

Wake after sleep onset, aging and, 206
Walking, readaptation to, 418–419
Water requirements, in elderly, 352
Welford, 220
"Weltoffenheit," 58
Werner syndrome, chromatin alterations in, 18
Wernicke's encephalopathy, 253, 277
Wild fowl, biosocial organization, 53
Wilson, 112–114
Wing's diagnostic system, 130
Woodward, K., 492

World Assembly on the Elderly, 215

X

Xenon-133 inhalation technique, 154, 156, 165
Xenobiotics, cancer and aging, 15–16

Y

Yahweh, 66
"Yield," definition, 47–48
Young-old, definition, 75

Z

Zeitgeist, 50
Zung Depression Scale, 236